The Speech Sciences

The Speech Sciences

Raymond D. Kent, Ph.D.
The University of Wisconsin-Madison
Madison, Wisconsin

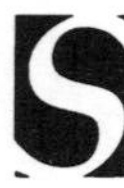

SINGULAR PUBLISHING GROUP, INC.
SAN DIEGO · LONDON

Singular Publishing Group, Inc.
401 West "A" Street, Suite 325
San Diego, California 92101-7904

Singular Publishing Group Ltd.
19 Compton Terrace
London, N1 2UN, U.K.

e-mail: singpub@mail.cerfnet.com
Website: http://www.singpub.com

Typeset in 10/12 Times by So Cal Graphics
Printed in the United States of America by McNaughton and Gunn

Library of Congress Cataloging-in-Publication Data
Kent, Raymond D.
The speech sciences / Raymond D. Kent
p. cm.
Includes bibliographical references and index.
ISBN 1–56593–689–2
1. Speech. I. Title.
QP306.K46 1997
612.7'8—dc21 97–9480
CIP

CONTENTS

PREFACE

> *"What we can put on our shelves we should not put into our brains."*
>
> (Auguste Forel)

An introductory text is a negotiation between the writer and the reader. The writer is responsible to present accurate information in a fashion that is reasonably coherent and concise, but is also reasonably complete. The introductory textbook is therefore a kind of information filter. For every fact or concept that is included, several are excluded. Some information that might be presented in the interest of completeness may not be highly relevant to the course for which the book is used or to the reader's eventual purposes. The writer must select the pieces of information that fit into a conceptual whole. The reader's task is to determine what is important to him or her. Rarely does the reader seek to memorize each and every fact. Rather, readers do their own kind of information filtering, separating the essential information from the nonessential, the interesting from the mundane. Writer and reader are then involved in a mutual process, and it is fortunate that readers frequently make up for the failings of the writer, occasionally filtering out the unnecessary information and integrating pieces of knowledge that have not been woven tightly in the book.

Few of us have photographic memories and we therefore learn selectively. Some things we commit to memory; others we merely acknowledge as being retrievable from some source should the need arise. The quotation from Auguste Forel that leads this preface is the pedagogical philosophy of this book. Some information should be shelved so that it can be retrieved when needed. Other information is intrinsic to the subject matter and serves as the conceptual framework for basic understanding. The attempt in this book is to deliver primarily the latter but to guide the reader's possible need for the former. In one sense, the book is an encyclopedia, but in another sense it is not. The word *encyclopedia* is derived from Latin and Greek roots denoting instruction in "the circle of the arts and sciences." An encyclopedia of speech therefore gives instruction in the circle of speech arts and sciences. *The Speech Sciences* aspires to be this kind of encylopedia, with an emphasis on the sciences. In common usage, the word *encyclo-*

pedia often is taken to mean an exhaustive and detailed account of knowledge. *The Speech Sciences* is not intended to plumb the depths of each and every bit of knowledge about speech. For those readers who seek to go deeper, advice is given on which shelves to look. This is one reason why references are cited in the text. Although these citations break the flow of writing somewhat, they are essential to validate the information given and to aid the reader who wants to study further.

Information about anatomy and physiology can be as detailed as one wants to make it. The assumption behind this book is that most readers will not need finely detailed information about anatomy and physiology so much as they will need concepts and frameworks for a functional understanding of speech. Certainly, some basic information is required before concepts and frameworks become interpretable. But a thorough exploration of anatomy and physiology not only would make the book much longer that it is, but it would, in its finer points, uncover inconsistencies and disagreements that encumber the introductory text with material of questionable value.

The plural form *speech sciences,* rather than the singular form *speech science,* is used as the title of this book to reflect the continuing expansion of the study of speech into a broad discipline that embraces several related specialties. The specialization results from the multidisciplinary nature of speech as scientific phenomena and also from the increasing applications of knowledge about speech. The attempt in writing this book is to survey these various sciences of speech and to consider their unity demonstrated in the distinctively human faculty of talking.

Texts on speech science often present a single version of the anatomy, physiology, and acoustics of speech, that version being modeled on the adult male. Sex and age differences are noted only in passing, if at all. But there are many important differences in speech science related to age and sex. This will come as no surprise to readers, who can often determine the gender and make a fairly accurate guess as to the age of a telephone caller even after hearing only the single word, "hello." Age and gender differences are discussed in this book by reference to boys and girls and men and women of different ages, proceeding from the newborn to the elderly. For most of us, speech is a lifelong partner. We hear it from the womb, develop it as children, perfect it in adulthood, and through it give voice to our thoughts. Humans are, as Dennis Fry named us, *homo loquens,* the talking animal. Because speech is produced with physiologic systems that change during our lifetimes, speech has a lifecourse story. Some basic aspects of this story will be told in this book.

The sciences of speech are distinct enough that some scientists work in a single slice of the large circle of speech. But the understanding of speech as a functional human behavior requires that these separate specialties be drawn together, placed in the circle of their mutual connectedness. This integration is attempted at several places in the book, but especially in the first and the final few chapters. There is much about speech that is general to the human species, but there is also much about speech that is specific to groups of people and much that is individual. The power of speech lies in both its general capacity for human interaction and its individuality of expression. Speech is public yet private. We speak so that others may hear us and that we may hear ourselves. Communication is a social and intellectual imperative; speech is the preferred and primary form of human communication. Let us examine how it is produced and perceived.

R.D.K.
Madison, Wisconsin

ACKNOWLEDGMENTS

Several people provided assistance, intervention, and encouragement that helped to bring this book to completion:

Thanks to my family—

my wife, Jane, for reading the manuscript and suggesting numerous improvements, as well as for putting in long hours in various chores to bring the manuscript to final form;

my son, Jason, for help with photography;

my daughter, Laurel, for diligent work with the initial stages of citation accuracy and text uniformity.

Thanks to colleagues—

Charles Speaks, for generously giving of his time to read several of the chapters and offering a number of important corrections and refinements;

Ronald Scherer, for careful reading and excellent suggestions on an early draft of some of the chapters;

Julie Liss and Christopher Moore, who responded promptly, charitably, and most effectively, to a call for chapter reviews;

Terry Wiley, for a critical reading of one chapter on short notice;

Michael R. Chial, who provided valuable reference material.

Kris Tjaden, for reviewing most of the chapters of the book.

Thanks to the people at Singular—

Sadanand Singh, for his zeal for this project from its inception to its completion;

Angie Singh, for her fine efforts to bring the book to production;

Marie Linvill, for frequent help along the way;

Pam Rider, for editorial precision, sensitive wordcraft, and being able to see both the forests and the trees;

Sandy Doyle, for overseeing the many details of production.

Thanks also to—

Betsy True, medical illustrator at the University of Wisconsin-Madison Hospitals and Clinics, for her talent in bringing my rough ideas to graphic reality.

The writing of this book began as a solitary venture but, as time and pages went by, more and more friends and associates offered their help and encouragement. I thank them all.

This book is dedicated to the memory of three scientists, in the hope that it reflects at least some small part of the broad and deep understanding that they brought to the speech sciences:

Harvey Fletcher
Dennis H. Klatt
Raymond H. Stetson

CHAPTER 1

Speech Communication and the Speech Sciences

> *"The capacity to speak is the chief distinguishing characteristic of the species* **Homo sapiens** *and the most common feature of our everyday lives. Except for breathing, there is nothing we human beings do more routinely and repetitively than communicate to one another."*
>
> (J. J. Lynch, *The Language of the Heart.* New York: Basic Books, 1985, p. 118.)

INFORMATIONAL SOURCES IN SPEECH

The sound signal of speech is rich in information. By hearing just a few syllables uttered by an invisible and unknown talker in a darkened room, we may reach a linguistic interpretation ("Is someone there?" we hear), an impression of the unknown talker's age and gender (a young woman), and a guess as to the talker's emotional state (surprise). The power of spoken language is demonstrated every day in telephone conversations, radio communications, public address systems, and ordinary chats among friends.

Traunmuller (1994) listed four kinds of information contained in the speech signal: phonetic, affective, personal, and transmittal qualities. They are illustrated in Figure 1–1 and are described in the following sections.

1. Phonetic quality refers to the linguistic content of the speech message. Phonetic quality is specific to humans and is defined in terms of the conventions of a particular language. The phonetic quality may be considered the essential material from which we derive the linguistic meaning of a message. Individual languages are tied to a distinctive phonetic system. Although some broad universals may apply to the different languages of the world, the differences among them are perhaps more readily apparent. Proficiency in a language includes competence in its phonetic aspects. Interestingly, the phonetic aspects are among the most challenging in attempts to become fluent in a nonnative language. Particularly when we try to learn another language after the age of puberty, there is a strong likelihood that the second language will be spoken with an accent that reflects the phonetic characteristics of the native language (Flege, 1987; Flege & Fletcher, 1992; Oyama, 1976, 1978). The native language seems to leave a strong imprint on our phonetic abilities, and this imprint is overcome only with considerable difficulty once we have passed childhood.

2. Affective quality (or emotional quality) is paralinguistic, meaning that it accompanies the linguistic message of speech and may contribute to the interpretation of that message. For example, an ironic or sarcastic message is typically one that carries a mismatch between the linguistic content and the accompanying affective content. The would-be golfer who says, "What a perfect day," while looking out the window at a thunderstorm is using irony. The golfer's words say one thing, but the paralinguistic message conveys something quite different. Affective quality communicates information and is not specific to humans. Humans and dogs can communicate information to one another through the affective quality of their vocalizations. Scherer (1981) wrote that emotion is the organism's interface to its outside world. He described three principal functions of emo-

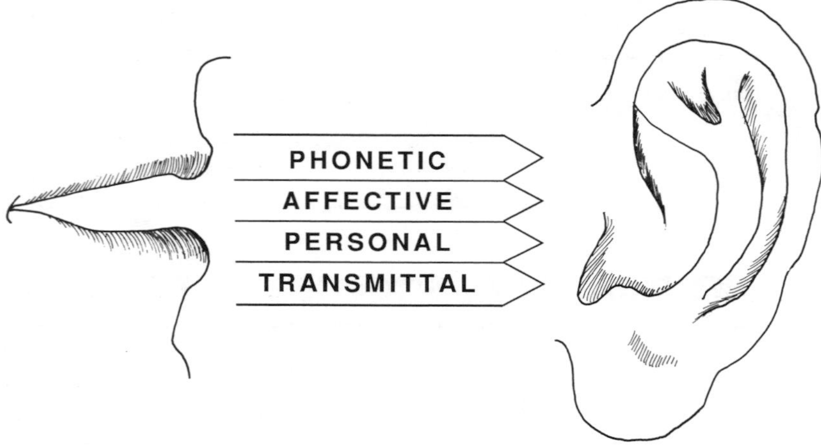

Figure 1–1. The four information sources in speech communication.

tions. First, emotions reflect an appraisal of the relevance and importance of stimuli. Second, emotions are the basis for physiological and psychological preparation for action. Third, emotions communicate an organism's state and behavioral intentions. It is the third function that is particularly relevant to spoken communication by humans. Speaking is a primary channel for human emotion.

Some vocalizations are strongly associated with emotional state but convey little or no phonetic information. Crying and laughter unmistakingly signal the emotion of the person who emits them. But both are very simple from a phonetic point view. Provine (1995) points out that a laugh typically takes the form of a series of short vowel-like notes or syllables. Each syllable is less than one tenth of a second in duration and the syllables are separated by a gap of about one fifth of a second. Laughter is not defined by any particular vowel, but the same vowel tends to be used repetitively to form the syllable sequence of laughter, as in: "ha-ha-ha," or "ho-ho-ho," or "hee-hee-hee." It is unnatural and unusual to form a laugh with varying vowels such as "ha-hee-ha-ho." Anyone laughing in such a manner will most likely attract quizzical reactions from others.

Speech can be affected by a number of stressing factors, including those in the physical domain (e.g., exercise, environmental noise, intense vibration), chemical domain (fatigue, sleep deprivation, medications, alcohol), and the physiological domain (illness, workload, anxiety, depression). Murray, Baber, and South (1996) offer a more complete taxonomy of stress factors that can influence speech. Suffice it to say that speech is potentially affected by a large number of common and uncommon circumstances. Listeners who are highly familiar with us will sometimes ask, "Is something wrong? You sound different." They are picking up subtle cues in our speech patterns.

3. Personal quality is extralinguistic, meaning that it is outside the ordinary linguistic aspects of speech. Personal quality is informative about the talker, but not the message. The information can include the talker's gender, age, and even state of health (Kent & Chial, in press). Our vast experience with speech enables us to make multiple inferences about the personal qualities of a speaker. The inferences sometimes can be mistaken, but it has been demonstrated that listeners can make fairly successful guesses about attributes such as age of a speaker. Many individuals are quite adept at speaker recognition and can identify entertainers, government leaders, and newscasters from even brief recordings of their voices. Most of us can recognize friends and family members from a single "hello" spoken over a telephone. Vocal individuality arises early in life, such that even the cries of infants can be discriminated (Gustafson, Green, & Cleland, 1994).

Experiments indicate that the perceptual representation of speaker gender is based on general auditory features and is qualitatively different from the representation of phonetic information (Mullenix, Johnson, Topcu-Durgun, & Farnsworth, 1995). It appears that recognition of speaker gender is less abstract than the recognition of phonetic information and relies on auditory information about acoustic voice parameters. If this conclusion can be generalized to other types of personal information, then it would appear that personal quality is represented perceptually in a fundamentally different way than phonetic quality.

4. Transmittal quality gives perspectival information, that is, information relative to perspective on the talker's location, including the distance from the one who hears the signal, orientation in space, presence of background noise, and influence of environmental acoustics that may introduce effects such as reverberation. Our recognition of this information is often useful in improving speech communication. For example, a listener who judges that speech is being transmitted over a noisy channel will make a number of adjustments in speaking pattern to promote the intelligibility of the spoken message. Increasingly, spoken messages are stored in computers in digital form, transmitted electronically over communication networks, and even altered in various ways for economical transmission. Transmittal quality is an important issue in communication technology.

Speech, therefore, is more than a linguistic message communicated by sound. Sound can carry many dimensions of information and speech is one of the richest sounds in our human experience. The power of these various dimensions is easily demonstrated. Think of how many times we say (or think) it is not *what* a person said, but *how* it was said. When we hear speech, we constantly weigh the various kinds of information available to us to draw interpretations, form opinions, and formulate our own responses. The sounds of speech are an invisible fabric of culture and connectedness. To live without these sounds is to live a radically different life. Helen Keller described the importance of speech in a letter to a Dr. J. Kerr Love:

> I am just as deaf as I am blind. The problems of deafness are deeper and more complex, if not more important, than those of blindness. Deafness is a much worse misfortune. For it means the loss of the most vital stimulus—the sound of the voice that brings language, sets thoughts astir and keeps us in the intellectual company of man. (From a letter dated March 31, 1910, from the souvenir program commemorating Helen Keller's visit to Queensland Adult Deaf and Dumb Mission in 1948; cited by Ackerman, 1990)

And yet we can tire of speech, especially the incessant sounds of an unwelcome and intrusive talker. Perhaps one of the most annoying things about this kind of situation is that we have almost no capability to refuse to understand the speech messages around us—short of plugging our ears or otherwise escaping the sounds on which speech is carried. The perception of speech seems automatic and mandatory. The psychologist Jerry Fodor (1983) recognized these properties in his discussion of speech in his book on the modular theory of psychology. He described the perception of spoken language as mandatory. There is something about speech that is undeniable—its message permeates into our consciousness. Some surgeons have been surprised to learn that an anesthetized patient can recall on waking up comments made by the surgical team during an operation. Speech understanding can occur even in the face of general anesthesia.

This book will have little to say of inner speech, or the way we use speech internally as part of our thinking process. This personal dialogue or monologue is part of common human introspection. Inner speech is not readily accessible to scientific investigation, at least not by contemporary laboratory methods. But the day may come when even inner speech may be monitored to some degree by machine and better understood through refined methods of scientific investigation. Science grows in breadth as well as depth. Issues that are today on the fringe of scientific research may be within the sphere of active research tomorrow. Perhaps different aspects of language will be discovered as language is studied in individuals with atypical communication. Individuals with autism are commonly thought to have communication impairments but one woman who wrote of her autistic life had this to say:

"I have also had the pleasure of being with others labeled 'autistic.' This was the only group who spoke my own language so well that I realized that much of what I had thought of as my personality was in fact my individual expression of many of the misunderstood and confusing symptoms of autism."

(D. Williams, *Nobody Nowhere*. New York: Avon Books, 1992, pp. 199–200.)

THE PHYSICS AND BIOLOGY OF SPEECH COMMUNICATION

"Talk is part of our very biological heritage by virtue of our membership in the human species. Talk is an imperative for us. It is an imperative for us to connect with others through talk, it is an imperative for us to to explore our worlds through talk, and it is an imperative for us to express our self-hood through talk."

(J. W. Lindfors: Speaking creatures in the classroom. In S. Hynd and D. L. Rubin (Eds.), *Perspectives on Talk and Learning*. Urbana, IL: National Council of Teachers of English, 1992, p. 21)

Many species of animals use sound for purposes of signaling. Furthermore, sound is produced in a variety of ways. One of the most common is the generation of sound by a pulmonary apparatus (such as the lungs of mammals) or air sacs (in many frogs). Insects such as grasshoppers or crickets produce a stridulation sound by rubbing together wing cases, legs, or shells. Gorillas produce a percussive sound by beating on the chest. Many species, including chimpanzees, goats, and rabbits, stamp with their feet. The whale flaps the water with its fin. The woodpecker taps with its bill. The porcupine shakes its body cover of quills. The rattlesnake rattles the appendages on its tail.

Sound is produced for many different purposes, including mating, maintaining contact with others in a group, cooperation in defensive activities, acquiring food, and recognition of young. One hallmark of mammals is the isolation cry of the young when separated from the parent. This cry is atypical of reptiles but common in mammals. The frequency and nature of sound production also varies with the habitat and living patterns of animals. Among the most vocal are animals that live in tall grass, reeds, scrub, or forests. Examples of vocal animals are birds, monkeys, squirrels, and many insects. Mobility also appears to be a factor, in that slowly moving creatures (like the sloth) or creatures with fixed habitats (like the rabbit) are quiet compared with faster or more mobile animals. With respect to activity patterns, nocturnal animals such as owls, nighthawks, and coyotes are often prolific sound producers, but diurnal species living in open terrain (vultures, giraffes, and antelope) tend to be quiet. The most vocal animals are those that travel extensively and quickly, and who are not readily visible to their comrades because of vegetation or darkness. Within-species comparisons bolster these principles. For example, the vocal chimpanzee is more mobile than the quieter orangutans and gorillas. Song birds frequently have dull plumage compared with the bright colors of many silent birds.

It is testimony to the appeal of speech as a means of communication that, almost without exception, human cultures have a spoken language. Only a minority of the world's languages have a written form, but virtually all of them have an oral form. Furthermore, despite the relatively frequent use of auxiliary sign languages among Native Americans and Australian Aborigines, spoken language is primary among all hearing communities (Meier, 1991; Umiker-Sebeok & Sebeok, 1978). Apparently, spoken language has a universal attractiveness. Certainly, speech communication offers a number of advantages: Talking frees our hands to do other things, speech can be carried out when the conversational partner is nearby but not visible, and speaking is easily accomplished with different numbers of listeners within earshot of the speaker.

Another advantage of speech is that it requires relatively little energy and therefore can be carried out with little risk of exhaustion. Certainly, marathon efforts at talking can eventually wear a speaker down. But the capacity for talk is considerable, as indicated by some examples cited by Fullerton (1975). The longest recorded speech was given by Senator Huey Long of Louisiana in a filibuster that began at 12:30 P.M. on June 12, 1935. He spoke for over 15 hours, until 4 A.M. the following day. His speech was 150,000 words long and filled 100 pages of the *Congressional Record*. But even this senatorial accomplishment pales in the face of the longest sermon on record, which was delivered by a minister in West Richland, Washington in 1955. The minister sermonized for 48 hours and 18 minutes. His listeners, eight of whom stayed for the entire sermon, probably deserve recognition for their forebearance. Both the senator and the minister may have been reduced to exhaustion through bodily fatigue. If their bodies could have been refreshed, who knows how long they might have continued to speak?

Speech usually is regarded as a kind of sound. Yet, speech can be understood at least partially by some individuals who cannot hear and by others who can neither see nor hear. Speech is sound in its typical form—but even if the sound is removed, by deafness or distance for example, speech remains as a pattern of movements. **Speech reading** (also called lip reading) is the visual understanding of spoken speech. Many groups of sounds can be distinguished from their visible characteristics. Sounds that have the same appearance are called **visemes**. For example, the sounds *b*, *p*, and *m* in the words *bay*, *pay*, and *may* are a viseme class. They share the visible feature of lip closure and, therefore, are visually similar. People with hearing impairment often learn speech reading as a means to improve their speech understanding. Fortunately, some of the weakest sounds in speech are also the most visible. For example, the sounds formed by the lips (*m* and *b* as in *maybe*) or by the lips and teeth (*f* and *v* as in *favor*) are typically weak in energy but their production is observable. Speech also has a potential tactual dimension. With proper training, we can understand speech from tactile information obtained by strategically placing a hand over the talker's face and neck. This method of speech reception, called **Tadoma** after two of its first users in the United States (Tad Chapman and Oma Simpson; Vivian, 1966), can be learned by persons with normal hearing and typical speech experience. And, interestingly, some aspects of speech may be relevant even to nonvocal activities such as reading and memorizing. Some theories of reading propose that readers convert letters they see to a phonological (sound) code. To understand speech, then, we must consider its various manifestations, audible and inaudible, visible and invisible.

THE LINGUISTIC ROLE OF SPEECH

> *"The subject [of language] is complicated by the fact that linguistics is the most ancient scholarly branch . . . and, most importantly, these ancient statements about language retain a peculiar interest; even nowadays, they have not become just a property of the archives of the history of science."*
>
> (V. V. Nalimov, *In the Labyrinths of Language: A Mathematician's Journey*. Philadelphia: ISI Press, 1981, p. 1.)

At the risk of being tautologous, one may say that speech is spoken or vocal language. Not every sound that a human makes is speech. The word *speech* is confined to those sounds that impart linguistic meaning. Not every language is spoken. A notable exception is American Sign Language (ASL) used by many individuals in the United States who are deaf. Speech is a sound system used to express language. Every competent speaker of a language has learned to produce sounds in a highly regular way that affords reliable communication.

Every language learner must acquire the **phonemes** of the language. These are the elemental sound units from which all words are formed. For example, the words *hill*, *pill*, *bill*, *fill*, and *kill* differ from one another in the initial sound segment, or phoneme. Phonemes are the sound distinctions by which different words in a language are composed. The number of phonemes varies across the world's languages, from fewer than 20 to more than 100. English is an average language in the size of its phonemic inventory, having about 44 phonemes. The way in which these sounds are actually used to make words is the subject of **phonology**, a branch of linguistics concerned with sound patterns. Another field, **phonetics**, is concerned with the ways in which sounds are formed. The general field of phonetics is introduced in Chapter 3. Phonetics can be subdivided into specialties, such as physiologic and acoustic phonetics, both of which are discussed in this book. Physiologic phonetics is concerned with the physiology of sound production, that is, the movements of muscles, bones, and cartilages that generate the sounds of speech. Acoustic phonetics deals with the acoustic signal that is heard as speech.

It is important to distinguish *alphabet* characters from phonemes. Although an alphabet ideally would represent each sound of a language by a separate written symbol, alphabets typically fall short of this ideal. Korean and Finnish come fairly close to having an alphabet that is nearly phonetic.

English does not fare as well, so there are many discrepancies between alphabetic representations and sound patterns. These discrepancies are a major source of difficulty in learning to read and write English. A given alphabet letter can represent several different sounds. For instance, the letter *s* can represent the quite different sounds in the words *see*, *sugar*, and *rise*. Another difficulty is that the same sound is associated with different alphabet letters. For example, the letter *c* can have the hard sound of *c* in *car* or the soft sound of *c* in *city*. Or, *c* can combine with *i* to form a "sh" sound as in the word *delicious*. The deficiencies of the English alphabet as a phonetic alphabet are notorious. For matters of phonetic description, it is preferable to use a special system, such as the International Phonetic Alphabet, which is summarized later in the book.

The 40 or 50 phonemes of the average language have a remarkable capability to form words. On average, languages have about 60,000 words, which are created from different combinations of the 40 or 50 phonemes that are the building blocks of spoken language. The words, in turn, can be used to produce an infinite number of sentences, given that any sentence can be made longer and longer by the addition of words ("I said that he reported that they knew that she said . . . "). As many linguists like to say, language uses finite means to achieve infinite possibilities.

Although languages differ in their phonemic inventory, some phonemes occur much more frequently than others across languages. For example, the vowel that occurs in the word *he* occurs in more than 90% of the languages examined by Maddieson (1984). For some reason, this vowel is highly favored by languages as they form their phonemic systems. Frequently occurring consonants include the stop consonants that begin the words *pill*, *till*, *kill*, *bill*, *dill*, and *gill*. The selection of phonemes does not appear to be a random process. For reasons discussed later in the book, certain sounds are preferred in the world's phonemic systems.

Speech has been described as a robust system, meaning that it survives various kinds of interference, especially the inevitable background noises that compete with the speech signal. The robustness derives in part because all natural languages are about 50% redundant. That is, about half of the spoken message can be deleted, with speech remaining fairly understandable. A graphic illustration of the redundancy of language is to print a message with some of the alphabet characters removed. In the example that follows, the alphabet letters corresponding to vowels have been deleted. The # symbol represents a word boundary.

c_____n # y_____ # r_____ d #
th_____ s # m_____ ss_____ g

You probably guessed that the example reads: "Can you read this message?" A personalized license plate reads: RTTWLR. What kind of pet do you think the driver owns?

To study even one language thoroughly is quite a challenge, given that its vocabulary may number some 60,000 words. English may have the largest vocabulary of any language: the *Oxford English Dictionary* lists about half a million words. But a far greater challenge is to study the world's languages in an effort to see how they differ and how they are similar. The number of languages spoken in the world is quite difficult to estimate with accuracy, but many sources use a figure of about 4,000 to 5,000. Only about 140 of these are spoken by more than 1 million people (Crystal, 1987). The 10 languages with the largest number of speakers are as follows (beginning with the language spoken by the largest number): Chinese, English, Spanish, Hindi, Arabic, Bengali, Russian, Portuguese, Japanese, German.

Although Chinese is spoken by the largest number of people (because of the huge population of China), English tends to predominate for business, scholarship, science, and technology. One language scholar commented, "Among the supranational languages there is one that occupies a very special position since in all supranational languages there are bilingual speakers who are also competent in this one language, which is therefore central to all central languages: and this supercentral language is, of course, English" (de Swaan, 1991, p. 17). As pointed out in the *Story of English* (McCrum, Cran, & McNeil, 1986), the linguistic ascendency of English is remarkable. The English language did not yet exist when Julius Caesar set foot on the British Isles some 2000 years ago. About 500 years later, a language called Englisc was spoken by a small number of people. During William Shakespeare's era, no more than 7 million claimed English as a native tongue and almost all of them lived in the British Isles. Today it may be spoken by as many as 1 billion people, perhaps only half of whom speak it as a first language. McCrum et al. (1986) summarize the linguistic potency of English: "English at the end of the twentieth century is more widely scattered, more widely spoken and written, than any other language has ever been. It has become *the* language of the planet, the first truly global language" (p. 19, emphasis in original).

This does not necessarily mean that English is spoken in the same way around the world. There are a number of dialects of English, and some scholars believe that these dialects will grow increasingly different, to the point that some of them will not be mutually intelligible a century from now. Other scholars take the contrary view that an international form of English will emerge that suffices for international communication. The renowned linguist David Crystal takes a middle-ground position in believing that the next generation of English speakers will be triglossic, "having command of the national standard, our own local standard, and an international standard" (Lockett, 1992). These various hypotheses about language change reflect a common view that spoken language is dynamic, subtly ever changing.

The majority of the world's languages do not have a printed form. Therefore, these languages depend on speech for their expression and for their continued existence. If speakers of the languages die, so do the languages. Such language death is occurring today at a rate that dismays interested people who would like to preserve at least some record of the disappearing languages. Toward this end, a group of linguists established the Endangered Languages Fund (Linguistics Department, Yale University, New Haven, CT). In the opinion of some linguists, the number of languages spoken in the world may diminish from the current several thousand to perhaps only a few hundred. As an example of the rate of disappearance of languages, only about 20 American Indian (Native American) languages survive of the hundreds that were spoken a few generations ago. The individual speech act is a perishable message—unless it is recorded, it is gone forever. The same is true for spoken languages that have no surviving speakers. When the last speaker of a language expires, he or she dies both a personal death and a linguistic death that reaches back to generations.

It is not only human languages that are disappearing from the face of the earth. As animal species become extinct, so do the sounds that the animals make. With the encroachment of humans on animal habitats, the acoustics of wild places are increasingly subject to human-caused sounds. In the interest of preserving the sounds of individual animals and the sounds of natural habitats, a number of people have begun to obtain recordings of natural sounds. The world's largest archive of these sounds is the Library of Natural Sounds at Cornell University, which has more than 100,000 recordings (see *Bulletin of the Library of Natural Sounds*).

Any sound signaling system, then, is at risk for extinction with no lasting record of its existence, if the users of that system disappear. Tape recordings can preserve a record of sounds produced by humans and animals. But speech is also fleeting on the more immediate temporal scale. As soon as we produce a word, it is gone. The medium of speech is highly perishable and this feature makes certain demands of both speaker and listener, if communication is to be successful. The speaker continues to talk on the assumption that the listener is comprehending the message. If the listener fails to understand part of the message, he or she may have little time to reconsider the matter if the speaker has gone on to new thoughts. Ordinary conversation places a premium on time, for the message must be understood as it is spoken, and new thoughts are quickly assembled into the next utterance.

Among the various communication systems devised by humans, speech is particularly efficient. Studies of human-to-human communication have compared the efficiency of different systems including typewriting, handwriting, video, voice, and their combinations (Ochsman & Chapanis, 1974). When voice was available to persons communicating in a problem-solving task, the time to a solution was reduced by more than 50% compared to typewriting. Similarly, in studies of equipment assembly tasks, interactive telephone speech had a three-fold speed advantage over keyboard communication (Cohen, 1984; Oviatt & Cohen, 1991). Spoken communication is not only natural but efficient. This is one reason for the keen interest in the development of voice communication between humans and machines. If humans could control computers with speech commands rather than keyboards, many cases of repetitive-use syndrome (such as carpal-tunnel syndrome) could be avoided. Voice control also would free the user's hands for other tasks.

BIOLOGICAL DIFFERENCES AMONG SPEAKERS

Gender Differences

Speech and voice are among the human behaviors that are most readily—almost insistently—labeled as male or female. The gender of adults is usually identified quickly from the sound of their voices, and gender distinction is possible even for children who have yet to cross the maturity divide of puberty. Gender distinctions are built on biology (sex differences in anatomy and physiology) and culture (different roles assumed by males and females in a particular society). Adult males and females have different physical systems for speech and voice, but these physical differences do not account for all the gender differences that occur in various cultures. Speech and voice also may be said to have a life course, or a pattern of developmental change from infancy to adulthood to the later years of life. Life course changes reflect physical changes in the speech production system that occur during development and aging. Our speech and voice patterns change as we age, like an acoustic mirror of our own life course.

A large number of sex differences have been described in studies of mammals (Glucksmann, 1981). These differences are important for several reasons, one of which is that they can help to explain how different diseases and disorders affect men and women in different proportions. For example, men are more likely to have gout and cancers of the oral and pharyngeal cavities. Women are more likely to have obesity with diabetes and thyroid tumors.

At least at the population level (i.e., when large numbers of subjects are involved), fairly consistent sex differences have been observed in several studies of spoken language abilities. First, girls generally lead boys in language acquisition (Bradshaw & Nettleton, 1983; Schachter, Shore, Hodapp, Chalfin, & Bundy, 1978). Boys also are more likely than girls to have disorders and delays in spoken language development (Bradshaw & Nettleton, 1981; Languis & Naouv, 1985; Fletcher & Ingham, 1995). Communication disorders in general show a sexual imbalance, with males showing the higher proportion of disorders such as childhood articulation disorders, developmental stuttering, specific language impairment, and adult aphasia (impairment of language owing to conditions such as cerebrovascular accident [CVA] or stroke). Sex differences are especially prominent in stuttering (fluency disorders) and specific language impairment. In the case of developmental stuttering (i.e., stuttering that appears in childhood), boys outnumber girls by ratios in the range of 3:1 to 5:1 (Peters & Guitar, 1991). When girls are diagnosed as stutterers, they have a greater likelihood for recovery than do boys (Ambrose, Yairi, & Cox, 1993; Seider, Gladstien, & Kidd, 1983). Acquired stuttering (i.e., stuttering that appears in adulthood typically as the result of neural damage) may have a sex ratio as high as 15 males for every female affected (Mazzucchi, Moretti, Carpeggiani, & Parma, 1981). These large sex ratios indicate that males are particularly at risk for disorders of speech fluency (and perhaps related sensory and motor abilities; Kent, 1984). Concerning specific language impairment in children, Robinson (1987) pooled data from 10 different studies and obtained an overall sex ratio (boys to girls) of 2.82, which is similar to the sex ratio for developmental stuttering.

Some evidence also points to a sex difference in the effect of aging on spoken language. It was concluded in one study of a large number of men and women that, "While males presented a steady and permanent decrease in spontaneous language production, evident since the 31–50 year-old range, language production in females was abundant even at the 51–65 year-old range" (Ardila & Roselli, 1996, p. 76).

Across the general facets of spoken language, females appear to have a lifelong superiority over males. Females learn to speak earlier, are less likely to have disorders of spoken language, have a better chance of recovery from at least some speech disorders, and maintain their linguistic competence more effectively into old age. Later chapters (7 and 13) explore some possible biological reasons for this female advantage. Sex-related differences in diseases and disorders are not necessarily due to biology alone, but sometimes also to cultural differences between males and females. Sex and gender differences will be taken up at various places in this book, primarily with an eye toward explaining differences in function and pathology. But it is well to underscore that individual variations in either sex are very large compared to the population means. Some boys acquire language very early and produce it very fluently, and some girls are slow to acquire language and lack fluency.

Age Differences

Age is a potent variable in speech, hearing, and language. In one sense, spoken language is acquired quickly, considering the large amount of information to be acquired and the poor understanding we have of how this process works. But in another sense, spoken language has a time course of several years before adultlike proficiency is attained. In this book, four general age periods are used in describing developmental processes: prenatal, infancy, childhood, and adolescence.

Prenatal Period

This period extending from conception to birth, or about 40 weeks, is subdivided into three stages: an embryonic period from conception to 8 weeks, a middle fetal period from 9 weeks through 24 weeks, and a late period from 25 weeks to birth. On occasion, reference is also made to trimesters, or 3-month periods, in gestation. These are called the first, second, and third trimesters. As we will see in later chapters, the human fetus swallows, hiccoughs, and hears (perhaps well enough to know the mother's voice at birth).

Infancy

Infancy, from the Latin for "incapable of speech," generally refers to the first 2 years of life. This period has three stages: the neonatal period (birth to 1 month), infancy proper (1 month to 1 year), and late infancy (the second year of life). Recent evidence indicates that, even in the first year of life, infants exhibit a number of important behaviors pertinent to speech. For example, even during the first year of life babbling begins to take on some of the phonetic characteristics of the parental language. Infant babbling has some properties that appear to be universal, insofar as babies the world over demonstrate certain common characteristics (Locke, 1983). But babbling also seems to be shaped in various subtle ways by the infant's language environment. Speech learning may be begin well before traditional accounts of development have noted it. The typical estimate is that a child's first words are produced at about 12 months. Children who are deaf learning manual communication with American Sign Language seem to be on roughly the same schedule. Possibly, signing children get off to a faster start than speaking children. In one study of 13 signing children born to parents who are deaf, it was reported that the children had a vocabulary of 10 signs by the age of 13.2 months (Bonvillian, Orlansky & Novack, 1983). By comparison, 18 children learning spoken English reached a vocabulary of 10 words at 15.1 months (Nelson, 1973). Is speech harder to learn than signs? More recent data, reviewed here, cast doubt on this conclusion.

A typical estimate of the first use of signs or words is near the end of the first year of life. According to data on spontaneous word production collected by Fenson et al. (1993), children typically have acquired 10 words by 13 months of age and over 300 words by 24 months of age. However, the range of vocabulary size was considerable, and the mean data should be regarded as a gross estimate. A child's comprehension vocabulary is much larger than his or her production vocabulary. For example, Fenson et al. (1993) estimated the comprehension vocabulary of a 13-month-old infant to be about 110 words (compared to a production vocabulary of only about 10 words). Sex differences in vocabulary acquisition were rather small in the Fensen et al. (1993) data, with girls having a slightly faster mean rate. However, this difference was very small compared to the wide individual variations within each sex. By the time infancy comes to a close, a child possesses a small but accelerating productive vocabulary and a considerably larger comprehension vocabulary.

Childhood

Childhood runs from 2 to 10 years for girls and from 2 to 12 years for boys. Because boys generally mature later than girls, the span of childhood differs for the two sexes. The preschool years are ages 2 to 6 years, and the school years are ages 6 to 10 years for girls and 6 to 12 years for boys. Of course, boys and girls generally are in the same grades, but the term *school* is used in this context to identify a developmental period. This period is an active period of language learning. It has been estimated that a child learns about *21 new words each day* (including weekends and holidays!) between the ages of about 6 and 8 years (Miller, 1977). That is a remarkable learning feat—all the more so because most parents would not be aware of deliberately teaching their children so many words in such a short period. Indeed, it may be better that parents do not set out to perform deliberate vocabulary instruction. The conclusion must be "that children learn a lot more words than we teach them" (Miller, 1977, p. 156).

Another particularly important aspect of childhood is the frequent speculation that the **critical period for language acquisition** falls during this period. Lenneberg (1967) believed that, "the primary acquisition of language is predicated upon a certain developmental stage which is quickly outgrown at the age of puberty" (p. 142). The critical period hypothesis maintains that language must be learned during a particular developmental period or it will not be learned effectively. Children who do not learn language during the critical period will suffer a lifelong deficiency in language. Scientists have studied children who have been deprived of language during all or part of the presumed critical period. Examples of reports on these children are Curtiss (1977), Davis (1947), Koluchova (1972), and Mason (1942). Although these studies are not necessarily conclusive proof of the existence of a critical period for language acquisition, they point at least to the existence of a "sensitive" period during which language acquisition is optimized. Although there are differing views on exactly what a sensitive period may be (Newport, 1991), many scientists who study human development remain convinced that a certain period in early childhood is the ideal time to learn a language. The developmental advantage seems to apply not only to the first language but to later languages as well. In one study of the accuracy of foreign language pronunciation, the ability of English-speaking children to pronounce words spoken by a native French speaker improved with age up to 8 and 9 years, but then diminished (Misrachi & Denney, 1979).

Adolescence

The adolescent period is from 10 to 18 years for girls and from 12 to 20 years for boys. The three periods of adolescence are: prepubescence (10 to 12 for girls, 12 to 14 for boys), pubescence (12 to 14 for girls, 14 to 16 for boys), and postpubescence (14 to 18 for girls, 16 to 20 for boys). Adolescence is particularly notable as a period when sex differences emerge. Speech is a sex-distinctive signal, and the roots of this distinctiveness can be found in the anatomy, physiology, and acoustics of speech. Adolescence is a period when males especially experience a number of changes that affect speech and voice. During this time, the male voice deepens and most of the structures of speech production increase in size.

In summary, the period of infancy is the beginning of speech, and a great deal is accomplished during the development period that has a name meaning "lack of speech." But speech maturation continues for a considerable time into early and even middle childhood. The mastery of sounds in English typically continues until 6 or 7 years of age and refinement of the movements for speech is evident until about prepubescence.

THEORIES OF SPEECH PRODUCTION AND SPEECH PERCEPTION

There are not only different theories about speech, there are different *kinds* of theories. Speech can be modeled in various ways for different purposes. Table 1–1 summarizes some major kinds of models. A neural model of speech production accounts for the nervous system processes that regulate the activities of speaking. Typically, this kind of model talks about neural regulatory loops, brain centers, or some other concept of neural organization. An articulatory model deals with the movements of the speech structures and how they relate to one another. This kind of model usually has the goal of describing articulatory positions, movements, or configurations. It may say little or nothing about neural processes or about the muscles that actually move the articulators. A vocal tract model concentrates on the shaping of the vocal tract (the pharyngeal, oral, and nasal cavities) as an acoustic tube. A functional model tries to describe global or general functions of speech. For example, an information-processing model describes how various types of information are used to regulate speaking. A motor control model is concerned with the activation of muscles and how muscle contractions result in articulatory adjustments. A complete theory of speech would encompass all of these separate theoretical attempts. This would be an ambitious undertaking. Little wonder it has seldom been done.

THE SPEECH TECHNOLOGIES

The term *speech technology* is legitimate. Thanks to developments in engineering and computers, speech has entered the technological age. A speaker's message at one site can be decomposed, converted to a compact code, transmitted along with numerous messages along a fiberoptic cable, and reconstituted as a high-fidelity signal at another site. Or a personal computer can be programmed to respond to voice commands and respond in kind with synthesized speech. One aim of the book is to survey this new technology, which has touched or will touch nearly every human

Table 1-1. Types of models of speech.

Type of Model	Purpose
Neural	Accounts for the nervous system processes that control speech
Articulatory	Describes and/or explains the movements in speech production
Vocal tract	Describes and/or explains the shaping of the vocal tract in speech production
Functional	Accounts for the general functions or events in the formulation and execution of speech events
Motor control	Accounts for the patterns of muscle activation in the speech production system

enterprise, including commercial, scientific, educational, clinical, and artistic. Technology has been humanized as machines are designed to have humanlike capabilities. One of the most remarkable efforts has been the development of human-machine communication through speech. Exciting strides have been made in the design of machines that recognize human speech and produce speechlike signals. Work continues on machines that will recognize a talker (with sufficient reliability as to afford first-line security access to protected systems), understand that talker's request for information, and speak the information requested.

The continuing development of human-machine speech communication may bring to reality things that were science fiction only a few years ago. It may soon be commonplace to speak with computers to exchange information. Moreover, it may come to pass that the computer will be a linguistic intermediary between people who speak different languages. A person may be able to speak to a computer in English, and the computer will immediately translate the message to a language such as French or German. For that matter, we may soon come to the time when one computer telephones a human, only to encounter a computer-controlled speech recognition device that responds to the call in lieu of the human owner. The calling computer may leave a message that is received and decoded by the receiving computer. Computer-to-computer speech communication is entirely plausible.

Some say that we live in the Information Age, but perhaps it is equally apt to say that we live in the Communication Age. Technology has given its power to the human voice, so that we can communicate easily over large distances, from city to city, from continent to continent, and even from Earth to its moon or to other planets. The speed and efficiency of speech communication is a technological revolution. The nearly instantaneous communication available today stands in marked contrast to the agonizingly slow communication of two centuries ago.

> ***"It seemed unlikely that one nation could govern an entire continent. The distances were just too great. A critical fact in the world of 1801 was that nothing moved faster than the speed of a horse. No human being, . . . no letter, no information, no idea, order, or instruction of any kind moved faster."***
>
> (Stephen E. Ambrose, *Undaunted Courage: Meriwether Lewis, Thomas Jefferson, and the Opening of the American West.* New York: Simon & Schuster, 1996, p. 52.)

APPLIED SPEECH SCIENCES

Basic science asks how or why a phenomenon occurs. Basic speech science investigates the fundamental questions pertaining to how speech is produced and how it is perceived. The objective is one of essential understanding, whether or not the question at hand has an immediate application. On the other hand, applied science seeks practical implementation of scientific knowledge. One reason for the study of the speech sciences is that knowledge in this area is fundamental to various applications, such as the speech technologies discussed in the preceding section. But there are several other areas of application, including the assessment and treatment of speech disorders, forensic purposes such as identifying criminal suspects from tape recordings of their voices, improving the clarity of speech signals in noisy or otherwise disruptive environments, and compressing the acoustic signal of speech in a form that can be economically stored or transmitted. These applications are maturing quickly and now form a very important part of the speech sciences. This book delves into both basic and applied aspects of the speech sciences. The basic aspects pertain to fundamental questions about speech, irrespective of any particular application. In its barest form, the question, "How do we produce speech?" is a question of basic speech science. The applied aspects of speech science cover practical problems involving speech production or speech perception. For example, trying to devise a way to make speech more intelligible over a noisy transmission system is an applied problem. Basic and applied aspects of speech science inform one another.

On The Reference Shelf

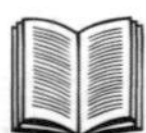

General references for readers who want deeper or extended discussions of selected topics

Crystal, D. (1987). *The Cambridge encyclopedia of language*. New York: Cambridge University Press.
Encyclopedia is an apt title for this comprehensive and entertaining look at language.

Fullerton, T. T. (1975). *Triviata: A compendium of useless information*. New York: Bell Publishing Company.
The information is perhaps without much use, but the book is a collection of interesting facts, some of which are cited in this chapter.

McCrum, R., Cran, W., & MacNeil, R. (1986). *The story of English*. New York: Viking Penguin, Inc.
A classic history of the English language, with information on its various dialects.

Chapter References

Ackerman, D. (1990). *Natural history of the senses*. New York: Random House.

Ambrose, N., Yairi, E., & Cox, N. (1993). Genetic aspects of early childhood stuttering. *Journal of Speech and Hearing Research, 36,* 701–706.

Ardila, A., & Roselli, M. (1996). Spontaneous language production and aging: Sex and educational effects. *International Journal of Neuroscience, 87,* 71–78.

Bonvillian, J. D., Orlansky, M. D., & Novack, L. L. (1983). Developmental milestones: Sign language acquisition and motor development. *Child Development, 54,* 1435–1445.

Bradshaw, J. L., & Nettleton, N. C. (1981). The nature of hemispheric specialization in man. *The Behavioral and Brain Sciences, 4,* 51–91.

Bradshaw, J. L., & Nettleton, N. C. (1983). *Human cerebral asymmetry*. Englewood Cliffs, NJ: Prentice-Hall.

Bulletin of the Library of Natural Sounds. Available from Cornell Laboratory of Ornithology, 159 Sapsucker Woods Road, Ithaca, NY 14850.

Cohen, P. R. (1984). The pragmatics of referring and the modality of communication. *Computational Lingistics, 10,* 97–146.

Crystal, D. (1987). *The Cambridge encyclopedia of language*. New York: Cambridge University Press.

Curtiss, S. (1977). *Genie: A psycholinguistic study of a modern-day "wild child."* New York: Academic Press.

Davis, K. (1947). Final note on a case of extreme isolation. *American Journal of Sociology, 52,* 432–437.

Fenson, L., Dale, P. S., Reznick, J. S., Thal, D., Bates, E., Hartung, J., Pethick, S., & Reilly, J. (1993). *The MacArthur communicative development inventories: User's guide and technical manual*. San Diego: Singular Publishing Group.

Flege, J. E. (1987). A critical period for learning to pronounce foreign languages? *Applied Linguistics, 8*, 162–177.

Flege, J. E., & Fletcher, K. L. (1992). At what age of learning (AOL) do foreign accents first become perceptible? *Journal of the Acoustical Society of America, 91*, 370–389.

Fletcher, P., & Ingham, R. (1995). Grammatical impairment. In P. Fletcher & B. MacWhinney (Eds.), *The handbook of child language* (pp. 603–622). Oxford, England: Blackwell.

Fodor, J. (1983). *The modularity of mind*. Cambridge, MA: MIT Press.

Fullerton, T. T. (1975). *Triviata: A compendium of useless information*. New York: Bell Publishing Company.

Glucksmann, A. (1981). *Sexual dimorphism in human and mammalian biology and pathology*. London: Academic Press.

Gustafson, G. E., Green, J. A., & Cleland, J. W. (1994). Robustness of individual identity in the cries of human infants. *Developmental Psychobiology, 27*, 1–10.

Kent, R. D. (1984). Stuttering as a temporal programming disorder. In R. F. Curlee & W. H. Perkins (Eds.), *Nature and treatment of stuttering: New directions* (pp. 283–301). San Diego: College-Hill Press.

Kent, R. D., & Chial, M. R. (in press). Voice spectrography ("Voiceprints"). In D. L. Faigman, D. Kaye, M. J. Saks, & J. Sanders (Eds.), *Modern scientific evidence*. St. Paul, MN: West Publishing Co.

Koluchova, J. (1972). Severe deprivation in twins: A case study. *Journal of Child Psychology and Psychiatry, 13*, 107–114.

Languis, M. L., & Naouv, P. (1985). Sex differences in neuropsychological function. In L. C. Hartlage & C. F. Telzrow (Eds.), *The neuropsychology of individual difference* (pp. 237–251). New York: Plenum Press.

Lenneberg, E. H. (1967). *The biological foundations of language*. New York: John Wiley.

Locke, J. L. (1983). *Phonological acquisition and change*. New York: Academic Press.

Lockett, J. (1992). Profile of a linguist: Professor David Crystal. *Language International, 4*, 36–37.

Maddieson, I. (1984). *Patterns of sounds*. Cambridge, England: Cambridge University Press.

Mason, M. K. (1942). Learning to speak after six and one half years of silence. *Journal of Speech and Hearing Disorders, 7*, 295–304.

Mazzucchi, A., Moretti, G., Carpeggiani, P., & Parma, M. (1981). Clinical observations on acquired stuttering. *British Journal of Disorders of Communication, 16*, 19–30.

McCrum, R., Cran, W., & MacNeil, R. (1986). *The story of English*. New York: Viking Penguin.

Meier, R. P. (1991, January/February). Language acquisition by deaf children. *American Scientist, 79*, 60–70.

Misrachi, E., & Denney, N. W. (1979). Developmental study of foreign language pronunciation. *Developmental Psychology, 15*, 458–459.

Miller, G. A. (1977). *Spontaneous apprentices: Children and language*. New York: Seabury Press.

Mullennix, J. W., Johnson, K. A., Topcu-Durgun, M., & Farnsworth, L. M. (1995). The perceptual representation of voice gender. *Journal of the Acoustical Society of America, 98*, 3080–3095.

Murray, I. R., Baber, C., & South, A. (1996). Towards a definition and working model of stress and its effects on speech. *Speech Communication, 20*, 3–12.

Nelson, K. (1973). Structure and strategy in learning to talk. *Monographs of the Society for Research in Child Development, 38*(1–2 Serial No. 149).

Newport, E. (1991). Contrasting conceptions of the critical period for language. In S. Carey & R. Gelman (Eds.), *The epigenesis of mind: Essays on biology and cognition* (pp. 111–130). Hillsdale, NJ: Lawrence Erlbaum.

Ochsman, R. B., & Chapanis, A. (1974). The effects of 10 communication modes on the behaviour of teams during co-operative problem-solving. *International Journal of Man-Machine Studies, 6*, 579–620.

Oviatt, S. L., & Cohen, P. R. (1991). The contributing influence of speech and interaction on human discourse patterns. In J. W. Sullivan & S. W. Tyler (Eds.), *Intelligent user interfaces* (pp. 69–83). Reading, MA: Addison-Wesley.

Oyama, S. (1976). A sensitive period for the acquisition of a nonnative phonological system. *Journal of Psycholinguistic Research, 5*, 261–285.

Oyama, S. (1978). The sensitive period and comprehension of speech. *Working Papers on Bilingualism, 16*, 1–17.

Peters, T. J., & Guitar, B. (1991). *Stuttering: An integrated approach to its nature and treatment*. Baltimore: Williams & Wilkins.

Provine, R. P. (1995, January/February). Laughter. *American Scientist, 84*, 38–45.

Robinson, R. J. (1987). Introduction and overview. *Proceedings of the first international symposium on specific speech and language disorders in children* (pp. 1–9). London: Association for All Speech-Impaired Children (AFASIC).

Schachter, F. F., Shore, E., Hodapp, R., Chalfin, S., & Bundy, C. (1978). Do girls talk earlier? Mean length of utterance in toddlers. *Developmental Psychology, 14,* 388–392.

Scherer, K. (1981). Speech and emotional states. In J. K. Darby (Ed.), *Speech evaluation in psychiatry* (pp. 189–240). New York: Grune & Stratton.

Seider, R., Gladstien, K., & Kidd, K. (1983). Recovery and persistence of stuttering among relatives of stutterers. *Journal of Speech and Hearing Research, 48,* 402–409.

Swaan, A. de (1991). The emergent world language system. *Language International, 3,* 17.

Traunmuller, H. (1994). Conventional, biological, and environmental factors in speech communication: A modulation theory. *Phonetica, 51,* 170–183.

Umiker-Sebeok, D. J., & Sebeok, T. A. (Eds.). (1978). *Aboriginal sign languages of the Americas and Australia.* New York: Plenum Press.

Vivian, R. (1966). The Tadoma method: A tactual approach to speech and speech reading. *Volta Review, 68,* 733–737.

Exercises

1-1. Select three episodes from your day in which you spoke with someone. Then analyze the three episodes by describing the following information sources for each: phonetic quality, affective quality, personal quality, and transmittal quality. Describe these information sources for both your speech and the speech of your communication partner.

1-2. Think of some tasks that you ordinarily accomplish by means of voice communication, such as scheduling an appointment, discussing a problem with someone, or asking for information on a particular subject. Then imagine how the pattern of communication would change if you accomplished the tasks by means other than voice communication. The alternative communicative means could include: typewriting, handwriting, manual gestures, and electronic mail.

1-3. Using an encylopedia or other source of information, describe the quantity of vocalizations typically used by the following animals: dog, canary, deer, porcupine, stumptail macaque (a kind of monkey), and giraffe. How do the variations in amount of vocalizations relate to each animal's habitat, visibility, and range of travel?

1-4. Analyze the vocal style of a prominent person (e.g., a news anchor, an actor or actress, or a government leader). What features of voice, speech, or language help to make this person distinctive by spoken language alone? Do you find it relatively easy or difficult to describe these distinctive features?

1-5. Find a television program that shows prolonged shots of a speaker's head (e.g., news programs or lectures). Turn the sound to a minimum so that no auditory information is available. Try to identify as many words as you can from visual cues. If you videotape the program, you can replay the segment with sound to verify your guesses (or you could simply use a videotaped lecture).

1-6. List some speech technologies that you have either used or benefitted from in the last year. Some possibilities are: tape recorders, telephones, voice mail, answering machines, machine speech, voice-activated or voice-controlled machines. What did you like or dislike about each form of technology? How might each technology be improved to make it more convenient and more useful?

1-7. View a science fiction motion picture and describe imagined improvements in speech technology used in the film. A particularly good one is Stanley Kubrick's *2001: A Space Odyssey* (United Kingdom, 1968), which features a talking computer (actually the human voice of actor Douglas Rains), voice identification for security access, and a televideo communication system between a space station and the astronaut's family on Earth. Another source of imaginative speech technology is the *Star Trek* television series or its successors.

1-8. If you have access to a computer with a CD-ROM and the multimedia *Encarta* software on a CD, you can gain some easy experience with different languages. Use the following procedure for *Encarta 1995*: Select *Arts, Languages and Literature* as the area of interest; then select *Language*; then select *World Languages InterActivity*.

CHAPTER 2

Basic Concepts from Physics and Mathematics

> *"There are however innumerable other local motions which on account of the minuteness of the moving particles cannot be detected, such as the motions of the particles in hot bodies, in fermenting bodies, in putrescent bodies, in growing bodies, in the organs of sensation and so forth. If anyone shall have the good fortune to discover all these, I might almost say that he will have laid bare the whole nature of bodies so far as the mechanical causes of things are concerned."*
>
> (Isaac Newton, in *Unpublished Papers of Isaac Newton*)

TOOLS FOR UNDERSTANDING

The basic sciences of physics, mathematics, chemistry, anatomy, and biology are tools for understanding various aspects of speech. Although these basic sciences cannot be considered here in any depth, selected issues in physics and mathematics are explored as preparation for their use in the following chapters. The fundamental questions addressed are:

1. What are the principles of air flow that can be applied to speech production? The answer to this question is found in the physics of fluids.
2. What are the basic issues in sound generation, acoustic resonance, and acoustic analysis? These issues are considered in a brief discussion of sound.
3. How can mathematics be used to (a) quantify the sounds we hear, (b) understand complex dynamic systems (like the biology of living organisms or the patterns of molecule movement in certain types of fluid motion), and (c) describe the geometry of certain complex systems found in nature? These questions lead to brief discussions of logarithms, decibels, chaos theory, and fractals.

> *This book will express physical quantities with the units of the modernized metric system, known as the* **Systeme International d'Unites (International System of Units)**, *which has the international abbreviation SI. The base units and derived units relevant to this book are listed in the Appendix to this chapter. For example, reference to this appendix shows that the quantity of length is expressed in terms of the* **meter** *(symbol* **m**).

THE PHYSICS OF FLUIDS

Gases and liquids are classified as fluids. This book is mostly concerned with gases, especially the air that is inspired and expired by the living human. This air supports life and also provides the basic energy of speech production. An understanding of the physics of gas flows is therefore essential to an understanding of how speech is produced. Some basic principles of the physics of fluids will be introduced here as background to subsequent discussions of air and liquid motion in the body.

Fluid mechanics is the physical science that studies the action of fluids at rest or in motion. The study of fluids at rest is called **fluid statics**, and the study of fluids in motion is called **fluid dynamics**. The term **hydrodynamics** refers to the flow of liquids or low-velocity gas flows in which the gas can be regarded as incompressible. The latter generally can be assumed for the gas flows in speech production and therefore hydrodynamics is the most relevant specialty of fluid mechanics.

HYDRODYNAMICS

A fluid can be conceptualized as consisting of innumerable tiny particles, each of which has a volume that is negligibly small compared to the total volume of the fluid. In general, the particles will have a motion, and this motion is fundamental to the study of both liquids and gases in human physiology. Fluid mechanics takes two primary approaches. The first is to focus on the behavior of a given particle of the fluid during its motion in a particular region. By analogy, one might observe one particular person in a crowd of pedestrians walking through a busy place like Times Square.

This is called the **Lagrangian method**, after the French mathematician and astronomer Joseph Louis Comte de Lagrange. The second is to consider the flow characteristics of particles as they pass in the neighborhood of a given point. Again by analogy, this approach is like counting the numbers of people who move around a particular corner of a city block. This method is the **Eulerian method**, named after the Swiss mathematician Leonhard Euler. Euler is regarded as the founder of the science of hydromechanics (Rouse, 1961). The Eulerian method leads to equations of motion that can be readily applied to practical situations. Although the Eulerian method is the basis for much of the following discussion, some later parts of the book also consider the behavior of individual particles.

Pressure, Volume, and Flow

Some basic quantities of fluid dynamics are **pressure**, **volume**, and **flow**. Pressure is the force per unit area acting perpendicular to a surface. Notice that this definition involves both the applied force and the area to which the force is applied. The formula for pressure, P, is

$P = F/A$, where F is force and A is area.

Force is defined by the equation

$F = Ma$, where M is mass and a is acceleration.

A particular force may be measured as the amount that it stretches a given spring. The unit of force is the **newton (N)**, which is the equivalent of one kilogram of mass with an acceleration of one meter per second squared ($1\ N = 1\ kg\ m/s^2$). The unit commonly used for pressure measurements in speech and hearing applications is the **pascal (Pa)**, named after Blaise Pascal. One pascal is equivalent to a force of one newton acting on a surface of one square meter. Because the pressure value of one pascal is very large compared to the pressures measured in most speech and hearing applications, it is typical to use the **micropascal** (μPa), which is one-millionth of a pascal. For example, the standard reference pressure used to determine levels for hearing is 20 μPa.

Volume is the quantity of air contained in a vessel or space. It is typically measured in liters (l) or milliliters (ml), but the physiology literature also frequently uses cubic centimeters (cc) as a unit of volume. An example of a volume measurement relevant to speech production is the maximum amount of air that can be inspired following a maximal expiration. This is known in respiratory physiology as **vital capacity** (abbreviated VC). The VC for adults varies from about 3.5 l to 6 l, with larger values for males. The liter is commonly used for volume measurements in Europe but not in the United States. Readers from the United States are most likely to see liters as the unit of volume for plastic containers of soft drinks. But for scientific purposes, the liter is preferred as a unit of measurement, as are the other units of the metric system.

Flow is the quantity of gas that moves through a given area in a unit of time. For speech applications, it is common to measure flow in units such as liters per sec (l/s), liters per minute (l/min), milliliters per sec (ml/s), or milliliters per minute (ml/min). Taking an example from speech, the average air flow during sustained phonation of a vowel at a moderate intensity is about 100 ml/sec for women and 110 ml/sec for men. As 1 l equals 1,000 ml, 100 ml is equivalent to one tenth of a liter. Therefore, if an adult man or woman phonates a vowel for 10 s, a total volume of about 1 l of air will be used.

In hydrodynamic systems, pressure and flow are closely related. Typically, air flows from a region of higher pressure to a region of lower pressure. This is the explanation for respiration. Air is inspired into the lungs because expansion of the chest wall or depression of the muscular diaphragm (which forms the floor of the thoracic cavity) increases the volume of the respiratory system. The increased volume causes a reduced air pressure within the lungs relative to atmospheric pressure. Consequently, air flows into the lungs. Expiration involves the inverse: the volume of the respiratory system is decreased so that air pressure within the lungs is greater than atmospheric pressure. This process is discussed in detail in Chapter 4. Put simply, air flows from one region to another because of pressure differentials. Pressure differentials can be created by adjusting the volume of one air space relative to another.

Types of Flow: Laminar and Turbulent

A major contribution that Euler made to the study of hydrodynamics was his recognition that simple and powerful laws for fluids could be derived if the fluid is assumed to be incompressible and ideal—that is, neglecting consideration of friction or viscosity. **Friction** is an opposition to flow and results in a loss of energy to heat. The laws so derived apply to a class of fluid flows called incompressible and frictionless flows. Such flows can be conceptualized as containing imaginary **streamlines** that connect the particles in the moving fluid (Figure 2–1). The streamlines are parallel to the direction of flow and represent the motion path of individual particles in a steady-flow condition. Daniel Bernoulli formulated an important principle about this kind of flow. His principle (**Bernoulli's principle** or **theorem**) states that the total mechanical energy of the fluid is constant along a streamline. Bernoulli's principle captured the balance between kinetic energy and potential energy over every part of a streamline in steady flow. It expresses an interrelationship among the effects of pressure, velocity, and gravity. An important aspect of Bernoulli's principle is that as velocity of flow increases, the pressure decreases (and vice versa). This relation is basic to the design of nozzles, the construction of flow measuring devices, the understanding of lift in aerodynamics, and—more to the point of this book—the vibration of the vocal folds in speech and song. Bernoulli's principle as it relates to velocity and pressure is illustrated in Figure 2–2. This drawing shows a fluid moving through a tube at a constant rate of flow. The total energy of the fluid is the sum of its potential energy and kinetic energy. Potential energy is also pressure energy. Total energy decreases from Region 1 to Region 2 to Region 3 because some energy is lost to friction (which converts energy to heat). At Region 2 (tube constriction), the fluid velocity increases, which leads to an increase in kinetic energy and a decrease in potential energy. Therefore, the pressure decreases at Region 2. At Region 3, where the tube widens, the fluid velocity decreases and kinetic energy is converted into pressure energy. The pressure energy is higher at Regions 1 and 3 than at Region 2.

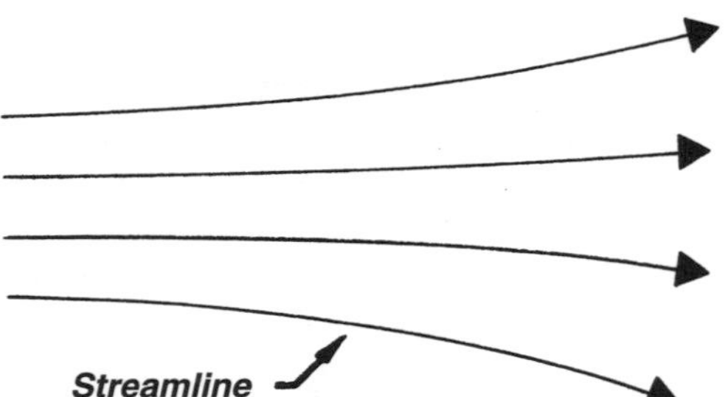

Figure 2–1. Streamlines of fluid flow within a pipe.

As shown in Figure 2–2, when fluids flow through a pipe, some of the mechanical energy of the flow is dissipated as the consequence of viscous friction. The energy loss can be expressed as a pressure drop along

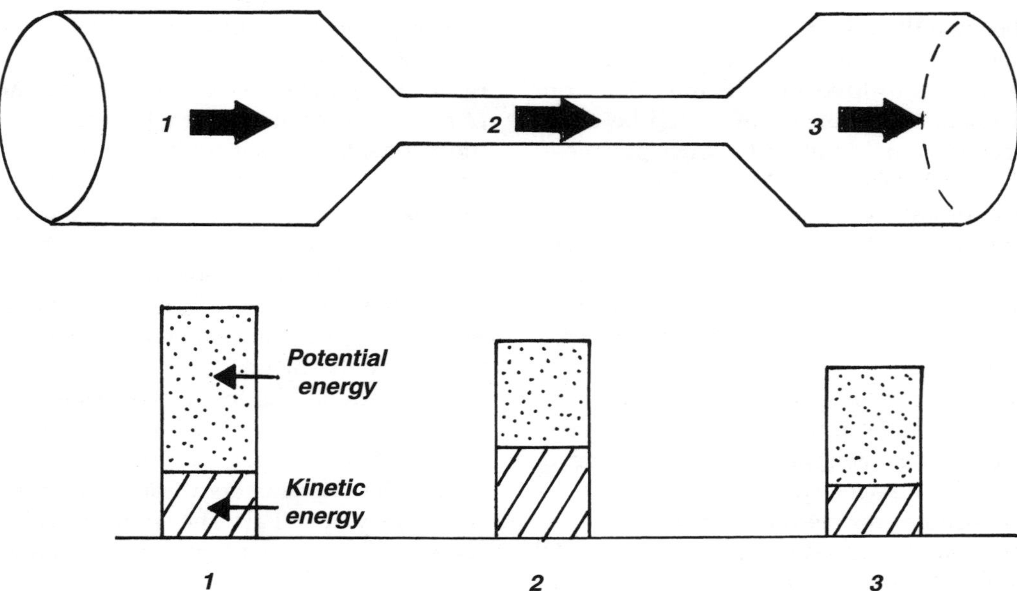

Figure 2–2. An illustration of the Bernoulli effect in which a fluid passes through a constriction in a pipe. In the constricted region, the velocity of flow increases and the pressure is reduced. The bar graphs at the bottom of the illustration show the relative changes in kinetic and potential energy corresponding to Regions 1, 2, and 3 in the pipe.

the pipe. To make this relevant to speech, consider that the air moving from the lungs up through the throat and out the nose or mouth loses some of its total mechanical energy to viscous friction.

It was discovered in experiments conducted in the 19th century that, for low velocities of flow, the pressure drop was linear with flow velocity, making for simple calculations of the relation between pressure and flow. But at high flow velocities, the relation changes: The pressure drop is more closely proportional to the square of velocity and the relation is therefore nonlinear. A British engineer named Osborne Reynolds put the problem into relief by demonstrating that viscous flows through pipes have two kinds of flow. In **laminar flow**, the particles of the fluid follow the streamlines (Figure 2–3). In **turbulent flow**, the particles have a much more complex behavior

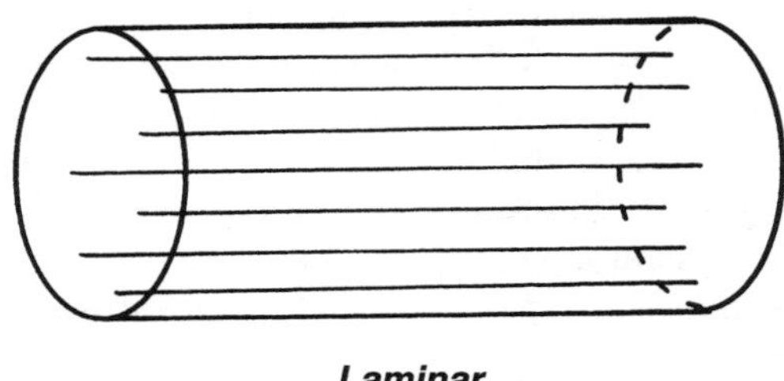

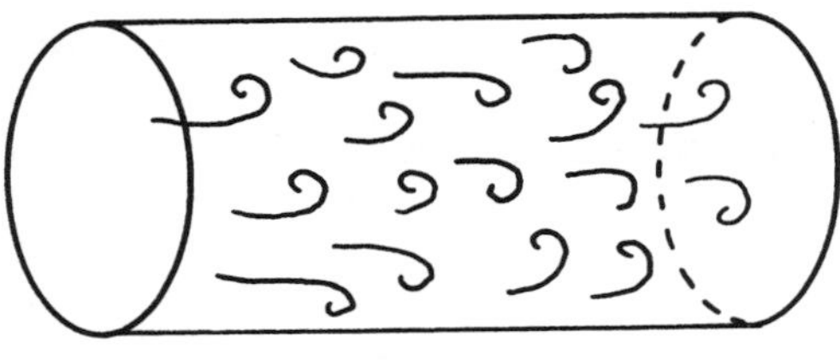

Figure 2–3. Illustrations of laminar and turbulent flow through a pipe.

because the flow produces eddies, or patterns of fluctuating velocity (Figure 2–3). Reynolds realized that the transition from laminar to turbulent flow could be determined from the value of a single parameter now called the **Reynolds number**, which is the product of velocity, fluid density, and pipe diameter, divided by the fluid viscosity. For a Reynolds number of less than 2,100, flow will be laminar. For values higher than 2,100, the flow typically will be turbulent.

In later chapters, the distinction between laminar and turbulent flow is important in discussing how speech sounds are formed. For the moment, two simple examples demonstrate the relevance of the flow patterns to speech. Vowels, such as the "ah" sound a physician asks a patient to utter during an examination of the throat, generally are modeled as having a laminar flow, so that particles can be assumed to move along the streamlines. The word laminar means layered. This kind of flow is typical of all sounds called **sonorants**, which are the resonant sounds including the vowels, nasals like the consonants in *man*, and liquids like the consonants in *real*. **Fricatives** such as the consonants in the word *sashes* are produced with a turbulent flow. Generally, any sound that has a conspicuous noisy quality has a turbulent flow as part of its generation. A sound that has the smooth resonant sound like that of vowels is primarily the result of laminar flow. An everyday illustration of laminar and turbulent flow is the smoke pattern from a cigarette or chimney in still air. The smoke initially rises in a laminar pattern, but eventually breaks up into the eddy patterns characteristic of turbulence. The laminar pattern continues until it is destabilized.

SOUND

Sound is a form of energy. In common usage, sound is a physical energy transmitted through air that can stimulate the sense of hearing. However, physicists often use the term to include physical phenomena occurring in solids and liquids as well. The term **sonic** is an adjective referring to sound. **Subsonic** means below the range of human hearing, and **supersonic** means above the range of human hearing. The terms "below" and "above" in the preceding sentence refer to the frequency of vibration (closely related to the perception of pitch). More precise physical definitions will be given later. For the present, it is sufficient to note that human hearing has a limited range and it is this range that is usually applied to define the term sonic.

Acoustics is the study of the physics of sound. **Psychoacoustics** deals with the psychological response to acoustic stimuli and includes topics such as loudness, pitch, and timbre. Modern acoustics began with the publication in 1894 of Lord Rayleigh's *The Theory of Sound*, which set forth basic principles still observed today.

Wave Motion

In most common experience, energy is transferred from one point to another in one of two ways. The first is the passage of matter from point to point, as with a bullet that is shot from a gun to a target. The second is the transfer of energy through a continuous physical medium, such as the ripples created when a stone is thrown in a quiet pool of water. In this second type of energy transfer, although the individual particles of the medium are displaced only a minute distance, those particles propagate the energy in a wavelike manner over a potentially large distance. This kind of energy transfer is called **wave motion**.

Like several types of energy, sound travels in waves. Other wave energies include light, radio waves, and electromagnetic radiation. They all share the transfer of energy through a medium even though the medium as a whole does not move from point to point. Sound differs from these other types of wave energy in that sound waves actually impart the physical motion to air particles, which move, however slightly, as part of the sound wave. As noted in the beginning of this chapter, air and other fluids can be conceptualized as consisting of innumerable tiny particles. Air particles can be further conceptualized as being elastically coupled, as though they were interconnected by tiny springs (Figure 2–4). Sound energy produces a displacement of the particles. If air were inelastic, any given displaced particle P_1 would simply remain in its new position. But because air is elastic, P_1 tends to return to its original position, as though it were drawn back by a spring. Before it returns to its original position, it collides with an adjacent particle P_2. P_2 in turn collides with P_3 before returning to its original position. In this way, sound energy is transmitted particle to particle even though the particles return to their original positions. Collision zones are called **condensations** because they are characterized by an aggregation of particles. The zones where particles have moved apart are called **rarefactions**. The wave motion is therefore a sequence of condensations and rarefactions. The sound wave can be likened to a domino effect action, with the important exception that air particles, unlike dominoes, return to their starting positions. Sound waves are an example of **longitudinal waves**, in which the energy is propagated as back and forth motions of particles, with the particle motion being parallel to the direction of wave motion. This is to be distinguished from **transverse waves**, in which particles move transversely to the direction of wave motion. An example of a transverse wave is the rippling created when a stone is thrown into a quiet pool of water. The transverse nature of the wave can be seen when another object in the pool, such as a floating leaf, bobs up and down as the wave passes.

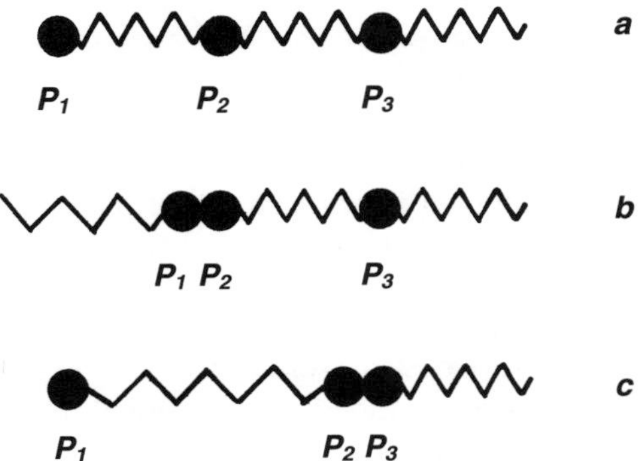

Figure 2–4. Schematic illustration of air particles considered as tiny spheres connected by springs. Wave motion causes a displacement of air particles in a kind of domino effect. See text for discussion.

The Slinky™ common coil toy also can be used to demonstrate longitudinal waves. If a Slinky is stretched out and a to-and-fro motion is introduced at one end, the coils of the Slinky will vibrate back and forth in the direction of the wave of motion. Notice that the Slinky is analogous to air in the sense that the coils are elastically coupled. The wave motion observed in the Slinky is analogous to the wave motion of sound in the air.

Sound energy, then, propagates as a wave in which adjacent air particles are moved to and fro in tiny displacements. The denser the air, the more closely spaced the particles are, and the spacing of particles can affect sound propagation. The speed of sound varies with atmospheric pressure and the temperature and humidity of air. In rarer air, such as at high mountain elevations, sound is not as efficiently transmitted. In an extreme case, such as the surface of the moon, it would be strangely silent, because the air particles are very widely scattered. Huge collisions of objects on the moon would be soundless.

At sea level and a dry air temperature of 0° centigrade, the **speed of sound** is 331 m/s (1,085.96 ft/s). The great physicist Isaac Newton is credited as being the first to measure the speed of sound. Unlike the speed of light, the speed of sound energy is highly dependent on the medium through which it travels. This is understandable given that sound energy involves innumerable small collisions between adjacent particles. The density of these particles and their elasticity determines the speed at which sound can be propagated. Because of its density and elasticity, water is an excellent transmitter of sound, which is why submarines can be detected by **sonar** (for SOund NAvigation Ranging). Engine noise from a submarine can travel for thousands of miles in the ocean, especially if it travels though what is known as a "deep sound channel" (Munk, 1993). Sound also travels faster in water than in air. The speed of sound in the ocean is about 1500 m/s, about five times the speed of sound in air. In 1960, depth charges (deep-sea explosions) set off at Perth, Australia, produced low-frequency sounds that were recorded 3.5 hours later off the coast of Bermuda, 20,000 miles from the source. The ocean, as one observer put it, is a concert hall of sound. Human-made sounds, such as those from ships, add greatly to the total mix of acoustic events in the watery environment.

To understand the analysis of sound, we now consider a sound that rarely occurs in nature. This unnatural sound is the means to a powerful analysis of a large number of complex sounds. The sound in question is the **sinusoid** (from the trigonometric sine function) and is the tone produced by an appropriately struck tuning fork ("appropriately" in this context basically means "not too hard"). A sinusoid is also described as projected uniform circular motion, also known as **simple harmonic motion** (the kind of motion produced by a particle that moves at a constant velocity in a circle). Figure 2–5 illustrates how the sinusoid is related to circular motion. A peg is attached to a point near the rim of a circular plate. The plate is then rotated around its diameter in a darkened room while a light source is placed on one side and a white screen on the other. As the plate revolves (performing uniform circular motion), the peg will cast a shadow that moves up and down on the screen. Now if the screen is moved away from the plate at a constant rate, a sinusoid will be traced on the screen. A very important thing about a sinusoid in acoustic analysis is that it can be specified by three physical properties, its **frequency**, **amplitude**, and **phase**. *Frequency* is the rate of vibration of a sound. *Amplitude* is the magnitude of vibration. *Phase* is the point on the sinusoidal function at which the waveform commences. To understand these quantities, it is helpful to consider further the example of the tuning fork.

Figure 2–6 shows how the to-and-fro movements of a tuning fork relate to the sine function. In this illustration, the periodic (occurring at regular intervals) movements of the fork cause the air particles to form regularly spaced regions of condensation and rarefaction. Note that the condensations and rarefactions are associated with the crests and troughs of the sinusoidal pattern. The graph of the sinusoid is an example of a **waveform**, which represents the shape of the wave over time. A complete to-and-fro vibratory cycle of the fork is equivalent to one complete cycle of sinusoidal motion. This sinusoidal cycle is the basic component used in acoustic analysis. The sinusoid is an example of how a pure mathematical function (in this case, a trigonometric function) finds important application in describing events in the physical world, even though the sinusoid rarely if ever occurs in natural systems. Mathematics is a powerful tool in the physical sciences.

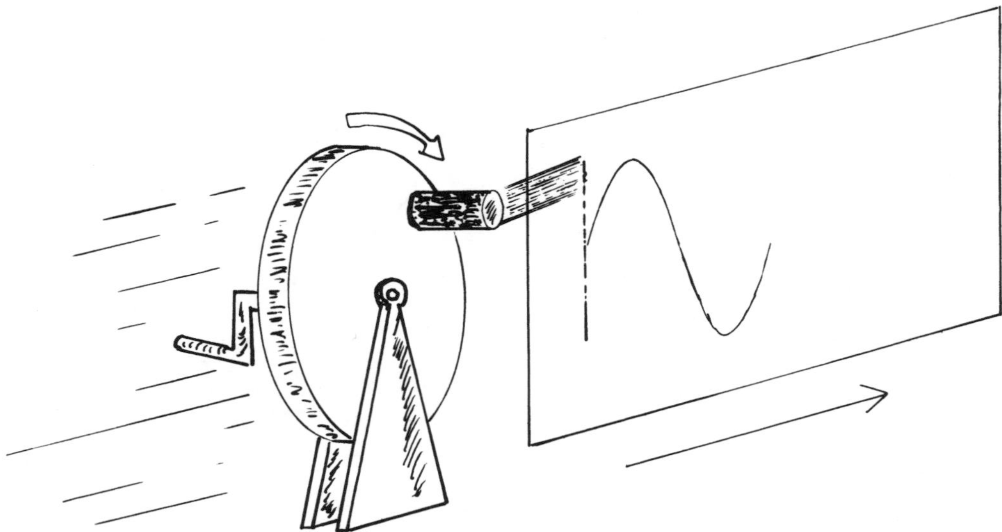

Figure 2–5. Illustration of an apparatus to show how uniform circular motion relates to a sinusoidal waveform. Imagine that the rotating wheel is positioned between a light source and a projection screen. As the wheel is cranked to turn at a constant speed, the peg attached to the rim of the wheel will leave a shadow on the screen. Now, if the screen is moved at a constant speed in the direction of the arrow, the peg's shadow will leave a sinusoidal waveform on the screen. Therefore, a sinusoid can be described as a linear projection of uniform circular motion.

Frequency

The effects of changing the frequency of sinusoidal vibration are illustrated in Figure 2–7. Notice that with increased frequency of vibration, more cycles of the sinusoid are completed in a unit of time. Frequency, then, is the number of cycles of vibration per second, typically expressed as hertz (Hz), after the physicist Heinrich Hertz. The total time required for one cycle of vibration is the **period,** t_0. Frequency and period are inversely related,

$$f = 1/t_0 \text{ and } t_0 = 1/f$$

A sinusoid with a frequency of 1000 Hz has a period of 1 ms. A sinusoid with a frequency of 100 Hz has a period of 10 ms. The lower the frequency of vibration, the longer the time needed for a complete cycle of vibration. Suppose that sinusoids were selected to match the voice pitches of a man and a woman. The average voice pitch for a man matches a sinusoid with a frequency of about 120 Hz. The period for this tone is about 8.3 ms. The average voice pitch for a woman matches a sinusoid of about 240 Hz. The period for this tone is about 4.2 ms. If a woman sings a note that is matched to a tone of 1000 Hz, then the corresponding period is 1 ms. (**Pitch** is the perceptual correlate of frequency, which is a physical quantity; however, in much of the speech literature pitch and frequency are used almost interchangeably, although they should not be.)

Human hearing has a frequency range from about 15 Hz to 20,000 Hz. Because the range is large, frequency values often are expressed in kilohertz, kHz (**kilo-** means one thousand; therefore 1 kHz is 1000 Hz). Several other frequency terms are used in the sciences and arts related to sound. **Har-**

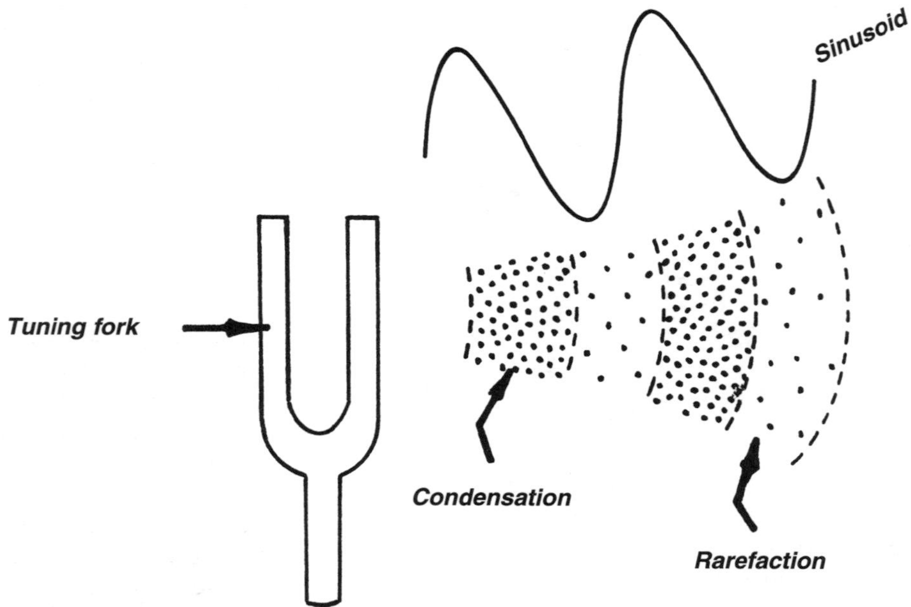

Figure 2-6. Relation between the to-and-fro movements of a tuning fork and the sinusoidal function of condensation and rarefaction.

monic deals with integer relations among elements. As applied to sounds, harmonics are components that are related to one another in a harmonic series. For example, three sounds have the harmonic relation 1, 2, 3, if they form a harmonic series in which the second tone is twice the frequency of the first, and the third tone is three times the frequency of the first. Many complex sounds in physics and the performing arts can be described as a **fundamental tone** (the lowest, or basic, frequency) and its harmonics. This is true for string instruments, for horns, and even the human voice. An **Octave** is a 2:1 relation between two sounds. The A above middle C on a piano typically is tuned to a frequency of 440 Hz. The next higher A on the piano is one octave above and has a frequency of 880 Hz. The piano note that is one octave *lower* than 440 Hz is a note with a frequency of 220 Hz. On average, men's speaking voices are one octave lower than women's. The average fundamental frequency of a man's voice is about 120 Hz, compared to the average woman's fundamental of 240 Hz. The terms introduced in this paragraph are particularly useful in describing the **quality** of sound.

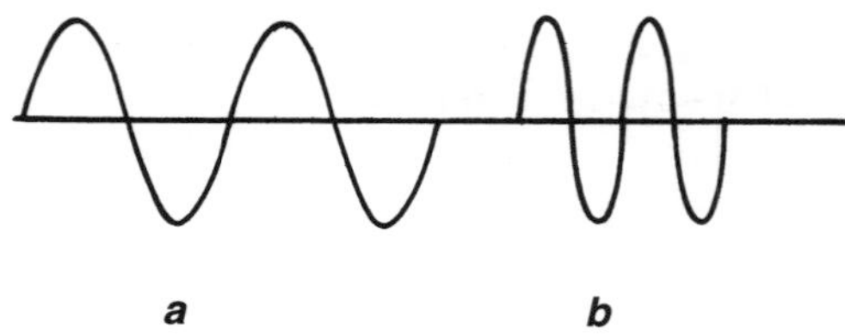

Figure 2-7. Example of two sinusoids of different frequency. The sinusoid labeled a has **a** lower frequency than the sinusoid labeled **b** because it has fewer cycles per unit of time.

Amplitude

Changes in amplitude of vibration are illustrated in Figure 2–8 for a tone of fixed frequency. The magnitude of displacement of the tuning fork determines the to-and-fro motions of air particles and therefore the amplitude of the corresponding sinusoidal wave. As displacement of the fork increases (larger to-and-fro swings), the amplitude of the sinusoid increases accordingly. The actual magnitudes of vibration are extremely small, so it is impractical to express the magnitude of a sound in this way. More practical measures of sound magnitude are **intensity** and **sound pressure**. Intensity is the sound energy per second over an area of 1 square meter and is typically expressed in the unit of watts per square meter. Hence, sound intensity is the rate of energy flow at a point. Although sound intensity was central to Lord Rayleigh's influential book *The Theory of Sound*, it was only quite recently that practical methods were available for the measurement of intensity (Rasmussen, 1989). Pressure, as noted earlier, is the amount of force per unit area. Humans are sensitive to a huge range of intensities or sound pressures. The range of intensities detected by the ear is at least 10 million million (1 followed by 13 zeros) to one. Such a number is inconveniently large. Therefore, intensities and sound pressures usually are expressed on a logarithmic scale that greatly compresses the numerical representation. This scale is the bel or decibel scale (**deci-** means one tenth; hence, decibel is one tenth of a bel) and is discussed in the final section of this chapter, Applied Mathematics, following a discussion of logarithms.

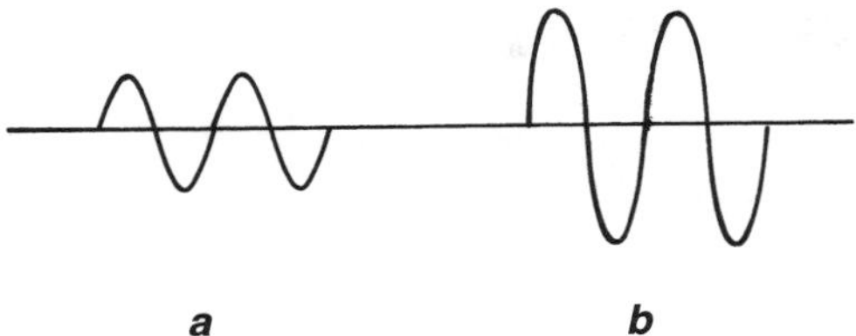

Figure 2–8. Differences in amplitude for a sinusoid of fixed frequency. Notice that the number of cycles per unit time does not change, but that the displacement (amplitude of the wave) is larger in **b** than in **a**.

Fourier Analysis

As mentioned earlier, the sinusoid is of particular interest because it can be regarded as the basic component of more complex sounds. The basic idea is that complex sounds can be considered as consisting of a combination of sinusoids of the appropriate frequencies, amplitudes, and temporal relation (called **phase**). This is the principle of **Fourier analysis**, according to which sounds can be analyzed as a number of harmonics. Fourier analysis is therefore the determination of the sinusoidal constituents of a sound. Figure 2–9 is an example of a Fourier analysis (also called an **amplitude spectrum**) in which three sinusoidal components are identified. Note that each sinusoid appears as a single vertical line along the frequency axis. The height of the line represents the amplitude of the component. Fourier analysis was developed from Fourier's discovery that any periodic waveform could be represented as a summation of sinusoidal vibrations. That is, a periodic waveform can be analyzed into a discrete number of individual sinusoids of appropriate frequency, amplitude, and phase.

Now if sounds can be analyzed as a combination of sinusoids, then we might ask: Is it possible to create complex sounds by combining an appropriate number of sinusoids? The answer is yes. The generation of complex sounds in this way is an example of **sound synthesis**. The basic idea can be extended to speech. **Machine speech**, or synthesized speech, frequently is generated by this principle.

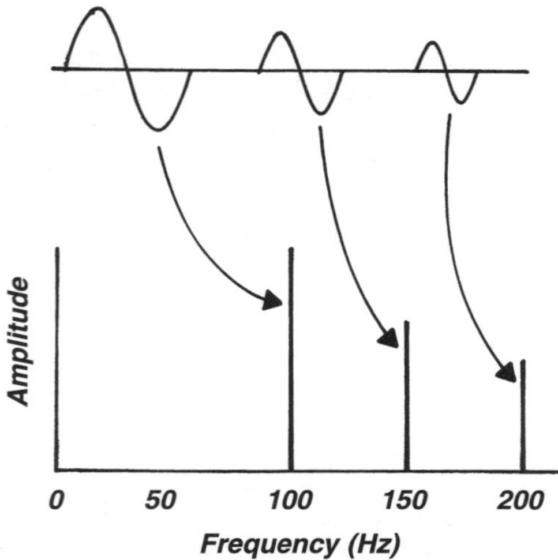

Figure 2–9. Example of a Fourier analysis of a complex sound. The graph shows the amplitude of sound components as a function of their frequency. The sound in this example has three components located at the frequencies of 100 Hz, 150 Hz, and 200 Hz. Each vertical line in the graph represents a sinusoidal component of the sound being analyzed; that is, each line is equivalent to one of the sinusoids shown above the spectrum.

> *"The importance of SHM [simple harmonic motion] in the study of physics cannot be overestimated, for it was shown by the great French mathematician Baron Jean Baptiste Joseph Fourier in the 19th century that any motion, however complex, can be expressed as, or broken down into, a sum of SHMs."*
>
> (L. Motz & J. H. Weaver, *The Story of Physics*. New York: Plenum Press, 1989, p. 65.)

Signal-to-Noise Ratio

Ambient means an environment. Ambient sound is the sound associated with a given environment. Because speech is ordinarily transmitted as an acoustic signal, speech competes with any background sound created in the environment. The quietest environment, such as the isolated areas in the Colorado plateau, are as quiet as a professional sound studio (Grasser & Moss, 1992). Even high-quality monitoring equipment can barely register the sound levels in such mountain quiet. Things can change markedly with the introduction of a sound source, such as a motorized vehicle or even buzzing insects. Much of our life is lived in the presence of readily audible environmental sounds. Therefore, we often have to pick out sounds of particular interest from a background of other sounds. This acoustic competition is a severely limiting factor for speech communication in many environments.

The relative intensity of a signal compared to the intensity of background noise is given by the **signal-to-noise ratio** (S/N). Large positive values of this number are preferable because they indicate a strong signal relative to the noise background. Small positive values or negative values are less favorable for detection of signals because the noise rivals or exceeds the signal in intensity.

Resonance

Galileo Galilei, the famous 17th century scientist, discovered principles of resonance from observations of simple systems such as a pendulum (Olenick, Apostol, & Goodstein, 1985). He noted that it was possible to increase the amplitudes of a swinging pendulum by the application of small, well-timed forces. A commonplace example is pushing someone on a swing. To achieve maximum benefit of the pushes, they should be timed to occur at the same point of each swing. This is an example of **forced oscillation**, in which vibrations are induced by an external driving force. Galileo further realized that, if the frequency of the external driving force was equal to the natural frequency of the system (i.e., the frequency at which the system will naturally oscillate), then the effect on the amplitude was remarkably large. **Resonance** is said to occur when a vibrating system is driven by a periodic force at the natural frequency of the system. Resonance is therefore frequency-dependent. The conditions at which resonance will occur can be specified by the characteristics of the vibrating object and the driving force. A child on a swing is a physical system with a particular natural frequency. The parent who pushes the child on the swing discovers the proper timing of pushes to achieve maximum amplitude of the back-and-forth swinging motions. In so doing, the parent is driving the swing at its natural, or resonant, frequency.

Consider the examples of resonance:

1. A tuning fork is struck in the vicinity of a piano. The piano seems to spontaneously produce a tone of the same frequency.
2. A string of cars passes over a long suspension bridge at close, regular intervals, ignoring a sign that warns drivers to maintain a minimum distance. The bridge begins to sway detectably.
3. A young girl moistens the lip of a crystal goblet and then runs her finger around the mouth of the goblet, adjusting the speed of her finger motion until the glass emits a loud, clear tone.
4. The case of an inexpensive plastic radio vibrates unpleasantly when certain sounds are played through its speaker.
5. A strong wind blows across telephone wires, causing them to "sing in the wind." The singing sound arises from both turbulence and resonance. Turbulence is generated when the air flowing across the wires produces eddies, like those in Figure 2–3. Under the right conditions, the turbulence effects will cause resonance in the wire, as vortices peel off the wire and set it into motion. This is the basis for the aeolian harp. (Aeolius was the Greek god of the winds.)
6. Scientists developed "air-ride" seats to protect the spines of drivers of trucks and heavy equipment from cumulative trauma disorders. Whole-body vibration trunk resonances fall in the range of 4 to 8 Hz, and continued exposure to driving forces in this frequency can damage the the spine (Wasserman, 1995).
7. The military has had an interest in intense energy sources that have a frequency close to the natural frequency of the human body. Imagine what would happen if the body as a whole were set into vibration. Enemy soldiers subjected to this phenomenon might be temporarily impaired.

In each example, an external periodic driving force causes vibration in a physical object. The vibration occurs because the external force was matched in its frequency to the natural frequency of the object. Resonance results in the reinforcement of sound energy at the natural frequency of the object. The result of the resonance can be desirable or not. Resonance is basic to the construction of musical instruments and can distinguish a good from a poor instrument. Perhaps the Italian violin maker Antonio Stradivari knew secrets of resonance when he changed the proportions of his violins to create instruments that are still regarded as exceptional. (Stradivarius is the Latin equivalent of his name and is typically used to identify his violins.) Some believe that Stradivari used a certain varnish that imparted remarkable acoustic qualities to his instruments. The real answer is unknown. Resonance also can be destructive, as when a suspension bridge is set into dangerous vigorous motion by an external force (as in example 2 in the list of resonance phenomena). A bridge in Manchester, England actually collapsed when soldiers marched over it while keeping cadence, and a bridge over the Puget Sound near Tacoma, Washington collapsed in response to a prevailing wind of about 42 mph. And, of course, there is the example of the vocalist who can shatter a crystal goblet by producing a note that matches the natural frequency of the goblet.

For simple physical objects, the natural frequency can be predicted from basic physical properties. The natural frequency of a string depends on its mass, length, and tension. The natural frequency of a jar depends on the volume of air contained in it and the diameter of its mouth. This second example has special relevance to a book on speech. Talking is in large part a matter of adjusting the natural frequencies of the talking instrument, the vocal tract. When talkers move their lips, tongues, and other speech organs, they create different resonant conditions. Speech is a matter of tuning an air-filled resonator to form distinctive sounds. The details of this process are covered in Chapter 9. For the moment, it is sufficient to note that a talker is, in part, an air-filled tube with adjustable dimensions and, therefore, tunable resonances.

Damping and Reverberation

Because sound is propagated by moving particles in the air, sound energy is dissipated in the process. The diminution of amplitude of vibration due to frictional resistance is called **damping.** A damped sinusoidal waveform is shown in Figure 2–10; notice how the energy "dies out." Friction was mentioned earlier in this chapter in connection with fluid mechanics. Friction also is relevant to acoustics. Friction is an opposition to motion. Sound energy is lost to frictional resistance and therefore sound waves do not last forever. In systems with low damping, sound waves continue for a relatively long time. In systems with high damping, sound waves tend to die out quickly. Damping is related to the **bandwidth** of the sound. Bandwidth is the frequency range of energy of the sound. A sound with a large bandwidth contains a wide range of frequencies, whereas a sound with a narrow bandwidth contains a small range of frequencies. The larger the damping, the greater the bandwidth. This issue is revisited in Chapter 9.

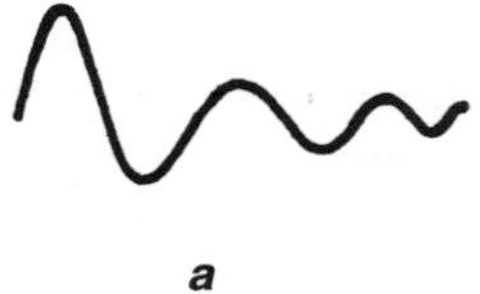

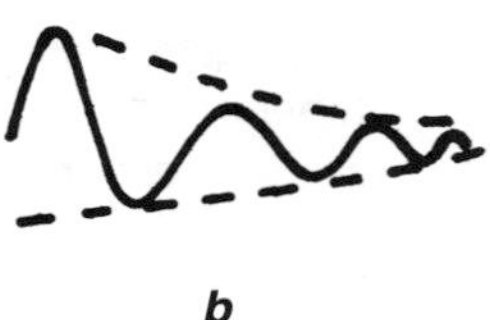

Figure 2–10. Example of a damped sinusoidal waveform. The amplitude of the waveform diminishes over time as shown in **a**. The dashed lines in **b** show the rate of decay of the damped waveform.

In most modern houses and buildings, sound is effectively absorbed by furniture, draperies, and wall coverings. If it were not so, then sounds would tend to **reverberate**, bouncing back and forth from wall to wall. Reverberation can interfere with speech communication and with music. The music of the Western world has been shaped by this principle. An echo that is not damped to inaudibility within 50 ms is likely to interfere with the next sound in the musical sample. What would music be like if it were produced in highly reverberant rooms? One answer is the Gregorian chant. These chants were first produced in medieval cathedrals made of stone walls. This highly reverberant environment interfered with all but very simple intonations. Therefore, Gregorian chants are a form of music adapted to a particular acoustic environment. More complex music requires acoustic environments that are less reverberant. Reverberent environments can hinder the understanding of speech, because the sound echoes create an interference effect. Unfortunately, some classrooms are highly reverberent and therefore less than ideal for ensuring intelligibility of speech throughout the room. This issue is revisited in Chapter 10 with reference to the difficulty that some children may experience in understanding speech in the typical classroom.

APPLIED MATHEMATICS

> *"Nature speaks with a thousand voices, and we have only begun to listen."*
>
> (Ilya Prigogine and Isabelle Stengers, *Order Out of Chaos.* Toronto: Bantam Books, 1984, p. 77)

This chapter certainly does not cover mathematics in any detail, nor does this book require a mathematics background. But it is convenient and helpful to discuss here some concepts that are important to later discussions of acoustics, anatomy, and physiology. These concepts offer effective, even startling, ways of understanding issues that arise.

Logarithms

Human sensation often has a nonlinear relation with the physical properties of a stimulus. For example, the auditory estimation of the loudness of a sound does not change in a linear relation with changes in the physical magnitude of the sound. Similarly, human judgments of the pitch of a tone are decidedly nonlinear. Nonlinear scales therefore are convenient to use in describing auditory function (and other sensations as well). The convenience is also related to the size of the numbers involved. If the human loudness response is expressed in linear relation to the physical magnitude of a sound, then the ratio of the loudest sound (just short of the pain threshold) to the softest sound we can hear is on the order of 10 million million to one. This vast range makes it awkward to quantify the values of individual sounds. The same range in physical magnitude can be greatly compressed with the use of **logarithms**. The actual problem of measuring sound magnitude will be taken up later. The present task is to consider what a logarithm is. The basic idea is to transform a number scale of vast range to a scale of a smaller, more convenient range.

Any number can be expressed as a power of 10. To take some examples, 100 is 10 to the second power of 10, or 10^2, and 10,000 is 10 to the fourth power of 10, or 10^4. The exponents become the means to a logarithmic scale. Instead of using the original large number, we can write only its **exponent**, or the value to which 10 must be raised to equal the original number. The number 10 is the **base** and logarithms to the base 10 are called **common logarithms**. They are used so frequently that the base often is omitted and logarithm is abbreviated to **log**. Therefore, someone might say that the log of 1,000 is 3. To be more precise, we could say that the log to the base 10 of 1,000 is 3. Notice that the same logarithmic interval can represent very different intervals of the original numbers (Table 2–1). For instance, there is a logarithmic interval of 1 between 10 and 100 but also a logarithmic interval of 1 between 100,000 and 1,000,000. Therefore, there is a greater compression for large numbers than for small numbers.

As mentioned, the base 10 is used quite frequently in general applications and when the base is omitted from notation, the base 10 usually is assumed. However, another very important class of logarithms is the so-called **natural logarithm**, based on the **natural number** *e*. The number *e* is like *pi* in its importance to mathematics. Like *pi*, *e* can be expressed as an infinite nonrepeating decimal fraction. The value of *e* to eight decimal places is 2.71828285. We will not concern ourselves with its mathematical derivation in this text. The interesting thing about *e* is that it appears repeatedly in diverse fields, such as the pure theory of numbers, geometry, physics, biology, astronomy, and a number of other areas of study. The discussion in this book only covers *e* in a few limited areas, rather like a quick glimpse at this extraordinary number. It reappears toward the end of this chapter. For the "story of *e*," see Maor (1994).

Table 2–1. Examples of the relations between numbers and their logarithms. The logarithm to base 10 (log_{10}) is the power to which 10 must be raised to yield the number shown. For example, 100 is 10^2, so the logarithm of 100 is 2.

Number	Logarithm (to base 10)
1	0
10	1
100	2
1,000	3
10,000	4
100,000	5
1,000,000	6
10,000,000	7

Bel and Decibel

The bel and decibel, as noted earlier in this chapter, are the units by which the magnitude or strength of a sound is typically expressed. The bel is simply the logarithm of a ratio. It is named in honor of Alexander Graham Bell, the inventor of the telephone. As discussed in the previous section, the logarithm is especially useful to express a large range of values, such as the magnitudes of sound energy to which the ear responds. These quantities can be expressed as a ratio in which the intensity of any given sound, I_1, is compared to a reference intensity, I_0. The bel, then, is a logarithm to the base 10 of a intensity ratio:

$$N\ (\text{bels}) = \log_{10} I_1/I_0$$

The bel is actually a very large unit—too large for most purposes in applied acoustics. Therefore, the decibel (dB) was adopted to represent one-tenth the ratio of a bel. The decibel is defined as follows for a intensity measurement:

$$N(\text{dB}) = 10 \log_{10} I_1/I_0.$$

For example, if I_1 were 1,000 times as great as I_0, the power ratio would be 1,000 and the equivalent value in decibels would be

30 (because the logarithm to the base 10 of 1,000 is 3 and 10 × 3 = 30).

In most acoustic applications considered in this book, sound magnitude is expressed either as intensity level (IL) or sound pressure level (SPL). Intensity level is a ratio in decibels of any given intensity to a reference intensity. The reference intensity of 10^{-12} watt/m^2 has been adopted for the expression of intensity levels. The formula for intensity level is given below for a reference intensity I_0 and a measured intensity I_1:

$$\begin{aligned} \text{IL (db)} &= 10 \log_{10} I_1/I_0 \\ &= 10 \log_{10} I_1/10^{-12}\ \text{watt/m}^2. \end{aligned}$$

Sound pressure level is frequently used in speech and hearing applications because microphones, most measurement devices, and the ear itself respond to sound pressure. Sound pressure level therefore is determined for a ratio of sound pressures. The standard reference sound pressure is 20 µPa, which is the pressure produced in air by a sound wave with an intensity of 10^{-12} watt/m^2 under specified conditions of atmospheric pressure and air temperature. The formula for SPL is:

$$\begin{aligned} \text{SPL (db)} &= 20 \log_{10} P_1/P_0 \\ &= 20 \log_{10} P_1/20\ \mu\text{Pa}. \end{aligned}$$

In comparing the formulas for IL and SPL in decibels, you can see that the multiplier is 10 for IL, but 20 for SPL. The reason for this change in multiplier is that intensity is proportional to the pressure squared. Therefore 10 is multiplied by 2 to obtain the multiplier for SPL.

The actual measurement of sound intensity or sound pressure level requires careful attention to details (Rasmussen, 1989; Rossing & Fletcher, 1995; Speaks, 1996). For present purposes, it is sufficient to be aware that standards exist for these measurement procedures.

The decibel is a practical unit of measurement because it is based on the logarithm. It is convenient for sound measurements because it expresses a large range of actual physical values (power, intensity, or sound pressure) as a relatively condensed range of numbers. The range of hearing is about 140 dB, from the faintest sound that can just be detected to the loudest sound that is nearly strong enough to cause pain. The decibel is just one example of a mathematical device that is usefully applied to nonlinear systems. In the following section, we turn to another type of nonlinearity, the class of nonlinear dynamic systems. These are of considerable interest in the science of physical and living systems because many of these systems turn out to be nonlinear.

Chaos

> ***A. A violent order is disorder; and***
> ***B. A great disorder is an order. These***
> ***Two things are one. (Pages of***
> ***illustrations).***
>
> (Wallace Stevens,
> *Connoisseur of Chaos*, 1942)

A new form of mathematics has emerged to deal with complex systems, such as systems with complicated dynamic properties or systems with complex geometric forms. This new mathematics has had a profound influence in physics, chemistry, physiology, biology, and anatomy. Because occasional reference is made to this form of mathematics in the remainder of this book, a few words of explanation are in order.

In their book *Order Out of Chaos*, Ilya Prigogine and Isabelle Stengers credit the French mathematician Baron Jean-Joseph Fourier for the birth of the "science of complexity." (It was the same Fourier who was responsible for the Fourier analysis used to determine the spectral composition of sound.) In 1811, Fourier received the prize of the French Academy of Sciences for discovering that heat flow is proportional to the gradient of temperature (i.e., as the gradient of temperature increases, so does heat flow). The remarkable thing about this law is its generality: It applies to all matter—solid, liquid, or gaseous—and it does not depend on the chemical composition of the body in question. Fourier's law helped to explain why power was lost from heat engines, making them less efficient. It also was the root of William Thomson's second law of thermodynamics, which states that some heat is irreversibly lost in all natural systems that produce effects of some kind. This law has extraordinary cosmological implications, given that the inevitable result of this heat loss on the vast scale is the heat death of the universe. The second law of thermodynamics leads to an eventual homogeneity of temperature and therefore the absence of any mechanical effect and the absence of life.

Chaos theory is a mathematical theory of the breakdowns of ordered systems into disorderly or chaotic ones. Fourier's observations about heat propagation were an intellectual seed that eventually flowered as chaos theory, which is now one of the most rapidly growing areas of theoretical physics and an important force in current thinking about living systems. Chaos theory differs from classical physics in that the former concentrates on ordered, predictable systems. But natural systems tend toward disorder, such as when a rising column of smoke breaks up into complex, seemingly irregular patterns.

Chaos theory is especially applicable to dynamic systems that are composed of many moving elements, such as a stream of water molecules, a column of smoke particles rising in the atmosphere, or a group of planets orbiting the sun. These dynamic systems are said to be deterministic (meaning that they follow laws such as those of Newtonian mechanics) but unpredictable (chaotic). One reason for the unpredictability is that slight variations in the initial conditions of the system can have profound effects on the system's course. In fact, it is the sensitivity to initial conditions that is almost a defining property of a chaotic system.

"This characteristic of chaos was described in the early sixties, in the context of fluid motion, by Edward N. Lorenz, a meteorologist at the Massachusetts Institute of Technology, who noted its influence on Earth's weather. Man never will be able to predict weather more than a few days in advance, Lorenz discovered, because it is impossible to know all the conditions affecting its course; the flap of a butterfly's wings stirring the air might generate conditions that eventually trigger a tornado. (It is because of Lorenz's insight that sensitive dependence on initial conditions is sometimes referred to as the butterfly effect.)"

(Bernardo A. Huberman, "An ecology of machines," *The Sciences*, Vol. 29, No. 4, July/August 1989, p. 42)

It was quite revolutionary to conceive of systems that are deterministic yet unpredictable. A major characteristic of these systems is that they exhibit elements of order. These elements can be observed in a **phase-space graph**, which is a diagram that shows the relation of two or more physical features, such as the position and velocity of a moving object. As an indication of how chaos might be applied to speech, think of the position and velocity of a speech organ such as the jaw. Some investigators have constructed phase-space graphs of jaw motion to see if elements of order can be observed. This issue is revisited in Chapter 11.

One of the clearest demonstrations of chaos theory is in hydrodynamics, especially the generation of turbulence. Turbulence is perhaps the epitome of disorder, yet as we shall see, the apparent disorder has an underlying orderliness. To inform our discussion, let us consider a pan of water placed over a gas burner. If the gas flame is set on low so that a small degree of heating occurs, the heat propagation in the water will be in a state called a **conducting regime**; that is, the heat is conducted through the water, which remains motionless. If we touch the water with a finger, we can confirm that the water is being heated. If the flame is turned up sufficiently high, the water begins to move. It has now entered into a **convection regime**. The transition from conduction to convection is an example of a **bifurcation**, or change in state. The amount of heating is a **bifurcation parameter**. Sometimes a very small change in the bifurcation parameter is sufficient to cause a change in the regime of the system under observation. This sensitivity to a bifurcation parameter is similar to the sensitivity to initial conditions, the idea that gave rise to the popularized example of a butterfly beating its wings causing a major meteorological disturbance elsewhere in the world. These changes in the system are typically described as **attractors.** (See Figure 2–11 for examples of attractors.) Attractors represent stable states of a system as observed in a phase-space diagram. The system may pass from one state to another as various conditions change. Turbulence is an example. Recall that the Reynold's number can be used to determine the transition from laminar to turbulent flow. When any of the variables that detemine Reynold's number are changed, a fluid may undergo this transition. It has been shown that the transition is toward an attractor state. Furthermore, as is discussed later, the attractor state has an underlying order that can be apprehended with a special kind of geometry.

Chaos theory will be important to some issues in this book because this theory is being used to explain characteristics of living systems. In general, these systems are

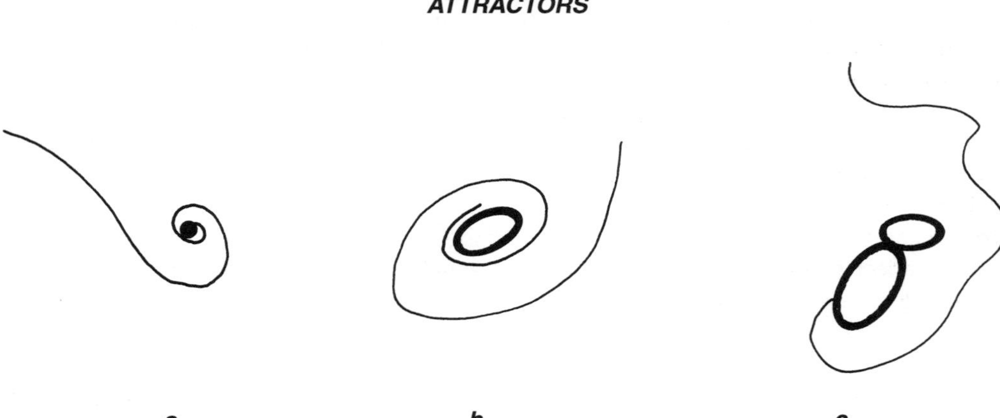

Figure 2–11. Examples of attractors drawn in a phase-space graph. The thick line represents the attractor (a point in **a**, an elliptical orbit in **b** and a more complex shape in **c**). The system is represented by the line in the phase-space graph that eventually converges on the attractor.

highly complex and therefore possess many degrees of freedom or possible actions. But the behavior of these complex systems can often be described fairly simply in terms of attractor states and variables that effect bifurcation. For example, a contemporary theory of motor control is based on the idea that movements have well-defined attractor states. As a horse changes its gait from trot to gallop, the transition can be explained as a bifurcation. The trot and gallop are each regimes of locomotion. Later we will ask what possible attractors for speech might be.

Some aspects of the theory of chaos are closely related to fractals, and fractals can make visible the orderliness that hides in chaos. For example, we will see below what order might lie in turbulence.

Fractals

Complex geometric forms are abundant in nature. Examples are trees (both deciduous and coniferous), snowflakes, cumulus clouds, mountain ranges, coastlines, coral formations, and several organs of the body (such as the respiratory and circulatory systems). Fractals are a concept developed by Mandelbrot (1982) to address complex geometric forms. Fractal structures may appear on initial observation to be highly complex and nonhomogenous. They represent difficulties in being pictured by more conventional mathematics, such as Euclidean geometry. When a fractal structure is examined with increasing levels of magnification ("zooming" in on smaller and smaller pieces of the structure), greater levels of detail come into view. But the structure at the small scale is similar to that at the large scale. There is a self-similar pattern at various levels of magnification, almost as though the whole structure is constructed from a basic geometric form that is repeated at various levels of size. An example is the coastline of England, which is rather ragged. Suppose that the coastline is viewed from a satellite high above the earth, then from a plane flying high above but not so high as the satellite, next from a plane flying low, then from an ordinary standing position, and finally through a magnifying glass trained on a small section where water meets sand and rock. Each of these views would reveal a rather similar ragged structure of the coastline.

Recognition of the basic self-similar pattern is the key to fractal geometry. By the application of this principle, complex systems that defy more conventional geometries yield to a powerful but simple understanding. Some examples of fractal geometry applied to human anatomy are: the pattern of blood supply to the heart and lungs, the branching of the airways in the lungs, and the structure of brain cells. The last two of these are considered in Chapters 4 and 7, respectively.

A more immediate example of fractal geometry is the turbulence in fluid motion, as discussed earlier in this chapter. Recall that turbulence is a condition in which the motion of the fluid becomes complex, with numerous eddies being formed in the flow pattern. At first look, the pattern may appear disorderly and random. But physicists realized that, at least under certain conditions, these patterns contain a certain orderliness (Frisch & Orszag, 1990). In particular, the turbulent flows are hierarchical and involve the generation of eddies of various sizes (Figure 2–12). At the top of the hierarchy are the largest eddies that are generated by the forces that drive the flow. Because these large eddies are unstable, they produce new eddies that are somewhat smaller. These, in turn, become unstable and produce still smaller eddies. This branching process continues until it is stopped by molecular viscosity, which gives a finite limit to the generation of eddies. The multiply branching effect is called **cascading.** This concept enables un-

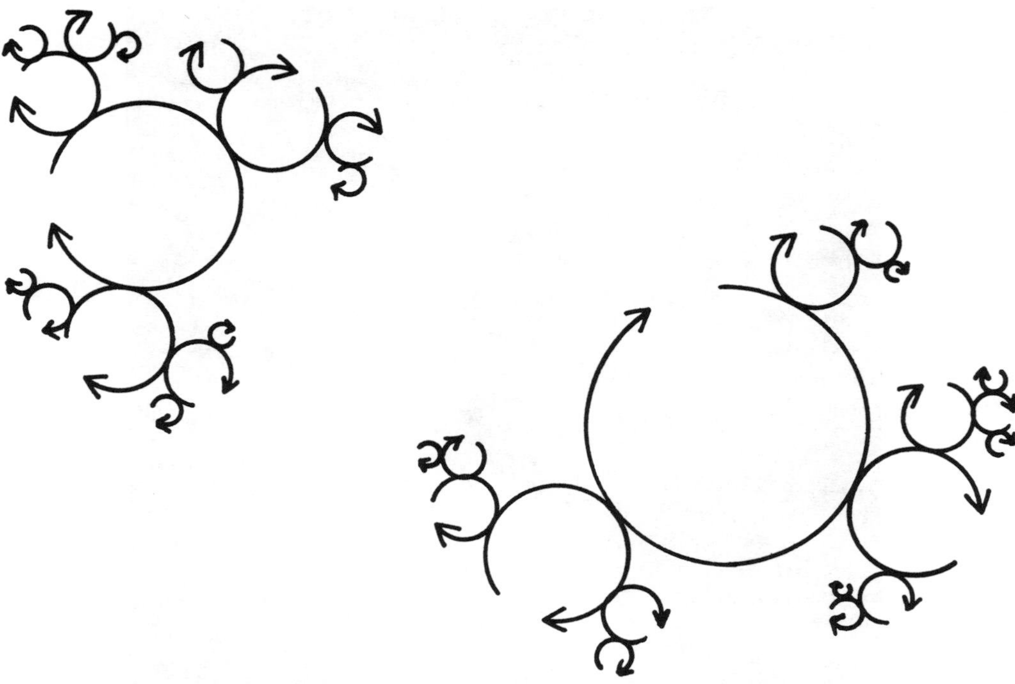

Figure 2–12. A schematic illustration of the formation of eddies in turbulent flow. The rotational elements appear as self-similar patterns of progressively smaller size. This is an example of fractal geometry.

derstanding of a complex, seemingly unorderly, process as one that involves a sequence of eddies of various sizes.

Self-similarity is found in many natural patterns. Among the most commonly occurring curves in nature is the logarithmic spiral, exemplified in the graceful curves of the nautilus shell (Figure 2–13). This spiral occurs in a variety of natural forms, including shells, horns, tusks, sunflowers, and the spiral galaxies of astronomy. Nature often has taken the logarithmic spiral as a blueprint. Artists and mathematicians also have been intrigued by this curved pattern. Jakob Bernoulli, one member of a highly talented family (including his nephew, Daniel Bernoulli, who was mentioned earlier in regard to fluid physics), was so fascinated by the logarithmic spiral that he called it the *spira mirabilis* (the marvelous spiral) and requested that it be engraved on his tombstone along with the inscription *Eadeam mutata resurgo* ("though changed, I shall arise the same"). This resurrection inscription must have been rooted in Bernoulli's discovery that the logarithmic spiral retains its shape under a number of geometric transformations (inversion, evolution, reflection, and refraction). Unfortunately, Bernoulli's request was not fully honored, as the stonemason commissioned to do the engraving produced an Archimedean or linear spiral (like the spiral formed by the grooves on a phonograph record) rather than the *spira mirabilis*.

What does the logarithmic spiral have to do with fractals? Like the fractals described above, it is self-similar. As the spiral is rotated by equal amounts, the distance from the pole increases by equal ratios. That is, the spiral grows by a geometric proportion. This esthetic property, no doubt a major

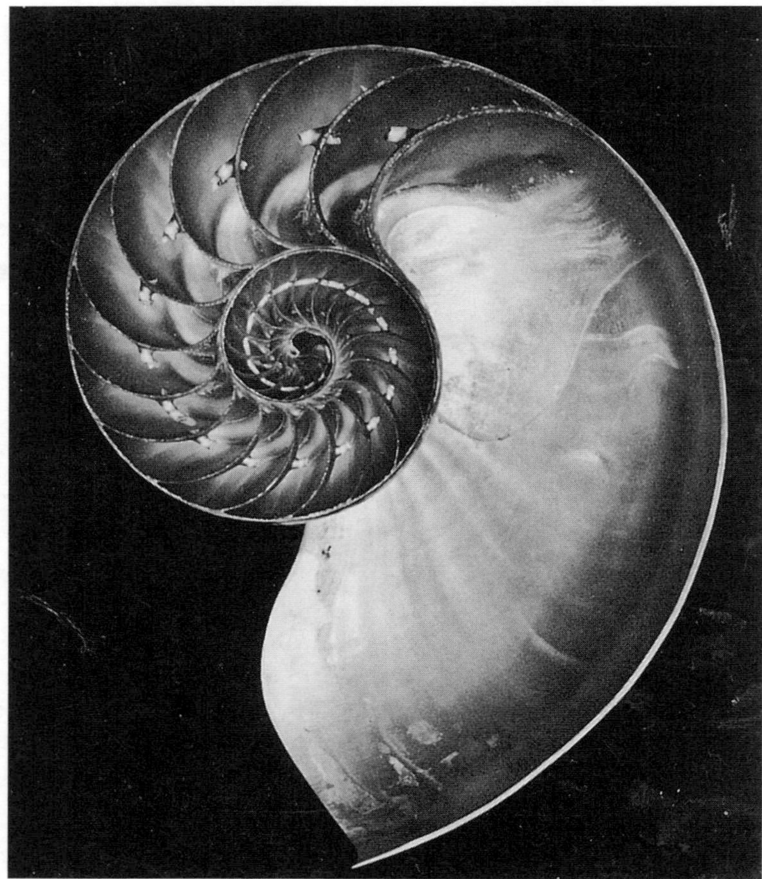

Figure 2–13. Natural example of a logarithmic spiral: the shell of the Chambered Nautilus.

reason for the artistic attraction of the logarithm spiral, also relates to that important mathematical constant, the number *e*, the base of higher mathematics. This number, so central to mathematics, is related to the logarithmic spiral in the following way:

$$r = e^{a\theta}$$

where r is the distance of a point P from the pole of a polar coordinate system (basically the center of a system of concentric circles),

e is the natural number,

a is a constant,

and θ is the angle between the line OP and the x-axis.

So far, it might seem that the logarithmic spiral would be more suited to a book on mathematics or the visual arts than to a book on speech and hearing. The relevance of this spiral will become clear in Chapter 6 (The Auditory System), where nature's elegant logarithmic spiral will be taken as the geometric form of the organ of hearing. This organ is called the **cochlea**, which means "shell." Nature has favorite forms that appear in various physical and biological systems. The logarithmic spiral is one example of such a favored design.

One can learn something about anatomy, physiology, and acoustics without going deeply into mathematics. But to study these subjects with total disregard of mathematics is to miss the powerful economy of mathematical description as well as the uncanny fit of mathematics to the natural world. Although this book is not a treatise on the mathematical modeling of the topics at hand, it will occasionally draw a connection between a natural phenomenon in speech and a mathematical concept. Fractals in particular will reappear in various patterns and various sizes in later chapters. That, of course, is their nature.

Hermann von Helmholtz was an outstanding scientist of the 19th century. One of his contemporaries, W. K. Clifford, wrote of Helmholtz as follows:

"In the first place he began by studying physiology, dissecting the eye and the ear, and finding out how they acted, and what was their precise constitution; but he found that it was impossible to study the proper action of the eye and ear without also studying the nature of light and sound, which led him to the study of physics. He had already become one of the most accomplished physiologists of this century when he commenced the study of physics, and he is now one of the greatest physicists of this century. He then found it was impossible to study physics without knowing mathematics; and accordingly he took to studying mathematics and he is now one of the most accomplished mathematicians of this century."

(Cited in R. A. Millikan, D. Roller, & E. C. Watson, *Mechanics, Molecular Physics, Heat and Sound.* Cambridge, MA: MIT Press, 1937, p. 417.)

On The Reference Shelf

General references for readers who want deeper or extended discussions of selected topics

Millikan, R. A., Roller, D., & Watson, E. C. (1937). *Mechanics, molecular physics, heat and sound*. Cambridge, MA: MIT Press.

An older physics text that contains many historical references.

Rossing, T. D., & Fletcher, N. H. (1995). *Principles of vibration and sound*. New York: Springer-Verlag

A general introduction to acoustics and vibration; a background in mathematics through calculus is recommended.

Speaks, C. E. (1996). *Introduction to sound* (2nd ed.). San Diego: Singular Publishing Group, Inc.

A systematic discussion of basic acoustics; comprehensive but approachable for students who do not have a background in mathematics or physics.

Chapter References

Frisch, U., & Orszag, S. A. (1990, January). Turbulence: Challenges for theory and experiment. *Physics Today*, 24–32.

Grasser, M. A., & Moss, K. (1992). The sounds of silence. *Sound and Vibration, 26*, 24–26.

Mandelbrot, B. B. (1982). *The fractal geometry of nature*. New York: W. H. Freeman.

Maor, E. (1994, July/August). The story of *e*. *The Sciences, 34*, 19–23.

Motz, L., & Weaver, J. H. (1989). *The story of physics*. New York: Plenum Press.

Munk, W. (1993, September/October). The sound of oceans warming. *The Sciences, 33*, 20–26.

Olenick, R. P., Apostol, T. M., & Goodstein, D. L. (1985). *The mechanical universe: Introduction to mechanics and light*. Cambridge, UK: Cambridge University Press.

Prigogine, I., & Stengers, I. (1984). *Order out of chaos*. Toronto: Bantam Books.

Rayleigh, J. W. S., Baron (1894). *The theory of sound*. Reprinted by Dover Publications, New York (1945).

Rasmussen, G. (1989, March). Intensity—Its measurement and uses. *Sound and Vibration, 23*, 12–21.

Rossing, T. D., & Fletcher, N. H. (1995). *Principles of vibration and sound*. New York: Springer-Verlag.

Rouse, H. (1961). *Fluid mechanics for hydraulic engineers*. New York: Dover Publications.

Speaks, C. E. (1992). *Introduction to sound*. San Diego: Singular Publishing Group, Inc.

Wasserman, D. E. (1995, April). Whole-body vibration exposure and the human spine. [Editorial]. *Sound and Vibration, 29*(4), p. 5.

Exercises

2-1. Scientists are not the only ones concerned with measurements of force, pressure, volume, and flow. Measurements of these quantities arise in everyday life. Consider the following examples and describe for each the units of measurement commonly used.

a. Air pressure in a tire
b. Gasoline from a service station pump
c. Capacity of a car trunk
d. Amount of water added to a recipe
e. Water used by a household during a billing period.

2-2. Floor coverings made of vinyl can be damaged by the force of walking. It has been discovered that the greatest risk of damage often comes not from large men but from women wearing pointed, high-heeled shoes. Why is this the case? *Hint*: Think of the force per unit of area.

2-3. Astronomers measure the vast distances in space in terms of light years, or the distance covered by light in 1 year. Why would measurement of distance in terms of "sound years" or even "sound minutes" not be as accurate as the light method?

2-4. School children often learn that the distance from a flash of lightning can be estimated by counting the number of seconds between the flash and the sound of the ensuing thunder. Then the number of seconds is divided by 5 to obtain the distance in miles. Explain why this estimation works.

2-5. Movies of the Old West sometimes show someone putting his or her ear to the ground to listen for the sound of approaching hoofbeats. Why would a person do this?

2-6. Fill a jug or bottle with water and then turn it upside down so the water runs out. Listen to the sound of the gurgling water. Does the pitch of the gurgle seem to change? If so, why? *Hint*: As water runs out of the container, the resonating chamber changes in volume.

2-7. Obtain two tuning forks of the same frequency. Place them next to one another and strike one so that it produces a tone. Does the other one begin to resonate? If so, why?

2-8. Look about you (even your own body) for natural objects that might be described in terms of fractal geometry. Try to imagine the self-similar pattern that might be used to create the larger, complex result.

APPENDIX

Base Units, Derived Units, and Prefixes of the Systeme International d'Unites (SI) Most Relevant to This Text.

Quantity	Unit Name	Unit Symbol
	Base Units	
length	meter	m
mass	kilogram	kg
time	second	s
amount of substance	mole	m
	Derived Units	
frequency	hertz	Hz
force	newton	N
pressure, stress	pascal	Pa
work, energy, heat	joule	J
power	watt	W
resistance	ohm	Ω
	Prefixes	
10^{9}	giga	G
10^{6}	mega	M
10^{3}	kilo	k
10^{2}	hecto	h
10^{1}	deka	da
10^{-1}	deci	d
10^{-2}	centi	c
10^{-3}	milli	m
10^{-6}	micro	μ
10^{-9}	nano	n

CHAPTER 3

An Overview of Anatomy, the Speech System, and Speech Sounds

> *"If a problem is too complex to be solved all at once, then break it up into problems that are small enough to be solved separately."*
>
> —advice from the philosopher René Descartes

This book discusses the speech system as a collection of subsystems. This analytic approach helps in the understanding of a complicated biological system that may include as many as 100 different muscles, several types of physiological variables, and a neural control that may involve extensive areas of the nervous system. For all its ordinariness, speech is still a challenge to the scientists who are trying to understand it. This chapter prepares the way for later chapters by charting the territory. It also presents some general concepts in anatomy, physiology, and phonetics that will be helpful later.

BASIC ANATOMIC TERMINOLOGY AND CONCEPTS

Anatomy is the science of body structure. Although interest in anatomy goes back to ancient times, the first accurate and complete description of human anatomy was *De Humani Corporis Fabrica Librorum Epitome* by the Flemish anatomist Andreas Vesalius (1514–1564). This work was a signal event and helped to usher in systematic studies of the anatomy of the human body. As knowledge grew, so did the need for specialization. In 1601, Julius Casserius published *De Vocis Auditusque Organis Historia Anatomica* (*On the Anatomy of the Voice and Hearing*), an illustrated text on the larynx and ear. Nearly four centuries have passed since Casserius' work, and knowledge has grown around the framework that he and others built.

Like any science, anatomy has developed a terminology and a set of basic concepts that are used fairly consistently by those who practice the science. The terms are especially helpful in describing the complex properties and relationships encountered in anatomic systems. Only a few of these terms are introduced in this book, but they are used frequently. In addition, a few basic anatomic concepts are introduced because of their central importance in the understanding of almost any bodily system.

Anatomists use specialized terms to describe the locations and orientations of parts of the body. These are illustrated in Figure 3–1 and are presented below as paired terms.

- **Anterior** refers to the front, **posterior** to the back.
  Example: The nose is on the anterior aspect of the head, and the nape of the neck is on the posterior aspect of the body.
- **Ventral** refers to the belly, **dorsal** to the back.
  Example: The chin is on the ventral aspect of the body; the nape of the neck is on the dorsal aspect. Readers who like to fish or cook may find it helpful to think of the ventral and dorsal fins of a fish.
  (Note that, for the human body in upright posture, anterior and ventral have the same meaning, as do posterior and dorsal. But if the human body assumes a posture on hands and knees, the terms would have a different reference. Particularly for nonhuman species, such as cats and dogs, the anterior-posterior and ventral-dorsal dimensions can have a different meaning.)
- **Superior** means to the top or upper part, **inferior** to the bottom or lower part.
  Example: When the body is in the upright position, the eyes are superior to the mouth, and the nose is inferior to the forehead.
- **Cephalad** refers to the head, **caudal** to the tail.
  Example: The tongue is cephalad to the neck, and the stomach is caudal to the esophagus.
- **Lateral** refers to the sides or margins, **mesial** or **medial** refers to the midline.
  Example: The ears are on the lateral regions of the head, but the nose is on the mesial portion of the face.
- **Proximal** means toward the midline or center, **distal** means toward the periphery.
  Example: The fingers are distal to the elbow, and the shoulder is proximal to the elbow.

Anatomists typically study a specimen by cutting it in various sections or slices, as follows.

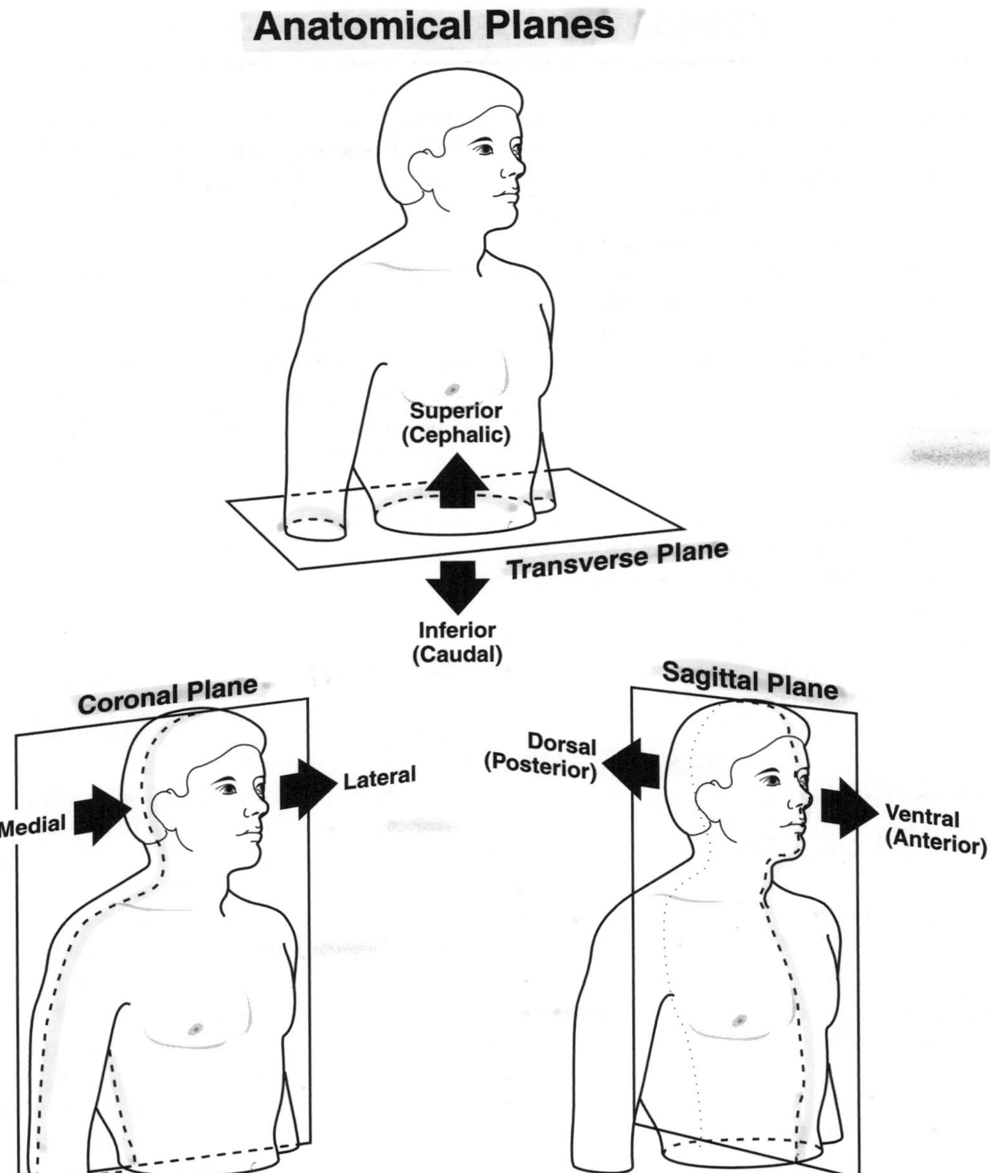

Figure 3–1. Planes, directions, and orientations used in anatomic descriptions.

- **Sagittal** is a vertical slice taken with an anterior-posterior orientation. A sagittal section cuts the specimen into right and left parts.
- **Coronal** is a vertical slice taken with a side-to-side orientation; it cuts the specimen into anterior and posterior parts.
- **Transverse** is a horizontal slice; it cuts the specimen into superior and inferior parts.

PRIMARY TISSUES OF THE BODY

The body is constructed of many tissues. But for purposes of gross anatomy of the speech system, this book focuses on bones, cartilages, connective tissues, muscles, glands, lymphoid tissue, various types of membranes, and nerve tissue. A few preliminary comments on these types of tissue sets the stage for an overview of the speech production system.

Bone

The skeleton of the body is its bony framework. A total of 206 bones make up the complete human skeleton, as first described in 1659 by Coiter. Bones are an efficient support system for the body. They make up 6–8% of the body weight of most adult mammals, compared to 37–46% of body weight for muscles (Glucksmann, 1981). The bones of birds are even lighter because weight is a disadvantage to flight. Bone is hard, but not dead. Healthy bone is living tissue that contributes to a number of important functions, including the support of the body, efficient movement, and production of blood cells. Furthermore, bone, itself, is constantly being broken down and rebuilt. This process, called **remodeling**, depends on a dynamic linkage between two kinds of cells, osteoclasts that absorb bone and osteoblasts that form new bone. Bones are continually being renewed by the processes of resorption and deposition. The bones of a baseball pitcher's throwing arm are larger and stronger than those of the nonthrowing arm. Use makes strength. These same processes of remodeling account in part for the growth of bones in children.

The growth phenomena were first described by scientists who fed animals materials containing the dye *madder* obtained from the plant *Rubia tinctorum*. The dye stained newly deposited bone in an animal's body and therefore allowed the scientists to see how bone is renewed. The discovery of this method is a good example of serendipity and eureka (as in "Aha!"). In 1736, John Belchier, a London surgeon, observed that the bones of the pork roast he was having for dinner were stained red but the meat was not. He inquired as to the cause of the red stain and learned that the pigs had been fed a diet containing madder, the dye described above. Belchier realized that the dye could be a tool for the study of bone development, and it was used for this purpose until the 20th century, when radiolabeling techniques were developed.

Cartilage

Cartilage is a tissue that is softer and more flexible than bone. This text is concerned with two primary types of cartilage. **Hyaline** cartilage is relatively dense and hard and therefore occurs in regions where rigid support is needed. With aging, hyaline cartilage is often **ossified** (turned to bone). **Elastic** cartilage is a more flexible cartilage and is suited to protective and cushioning functions. Elastic cartilage normally does not become ossified, even in old age. As we will discover in later chapters, ossification of hyaline cartilage is one index of aging. Although cartilage is encountered in many areas of the anatomy to be reviewed in Chapters 4 and 5, it is particularly important to the larynx (voice box) discussion in Chapter 4. The instrument of voice is constructed largely of muscle and cartilage.

Connective Tissue

Connective tissue gives integrity to the cells of various organs. We are concerned with two major types. **Ligaments** are strands, or sheets, of tough, flexible material that are used to connect bones at joints. **Tendons** are tough but nonstretching bands that connect muscles and bones. One tendon with which many people are familar is the Achilles tendon, which attaches the muscles of the calf to the heel bone. The myth of Achilles was that he was vulnerable at only one point in his body—his heel.

Muscles

All movement is the result of the contraction of muscles. Therefore, muscles can be regarded as providing the "motor" function of the body, and, in fact, muscle function is often termed **motor** function. Muscles consist of three types of tissue. **Striated (skeletal)** muscle (striated means striped) is the type of muscle used to move the bones and cartilages of the skeleton. It serves rapid voluntary motions, such as walking, throwing, and speech. It consists of long fibers that are encased in a membranous sheath called the sarcolemma. **Unstriated (smooth,** or **visceral)** muscle tends to be used for slow involuntary movements, such as those in the viscera (stomach, intestines, and lungs). It is composed of spindle-shaped cells. **Cardiac** muscle is the specialized muscle of the heart that performs continuous rhythmic contractions.

In anatomic descriptions of striated muscle, the following conventions are used and followed in this book. The **origin** of a muscle is the attachment that is fixed or at least relatively so. Ideally, the origin is the *anchor* point of a muscle. The **insertion** of a muscle is the attachment that is relatively movable. Therefore, the **action** of a muscle is its effect and is typically described in terms of the movement performed at the insertion when the muscle contracts. The **course** of a muscle refers to the orientation of its fibers. The names of muscles may seem formidable at first appearance, but they permit a fairly ready understanding if the reader asks, "What is the origin and what is the insertion?" For example, in later chapters we consider muscles called the **sternohyoid** (Chapter 4) and the **palatoglossus** (Chapter 5). Like most of the muscles we will encounter, the names of these muscles are derived from their attachments. The origin (less movable attachment) is named first, and the insertion (more movable attachment) is named second. Although not all muscles are named according to attachments, many are. So the muscle name often can be analyzed as [origin] + [insertion]. **Sterno-** refers to the sternum (breastbone) and **hyoid** refers to a bone in the neck. Therefore, sternohyoid is the name of a muscle that originates on the breastbone and inserts on the hyoid bone. Sternohyoid = [breastbone] + [hyoid bone]. Similarly, palatoglossus is the name of a muscle that runs from the palate (the roof of the mouth) to the tongue (glossus). Palatoglossus = [palate] + [tongue].

Frequently, striated muscles are organized as opposing pairs called **agonists** and **antagonists**. The Latin root *agonista* means "competitor." Agonists and antagonists have competing effects. An antagonist has the opposite action of an agonist. To appreciate a simple example, extend your forearm in front of you in a pointing motion and then bend it toward you so that your hand approaches your face. The muscle that performs this flexion (the backward bending) is an agonist. The antagonist muscle would perform the opposite action of extension. Alternating movements of flexion and extension are examples of agonist-antagonist muscle actions.

Glands

This term means any tissue that produces chemical secretions or excretions. The two primary types of glands are the **endocrine**

glands, which produce internal secretions, and the **exocrine glands,** which produce external secretions. The endocrine glands are ductless glands that secrete directly into the bloodstream. Hormones are one example. The exocrine glands, such as the salivary glands and the sweat glands, secrete into a duct that carries the chemical substance to the site of intended action. More is said about the salivary glands in Chapter 5. Some glands, such as the pancreas, have both endocrine and exocrine functions.

Glandular secretions are part of the body's internal clock, its **circadian rhythm** (*circa* means "about" and *dia* means "day"). Many body functions exhibit a daily cycle (Ralph, 1989; Takahashi & Hoffman, 1995). Body temperature slowly increases during the day to a high as great as 99° at 4 P.M. It then falls slowly for the next 12 hours, sometimes reaching a low of 96.6°. Prolactin, which regulates the production of milk in nursing mothers, peaks at about 3 A.M., just in time for an early morning feeding. The male hormone testosterone reaches its highest level at about 9 A.M. Even tolerance for pain has a circadian cycle. Dental patients can withstand pain better in midafternoon than at other times (a useful point to remember if you have to schedule a potentially unpleasant dental procedure). Possibly, all organisms—animals, plants, and bacteria—have circadian cycles. This cycle is a "biological imperative" (Takahashi & Hoffman, 1995) and may be regulated by individual genes, the first of which was discovered in the fruit fly. As is discussed in Chapter 7, even the brain acts like a gland in some respects.

The muscles and glands are sometimes called the **effectors** because they effect action in the body. All behavior is the result of activities of the muscular or glandular systems. Anything we would do to act directly on the world around us is the consequence of muscular or glandular activities, primarily the former.

Lymphoid Tissue

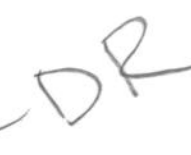

Lymphoid tissue is related to the **immune system,** which is the body's defense against **pathogenic** (disease-causing) agents that enter the body. These foreign substances are called **antigens**. The lymphoid tissues counteract antigens by manufacturing specific agents of defense called **antibodies,** which neutralize the antigen's harmful potential. The lymphoid tissues include the tonsils, adenoids, thymus, spleen, and lymph nodes distributed throughout the body. When a person detects swelling in certain regions of the neck and says, "My glands are swollen," it is actually the lymph nodes that are typically swollen as a response to invasion by a pathogenic agent. The bone marrow participates in the immune system by producing **leukocytes** (white blood cells) and **lymphocytes**. The primary concern in this book is with the tonsils and adenoids, which are discussed in Chapter 5. These are lymphoid tissues that form a kind of protective circle near the entrance to the throat. They tend to reach their maximum size in early childhood and then gradually shrink.

Membranes

A membrane, from the Latin *membrana* (parchment), is any thin layer of connective tissue that coats cells or organs or lines the various joints, ducts, tracts, and cavities of the body. Membranes are readily found, as every organ is surrounded by a membrane. In this book, we examine in particular the membranes associated with the mouth, nose, throat, lungs, and brain. In addition, two general membranes are of interest. **Serous membranes** contain a serumlike fluid and line a number of body cavities. The lungs are contained in serous membranes. **Mucous membranes** secrete mucus and typically are found as the lining of hollow tracts such as the mouth and nose.

Neural Tissues

The nervous system is discussed in Chapter 7. The chief concern is with nerve cells or neurons, but other nourishing and supportive cells also are considered. The nervous system is extraordinarily complex, so the approach in this book is to identify major structures of the brain and spinal cord and to outline the peripheral nerves by which these central organs are connected to the rest of the body. Selected issues in microanatomy and macroanatomy are included.

A general discussion of neuroanatomy pertinent to speech is given in Chapter 7. In the meantime, it will suffice now to comment briefly on the following major levels of the nervous system. The brain and spinal cord constitute the **central nervous system** or **CNS**. The CNS communicates with the body through the **peripheral nerves**, which make up the **peripheral nervous system** or **PNS**. The brain can be divided into a **brainstem**, the **cerebral hemispheres**, and the **cerebellum**. The brainstem controls basic body functions, whereas the cerebral hemispheres are classically regarded as the seat of intelligence, judgment, and planning. The term **cortical** often is used to refer to the outer rind of the cerebral hemispheres, because this outer covering is heavily invested with nerve cells or **neurons**. The term **subcortical** can cover a number of structures located below the level of the cortex. The cerebellum is a rather large brain structure that interacts with structures of the brainstem and cerebral hemispheres. The cerebellum appears to play an important role in the control of movement, but this is by no means its only function. Recent scientific reports indicate that the cerebellum also may be involved in sensory processing and perhaps even in language.

This general background on anatomical terminology and concepts can be used to discuss the anatomy relevant to the speech sciences. The following discussion is an overview of this anatomy. Details are covered in later chapters. The purpose of this chapter is to sketch the overall anatomy and to describe its subsystems. Because the overall anatomy of speech production is complex, the task of description is facilitated by employing a subsystem approach in keeping with the suggestion by Descartes quoted at the beginning of this chapter.

THE BODY SYSTEMS OF SPEECH PRODUCTION

Respiratory System

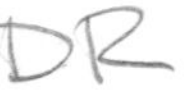

The respiratory system basically consists of the lungs, chest wall, abdomen, and the respiratory airway that extends to the mouth and nose. This system, pictured in Figure 3–2, is also called the pulmonary, or ventilatory, system. It is the means by which oxygen and carbon dioxide are exchanged in the blood. Fresh air is inspired into the lungs to supply oxygen. Carbon dioxide produced as a waste product by metabolic processes is expelled during expiration. The actual gas exchange occurs in millions of small sacs contained in the lungs. Ventilation is necessary to life, but it also is important for thermoregulation (body temperature control), the sense of smell (respiration drives the air currents past the olfactory receptors in the nose), and sound production (air movement is used to produce acoustic energy). The last of these is central to this book, given that the respiratory system supplies the basic energy of speech production. Sounds are produced on either the **ingressive** (inward flowing) or **egressive** (outward flowing) air. English is normally produced on egressive air only, but other languages make use of both directions of airflow. To judge the difference

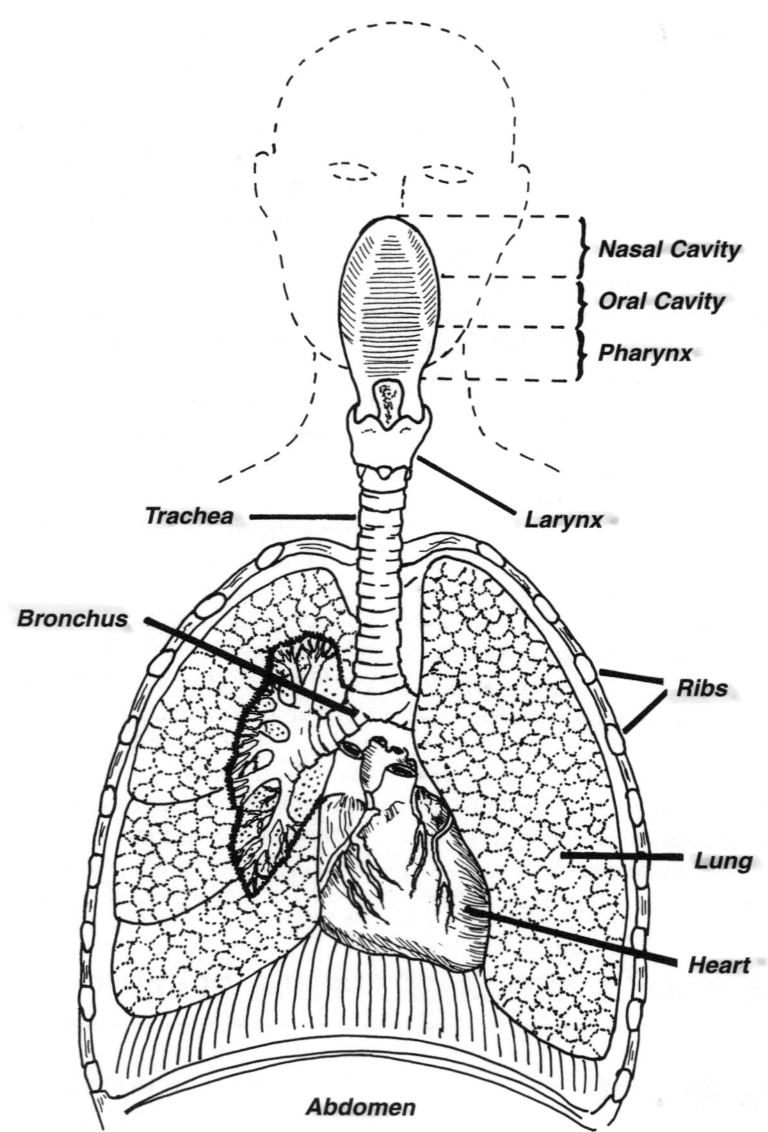

Figure 3–2. The respiratory system extending from the lungs to the mouth and nose.

between ingressive and egressive sounds, produce the vowel "ah" in the normal way and then again while inhaling. With some practice, you probably will be able to phonate on both inhalation and exhalation.

For the purposes of this book, the respiratory system is discussed primarily as the energy source of speech. Because the respiratory system moves air into and out of the lungs, the description of this system involves issues in aerodynamics (the discipline that deals with the physics of air). Respiratory anatomy and physiology are discussed in Chapter 4; aerodynamics is considered in an introductory fashion in Chapter 2 and with respect to speech physiology in Chapter 8.

Laryngeal System

The **larynx** (voice box) is an arrangement of cartilages, muscles, and other tissues that could be, and often are, considered part of the respiratory system. However, because of the special role of the larynx in speech in this text, it is accorded a separate status as a major system of speech production. The various muscles and cartilages of the larynx are discussed as they relate to the critical component, the vocal folds. The vocal folds are muscular cushions that can be set into vibration to produce the sound of voice. Figure 3–3 shows the appearance of the vocal folds when viewed from above (superior perspective). They are shown in color photographs in color plates 1 and 2 at the back of the book. Although the larynx is capable of highly refined muscular adjustments, its basic roles can be introduced as related to four functions of the vocal folds: complete opening, complete closure, vibration, and narrow opening. These functions are shown in schematic form in Figure 3–4. Complete opening is the condition of normal respiration in which the larynx minimally impedes the flow of air into and out of the lungs. Complete and forceful closure is desired to perform certain physically demanding activities, such as lifting a heavy object, pushing a stubborn door, defecating, and giving birth. Vibration is the condition that underlies phonation and is accomplished as a self-sustaining oscillation when the vocal folds are properly posi-

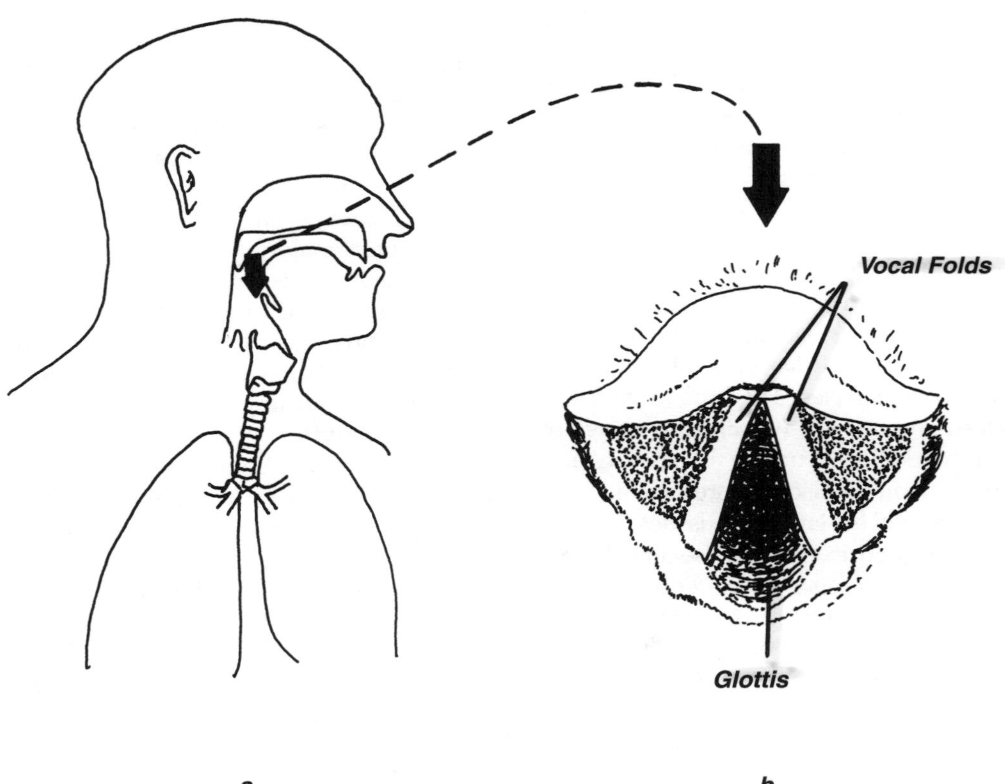

Figure 3–3. Drawing of the vocal folds as viewed from above, as though we were looking down in the direction of the arrow shown in part **a**. The vocal folds are shown in an open configuration in part **b**. The opening between them is the glottis.

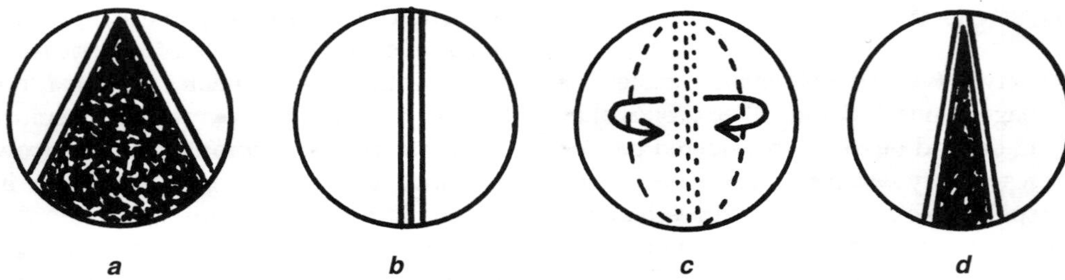

Figure 3–4. Drawing of several vocal fold configurations: (**a**) complete opening, (**b**) complete closure, (**c**) vibration, and (**d**) narrow opening.

tioned and a suitable aerodynamic force is present. Narrow opening is appropriate for an activity such as whispering in which air is forced through a constriction. Speech involves several adjustments, including at least three of these basic conditions, excluding only complete forceful closure. The anatomy and physiology of the larynx are two of the main topics of Chapter 4. Aerodynamic and acoustic aspects of laryngeal function also are mentioned in Chapters 8 and 9, respectively.

This highly simplified introduction to the larynx misses an important point that will be developed in Chapter 4. The human larynx has an unusual complexity when compared against the larynges of just about every other species. The human larynx is indeed special, and we take advantage of its remarkable structure in speech and song. Chapter 4 also explores age and sex differences in the laryngeal tissues. The larynx is a good example of **sexual dimorphism**, or sex-related differences in anatomical structure. It is also a good example of **ontogenetic** (developmental) differences in anatomy. As we will see, the larynx of an infant or young child is quite different from that of an adult man or woman. The larynx also undergoes change with aging, which is one reason why popular vocalists can eventually lose the artistry that they mastered in their youth.

Upper Airway (Supralaryngeal) System

The term **upper airway** is a rather inelegant expression for the **supralaryngeal** structures of pharynx, oral cavity, and nasal cavity (Figure 3–5, which also includes the systems already discussed). This complex system also is called the **pharyngeal-oral-nasal system** and the **vocal tract** (a simple term that reflects its acoustic function). This upper airway comprises many bones, muscles, and specialized tissues. It is here that the great majority of speech sounds in English are formed. Sound formation is the result of two basic processes: articulation, which is movement of structures to form strictures and shapes, and resonance, which is a matter of adjusting the length and shape of air-filled cavities to reinforce certain frequency regions of sound energy (as discussed in Chapter 2). Actually, articulation and resonance are related in the sense that articulation gives rise to characteristic resonator shapes of the vocal tract.

The human vocal tract changes remarkably in its size and shape from infancy to adulthood. The discussion of vocal tract anatomy reviews some of these developmental changes and their implications for speech development in childhood. Differences between male and female vocal tracts are also discussed. Although one can write a gener-

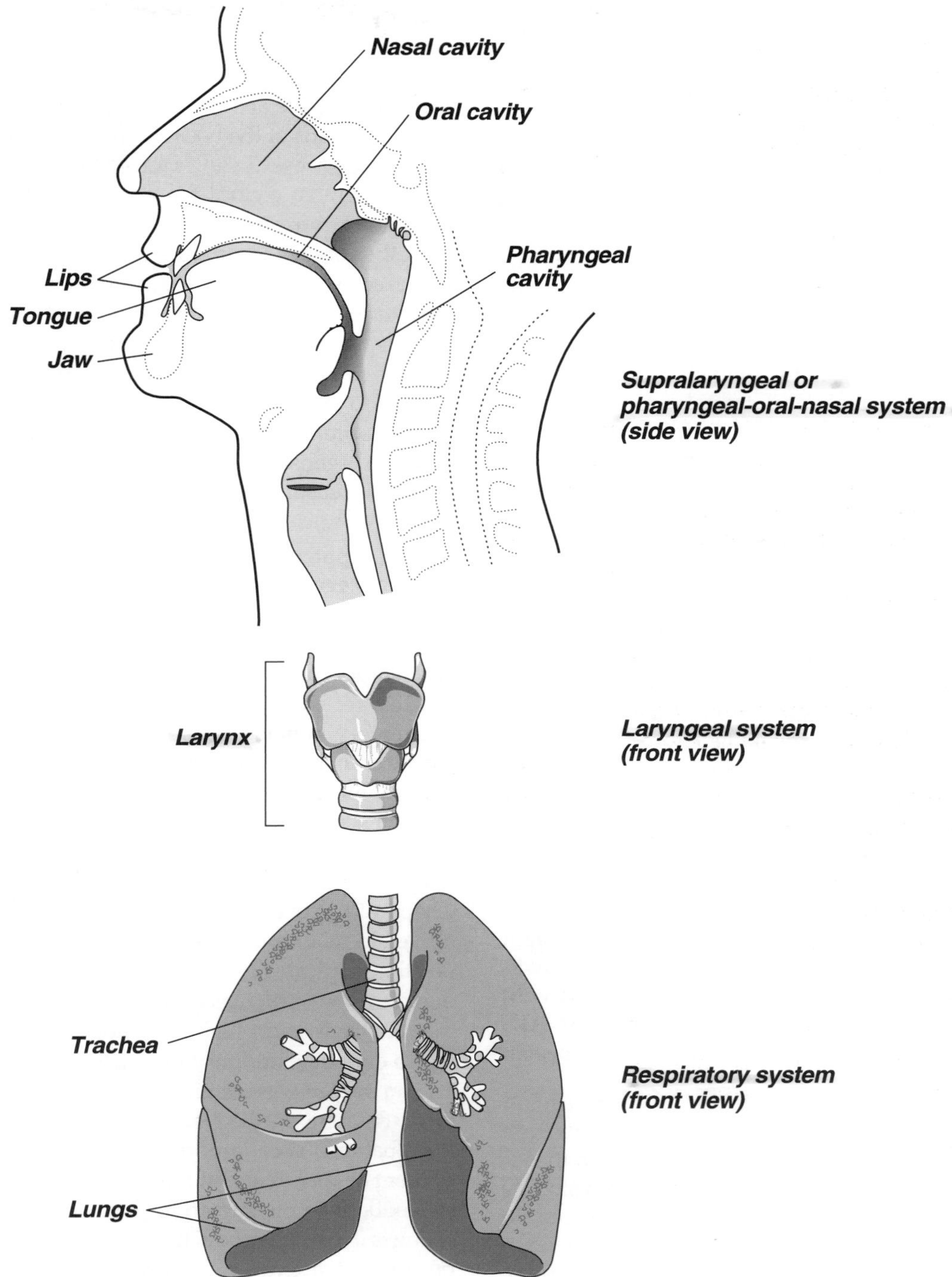

Figure 3–5. The supralaryngeal system (upper airway) of speech production shown with the respiratory and laryngeal systems.

al description of a vocal tract, variations attributable to age and sex have to be taken into account to draw an accurate picture of an individual's upper airway system of speech production.

The upper airway is the site of speech production insofar as individual sounds are concerned. If someone had a paralyzed upper airway, then speech would be impossible, even though the individual might be able to phonate (produce voice). Phonation alone does not produce many distinctive sounds in the English language. Paralysis of the vocal tract is not merely an abstract example for the sake of textbook discussion. It does, in fact, occur in a number of individuals with neurological diseases. One of these is amyotrophic lateral sclerosis, or ALS. It is known more commonly as Lou Gehrig's disease—named after the famous baseball player whose final years of baseball statistics charted the unrelenting progress of his disease. It has been estimated that about three-quarters of patients with amyotrophic lateral sclerosis (ALS) are nonspeaking before they die. The disease destroys the ability to control muscles and the muscles themselves atrophy (shrink). In the final stages of the disease, individuals often can barely phonate a weak sound, let alone articulate the sounds of speech. Their intellect may remain untouched. In fact, one of the most brilliant theoretical physicists ever, Stephen Hawking, continues to astonish the world with his ideas, even as a disease similar to ALS has robbed him of locomotion and speech.

The upper airway is discussed in relation to the formation of most sounds, both from the point of view of articulation and that of acoustics. Basic anatomy and physiology of the upper airway are considered in Chapter 5. Speech physiology and speech acoustics are covered in Chapters 8 and 9, respectively. The final section of this chapter discusses some basic aspects of phonetics, or the science that pertains to the production of speech sounds.

Neural Bases of Speech

For all the apparent ease of speaking, it is, in fact, a formidable activity because of its use of major organs of the body. Merely to utter the simple phrase "hello, is anyone home?" a speaker must control the chest wall, diaphragm, larynx, tongue, lips, velopharynx and other organs to produce a coordinated sequence of movements. How the brain accomplishes this feat is the area of study called speech motor control. Actually, it is better to say sensorimotor rather than motor, if only to remind ourselves that sensory functions are closely related to motor regulation. The organs of speech are spectacular in both their sensory and motor regimes.

Speech is plurimodal in the sensory information it generates. The sensory information includes: air pressures detected by mechanoreceptors in the respiratory tract, articulatory movements monitored by specialized receptors called muscle spindles, articulatory contacts sensed by mechanoreceptors in the soft tissues, and acoustic signals analyzed by the ear. What happens if the rich sensory flow is interrupted? If the interruption is brief, surprisingly little. In one experiment (discussed in some detail in Chapter 7), speakers were given trigeminal nerve blocks to minimize sensation for jaw position, topical anesthesia to reduce information about articulatory contacts within the oral cavity, and high-level noise masking to eliminate auditory feedback. The result on speech was minimal. But this is not to say that sensory feedback is unimportant. It probably is very important in the development of speech in children, and, if sensory feedback is interrupted for long periods, changes in speech production can occur. Experimental attempts to disrupt sensory feedback for speech cannot affect all of the sensory channels that might be used, so these experiments reveal the effects of only selective alterations.

Several different parts of the nervous system are involved in the neural regulation of speech. A simplified view of the nervous system is shown in Figure 3–6. This view shows that the nervous system is divided into two major parts, the central nervous system (brain and spinal cord) and the peripheral nervous system (cranial nerves and spinal nerves). The discussion in this book focuses on the representation of speech in the brain (Where in the central nervous system is language stored?) and how the nervous system controls the precise movements of speech by issuing commands along the peripheral nerves. Knowledge in this area has grown immensely with the introduction of modern brain imaging procedures, some of which enable the scientist to observe the regions of the brain that become most active when a subject performs a given task such as passively listening to speech, repeating words, or generating antonyms of words. Chapter 7 highlights the parts of the human nervous system most relevant to speech production and perception. A major question to be addressed is whether speech and language can be assigned to isolated parts of the brain or whether they are widely represented in the brain.

Aerodynamic Events in Speech

One path to understanding the production of speech is to study the aerodynamic events associated with it. The variables of

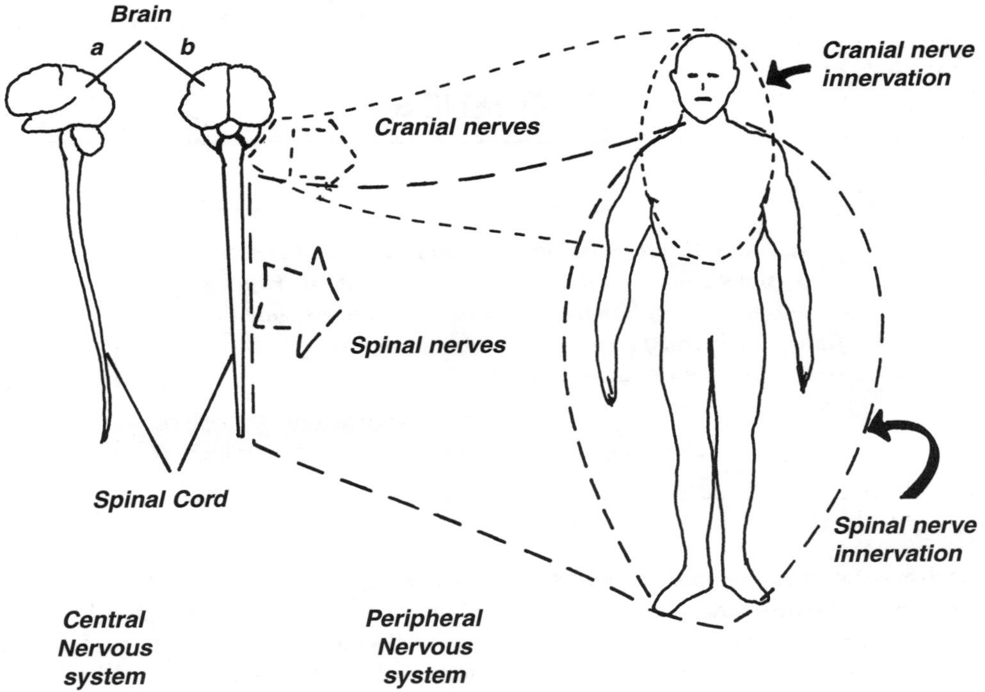

Figure 3–6. A simplified drawing of the major structures of the nervous system divided into the central nervous system and the peripheral nervous system. General innervation regions are shown for the cranial and spinal nerves.

interest are air volumes (such as the amount of air used in speaking), air pressures (such as the air pressure impounded in the mouth during the consonants in the word "speak"), and air flows (such as the air that flows through the mouth during phonation of a vowel). Aerodynamic energy provides the fundamental power of speaking. The respiratory system is the essential engine that supplies the air volumes, pressures, and flows. Although we may commonly think of speech in terms of acoustics (that is, sounds), it can also be understood in terms of aerodynamic variables. Some examples of aerodynamic information on speech are included in Chapter 8.

Acoustic Events in Speech

Raymond H. Stetson, an early pioneer in speech research at Oberlin College, wrote that "speech is movement made audible." Perhaps this crisp definition should be expanded somewhat to read, "speech is movement made audible for the purpose of language communication." Many movements are audible (snapping fingers, cracking joints, tongue clucking) but all are not speech. A variety of movements can communicate language. The manual sign languages of the deaf are "movements made visible for the purpose of language communication." Speech in its most common sense is a pattern of sound created by movements of a set of structures especially recruited for this purpose.

Modern speech science has made sufficient progress in understanding the acoustics of speech that computers can be programmed to produce speech (machine speech or synthetic speech) or to understand speech (machine speech recognition). Some of the most refined speech synthesis systems are such a good match to natural speech that listeners may not realize that they are hearing speech produced by machine.

PHONETICS

> ***"But a new interest and an added value have been given to it [the study of pronunciation] by the recent rapid development of phonetic science. What once seemed a field of arbitrary custom is now coming into view as an orderly realm of natural science."***
>
> (From the Preface, p. 3, of Albert Salisbury, *Phonology and Orthoepy*, Wm. J. Park & Sons, Madison, WI, 1897)

Phonetics is the study of speech sounds—how they are formed and how they are used in language. Much of the research effort in the speech sciences relates to fundamental issues in phonetics, and phonetics is therefore a centerpiece of speech science. An immediate obstacle that one confronts in talking about speech sounds is giving them labels that are unambiguously understood. Because different languages have different phonetic systems and different alphabet systems, there is no universal convention for the symbolic representation of a particular sound. As explained in Chapter 1, the majority of languages do not even have a written alphabet. To make matters worse, sound representation within even a single language can be complicated because of poor correspondence between phonemes (sound units) and graphemes (alphabet characters). English is particularly troublesome. The grapheme *s* can be pronounced as *s* in "see," *sh* in "sugar," or *z* as in "raise." Occasionally, highly similar sequences of graphemes are pronounced quite differently. Consider, for example, the words *daughter* and *laughter*. If English were completely consistent in its grapheme-to-phoneme correspondence, these two words should rhyme. Of course, they do not.

What is needed is a system that systematically and reliably assigns symbols to sounds. Ideally, this system should be universal and thereby apply to all of the world's languages. Such a system has been developed. It is called the **International Phonetic Alphabet** (IPA). It is an important system for phonetic studies and is a fundamental tool of linguists, psycholinguists, speech-language pathologists, and others. In most universities that offer instruction in the area, phonetics is a semester-long course that includes transcription practice. This book does not attempt to teach phonetics as a skill, but occasional references are made to phonetic principles and to various phonetic classes of sounds. A primary reason to introduce phonetics at this point is to define important concepts that will be used throughout the book. The following is a brief account of the phonetic system of American English. The IPA symbols are listed for readers who want to learn them, but they are not necessary for reading the other chapters of this book. In writing about speech, it is most convenient to refer to specific speech sounds in an unambiguous way. The IPA was developed for this purpose. However, other symbol systems can also be used. This book refers to individual speech sounds in two ways, the IPA symbol and a **UNIBET** symbol (a slightly modified version of the PHONASCII system; Allen, 1988; also see Bernstein Ratner, 1994). The UNIBET symbols can be printed using an ordinary keyboard. The disadvantage of the IPA symbols is that many of them are special symbols that are not represented on typewriters or computer keyboards unless a special font is used. For example, the symbol for the first sound in the word *thin* has the IPA symbol /θ/. The virgule, or slash, /, typically is used to denote a phoneme symbol in the IPA. An alternative way of representing this sound with the letters available on a keyboard is to use the letter T. For convenient reference, both the IPA symbols and keyboard-coded symbols are included, along with keywords, on the back inside cover of this book. The reader should be forewarned that phonetics books differ somewhat in their use of symbols and definition of phonetic classes. The following discussion is consistent with Shriberg and Kent (1994). The information that follows is a brief introduction to some aspects of phonetics, especially the classification of speech sounds into major groups.

Vowels

Vowels are sounds that are produced with a relatively open vocal tract. This means that there are no major obstructions along the passage from vocal folds to the mouth opening. Under typical circumstances, vibration of the vocal folds produces the sound energy of vowels. The shape of the vocal tract determines the resonance pattern for a particular vowel, as is discussed in Chapter 8. It is convenient to list the vowels in three general groups as illustrated in Figures 3–7, 3–8, and 3–9: front vowels, central vowels, and back vowels.

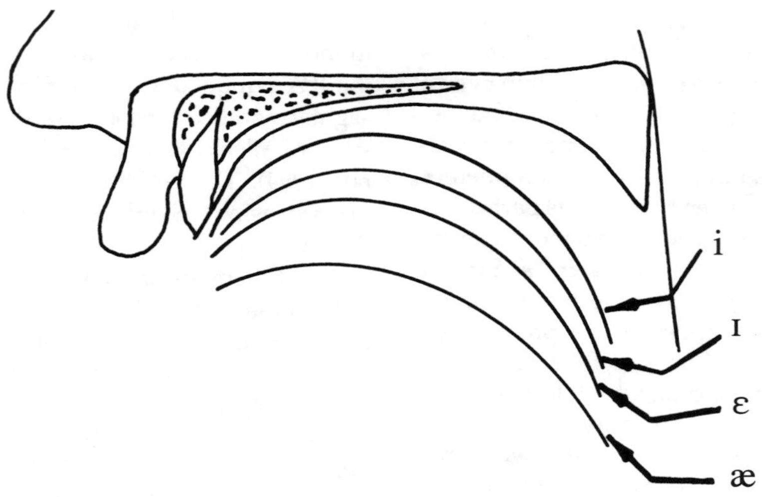

Figure 3–7. Schematic drawing of the articulatory configurations for four front vowels.

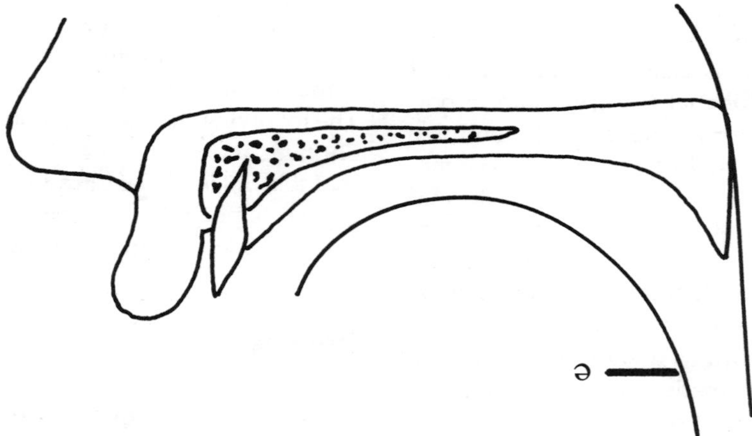

Figure 3–8. Schematic drawing of the articulatory configuration for a central vowel.

1. Front vowels

IPA symbols, UNIBET symbols, and keywords: /i/, /i/ — beat; /I/, /I/ — bit, /e/, /e/ — bate, /ε/, /E/ — bet, /æ/, /&/ — bat.

Phonetic features: front tongue position; various degrees of tongue height.

Figure 3–7 shows a diagrammatic representation of some of the front vowels.

2. Central vowels

IPA symbols, UNIBET symbols, and keywords: /ʌ/, /A/ — bud; /ə/, /6/ — first vowel in abut; /ɝ/, /3/ — bird.

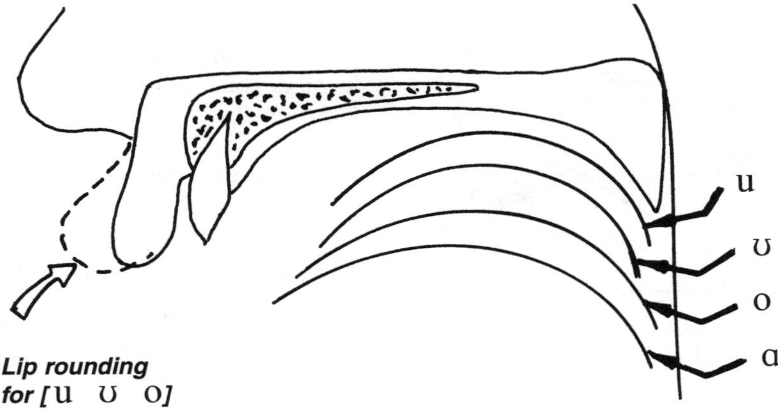

Figure 3–9. Schematic drawing of the articulatory configurations for four back vowels.

Phonetic features: Central tongue position (Figure 3–8).

3. **Back vowels**

IPA symbols, UNIBET symbols, and keywords: /u/, /u/ — boot; /U/, /U/ — book; /o/, /o/ — boat; /ɔ/, /O/ — bought, /ɑ/, /a/ — pot.

Phonetic features: Back tongue position; various degrees of tongue height; many back vowels have lip rounding. Figure 3–9 shows a diagrammatic representation of some of the back vowels.

Diphthongs

The diphthongs are vowel-like sounds that are produced as a slow gliding movement from one vowel (the **onglide**) to a following vowel (the **offglide**). Therefore, the IPA symbols for diphthongs are a **digraph**, or combination of two vowel symbols.

IPA symbols, UNIBET symbols, and keywords: /aɪ/, /ai/—bye; /aU/, /au/—bough; /ɔɪ/, /oi/—boy; /eɪ/—bay.

Phonetic features: Gradual change in position of tongue, jaw, and lips from one vowel configuration to another. An illustration of a diphthong articulation is given in Figure 3–10.

Stop Consonants

Stop consonants are formed by completely occluding the vocal tract at some point between vocal folds and lips. In American English, stops are formed at four places: glottal (closure of the vocal folds), velar (closure between the back of the tongue and the roof of the mouth), alveolar (closure between the tongue tip and the alveolar ridge), and labial (closure between the two lips). However, the glottal stop is not typically considered to be a phoneme and is not discussed further in this chapter. The remaining places of articulation are illustrated in Figure 3–11. Stops are classified as voiced or voiceless, depending on whether the stop is associated with voicing energy.

IPA symbols, UNIBET symbols, and keywords: BILABIAL /b/, /b/—bill; /p/, /p/—pill; LINGUA-ALVEOLAR /d/, /d/—dill; /t/, /t/—till; LINGUA-VELAR /g/, /g/—gill; /k/, /k/—kill. (The glottal stop /ʔ/ (UNIBET /7/) is not truly phone-

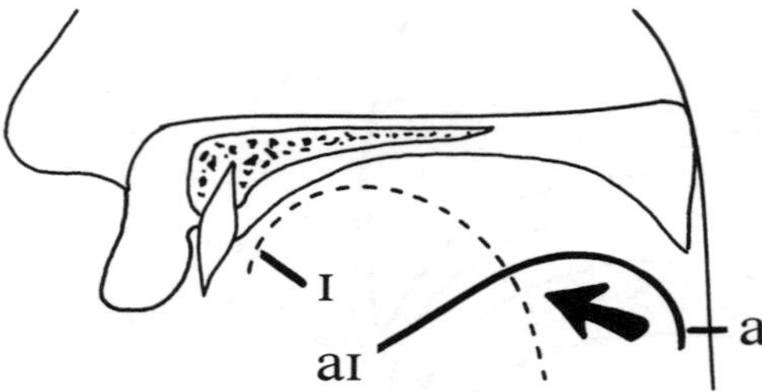

Figure 3–10. Example of the articulation of diphthong /aɪ/. The arrow indicates the direction of tongue movement.

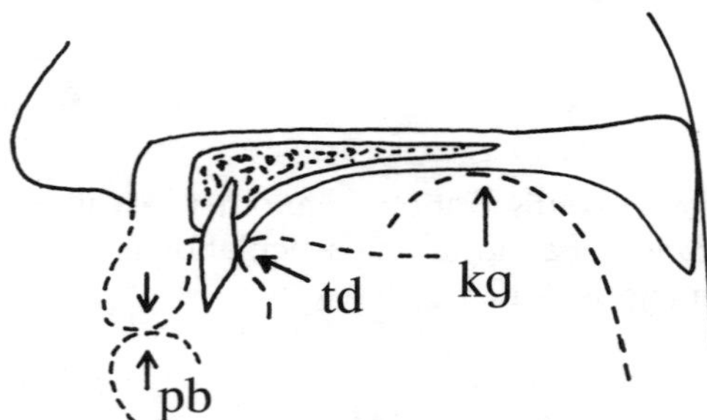

Figure 3–11. Schematic drawing of the places of articulation for the stop consonants. The arrow indicates the location of the obstruction for each place of articulation: bilabial, lingua-alveolar, and lingua-velar (dorsal).

mic in American English, but it occurs frequently as a kind of boundary marker, especially to separate adjacent vowels in a phrase such as Anna—Adams or co—own.)

Phonetic features: Complete closure of the vocal tract. Depending on position in the word, the closure may be followed by a brief burst of air, called the stop release.

Nasal Consonants

These sounds are formed by occluding the vocal tract in essentially the same way stops are formed, but the velopharyngeal port is open so that sound is transmitted through the nasal cavities. The nasal consonants in English are formed at the same places of articulation where stops are formed—bilabial, alveolar, and velar. See Figure 3–12.

IPA symbols, UNIBET symbols, and keywords: BILABIAL /m/, /m/—may; LINGUA-ALVEOLAR /n/, /n/—no; LINGUA-VELAR /ŋ/, /N/—hang.

Phonetic features: Open velopharyngeal port and occlusion of the oral cavity.

Fricative Consonants

Fricatives are distinguished auditorily by their sustained noisy quality. The noise is generated when air is forced through a narrow constriction. Therefore, the articulatory property of fricatives is a narrowing of the vocal tract at some point along its length. Fricatives are classified as voiced or voiceless. See Figure 3–13.

IPA symbols, UNIBET symbols, and keywords: LABIODENTAL /f/, /f/—fan; /v/, /v/—van; LINGUA-DENTAL /ð/, /D/—this; /θ/, /T/—thick; LINGUA-ALVEOLAR /s/, /s/—see; /z/, /z/—zoo; LINGUA-PALATAL /ʃ/, /S/—she; /ʒ/, /Z/—rouge; GLOTTAL /h/, /h/—he.

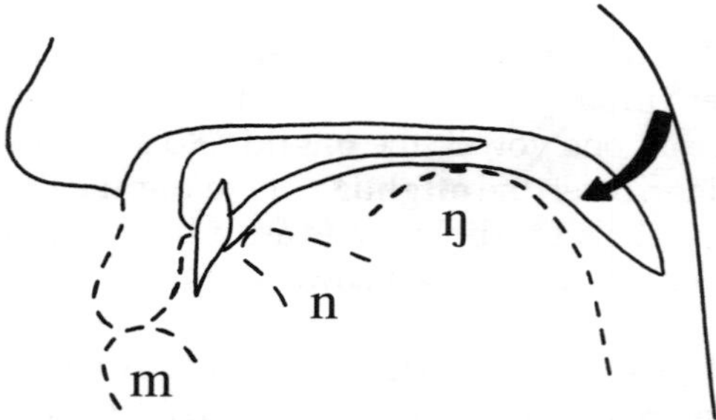

Figure 3–12. Schematic drawing of the places of articulation for the nasal consonants: bilabial, lingua-alveolar, and lingua-velar. The velum is lowered for nasal manner of production.

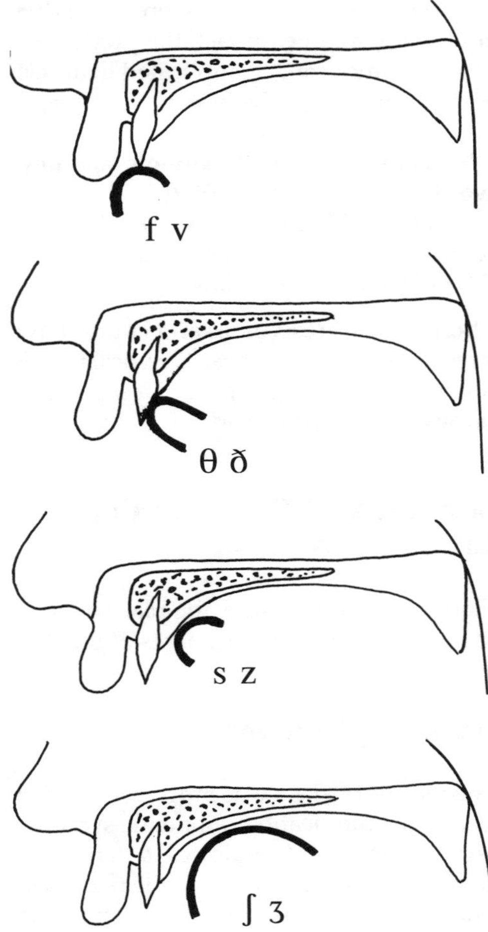

Figure 3–13. Schematic drawing of the places of articulation for the fricative consonants: labio-dental, lingua-dental, lingua-alveolar, and lingua-palatal. The glottal /h/ is not shown.

Phonetic features: Formation of a narrow constriction along the vocal tract and generation of noise as air passes through the constriction.

Affricate Consonants

Affricates are two-phase sounds formed initially as a stop (complete occlusion of the vocal tract) and secondly as a brief fricative (narrowing of the vocal tract). The two-phase production is represented by a combination of two symbols. See Figure 3–14.

IPA symbols, UNIBET symbols, and keywords: /tʃ/, /tS/—church; /dʒ/, /dZ/—judge.

Phonetic features: Two-phase production beginning with a stop articulation and ending with a fricative articulation.

Glide and Liquid Consonants

Glide and liquid consonants are sometimes grouped with the nasals as **sonorants,** or consonants that have a pronounced resonant quality. The sonorants are unlike stops, fricatives, and affricates, which tend to have a noisy rather than resonant quality. The glides are produced with a gradual movement of the articulators. Because of their similarity to vowels, the glides are sometimes called **semivowels.** The liquids tend to have a faster articulatory movement. The glides are initial sounds in *you* and *way*. The liquids are the initial sounds in *raw* and *law*. See Figure 3–15 for the glides and Figure 3–16 for the liquids. It should be noted that Figure 3–16 greatly oversimplifies the articulation of /r/, which is not produced with a single articulatory configuration. Different speakers sometimes produce the /r/ in dissimilar ways,

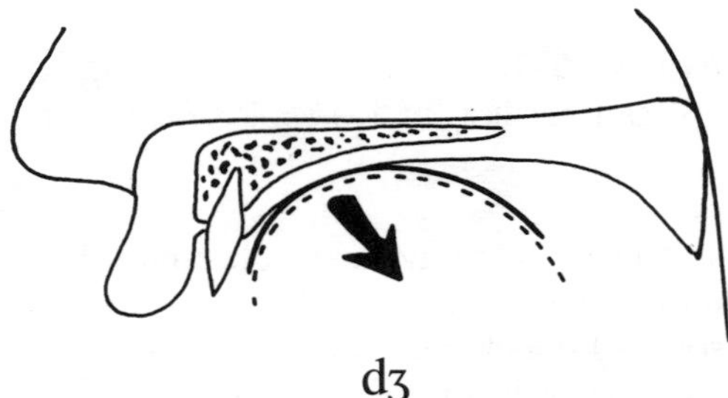

Figure 3–14. Schematic drawing of the articulation for the affricate /dʒ/. The arrow represents a movement from an obstruction (stop phase) to a narrow constriction (frication phase).

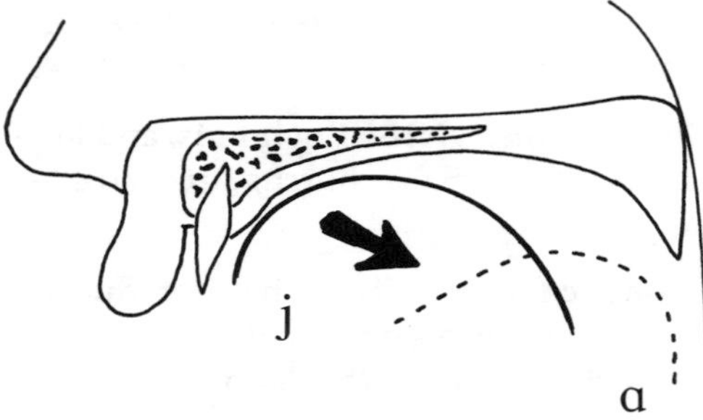

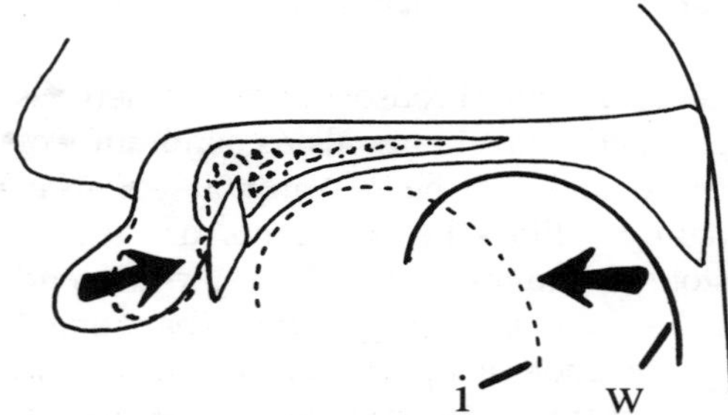

Figure 3–15. Schematic drawing of the articulation of the glides /j/ and /w/. The arrows indicate the direction of movement for the tongue or lips.

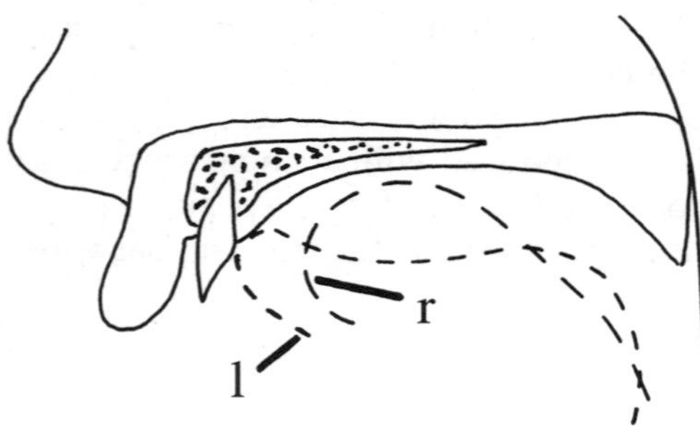

Figure 3–16. Schematic drawing of the articulation of the liquids /l/ and /r/.

and even an individual talker may have more than one way of producing this sound. Phonetics books typically recognize two major forms of /r/. One is the so-called **retroflex** /r/, which is made with a backward turning of the tip of the tongue. The other is the **bunched** /r/, which is made with a bunching motion of the dorsum of the tongue. In fact, the production of /r/ is much more complicated than this, and the story is still being told.

IPA symbols, UNIBET symbols, and keywords: PALATAL GLIDE /j/, /j/—you; LABIO-VELAR GLIDE /w/, /w/—way; RHOTIC LIQUID /r/, /r/—raw; LATERAL LIQUID /l/, /l/—law.

Phonetic features: Glides and liquids have a resonant quality because the vocal tract is not narrowed to the degree that significant noise energy is produced.

Summary of Consonantal Articulation

Figure 3–17 summarizes the place of articulation used for the consonants of English.

Note on Conventions

The virgule or slash was introduced earlier as a way of indicating phonemic symbols. For example, /t/ indicates a family of sounds considered to be a single phoneme. The various sounds in the family may differ from one another, but they have a common phonemic function in the language. These separate sounds may be **tokens** (individual samples of a sound) or **allophones** (a subtype within the phoneme family). To distinguish these phonetic elements from phonemes, the brackets [ ] are used to indicate tokens or allophones. For example, [t] denotes one particular sound token. Special symbols called **diacritics** can be used to distinguish sounds within a phoneme family, but this level of detail goes beyond the purpose of this book. The general rule, then, is that the slashes / / represent the phoneme (a large family of sounds) and the brackets [ ] represent a narrower phonetic class, often even an individual speech sound event.

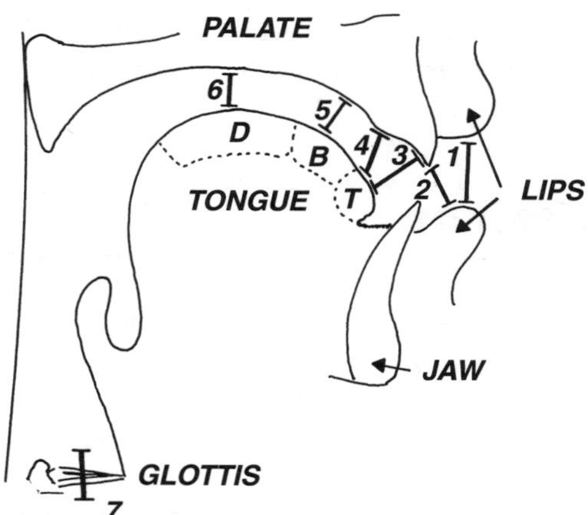

Figure 3–17. Schematic drawing of the vocal tract showing approximate place of production for most of the consonants in English. The divisions shown for the tongue are: T = tip, B = blade, and D = dorsum. The places of articulation are: 1 = bilabial, 2 = labio-dental, 3 = lingua-dental, 4 = lingua-alveolar, 5 = lingua-palatal, 6 = lingua-velar, 7 = glottal.

Cross-Language Perspectives on Phonetics

American English has selected for its phonemic inventory some of the most frequently used sounds in the world's languages. Crystal (1987) determined the 20 most frequently appearing consonants in a database of over 300 languages (UPSID, The University of California, Los Angeles Phonological Segment Inventory Database). Among the frequently used consonants are the following expressed in UNIBET:

Stops: / p b t d k g /

Fricatives: / f s S /

Nasals: / m n N /

Liquids and glides: / w l r j h / (some linguists classify /h/ as a glide rather than a fricative).

American English appears to be typical not only in the number of phonemes it uses (44) but also in its selection of consonants for its phonemic inventory.

According to George Bernard Shaw, his comic masterpiece *Pygmalion* (the basis for the musical *My Fair Lady*) was a didactic play about phonetics. Audiences may disagree about the central theme of the play, which also deals with the subjects of romance and duplicity. At any rate, phonetics does play a role as the young lady Liza Doolittle is schooled in the matter of pronunciation. A more modern story with a similar theme is Richard Powers' *Galatea 2.2*, in which a connectionist system (a neural network simulated on a computer) is taught to prepare for a comprehensive examination on the Great Books. The tutoring of the computer has some interesting parallels to the story of Liza Doolittle. Although the emphasis is on equipping the

> *"Speech itself, necessitating the steady retrieval of suitable language, is possibly even more astonishing. That particular sentence, one assortment of fourteen words, can be spoken far more speedily than written. A fast talker uses three words a second, which all pour forth in a logical, grammatical and meaningful manner."*
>
> (Anthony Smith: *Mind.* New York: Viking Press, 1984, p. 165)

computer system with language and cognition, speech recognition and speech synthesis are employed to give the system input and output capabilities. These technologies are examined in more detail in Chapter 12.

Chapter References

Allen, G. D. (1988). The PHONASCII system. *Journal of the International Phonetic Association, 21*, 11–17.

Bernstein Ratner, N. (1994). Phonological analysis. In J. Sokolov & C. Snow (Eds.), *Handbook of research in language development using CHILDES*. Hillsdale, NJ: Lawrence Erlbaum.

Casseri, G. C. (1601). *Iulii Casseri Placentini philosophi-atque medici patavii vtranqve medicinam exercetis De vocis avditvsque orgajnis historia anatomica singvlari fide methodo ac indvstria consinnata tractatibvs dvobvs explicata ac variis iconibvs ure excvsis illvstrata.* Colophon: Ferrariae, excudebat Victorius Baldinus typographus cameralis.

Crystal, D. (1987). *The Cambridge encyclopedia of language*. Cambridge, England: Cambridge University Press.

Glucksmann, A. (1981). *Sexual dimorphism in human and mammalian biology and pathology*. London: Academic Press.

Powers, R. (1995). *Galatea 2.2*. New York: Farrar Straus Giroux.

Ralph, M. R. (1989, November/October). The rhythm maker. *The Sciences, 29*, 40–44.

Shriberg, L. D., & Kent, R. D. (1994). *Clinical phonetics*. New York: Allyn & Bacon.

Takahashi, J. S., & Hoffman, M. (1995, March/April). Molecular biological clocks. *American Scientist, 83*, 158–165.

Vesalius, A. (1969). *De humani corporis fabrica librorum epitome* [*The epitome of Andreas Vesalius*] (L. R. Lund, Trans.). Cambridge, MA: M.I.T. Press. (Original work published in 1543).

Exercises

3-1. Match the terms in the left column with the corresponding definition in the right column.

anterior	away from midline
caudal	toward the front
cephalad	below
distal	above
dorsal	toward the tail
inferior	toward the midline
lateral	toward the rear
medial	toward the periphery
posterior	toward the belly
proximal	toward the center
superior	toward the head
ventral	toward the back

3-2. Using three pieces of roughly spherical fruit such as apples, carve simple facial features such as eyes and mouth on one side to make a face. Then cut the fruit to demonstrate the following sections: sagittal, transverse, and coronal.

3-3. Identify by phonetic classification the sounds in the words *spyglass*, *loudspeaker*, and *moonbeam*. The following categories should be used (possibly more than once in a given word): stop, nasal, fricative, affricate, glide, liquid, vowel (or diphthong).

3-4. Say the word *nonsense* to yourself and note where the tongue makes a contact for the consonants [n] and [s]. This is called an **alveolar** contact. Then select a long paragraph from any convenient book or magazine and read it aloud. As you do so, place a mark over every letter that corresponds to an alveolar contact. Repeat this exercise with two more places of articulatory contact: **bilabial** (the contact for the consonants in the word *bump*) and **velar** (the contact for the consonants in the word *king*). Does one kind of contact occur more often than the others?

3-5. Guess the number of phonemes in the following words (remember that alphabet letters do not always correspond to phonemes):

ox	oxen	people
through	speech	earn
thick	thing	sample
twice		

3-6. Using the same words listed in Exercise 3–5, transcribe each word using either the IPA or UNIBET. For example, the UNIBET transcription of *ox* is /aks/.

CHAPTER

4

The Respiratory and Laryngeal Systems

"Syllables govern the world"

— John Selden

It is perhaps ingenious, but certainly convenient to us as talkers, that speech is produced on exhaled air. So long as air must be moved into and out of the lungs for ventilation, it is eminently sensible to exploit the expended air to make the sounds of speech. Talking rides on ventilation. Overall, the process is quite efficient. Conversational speech produced at a moderate level of loudness essentially requires approximately the same volume of air that is used in normal rest breathing, at least for adults. In other words, speech is not hard work as far as the respiratory system is concerned. This is one reason why lectures, speeches, sermons, and conversations can go to great lengths, as pointed out in Chapter 1. The major modification that speech requires beyond rest breathing is extension of the expiration phase, so that several words can be uttered before the next inspiration. The basic pattern of speech breathing is: inspire (preferably quickly, to avoid long pauses in the stream of speech) and slowly expire while producing speech.

Because speech is superimposed on the ventilatory process, utterances take on the temporal boundaries of the **breath group**, which is the number of syllables produced on one expiration. Descriptions of speech production frequently assume the breath group as a fundamental unit of organization. In this respect, speech is unlike writing or manual signing, both of which can be carried out quite independently of the temporal pattern of respiration (so long as respiration occurs at all!). Talking must be interrupted by ventilatory requirements—unless we decide to talk on both inspiration and expiration, which does not seem an attractive concept in most natural languages. By necessity, speech is interrupted by inhalation pauses. As discussed in Chapter 3, phoneticians describe the sounds of English as egressive, meaning that they are produced on outflowing air (ingressive means inflowing air). An essential requirement of speaking is to generate an outward flow of air that can be shaped into the sounds of speech. But to make this outward flow possible, the speaker must first get air into the respiratory system. To use a very simple analogy, one can think of the respiratory system as a bidirectional air pump. It is the most massive of the subsystems of speech production, as it consists of a number of bones, muscles, and tendons, some of which are quite large. It also consists of a variety of membranes and other soft tissues. The immediate objective of this chapter is to discuss how the structures of respiration accomplish their tasks of getting air into and out of the lungs.

RESPIRATORY ANATOMY AND PHYSIOLOGY

To understand speech breathing, we must explore the basic anatomy of respiration and the fundamentals of aerodynamics. The relevant anatomy consists of the lungs, chest wall, and abdomen. Aerodynamics is the physics of air movement. Basic principles of aerodynamics are discussed in Chapter 2 under the heading of *fluid mechanics*. Reference to that chapter may be helpful in understanding air movement in respiration. At its simplest, speech breathing is the regulation of the exhaled airstream to support the processes of phonation and articulation and to insure the timely inspiration of air to support life and the next speech event.

Although the lungs are often likened to balloons, it is anatomically more correct to think of the lungs as a tree-like structure of multiple air-filled branches that terminate in tiny elastic sacs (Figure 4–1). The branchings begin with the **trachea** (windpipe), which divides into two **bronchi** (singular form *bronchus*) (Figure 4–2). Each of the bronchi further subdivides into **bronchioles**. These bronchioles subdivide into still smaller bronchioles and so on. The principle that is maintained is one of simple bifurcation—each branch subdividing into two other branches. The complex structure of the airways therefore arises from successive bifurcations, from largest to smallest airways. The entire tracheobronchial tree involves more than 20 generations of bifurcation. The design of this reiteratively bifurcated system has a geometry that is not easily described by classical geometry. But it does lend itself quite readily to fractal geometry in which a basic structure is repeated over and over in various sizes. (Fractals were introduced in Chapter 2.)

Figure 4–3 shows a very simple fractal representation of the design of the respiratory airway. Panel **a** in this figure can be taken as the trachea dividing into the left and right bronchi. Panel **b** adds another bifurcation (bronchioles), panel **c** still another, and panel **d** several more. The terminal twigs in panel **d** resemble some of the narrower bronchioles in the respiratory sys-

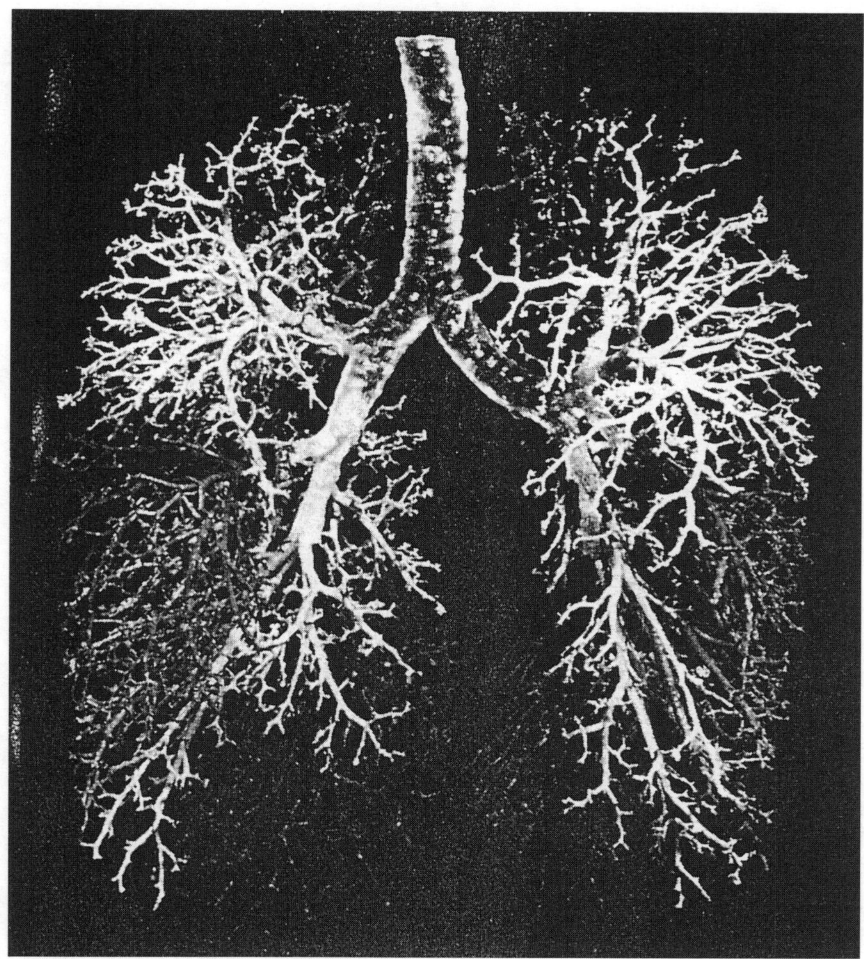

Figure 4–1. The air passages of the tracheobronchial tree and the lungs.

tem. In real lungs, the branching continues to include at least 20 and perhaps as many as 27 generations (Leff & Schumacker, 1993). In addition, to make Figure 4–3 more anatomically correct, the right side should have slightly shorter branches than the left, because the lungs are asymmetric in size.

The fractal pattern schematized in Figure 4–3 offers some important advantages. Because the bifurcations involve progressively smaller fractals, the elements in one generation of bifurcation are shorter and thinner then those in the preceding generation. Narrow tubes offer more frictional, or viscous, resistance to airflow than do wider tubes. The greater the resistance, the harder it is to move air. The resistance is proportional to the length of the narrow tubes. Therefore, it is best to keep the narrow tubes short. The fractal design provides the desired structure of multiple branching and also keeps the frictional losses low, because most of the distance of fluid transport occurs in large-diameter tubes. That is, the fractal design provides an aerodynam-

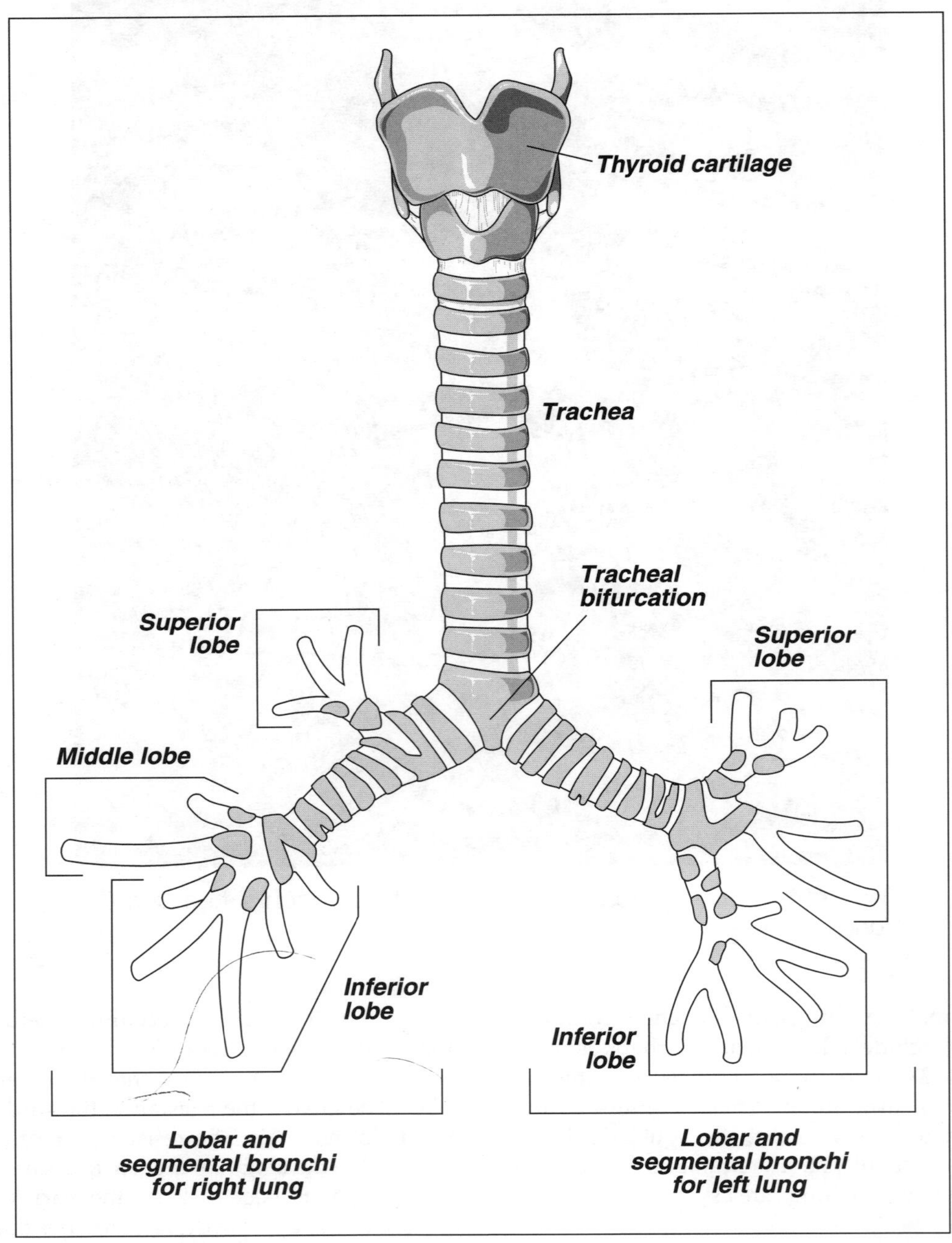

Figure 4–2. The larger structures of the respiratory airway: larynx (thyroid cartilage), trachea, and bronchi.

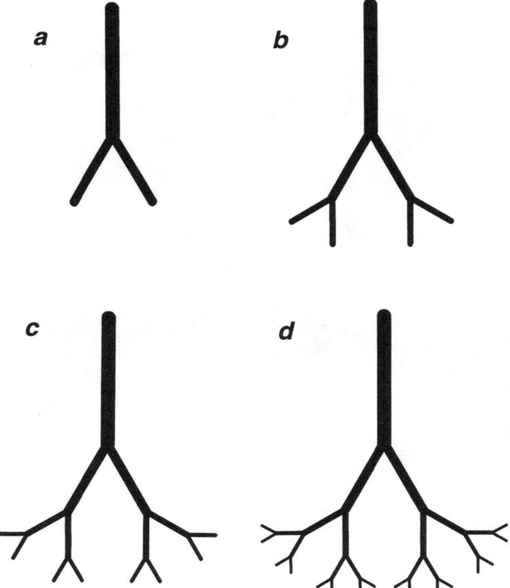

Figure 4–3. A simple fractal model of the respiratory airways. Progressive bifurcations are shown in panels **a, b, c,** and **d**.

ic advantage for ventilation by the lungs. Moreover, the rapidly branching airways actually increase the total cross-sectional area of the passages across generations of branching. For example, the tenth branching generation has a greater overall cross-sectional area (adding up all the cross-sectional areas in individual passages) than the eighth or ninth branching generation.

The respiratory tree is inverted, so that its trunk, the trachea, is the top, and its smaller branches, the bronchioles, spread out to the bottom and sides. Alternatively, one might think of it as a main root with its branching rootlets. The branching continues until narrow passages called **alveolar ducts** connect to tiny **alveolar sacs** in the lung tissue (Figure 4–4). The actual exchange of gases takes place in minute bubble-like spaces called **alveoli**. It is in these terminal air sacs, numbering 300 million, that oxygen and carbon dioxide are exchanged in the ventilatory process. The presence of these sacs and the rich network of blood vessels in the lungs was described in 1660 by the Italian scientist Marcello Malpighi. His descriptions complemented the pioneering work on blood circulation by William Harvey in 1628. Their combined work led to a basic understanding of the relationships between circulation and respiration.

As Figure 4–1 shows, the lung is not simply an empty vessel like a toy balloon but is rather a complex branching network of air passages that terminate in the spongelike air cells of the lungs. The proportion of the weight of the lungs to total body weight is larger in men than women (Comroe, Forster, Dubois, Briscoe, & Carlsen, 1957). The sex ratio (male:female) for surface area of the human lung is 1.25 to 1. The ratio for total lung capacity is 1.41.

The paired lungs are separated by a structure called the **mediastinum**, which consists of the heart, esophagus, trachea, and blood vessels. The lungs are encased in the rib cage and are bounded inferiorly by the **diaphragm**, which is a large, dome-shaped muscle that separates the thoracic and abdominal cavities (Figure 4–5). The diaphragm is a primary muscle of inspiration. Its curvature is not incidental: Its geometry contributes to a pressure differential between the thorax and the abdomen, with the abdominal contents depressed as thoracic volume increases. As a result, diaphragmatic contraction is highly effective in increasing the thoracic volume.

The diaphragm is a muscle common to mammals. This large muscle has openings for the passage of the esophagus, aorta, blood vessels, and nerves (some openings are illustrated in Figure 4–6). The lungs are enclosed by a membrane, or sac, called the **visceral pleura** (*pleura* from the Greek for rib, or side). The chest wall is lined with a similar membrane called the **parietal pleura**. We can say, then, that the lungs are contained in one sac, and this sac is contained in another sac, and the whole arrangement

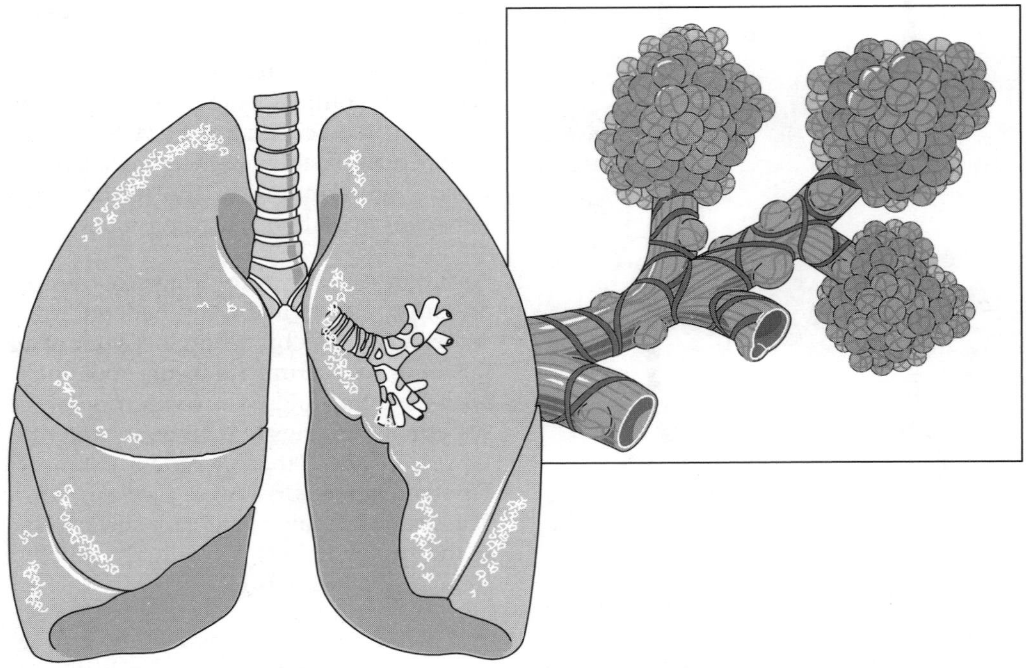

Figure 4–4. The lungs, and, in the inset, an enlargement showing the alveolar sacs.

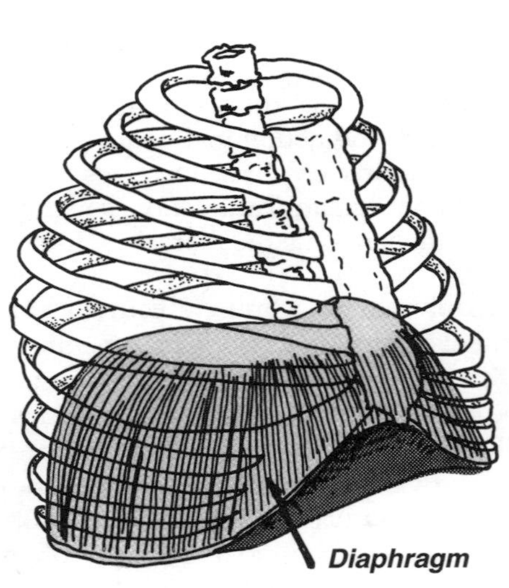

Figure 4–5. The bowl-shaped diaphragm and the rib cage.

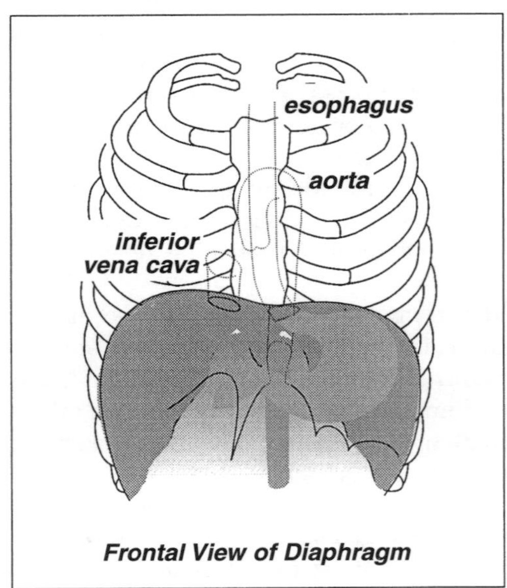

Frontal View of Diaphragm

Figure 4–6. A frontal view of the diaphragm, showing openings for esophagus, inferior vena cava, and aorta.

is contained within the chest wall. The pleura are separated by a space that is more functional than visible. It is sometimes called a *potential* space. The reason it is not visible as an actual space or separation between the membranes is that it is a region of negative air pressure that causes the visceral and parietal pleurae to stick closely together. This **intrapleural space** is at the heart of the mechanics of breathing for it enables the lungs and rib cage to work as an integrated unit. Essentially, this space serves as a kind of "glue" that maintains a functional unity between the lungs and rib cage. To see how this unit works, some additional anatomy information is needed.

The rib cage is literally a cage built of bones. It is attached anteriorly and posteriorly to the other bones of the upper body. Figure 4–7a shows the rib cage in relation to the vertebral column and pelvic bones. Figure 4–7b shows the relationship between the rib cage and the **clavicle** (collar bone) and **scapula** (shoulder bone). The 12 ribs on each side of the body form arcs that reach from the spinal vertebrae at the back to meet at or near the **sternum** (breastbone) at the front of the body. The sternum is shown in Figure 4–8. The sternum connects superiorly with the **manubrium** and inferiorly with the **xiphoid process**. The manubrium and xiphoid become fused with the sternum in adulthood, with some consequent loss in flexibility. The vertebrae, illustrated in Figure 4–9 are grouped as follows: seven cervical, twelve thoracic, five lumbar, one sacral, and one coccygeal. An abbreviated reference system to identify particular vertebrae uses a letter (C for cervical, T for thoracic, L for lumbar, S for sacral, and Cg for coccygeal) and an appropriate number counting from the skull end. For example, C3 indicates the third cervical vertebra and L5 indicates the fifth lumbar vertebra. Interestingly, all mammals have the same number of cervical vertebra, from short-necked creatures such as the shrew to long-necked ones like the giraffe.

Additional anatomic features are shown in Figure 4–10. The upper seven pairs of ribs individually connect to the sternum by means of a small cartilaginous insert called the **costal cartilage** (the term *costal* refers to the ribs). These are called the **true ribs**. The next three pairs of ribs jointly connect to a cartilage that attaches to the sternum. These are called **false ribs** and they have greater mobility than the true ribs. The lowest two pairs of ribs, called **floating ribs**, project to the front of the body, but do not attach to the sternum. The floating ribs have the greatest mobility of the three sets of ribs. The cartilaginous connections between the ribs and sternum are important, because they allow movements of the ribs during respiration. The flexibility afforded by the costal cartilage may decrease somewhat with age. In their connections with the vertebrae and sternum, the ribs are under a tension that can be appreciated during surgical disconnection of the ribs from the sternum. Surgical detachment causes the ribs to move apart as the tension is released. The tension is created by two major factors: First, the shaft of most ribs is twisted along the long axis, which creates a torsion; second, the ribs have a sharp bend (the **costal angle**) in their lateral aspect. The torsion can be demonstrated with a flexible plastic ruler. Take one end of the ruler in each hand and gently twist one end of its length relative to the other, such that its opposite ends have a twisted relationship. Now if you bend the ruler to form an arc while maintaing the torsion, you have a simple mechanical model of a typical rib.

The ribs are interconnected by sets of muscles called the **intercostal muscles** (literally, "between the ribs" muscles). These are divided into two sets, the **external intercostal muscles** and the **internal intercostal muscles**, as discussed next and illustrated in Figure 4–11a and 4–11b.

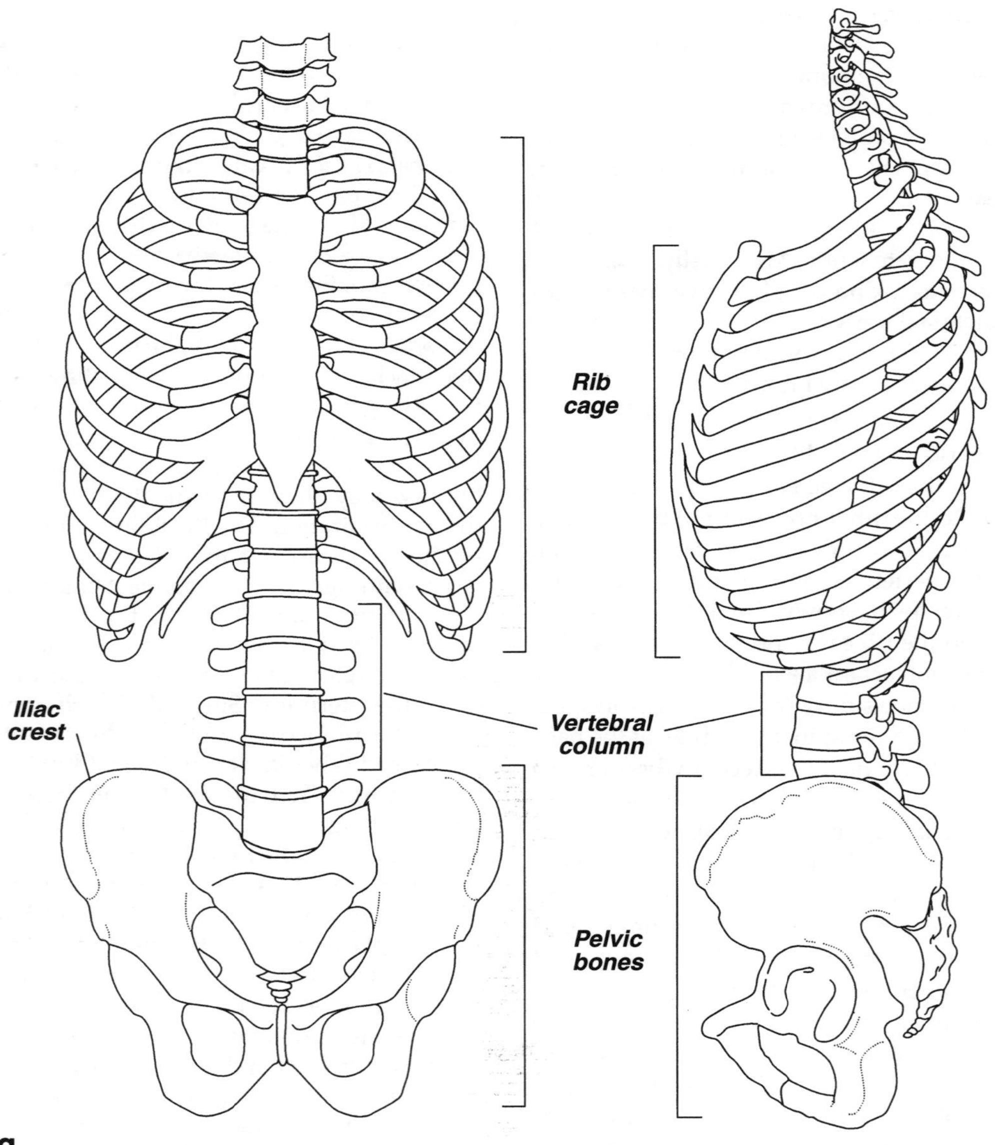

Figure 4–7. **a.** Anterior and lateral views of the skeletal framework of the neck, thorax, abdomen, and pelvis. The ribs form a cage that has anterior and posterior attachments. **b.** The rib cage shown with clavicle and scapula.

(continued)

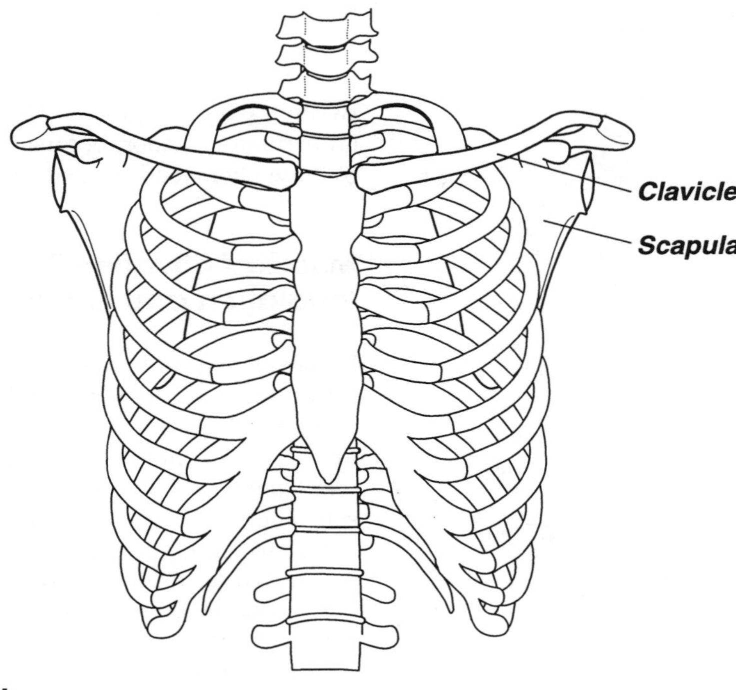

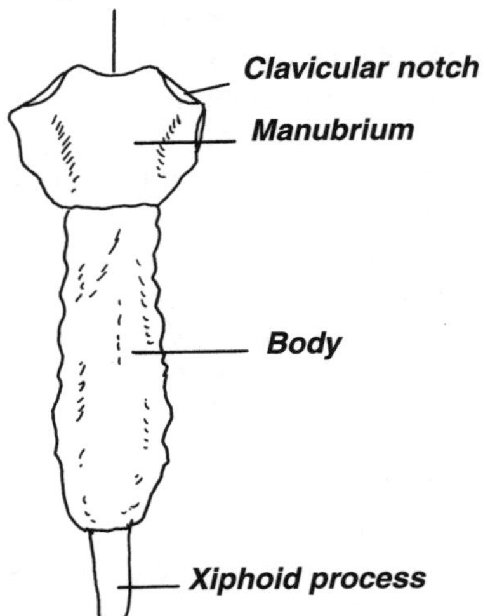

Figure 4–8. The sternum or breastbone.

External Intercostal Muscles

The external intercostals are thin fibers that arise from the lower margin of one rib and descend to insert on the upper margin of the next lower rib. These fibers extend from the vertebral column anteriorly to insert on the costal cartilages. One function of the external intercostals is to keep the intercostal tissue from being displaced during respiration. Such a displacement would reduce the efficiency of ventilation. They also are an important muscle of inspiration because they serve to elevate the ribs.

Note: Any muscle that acts to elevate the ribs will have an inspiratory effect. Any muscle that acts to depress the ribs will have an expiratory effect. This general rule is helpful in understanding the role of many of the muscles of respiration.

Internal Intercostal Muscles

The internal intercostals arise from the lower margin of each rib and insert on the

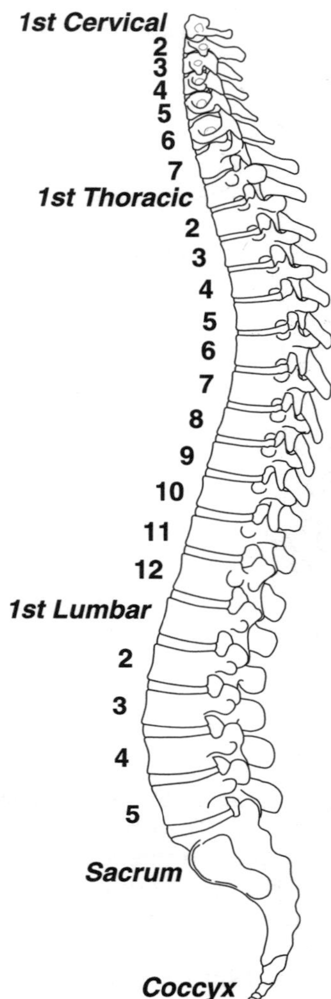

Figure 4–9. The vertebral column with numbered vertebrae.

upper margin of the next higher rib. The fibers extend from the sternum nearly to the vertebral column. The internal intercostals serve to prevent a collapse of the intercostal walls. The function of the internal intercostals differs between its two major portions. The intercartilaginous portion (the part of the muscle located between the costal cartilage) has an inspiratory action, because contraction of these fibers tends to elevate the ribs. The interosseous portion (the part of the muscle located between the bony segments of the ribs) has an expiratory action because contraction of these fibers tends to depress the ribs.

Muscle Activation During Inhalation and Exhalation

It may be helpful to discuss some general principles of respiration before further discussion of the muscles of this system. Figure 4–12 is a simplified illustration of how selected muscles function in inhalation and exhalation. During inhalation, the rib cage is elevated and expanded by contraction of the intercostal muscles and the pectoralis minor muscles (more is said about the pectoralis minor muscle later in this chapter). At the same time, the diaphragm contracts and flattens, which increases the size of the thoracic cavity in an inferior direction. During exhalation, the intercostal muscles, pectoralis minor muscles, and diaphragm all relax, which causes a contraction of the lung volume. Figure 4–13 is a schematic view of the rib cage and diaphragm in three respiratory states: (a) relaxed, (b) deep inspiration, and (c) maximal expiration. This illustration shows how the rib cage and diaphragm cooperate for respiratory actions. The reader might find in helpful to perform the actions in Figure 4–13 (e.g., inspire deeply) and try to sense the relative functions of the rib cage and diaphragm.

A number of other muscles are involved in respiration and are covered only generally. Their participation varies with individuals and with details of the respiratory pattern. These muscles are grouped as follows: neck muscles, anterior thoracic muscles, posterior thoracic muscles, and abdominal muscles. Within a given body region, these muscles frequently overlap one another

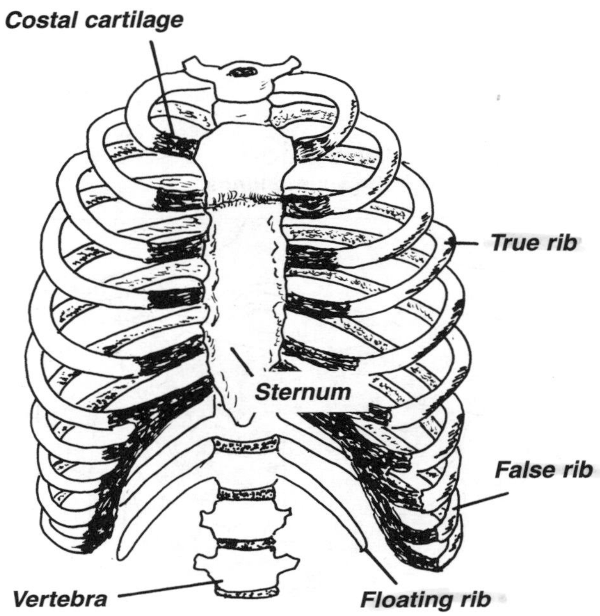

Figure 4–10. Anterior view of rib cage showing three types of ribs.

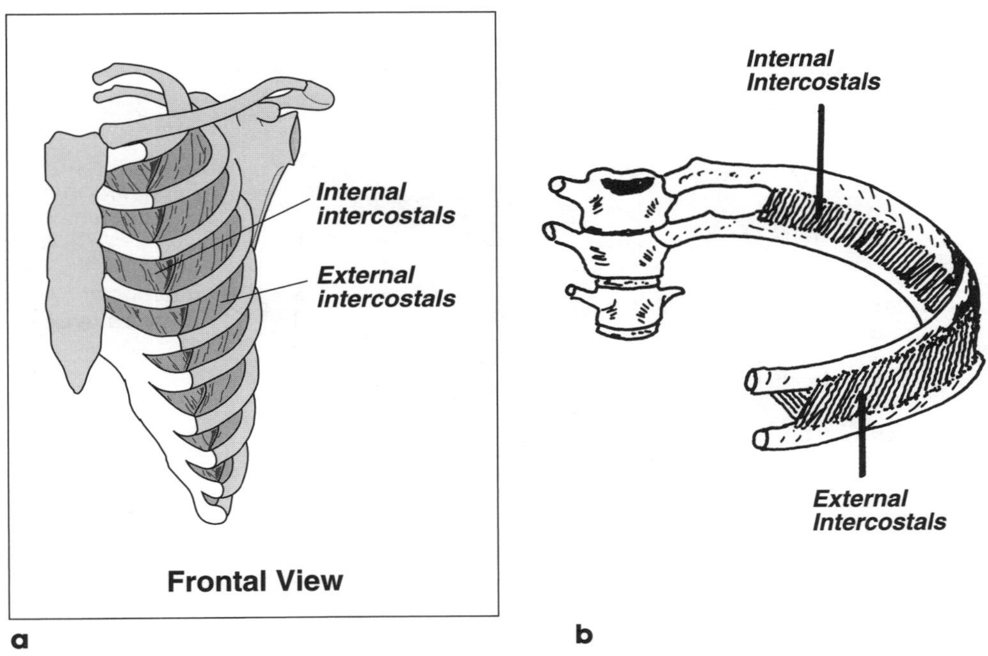

Figure 4–11. The internal and external intercostal muscles shown in (**a**) arrangement in rib cage, and (**b**) isolation of two ribs.

Inhalation

Air drawn into lungs

Pectoralis minor muscles contract

Intercostal muscles contract

Lungs expand

Diaphragm contracts and flattens

Exhalation

Air forced out of lungs

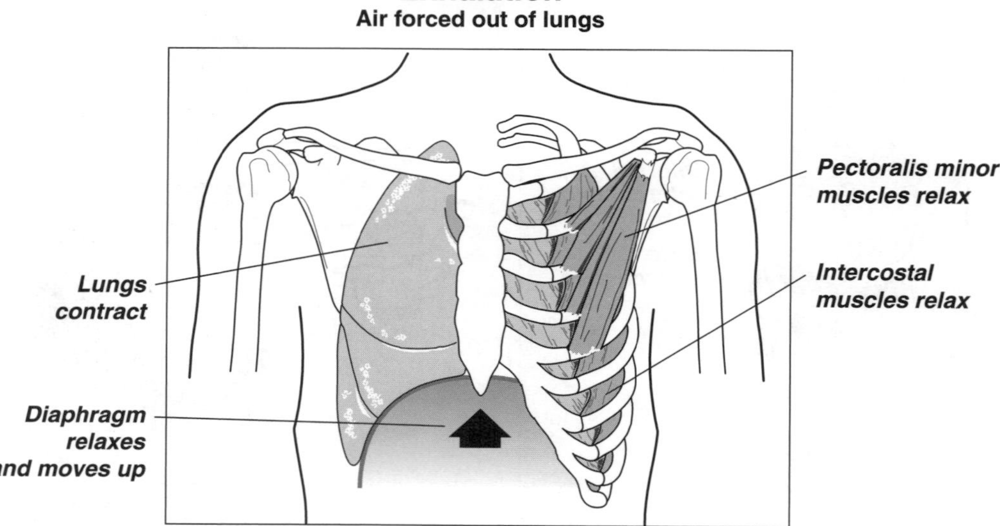

Figure 4-12. Simplified patterns of muscular action in respiration. The diagram shows the action of the intercostal muscles, diaphragm, and one accessory muscle, the pectoralis.

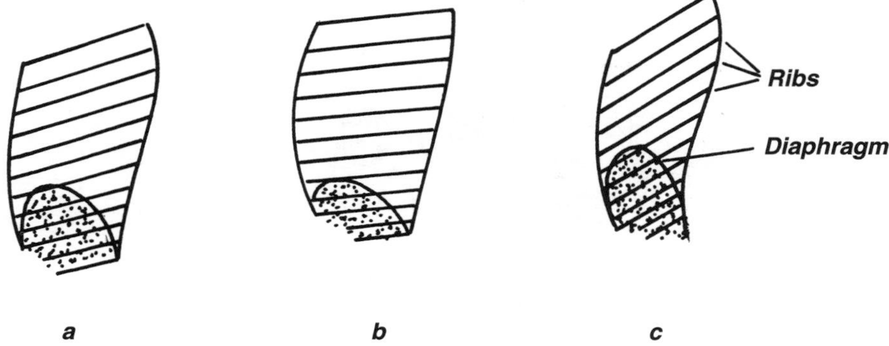

Figure 4–13. Schematic drawing of adjustments of the rib cage and diaphragm in three respiratory states: (**a**) at rest, (**b**) maximal inspiration, and (**c**) maximal expiration.

and several of them have an extensive course (considerable length or mass, and complexity of attachments). Some of them have a variable or minor participation in respiration, but they are included for completeness. Reference to Figure 4–7 is helpful in locating skeletal attachments.

Neck Muscles

The two neck muscles are the **sternocleidomastoid** (Figure 4–14) and the **scalenus** (Figure 4–15) (actually a group of muscles: anterior scalenes, medius scalenes, posterior scalenes, and minimum scalenes; the Latin root means *uneven*). The sternocleidomastoid muscle origin has two heads, one at the manubrium of the sternum and the other at the sternal end of the clavicle. This dual origin is reflected in the muscle name (*sterno-* plus *cleido-*). It inserts on the side of the skull posterior to the ear, partly on the mastoid process of the skull (skull anatomy is discussed in Chapter 5). Assuming that the skull is stabilized, contraction of the sternocleidomastoid muscle would elevate the rib cage. The sternocleidomastoid can be palpated by placing your fingers on the back sides of your neck as you nod your head toward your chest. The scalenes are a complex muscle group, but they share an origin on the cervical vertebrae and an insertion on the lateral regions of the first and second ribs. If the head is fixed in upright position, the scalenes function to elevate the first two ribs.

In summary, the neck muscles can assist respiration by elevating the upper ribs. Accordingly, they are primarily inspiratory muscles.

Anterior Thoracic Muscles

Several muscles are included in this classification (Figure 4–16), including the external and internal intercostals discussed previously as intercostal muscles. There are two pectoral muscles, the **pectoralis major** and the **pectoralis minor** (*pectoralis* is Latin for "pertaining to the chest"). The first of these originates from the clavicle and sternum (along with the neighboring costal cartilages). It runs laterally to insert onto the **humerus** (the long bone of the upper arm). Its primary function is for arm movement, but it can assist in lifting of the thorax, especially if the arms are raised. The

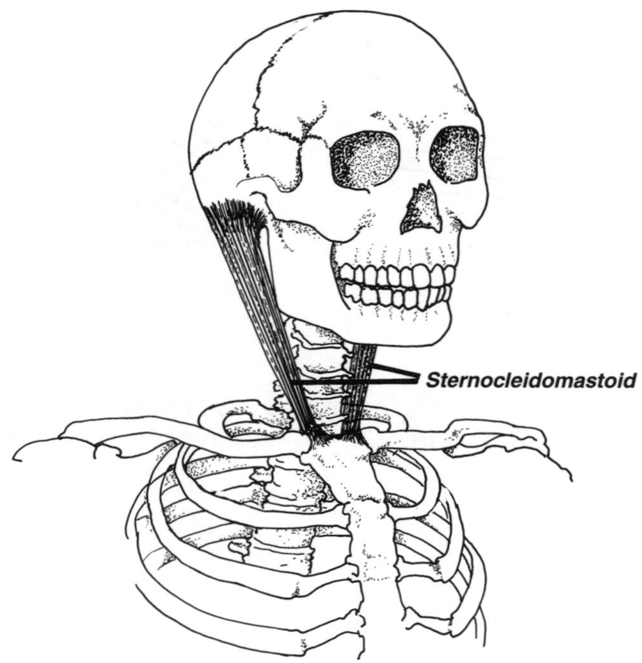

Figure 4–14. The sternocleidomastoid muscle, one of the neck muscles that can assist respiration.

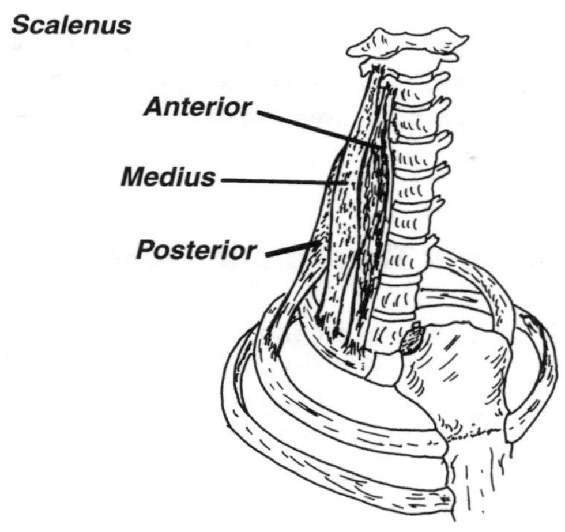

Figure 4–15. The scalenus muscle, with anterior, medius, and posterior bellies. This neck muscle can assist respiration.

pectoralis minor is situated beneath the pectoralis major. It originates on the anterior surfaces of the third through fifth ribs and inserts onto the scapula. This muscle can lift ribs three through five if the shoulder is stabilized. The pectoralis muscles are the "pecs," whose development is important to muscle builders. The **subclavius** muscle is a cylindrical muscle that runs beneath the pectoralis minor from the region of the first rib to the lateral part of the clavicle. It does not appear to have a role in respiration. The **serratus anterior** muscle is broad and thick. Its name *serratus* means saw-toothed and describes its origin as multiple slips of muscle attached to the upper eight or nine ribs. It courses posteriorly and medially to insert onto the scapula. It may exert a lifting action on the lower ribs. The **transversus thoracis** muscle is a deep muscle that arises from the sternum and inserts onto the costal cartilages and intercostal fascia of the upper ribs. Although this muscle has some potential to depress the costal cartilages, it is doubtful that it contributes much to respiration.

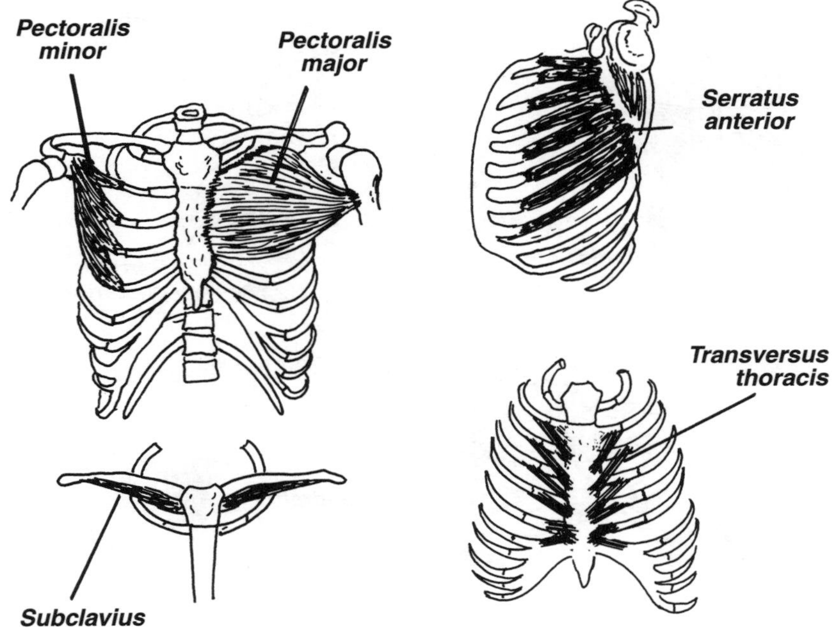

Figure 4–16. The anterior thoracic muscles: pectoralis minor and major, serratus anterior, subclavius, and transversus thoracis.

Most of the anterior thoracic muscles help to elevate the ribs and are, therefore, inspiratory in their effect.

Posterior Thoracic Muscles

The posterior thoracic muscles are sometimes referred to as back muscles. Only a brief description is given for each muscle; the major ones are shown in Figure 4–17. The **latissimus dorsimus** (*Latus* is Latin for wide) is a paired muscle with attachments between the lumbar and lower thoracic regions. It has a complex and broad origin including the lowest thoracic vertebrae, the lumbar fascia, and the external aspects of the lowermost three or four ribs. The fibers insert on a tendon that connects to the humerus (long bone of the arm). A potential respiratory action of this muscle is to raise the lower three or four ribs. The **serratus posterior superior** is located on the dorsal region of the upper thoracic wall. The fibers take their origin from a tendon that attaches to the lower cervical and upper thoracic vertebrae. They course laterally and inferiorly to insert on the posterior aspects of the ribs. The **serratus posterior inferior** takes its origin from the lower thoracic and upper lumbar vertebrae. It inserts on the posterior part of the four lowest ribs. Its action is to pull these ribs inferiorly during exhalation. The **sacrospinal muscles** are a complex set of fibers situated on either side of the vertebral column. Although they serve primarily to make adjustments of the vertebral column, they can assist respiratory function and therefore are included among the respiratory muscles. The **costal elevators** (**levatores costarum**) are paired muscles lateral to the vertebral column. The fibers reach from the lowest cervical and upper thoracic vertebrae to either the next lowest rib or to the second lowest rib. The action of this muscle is to raise the ribs during inspiration. The **quadratus lumborum** is a paired muscle found on the dorsal abdom-

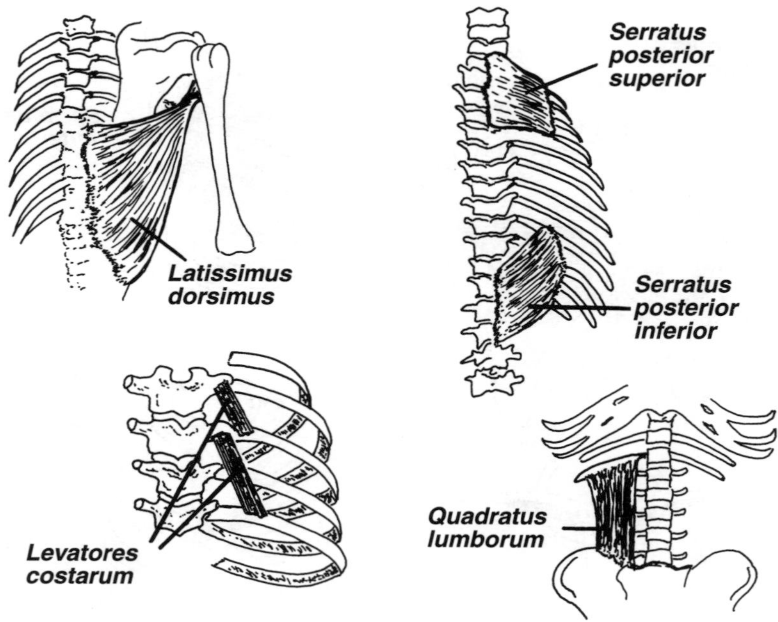

Figure 4–17. The posterior thoracic muscles: latissimus dorsimus, serratus posterior superior, serratus posterior inferior, levatores costarum, and quadratus lumborum.

inal wall. It arises from a structure called the iliac crest (the top of the hip bone) as well as the ligaments of the lumbar vertebrae. It inserts on the twelfth rib and on the upper lumbar vertebrae. An action of this muscle is to depress the last rib and thereby fix its position as the diaphragm pulls against it during respiration.

Abdominal Muscles

The diaphragm muscle, mentioned earlier because of its importance in respiratory function, is the major abdominal muscle. The diaphragm forms a muscular boundary between the thoracic and abdominal cavities. Its fibers have a broad circular origin, essentially the perimeter of the lower bony thorax, including the lumbar vertebrae, the lower six or seven ribs, and the xiphoid process (the inferior extension of the sternum). The fibers converge to form two central tendons. The diaphragm is unique among muscles because it inserts on its own central tendons, rather than on bone or some other external structure. In its relaxed state, the diaphragm has the shape of two elevated semicircular domes. Imagine a large inverted bowl just large enough to fit within the body at the thoracic-abdominal junction. The bowl is divided into halves, forming the semicircular domes just described. The base of each lung rests on either half of the bowl. Contraction of the diaphragm causes a flattening of the bowl, thereby creating a potential space between the diaphragm and the base of the lungs. The result is a decreased pressure within the lungs (alveolar pressure). If the respiratory airway is open to atmosphere, the decreased alveolar pressure draws air into the lungs. If the diaphragm is relaxed, it returns to its bowl-like shape and pushes air out of the lungs.

Contraction of the diaphragm is, therefore, an inspiratory action and relaxation is an expiratory action. During inspiration, the top of the diaphragmatic dome is at the level of the sixth intercostal space. During expiration, the top of the dome is at the level of the fourth intercostal space. That is, the diaphragm moves over a distance equal to two ribs. The lungs attach to the superior surface of the diaphragm. The diaphragm can be understood as a mechanical connection between two different cavities. The abdominal cavity can be likened to a liquid-filled container that can change in shape but not volume. The thoracic cavity can be likened to a gas-filled container that can change in both shape and volume. The diaphragm connects these two containers and provides them with a functional unity.

The diaphragm is involved with two other functions. First, it is a major muscular force behind the sneeze, which is basically an inflation of the lungs followed by a forceful expiration. The expiration propels air out of the respiratory airway at high velocities and is one means of expelling irritants from the passages. The second function is the hiccough, which is rather like a spasm of the diaphragm.

The other abdominal muscles are briefly discussed and are shown in Figure 4–18. Their principal action is upon the contents of the abdomen, the viscera. These actions can contribute to respiration, because the viscera can exert upward forces on the thoracic cavity. The **rectus abdominis muscle** is a paired muscle that extends vertically on either side of the midline. It can be conceptualized as two strips of muscle that begin at the pelvic girdle and run superiorly to the middle of the rib cage. The origin is on the **pubis bone** (part of the pelvic girdle) and the insertion is on the xiphoid process and the fifth, sixth, and seventh ribs. Its action is to compress the abdominal viscera and it can therefore contribute to expiration.

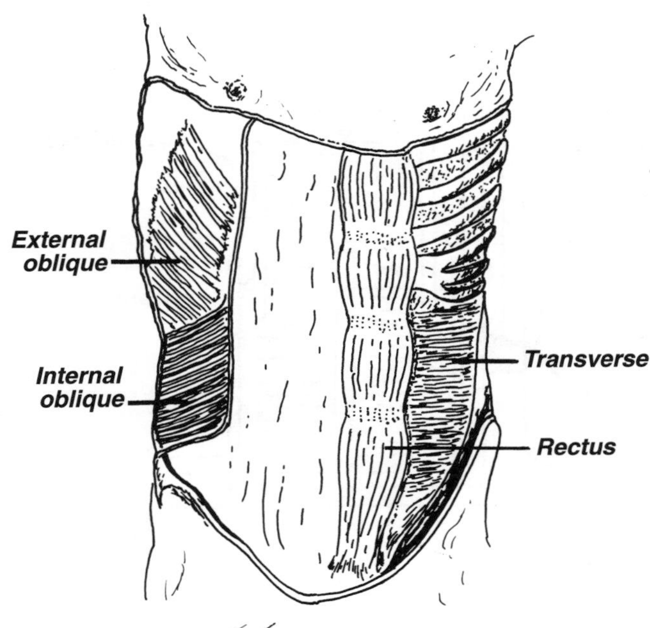

Figure 4–18. The abdominal muscles: external oblique, internal oblique, transverse, and rectus.

The remaining three muscles form three layers of the abdominal wall. The **external abdominal oblique** and **internal abdominal oblique** muscles can be conceptualized as fibers that run diagonally on either side of the abdominal wall. The external oblique is the outermost muscular layer and originates on the outer borders of the fifth through twelfth ribs. It inserts on the pubis, the iliac crest, and the inguinal ligament. The internal oblique originates on the iliac crest, the lumbar fascia (fascia are dense fibrous connective tissues similar to tendons or ligaments), and the inguinal ligament. It inserts largely on the abdominal aponeurosis and the cartilages of the 8th through 10th ribs. Finally, the **transverse abdominis muscle** lies within the other abdominal muscles. As its name suggests, it is a horizontally oriented muscle. Its widely spreading origin includes the inguinal ligament, iliac crest, lower borders of the sixth through twelfth ribs, and the lumbar fascia. It inserts primarily on the xiphoid process and the crest of the pubis.

All four of these muscles have the similar action of supporting and compressing the viscera. In addition, the external abdominal oblique muscle may assist with depressing the thorax (Palmer, 1993).

Spirometry

Spirometry is the measurement of air volumes and capacities. The measures typically are derived with a **spirometer** (also called a respirometer or wet spirometer), an instrument that records the volumes of air used in respiratory maneuvers. Figure 4–19 is a diagram of a wet spirometer. It es-

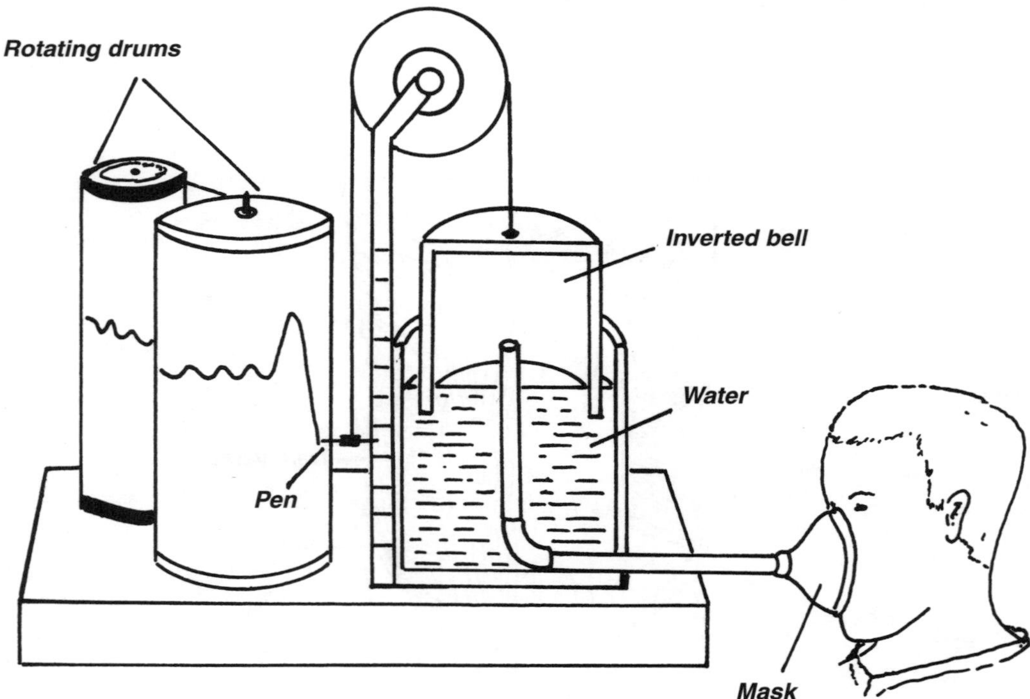

Figure 4–19. The spirometer, used to record the movement of air during respiration. Air from the lungs flows into and out of the inverted bell that is immersed in water. As the bell rises and falls with respiration, the stylus traces out a pattern on paper attached to the rotating drums.

sentially consists of an inverted bell that fits into a water-filled container. The subject breathes into a mask fitted with a tube that leads to the spirometer. As air is exchanged into the bell, it rises and falls relative to the water. A stylus or pen records the respiratory pattern on a sheet of paper attached to a rotating drum. Patterns of respiration are traced in a **spirogram** (Figure 4–20). From different respiratory tasks displayed on a spirogram, a number of different **volumes** and **capacities** can be determined. A volume is a primary subdivision of the total amount of air that can be contained in the lungs. A capacity is the sum of two or more volumes. Some specific volumes and capacities are:

Tidal volume (TV) is the volume of air exchanged during a specified task. A particularly important measure of TV is the value obtained for at-rest breathing. Resting tidal volume averages about 500 ml for an adult male. As exertion increases, TV increases to meet the respiratory demands of the task. Therefore, the tidal volume trace in Figure 4–20 has different magnitudes, as might be seen with changing task demands. But the resting tidal volume has special significance, as we will see later.

Inspiratory reserve volume (IRV) is the volume of air that can be inspired with a maximal effort above the end-inspiration phase of tidal breathing. That is, assume that a subject has just reached the inspiration peak of tidal breathing. Then, if the subject inspires maximally from this point, the volume of air taken in is the IRV. It represents the volume of air that potentially can be inspired beyond the inspiratory needs of rest breathing.

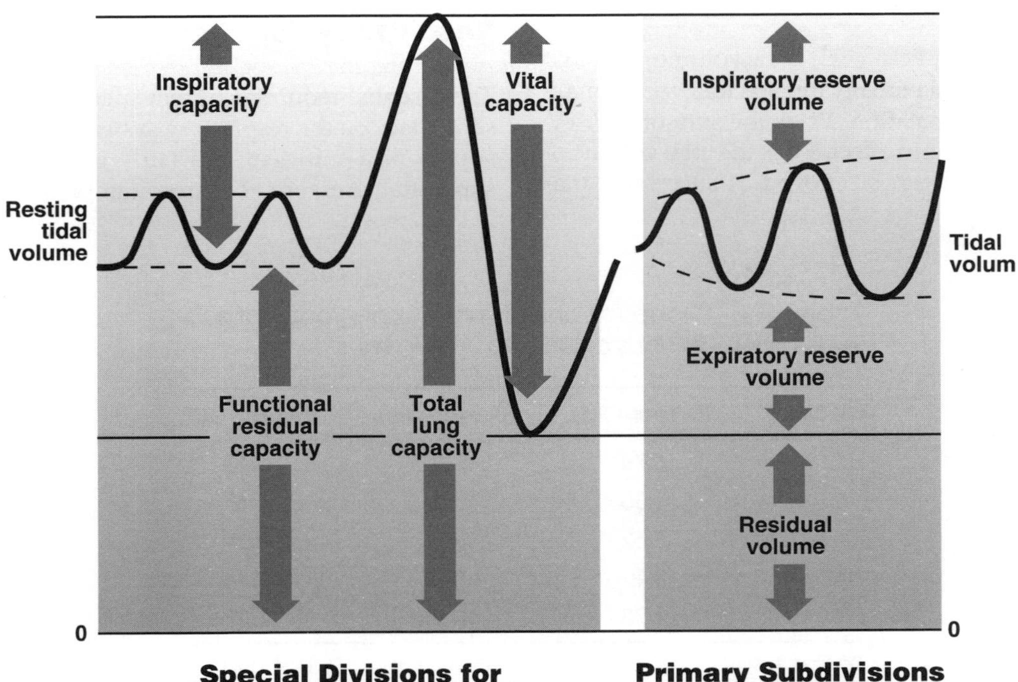

Figure 4–20. Patterns of respiration shown on a spirogram. See text for definition of volumes and capacities.

Expiratory reserve volume (ERV) is the volume of air that can be forced out of the respiratory system with a maximal effort below the end-expiration phase of tidal breathing. In other words, if a subject reaches the end of an expiration during tidal breathing and then forcefully expires all of the remaining air in the lungs, the ERV is the volume of this forceful expiration below the end-expiratory phase of tidal breathing. The ERV is the volume of air that potentially can be expired below the expiratory valleys of rest breathing.

Residual volume (RV) is the volume of air that remains in the lungs after a maximal expiration. The RV cannot be measured directly, because it refers to air that must be in the lungs for the organism to be alive. Under special circumstances it is possible to expel air from the RV. For example, if a person has expired to ERV and is then subjected to a push in the stomach, some of the air in RV will be expelled as a result of the mechanical deformation.

Vital capacity (VC) is the volume of air that can be maximally inhaled following a maximal exhalation. VC is the sum of IRV, TV, and ERV. In effect, VC is the total volume of air that can be moved in successive maneuvers of maximal expiration and inspiration. It is often used as an index of a person's pulmonary capacity.

Inspiratory capacity (IC) is the volume of air that can be inspired at the end-expiratory point of rest tidal breathing. It is the sum of IRV and TV.

Functional residual capacity (FRC) is the volume of air contained in the lungs after the expiration phase of normal rest breathing. It is the sum of ERV and RV.

Total capacity (TC) is the total volume of air that can be contained in the lungs. It is the sum of IRV, ERV, and RV.

Table 4–1 gives mean values for some subdivisions of lung volume for three age groups of individuals: 25-year-olds, 50-year-olds, and 75-year-olds.

Passive and Active Forces in Respiratory Function

The essential requirement that speech and song place on the respiratory system is the supply of a sufficient and fairly constant subglottal pressure. The respiratory sys-

Table 4–1. Group means of three age-groups of subjects for subdivisions of lung volume in liters.

Measure	25-Year-Olds	50-Year-Olds	75-Year-Olds
TLC	6.74	7.05	6.63
VC	5.35	5.09	4.47
IC	3.62	3.59	3.19
FRC	3.12	3.46	3.44
ERV	1.73	1.50	1.28

Source: From "Age and Speech Breathing," by J. D. Hoit and T. J. Hixon, 1987, *Journal of Speech and Hearing Research, 30*, p. 357. Copyright 1987 by the American Speech-Language-Hearing Association. Reprinted with permission.

tem satisfies this requirement through a combination of **active muscular forces** and **passive muscular forces**. The active muscular forces result from the active contraction of the muscles of the rib cage, diaphragm, and abdomen. The passive muscular forces are the forces generated by the elastic properties of the respiratory tissues (including the lungs, muscles, and tendons of the rib cage) as they return from an inflated or deflated state to a resting position. These are recoil forces and can be compared to the elastic forces at work when an inflated balloon begins to deflate. Figure 4–21 shows that the chest wall and lung have different recoils. At a very high lung value, both the chest wall and lung tend to collapse, because both are extended beyond their rest position. At a lower lung volume (about 50% of vital capacity), the chest wall is essentially neutral, but the lungs tend to collapse. At FRC (functional residual capacity), the tendency of the chest wall to expand is equal and opposite to the tendency of the lungs to collapse. Therefore, at FRC, the lung-chest wall unit is balanced. At a very low lung volume, the chest wall tends to expand and the lungs tend to collapse.

The passive recoil forces are modulated by active muscular forces for an efficient regulation of subglottal pressure during a sustained activity, such as speech or song. Therefore, breathing for the purposes of vocalization should be understood as a combination of passive recoil forces and active muscular forces. With this thought in mind, let us turn to a more explicit discussion of how the respiratory system meets the aerodynamic requirements of speech and song.

This discussion concentrates on two diagrams that are fundamental to the understanding of respiratory function. These are the **relaxation-pressure curve** (Figure 4–22) and the **pressure-volume diagram** (Figure 4–23). These two graphs are closely

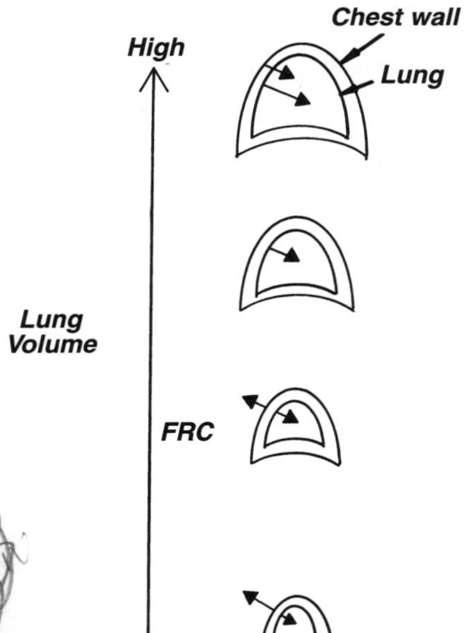

Figure 4-21. Diagram showing recoil properties of chest wall and lung as a function of lung volume. Arrows indicate direction of recoil: expansion (outward) or contraction (inward).

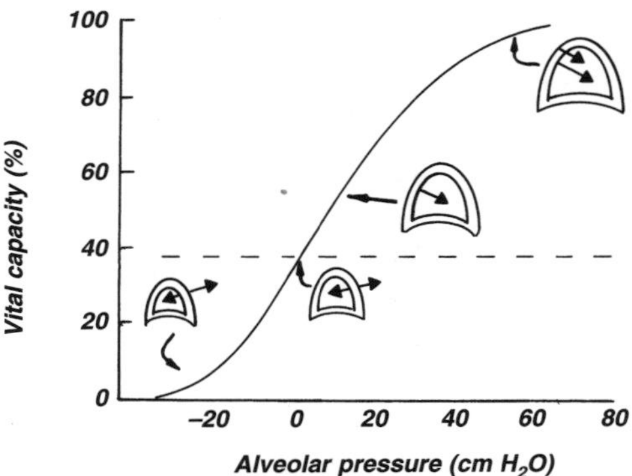

Figure 4-22. The relaxation-pressure curve which shows the alveolar pressure when the respiratory muscles are inactive at different levels of lung volume (expressed as a percentage of vital capacity). Recoil properties of the lung and chest wall are summarized in the sketches (compare with Figure 4–21).

related. The fundamental difference is that the relaxation-pressure curve pertains to *passive* conditions—that is, an absence of muscular (active) forces. The pressure-flow diagram combines the relaxation-pressure curve with the *maximum* expiratory and inspiratory pressures that can be developed with muscular activity.

The relaxation-pressure curve is useful because it tells us the passive alveolar pressures that are generated at particular volumes of air in the lungs. Recall that the lungs and chest wall function as a unit by virtue of their anatomic-physiologic coupling. At a particular lung volume, the relaxation (passive) pressure is determined by the combination of forces developed by the lungs and chest wall. This was discussed in relation to Figure 4–21. Figure 4–22 is based on the same information shown in Figure 4–21, but graphs the results as a relation between alveolar pressure (the pressure contained in the lungs) and the lung volume (expressed as percentage of vital capacity). Some basic principles are:

1. At high lung volumes (above 55% of vital capacity), both the lungs and chest wall tend to recoil to smaller sizes. In effect, at high lung volumes, both are stretched beyond their rest position. Therefore, the combined recoil forces contribute to a high alveolar pressure.

2. At a lung volume of 38%, the tendency of the chest wall to expand is *equal and opposite* to the tendency of the lungs to collapse. This is an equilibrium point on the relaxation-pressure curve and it corresponds to an alveolar pressure of zero. This lung volume corresponds to the functional residual capacity, as mentioned earlier.

3. At lung volumes that are above 38% of vital capacity, the relaxation pressure is positive, meaning that the air contained in the lungs has a higher pressure than the atmosphere. This being the case, expiratory forces are passive. The effect of relaxation would be an outflow of air. To inspire at these lung volumes, active (muscular) forces must be generated.

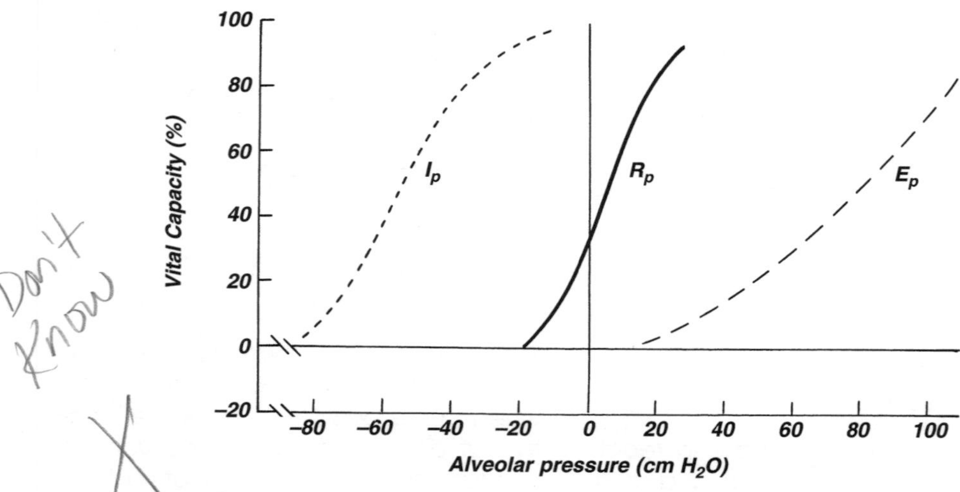

Figure 4–23. The pressure-volume diagram with curves to represent the relaxation pressure, R_p (from Figure 4–22), maximal inspiratory pressure, I_p, and maximal expiratory pressure, E_p.

4. At lung volumes that are below 38% of vital capacity, the relaxation pressure is negative, meaning that the air contained in the lungs has a lower pressure than the atmosphere. Therefore, inspiratory forces are passive. Relaxation at these volumes results in an inflow of air. Expiration requires active forces.

The relaxation-pressure curve may be thought of as the passive characteristic of the respiratory system, that is, the status of the system without muscular activity. Breathing for speech and song takes this characteristic into account in determining the need for muscular activity for a particular task. For example, at a lung volume of 80% of vital capacity, a task of conversational speech can be essentially carried out with passive forces, given the availability of a relatively high alveolar pressure. On the other hand, if the task is to inspire, then rather vigorous muscular forces are required to overcome the positive relaxation pressure. But at a low lung volume of 20% of vital capacity, conversational speech would require muscular forces because the relaxation pressure is negative. At this same lung volume, inspiration could be accomplished with passive forces.

The overall relationship between volume and pressure is shown in pressure-volume diagrams, which add maximum expiratory pressures and maximum inspiratory pressures to the relaxation-pressure curve. A common form of the pressure-volume diagram is shown in Figure 4–23. It contains three curves:

R_p = relaxation-pressure curve, as described earlier;

I_p = maximum inspiratory curve, which is the pressure obtained after a subject inspires to a given lung volume and then inspires again.

E_p = maximum expiratory curve, which is the pressure obtained after a subject exhales maximally, inflates to a specified lung volume, and then exhales maximally again.

Essentially, the pressure-volume diagram maps the physiologic limits of respiration as an aerodynamic system. For any given lung volume, it shows the relaxation (passive) pressure, the maximal (active) inspiratory pressure, and the maximal (active) expiratory pressure. The diagram allows determination of passive and active forces for various lung volumes and desired respiratory tasks.

Suppose that a speaker inspires to about 90% VC (a considerable inflation of the lungs) and then begins to phonate a sustained vowel. If the speaker simply relaxed all the respiratory muscles immediately after lung inflation, what would happen? The passive recoil forces would expel air from the lungs, much as an inflated balloon would collapse after the neck of the balloon is opened. Obviously, if the speaker wants to sustain the vowel phonation for a longer time, then the thorax-lung recoil must be abated. To accomplish this, the speaker can use the inspiratory muscles to control the rate of lung deflation. This process, called a **checking action**, allows the speaker to control the rate at which air is expired after the lungs are inflated. Checking action is used whenever expiration needs to be regulated, such as in conversation or singing.

Another diagram that is useful for describing respiratory function is the **flow-volume loop** (Figure 4–24). This diagram shows the relation between rate of airflow and lung volume for inspiration and expiration. The loop is asymmetric in two important ways. First, the expiration phase shown in the top half of the flow-volume loop indicates that the peak expiratory flow rate is achieved at a low lung volume of approximately 30% of vital capacity. Second, the peak rate of air flow is greater for expiration than inspiration.

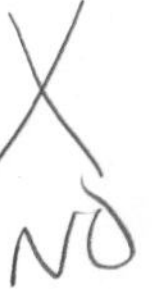

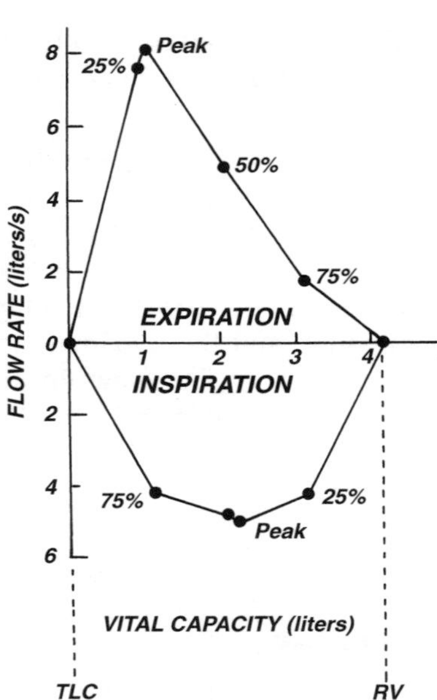

Figure 4–24. The flow-volume loop. Note the asymmetry in the expiration and inspiration phases.

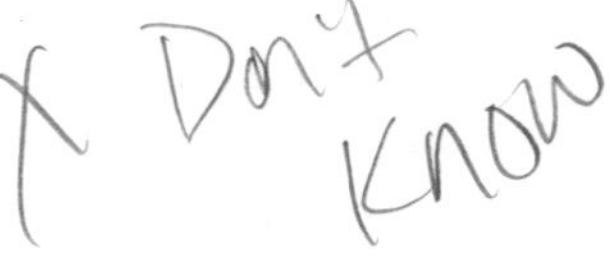

The measurement of lung volumes, the flow-volume loop, and other indices of pulmonic function can be important in the assessment of pulmonary disease (Leff & Schumacker, 1993). For example, **obstructive lung diseases** are associated with low values of FEV_1/FVC (i.e., the ratio of the forced expiratory volume in 1 second to the forced vital capacity). Low values of this ratio indicate a limitation of expiratory flow at relatively low flow rates. Obstructive lung disease often results from emphysema, asthma, chronic bronchitis, and cystic fibrosis. **Restrictive lung diseases** are diseases that restrict the extent of lung inflation and are, therefore, associated with low values of TLC. This kind of pulmonary disease can result from interstitial fibrosis, obesity, or myasthenia gravis (a neurological disease that interferes with the control of muscles).

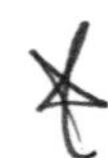

Breathing for Speech and Song

New knowledge has been gained about how the active and passive forces interact during speech and song. Recent research has led to a revision of a widely accepted idea about respiratory control for talking and singing. In the earlier view, based on work by Draper, Ladefoged, and Whitteridge (1959), the active muscular forces were thought to be shut off whenever the passive recoil forces were sufficient to generate the desired subglottal pressures. The more recent concept (Hixon & Weismer, 1995) is that the muscular forces are active *throughout* the speech breathing cycle. This continuous muscular activity during speech breathing is more efficient than an alternating on/off regulation of muscular forces. The key to efficient regulation is for the respiratory system to be tuned to a posture that is optimally suited to produce the rapid and small adjustments in subglottal pressure that may be needed for speech and song. The respiratory system is maintained in a dynamic balance of active and passive forces.

Another change in the understanding of how the respiratory system functions in speech pertains to the muscular forces used during the expiratory phase of speech breathing. The early view was that the muscles of the rib cage (internal intercostals) were the primary motor elements and that the abdominal muscles contributed to the muscular forces only during loud speech or near the end of the expiratory phases of speech breathing. The more recent view is that the abdominal muscles maintain activity *throughout* the expiratory phase of speech breathing and therefore help to regulate the subglottal pressure for speech and song. There apparently is an efficiency advantage to the relatively continuous abdominal activity during speech. First, this activity supplies a kind of platform for gaining maximal advantage from the expiratory actions of the rib cage. If the abdominal muscles were switched off, then the expiratory actions of the rib cage would result in an abdominal expansion that would absorb some of the force generated by the rib cage muscles—that is, there would be a net loss of effective forces for expiration. Second, the continuous activity in the abdominal muscles could help to keep the diaphragm at an optimal length to generate rapid inspirations as needed. The contributions of the rib cage and abdomen are schematically shown in Figure 4–25. The rib cage and abdomen are represented as pistons that cause the lungs (balloon) to expand or compress. The air can be valved at the larynx or at some point of articulatory constriction. The motions of the rib cage and abdomen can be shown on the **relative motion graph** (right side of Figure 4–25). This graph is a convenient and simple way of summarizing the contributions of the rib cage and abdomen to voice and song.

The capsule summary of speech breathing is: The inspiratory and expiratory muscles are continuously active during the expiratory phase that supports speaking and singing. The balanced activity of these two sets of musculature provides the constant subglottal pressure for phonation. This concept is different from one based on the work of Draper, Ladefoged, and Whitteridge (1959) that continues to be highly influential in descriptions of speech breathing. (See Exercise 4–3 for an opportunity to examine this issue in more detail.)

This general picture of the actions of the chest wall and abdomen during speech breathing probably has to be modified in

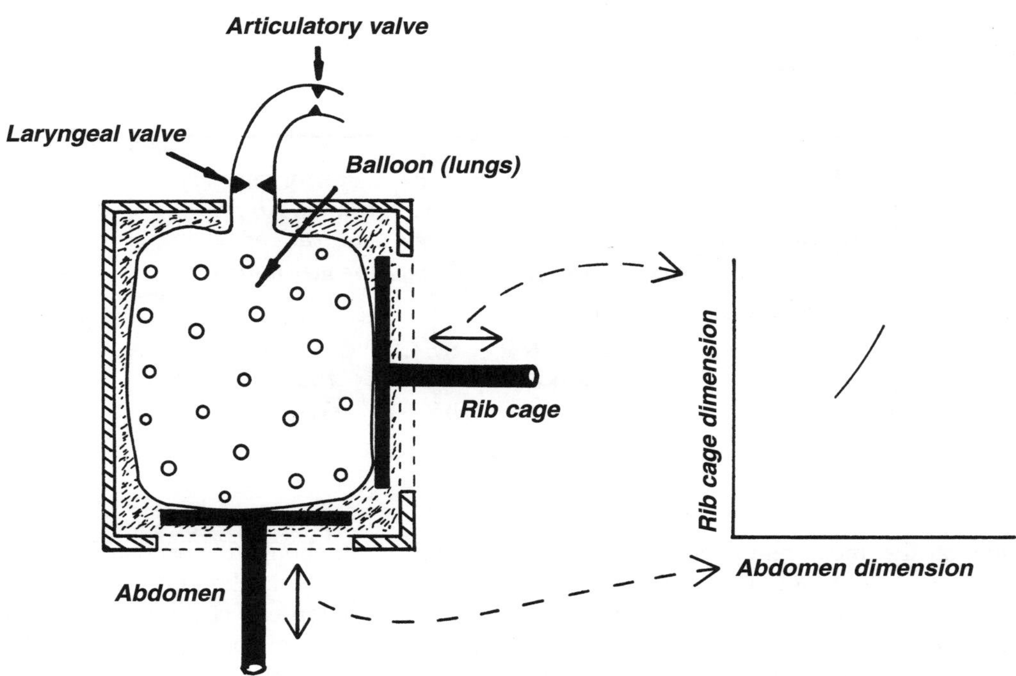

Figure 4–25. Schematic illustration of respiratory function, with rib cage and abdomen modeled as pistons and lungs modeled as a balloon. The relative motions of rib cage and abdomen are shown in the graph at the right side of the illustration. The trace shows relative motions for a spoken sentence.

some ways to account for individual situations. When detailed observations are made of different subjects engaged in different tasks, it appears that speech breathing patterns vary with the age, sex, and body type of a subject; with the nature of the spoken material; with the subject's body position; and with the loudness of speech.

Drawing on the conclusions of several recent studies, it is possible to give a general description of respiratory function related to various speaking tasks. First, it appears that speech breathing is little affected by the cognitive-linguistic planning requirements of an utterance (Mitchell, Hoit, & Watson, 1996). This conclusion was reached by comparing breathing patterns in two speaking tasks, one requiring the subjects to speak extemporaneously on a designated topic and another allowing the subjects to use an outline while speaking. But speech breathing did differ with respect to fluency-related measures of the speaking tasks. In the extemporaneous speaking task, a smaller number of syllables was produced per breath group, the average speaking rate was slower, and the average lung volume expended per syllable was greater.

During spontaneous speech, inspirations typically precede clause boundaries and the amount of air inspired is related to the length of the next breath group (Winkworth, Davis, Ellis, & Adams, 1995). The lung volume at speech initiation typically is in the range of about 10 to 14% VC above FRC (Hodge & Rochet, 1989; Hoit, Hixon, Altman, & Morgan, 1989; Winkworth et al., 1995). As a general rule of thumb, we can say that speech is initiated at a lung volume of about 45 to 55% VC.

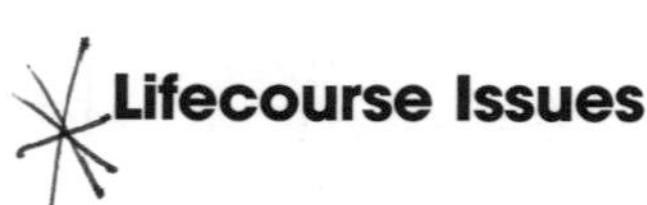

Lifecourse Issues

> ***"The shape, size and composition of the respiratory system changes dramatically from infancy to adulthood. All of these anatomic changes, as well as the maturation of pulmonary tissues, are likely to influence the mechanical properties of the respiratory system."***
>
> (C. J. Lanteri & P. D. Sly: Changes in respiratory mechanics with age. *Journal of Applied Physiology, 74,* 1991, p. 368.)

One of the most remarkable events in respiration occurs at birth. The lungs of the fetus are nonfunctional, as the respiratory needs of the fetus are accomplished by placental diffusion. But at birth, the neonate must quickly adapt to an entirely different mechanism of respiration: the direct exchange of gas with the atmosphere. The critical transition usually is made successfully, even though the neonate has relatively few alveoli in the lungs (the alveoli begin to develop especially in the second month postpartum, but the full complement of about 300,000 is not established until the age of 8 years). The birth cry is a vocal announcement of significant respiratory accomplishment. It is sufficiently important that it is one of 5 factors considered in calculation of the **Apgar score**, a 10-point scale used to assess neonatal health. The Apgar score is discussed in more detail in Chapter 14. (The neonate does not always begin life outside the womb with a cry. The author's daughter emitted a series of coos after she was born. Crying came later. The author's son announced his arrival with a robust cry.)

During human development, several changes occur in respiratory anatomy and physiology. A selected chronology is given in Table 4–2. Some of the major changes related to speech are that breathing rate decreases, capacities and volumes increase, and the size of the respiratory structures increases. It was noted at the outset of this chapter that speech is not hard work for the respiratory system. But this statement should be modified somewhat for children. Research on 4- and 8-year-old children has shown that for comparable levels of loudness, children generate subglottal pressures that are 50 to 100% greater than those used by adults (Stathopoulos & Sapienza, 1993). This research also demonstrated that children move their rib cages relatively more than adults to effect the same volume displacement of the lungs. Additional evidence that children's respiratory systems work harder than those of adults is that children have a shorter **maximum phonation time**, or the maximum duration of vowel phonation following a maximal inspiration (Harden & Looney, 1984; Kent, Kent, & Rosenbek, 1987). This issue is considered in more detail later in this section. Children also take breaths more frequently than adults (Hoit, Hixon, Watson, & Morgan, 1990). Adultlike function of the respiratory system is achieved at about 10 years of age (Hoit et al., 1990).

Typically, respiratory volumes and capacities reach their maxima in young adulthood. They change relatively little until middle age, when they begin to decrease. In some older individuals, the loss of air volume can be considerable. In general, vital capacity is related to sex and body size. The reduction of vital capacity in old age is linked to the loss of stature that often occurs in the elderly. With age, humans tend

Table 4–2. Developmental milestones in the respiratory system.

Age	Typical Event or Pattern
Birth	Diaphragm of newborn has a bellowslike displacement, unlike the pistonlike effect in adults. Rest breathing rate is 30–80 breaths/min. Frequent paradoxing occurs in early infancy; for example, the rib cage makes an expiratory movement as the abdomen performs an inspiratory action. Very few alveoli are present in the lungs of the newborn.
3 yrs	Respiratory function not closely geared to linguistic requirements until this age. Rest breathing rate is 20–30 breaths/min. Functional maturation is especially evident during the period of 3 to 7 yrs.
7 yrs	Essential convergence on adultlike patterns, but children use greater subglottal air pressures than adults for speaking. Number of of alveoli is approaching the adult value of about 300,000.
10 yrs	Refinement of respiratory patterns; functional maturation achieved. Rest breathing rate is 17–22 breaths/min.
12–18 yrs	Increase in lung capacity, especially in boys.

to lose stature and to have some reduction in vital capacity. A reduction of standing and sitting height begins at about age 40 in males and around age 43 in females, with a lifetime loss of standing height of about 1¼ inches for men and about 2 inches for women (Hayflick, 1994). Much of the loss in height in women is from osteoporosis and may be somewhat preventable by appropriate nutrition and exercise.

A phonatory function related to vital capacity is the maximum phonation time just described. The typical procedure used to estimate maximum phonation duration is to ask the subject to take a maximal inhalation and then to phonate as long as possible on the exhalation. It is important to note that maximum phonation duration is affected by two factors: the amount of air in the lungs and the efficiency of vocal fold vibration. Therefore, maximum phonation duration is not a simple and direct reflection of lung volume alone. But mean values of maximum phonation duration over a lifecourse show a pattern that presumably relates to changes in vital capacity. As shown in Figure 4–26, maximum phonation duration increases at the rate of approximately 1.4 sec per year during childhood. With aging, the phonation duration diminishes. Figure 4–25 also shows that the intersubject variability of maximum phonation duration is considerable (see Exercise 4–1).

With aging, the adult's respiratory system undergoes changes in structure and function. Rochet (1991) lists several examples of

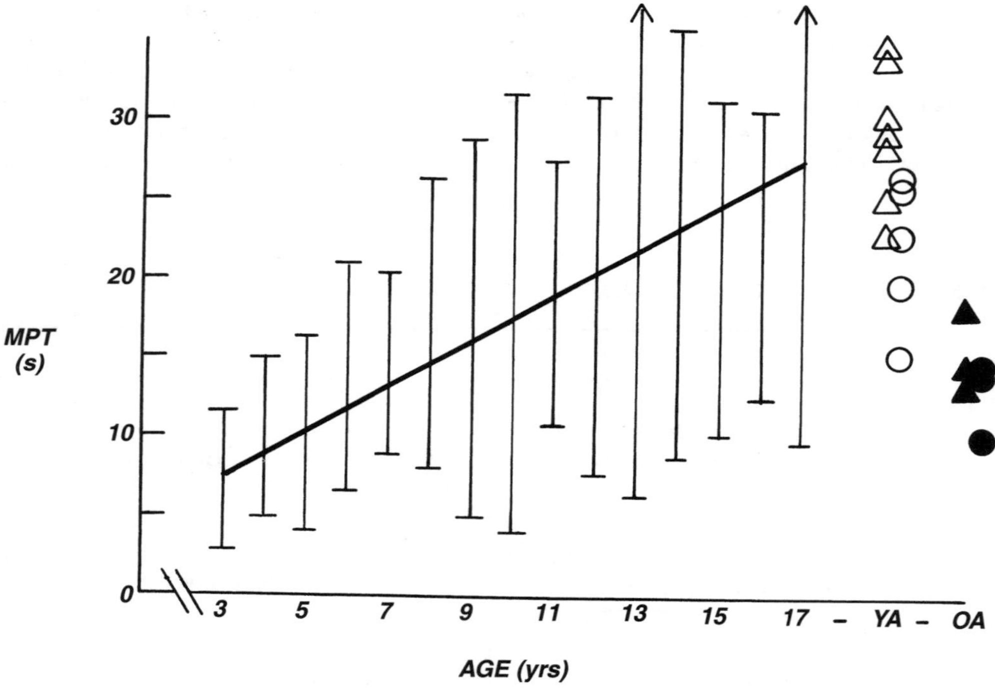

Figure 4–26. Maximum phonation time (MPT) for children aged 3 to 17 years. The vertical lines show the range of values for a given age. Data are included for boys and girls at each age. Mean data also are shown at the right side of the illustration for young adults (YA) and older adults (OA). Triangles represent data for males, and circles represent data for females.

changes in function: decrease in vital capacity, increase in residual volume, increase in functional residual capacity, and reduction in forced expiratory volumes and flow rates. These functional changes reflect several physical modifications, such as decreased elastic recoil of the respiratory tissues and decreased mass and strength of the respiratory muscles.

Respiratory function is affected by exercise, health, gender, and smoking as well as by age. In a study that examined the effects of smoking and age in men and women, Britt et al. (1981) estimated that the loss of pulmonary function in ml/yr was 16.7 in nonsmoking young men and 22.0 in nonsmoking young women. For smokers, the loss rate was 41.7 ml/yr for young men and 21.4 ml/yr for young women. For older nonsmoking men the loss rate was 42.8 ml/yr compared to 49.5 ml/yr for older men who smoked. For older nonsmoking women the loss rate was 27.7 ml/yr compared to 51.7 ml/yr for older women who smoked. The loss rate of about 50 ml/yr for older smoking individuals would lead to a cumulative loss of 500 ml in a decade.

Note on Clinical Application

The following questions point to clinical applications of some common measures of respiratory function discussed in this chapter.

1. Which *single* measure (of the capacities and volumes discussed in this chapter) would be suitable to evaluate the control of the inspiratory muscles? Explain why.

Answer: The best measure is the *inspiratory capacity,* because this capacity reflects the activation of the inspiratory muscles to bring air into the lungs, beginning at the resting expiratory level. The inspiratory reserve volume could also be used, but it does not reflect the inspiratory muscle activation deployed during tidal breathing.

2. A colleague suggests that the control of the expiratory muscles can be assessed by examining the exhalation phase of the resting tidal volume. Would you agree? Why or why not?

Answer: In general, expiration during rest breathing can be accomplished passively as the result of recoil forces. Therefore, the exhalation phase of resting tidal volume may not reflect activation of the expiratory muscles. A better measure to examine the expiratory muscles would be the expiratory reserve volume. Because this division of lung volume is below the resting expiratory level, it reflects expiratory muscle activity.

3. Explain the instructions that you would give to a person to obtain a vital capacity maneuver. That is, what would you ask him or her to do to get a VC estimate?

Answer: The general instruction is to ask the individual to take in as much air as possible, and then to expel as much air as possible. That is, the VC maneuver is a maximal inspiration followed by a maximal expiration. Typically, the examiner would ask the subject to produce at least two or three VC maneuvers and then to take the largest of the three as an estimate of the true VC. A mean of the attempts is not appropriate because the objective is to estimate the *maximal* effort. A precaution to be noted is that maximal efforts such as the VC maneuver can be taxing to individuals with impaired health.

Summary

The respiratory system provides the aerodynamic energy needed for voice and speech. It is a large system composed of a number of bones, cartilages, muscles, and related tissues. However, the function of this system can be understood in a simplified way by recognizing the motions of two major parts, the abdomen and the chest wall. The actions of the various muscles can be understood as how they affect these two parts of the system. For speech and song, the major adjustment from normal rest breathing is to extend the expiratory phase of respiration. It is during this phase that sound is usually produced. Air from the lungs is forced through the larynx and the supralaryngeal cavities. The tissues of the larynx include the vocal folds, which will vibrate under certain conditions. This vibration is the source of voice. The next section discusses how voice is produced.

LARYNGEAL ANATOMY AND PHYSIOLOGY

The larynx is a complex structure composed of cartilages, muscles, and various related tissues. It is popularly known as the voice box, in recognition of its generation of the sound of the voice. The Renaissance scientist and artist Leonardo Da Vinci was one of the first to provide systematic descriptions of the anatomy, physiology, and pathology of the larynx. This material was included in his book *Quaderni d'Anatomia* published in 1500. Among the various experiments that he performed was squeezing the lungs of a goose to generate laryngeal tones, an experiment that apparently was not repeated until almost two and one-half centuries later (Abitbol, 1995). As we will see, the simple experiment performed on the goose reveals a great deal about the mechanics of phonation.

The larynx sits on the top of the trachea and opens superiorly into the pharynx. The isolated intact larynx (anterior view) is pictured in Figure 4–27 and a series of schematic dissections (actually a progressive assembly of the larynx) is shown in Figure 4–28. Reference to these illustrations will be helpful in the following discussion.

Cartilages of the Larynx

The larynx consists of a framework of nine cartilages, three of which are large unpaired cartilages and three of which are small paired cartilages. The larger cartilages are pictured in Figures 4–27 and 4–28. The unpaired cartilages are the **thyroid**, **cricoid**, and **epiglottis**. The smaller paired cartilages are the **arytenoids**, **corniculates**, and **cuneiforms**. The unpaired cartilages are discussed first, with their combination giving overall shape to the larynx. The arytenoids are the only smaller cartilages to receive much attention here. The cartilages of the larynx are larger in men than women (by about 40%).

The large shield-like thyroid cartilage protects the inner components of the larynx. It is formed by the union of two quadrilater-

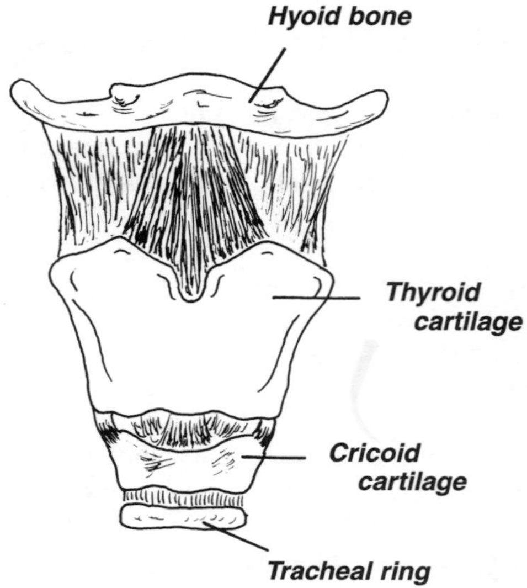

Figure 4–27. Anterior aspect of the larynx and first (most superior) tracheal ring.

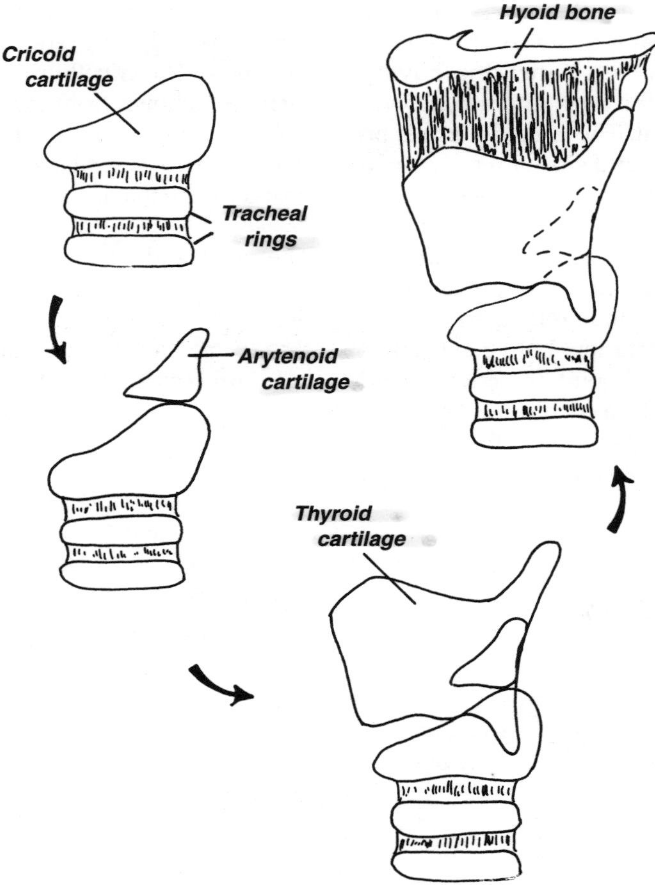

Figure 4–28. Assembly of the major cartilages and bones of the larynx, moving counter-clockwise from upper left: beginning with cricoid cartilage and trachea, adding arytenoid cartilage, adding thyroid cartilage, and, finally, adding the hyoid bone.

al plates into a V-shaped structure, with its vertex at the front and its open aspect at the rear (Figure 4–29). It might be likened to the angular bow of a ship or a V-plow. The V-like junction can be palpated at the front of the neck. The angle is narrower in men than women (Figure 4–30). Verhulst (1987) reported that the anterior angle of the thyroid cartilage was about 90° in adult males, compared to about 120° in females. Another gender difference is that the anterior junction usually is more noticeable in men and often can be seen through the skin of the neck. This anterior region is named the **laryngeal prominence**, or **Adam's apple** (a term from the Biblical book of Genesis). The thyroid plates do not completely join together along the anterior junction, but leave a small notch at the superior region. This is the **superior thyroid notch**. The posterior border of each thyroid plate extends upward and downward to form two **cornua** (horns). These are called the **superior and inferior thyroid cornua**. The superior cornua has a ligamentous attachment to the hyoid bone. The inferior cornua articulate with **facets** (tiny faces) on the cricoid cartilage.

The cricoid cartilage (Figure 4–31) is the only cartilage that forms a complete ring. It is said to resemble a signet ring, having a large plate at the back and a narrower region at the front. The cricoid perches on top of the trachea and sits within the open space formed by the thyroid plates. The cricoid attaches to other cartilages by means of four facets. Two concave facets are the attachments to the thyroid and two convex facets are the attachments to the arytenoids. The attachment between thyroid and cricoid is a true joint, the **cricothyroid joint**, constituted by a **cricothyroid capsule**. By virtue of this capsule's **cricothyroid ligament**, the thyroid can rock and glide relative to the cricoid. That is, this joint permits both translational (gliding) and angular (rocking) movment. The cricothyroid and other ligaments are shown from the anterolateral (a) and posterior (b) views in Figure 4–32. Note that the cricoid cartilage is the only laryngeal cartilage that is fixed in place.

The arytenoid cartilages are shaped like small pyramids placed on the signet portion of the cricoid ring. Each arytenoid has three projections: an **apex** at the top, a **muscular process** at the side, and a **vocal pro-**

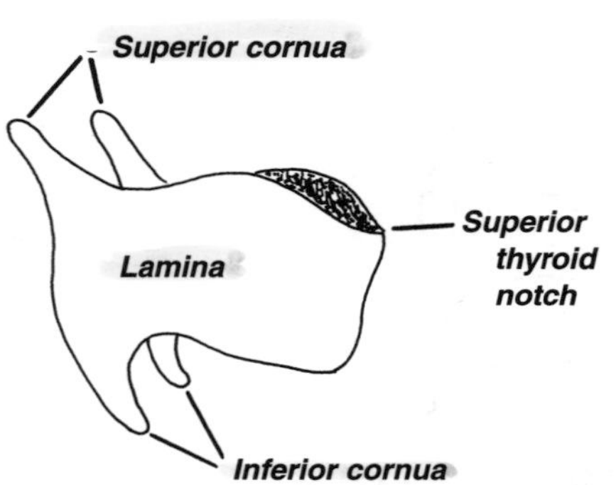

Figure 4–29. The thyroid cartilage in oblique anterolateral perspective. The two lamina that form its sides come together in a V-plow shape.

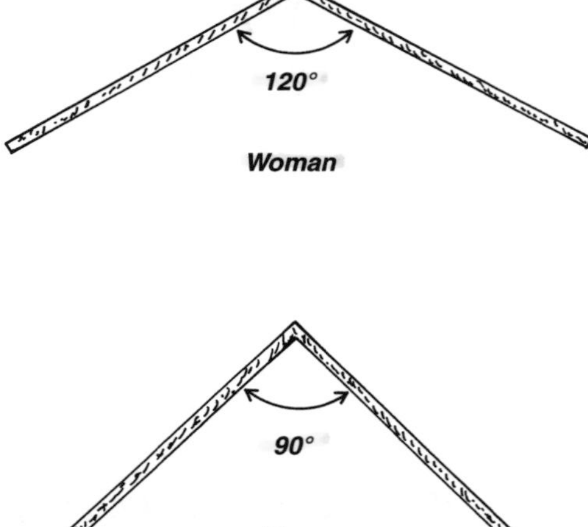

Figure 4–30. Sex differences in the thyroid angle, or the angle at which the two thyroid lamina meet.

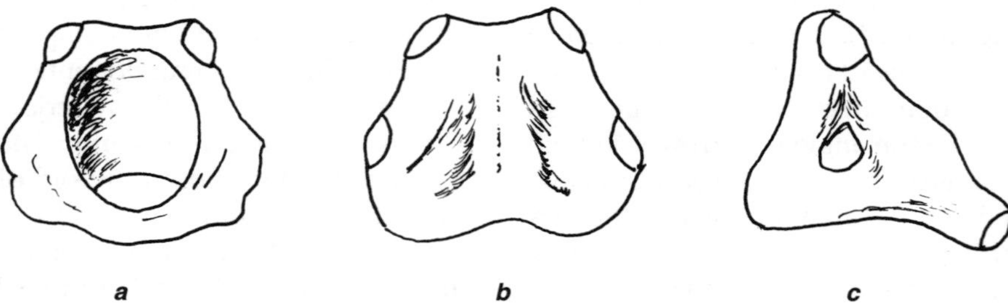

Figure 4–31. The cricoid cartilage: **a.** Anterior aspect, **b.** Posterior aspect, and **c.** Lateral aspect.

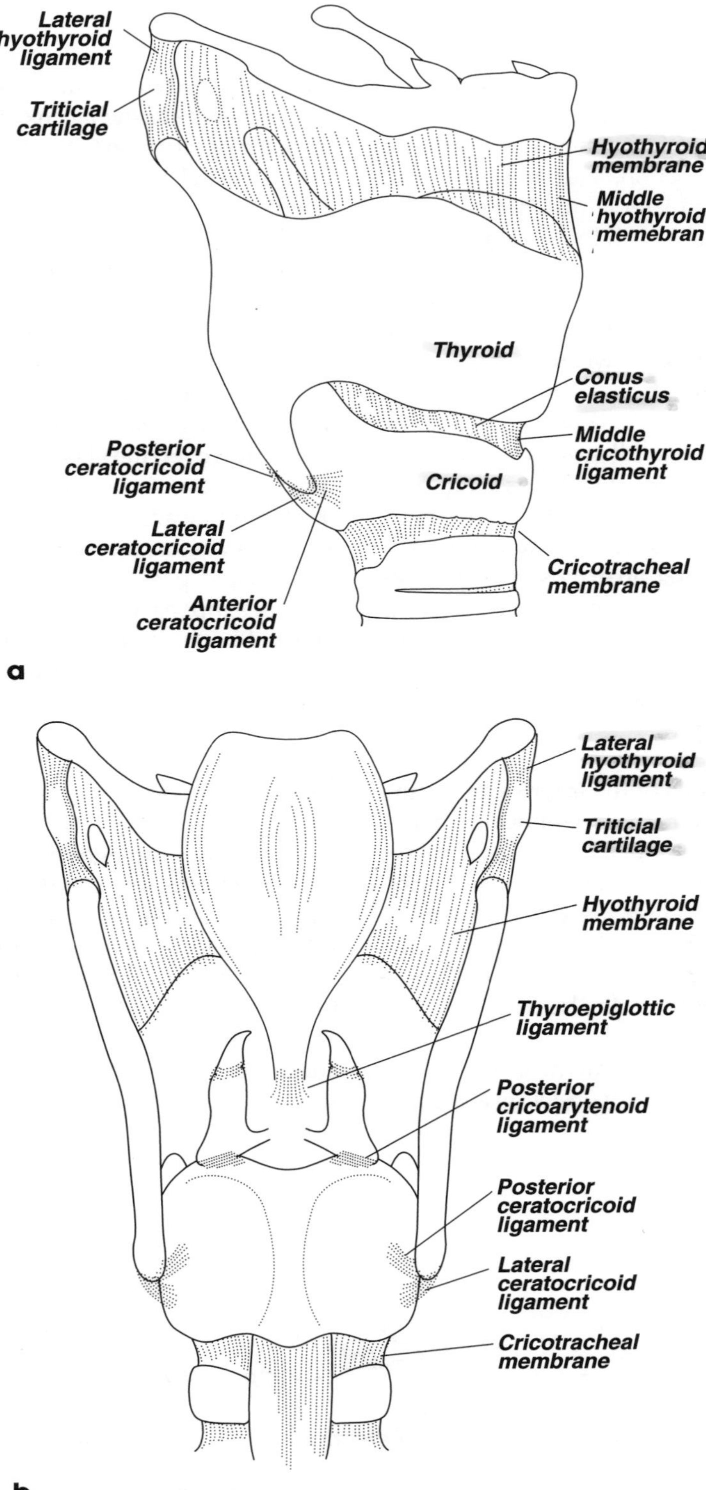

Figure 4–32. Ligaments and membranes connecting the hyoid bone, thyroid cartilage, and cricoid cartilage, shown in (**a**) anterolateral and (**b**) posterior perspectives.

cess that points toward the front (Figure 4–33). These processes are points of attachment that are of fundamental importance in laryngeal function. The muscular process is discussed later as an attachment for laryngeal muscles, and the vocal process is described as an attachment for tissues that constitute the vocal folds. The **cricoarytenoid joint**, a true joint, permits a rocking and gliding motion between the cricoid and arytenoid cartilages.

The other paired cartilages are quite small and are mentioned only in passing. The corniculate (meaning hornlike) cartilages are tiny structures that sit atop the arytenoids, almost like an extension of the arytenoids' apices. The cuneiform (meaning wedge-shaped) cartilages are located anterior and lateral to the corniculates and are buried in soft tissues that constitute the entry to the larynx.

The major actions of the larynx can be understood through the relationship of the thryoid, cricoid, and the two arytenoids. These cartilages are connected by an intrinsic membrane called the **conus elasticus** (Figure 4–32a). The epiglottis is not directly involved in normal phonation, but it helps to protect the entry to the larynx.

There is some disagreement in the literature about the histology (*histology* is the microscopic study of structures) of the various cartilages of the larynx. This book follows the descriptions of Kahane (1983) and Sato, Kurita, Hirano, and Kiyokawa (1990): The thyroid and cricoid consist of hyaline cartilage, the epiglottis of elastic cartilage, and the arytenoid of both hyaline and elastic cartilage. Histologic properties are important in understanding laryngeal function throughout life. As mentioned in Chapter 3, hyaline cartilages ossify with age, meaning that the cartilage becomes bone. However, the elastic cartilages never ossify. The presence of hyaline cartilage in the larynx means that one consequence of aging is an ossification of the thyroid, cricoid, and possibly arytenoid cartilages. As this happens, laryngeal function can be affected because of a loss of flexibility. Sex differences in ossification are discussed in a later section on **Lifecourse Issues**.

Vocal Folds

Now that the cartilages of the larynx have been described, we can turn to the essential tissues of laryngeal vibration, the **vocal folds**. The term *folds* is used in preference to the term *cord*, because the former is a better description of the anatomic structure. That is, the structure has a folded appearance. Although both words are used by specialists and laypersons, alike, the term

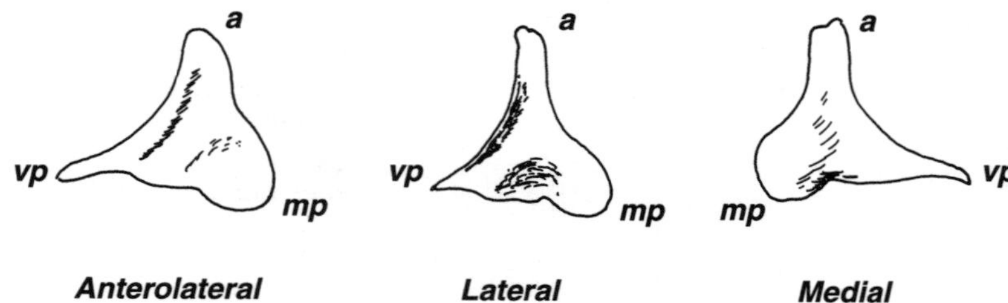

Figure 4–33. The arytenoid cartilages, shown in three perspectives. *Key:* a = apex, vp = vocal process, and mp = muscular process.

vocal folds is more apt. The vocal folds of the human apparently are unique in structure and this uniqueness may account for the virtuosity of human speech and song. More is about this later. But first, vocal fold anatomy is addressed. An understanding of the vocal fold anatomy is critical to an appreciation of modern theories of vocal fold vibration.

There are actually two pairs of vocal folds: the **true vocal folds** and the **false vocal folds**. The true folds lie inferiorly to the false folds. As can be seen in Figure 4–34, the two pairs of folds are parallel, both stretching from anterior to posterior across the airway. Therefore, in a coronal section, the false vocal folds appear as two shelves of tissue situated superiorly to the true vocal folds. The true vocal folds are more important in normal phonation. The false and true folds are separated by a small cleft called the **ventricle** (or **ventricle of Morgagni**), which, like the folds, runs anterior to posterior along the lateral wall of the airway. The true vocal fold, ventricle, and false vocal fold define major anatomic regions of the larynx: the **subglottic**, **glottic**, and **supraglottic regions**. The subglottic region extends from the lower margin of the true vocal fold to the inferior border of the cricoid cartilage. The glottic region is the true cord. The supraglottic region lies superior to the ventricle. The arytenoid cartilage spans the distance from the true vocal fold to the false vocal fold. The vocal process of the arytenoid is at the level of the true vocal fold, and the apex of the arytenoid is at the level of the false vocal fold.

A color photograph of the true and false vocal folds is shown in Color plate 1 at the back of the book. This photograph also shows the positions of the arytenoid cartilage, as viewed from above. Color plate 2 shows the vocal folds in states of breathing and phonation. During breathing, the folds are separated to allow the ready movement of air between lungs and the supralaryngeal cavities. During phonation, the folds are approximated (brought together) to enable vibration, as is discussed in a later section.

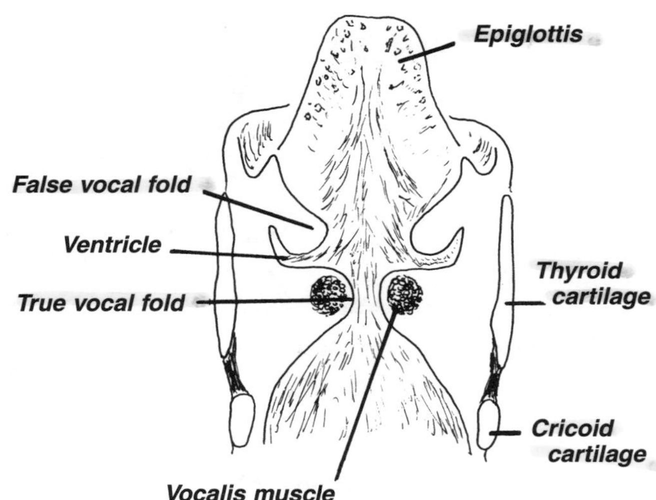

Figure 4–34. Coronal section of the larynx, showing true and false vocal folds separated by the ventricle of Morgagni. Vocalis muscle is the bulk of the true folds.

Note: In the remainder of this chapter the term *vocal fold* refers to the true vocal fold, unless stated otherwise.

The drawing of the adult vocal fold in Figure 4–35 shows that it has a five-layered structure. The outermost layer is a thin cap-

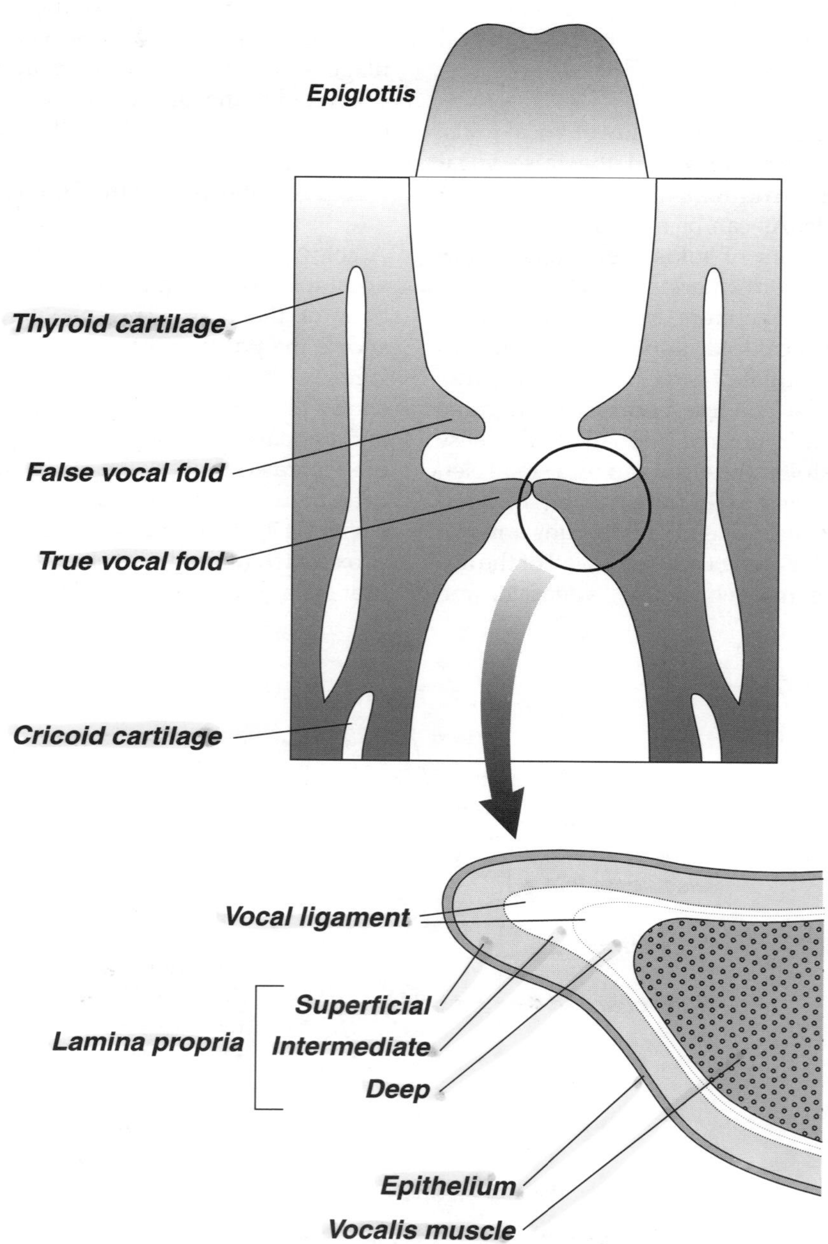

Figure 4–35. The vocal fold, shown in coronal section and an enlargement to represent the layered structure.

sule of **epithelium**, less than 0.1 mm in thickness. Underlying the epithelium is a composite structure called the **lamina propria**. This structure consists of three layers: **superior**, **intermediate**, and **deep**. The loose and pliant superficial layer is rather like soft gelatin in consistency. This layer, about 0.5 mm in thickness, is the most active in vocal fold vibration. The intermediate layer is mainly elastic and can be likened to a soft rubber band. It is about 1–2 mm thick. The deep layer contains a great deal of collagen and is rather like thick cotton thread. This layer is about 1–2 mm thick. Therefore, the lamina propria is a three-part structure that can be conceptualized as a layer of gelatin upon a layer of rubber upon a layer of thick thread. The intermediate and deep layers together constitute the **vocal ligament**. Lying beneath the vocal ligament is the **vocalis muscle**, which makes up the bulk of the vocal fold.

The layered structure of the vocal folds can be further described by histological properties and by mechanical properties that affect vibration (Hirano, 1974; Hirano & Kakita, 1985; Hirano & Sato, 1993). By histologic examination, the vocal fold has two major parts: the **mucosa** (epithelium and lamina propria) and the vocalis muscle. By mechanical properties, the five layers described earlier can be classified into three parts: the **cover** (the epithelium and superficial layer of the lamina propria), the **transition** (the intermediate and deep layers of the lamina propria; also known as the vocal ligament), and the **body** (vocalis muscle). Figure 4–36 summarizes the relations among the various terms used to describe the layered structure of the vocal folds. This terminology can be rather confusing on first look, because different layers are subsumed under different names, depending on whether the approach is histological or functional.

Color plates 3 and 4 in the back of this book show enlarged coronal sections of the vocal folds of an adult male and an infant, respectively. Color plate 3 shows the layered structure described. But Color plate 4 does not, because the layered structure is a developmental phenomenon and is not evident in the infant's vocal folds (more is said about this later).

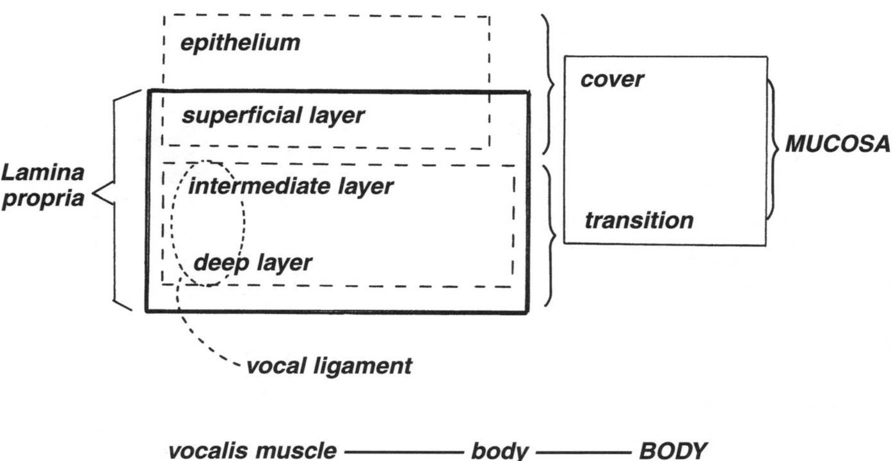

Figure 4–36. A schematic representation of the layered structure of the vocal folds.

Figure 4–37 illustrates the major cartilages and vocal ligament when viewed from above, that is, looking down into the larynx. The arytenoids are at the posterior part of the illustration and the thyroid angle is at the anterior portion. The vocal ligament (the structure composed of the intermediate and deep layers of the lamina propria) runs from the vocal process of the arytenoids to the inner aspect of the thryoid angle.

Especially in women, the vocal folds do not make uniform contact along their lengths during abduction. Rather, a triangle-shaped gap may persist in the posterior region (between the tips of the vocal processes of the arytenoids and the posterior wall of the glottis). This feature is called the **posterior glottal chink**, or **posterior glottal gap** (Figure 4–38). Studies show that the majority of women have a posterior glottal gap, but it is uncommon in men (Sodersten & Lindestad, 1990). A number of sex differences in laryngeal anatomy might account for the likelihood of the posterior glottal gap in women. Specifically, women have a larger ratio of cartilaginous to membranous glottis, a larger angle of the vocal folds at the anterior commissure, a relatively greater distance between the cricoarytenoid joint and the glottis, and a relatively greater increase in vocal fold length during abduction of the folds (Hirano, Kiyokawa, Kurita, & Sato, 1986).

The posterior glottal gap is one explanation for the observation that women's voices tend to be more breathy than men's voices. Because the vocal folds do not completely approximate during the closed cycle, turbulence noise is generated along with the periodic voice signal. This noise is heard as a breathy voice quality. However, the degree of breathiness in women's and men's voices may be influenced by cultural factors and not simply by anatomic differences. Trittin and Lleo (1995) reported that both men and women speakers of Spanish have a similar breathy quality. It is unclear if any cultures are associated with breathiness in men's voices, but lack of breathiness in women's. It appears that either the two genders are similar in breathiness or that women have greater breathiness than men. Perhaps both physiological and cultural factors need to be considered to explain gender differences in vocal quality. It is likely that age and gender interact in their influence on voice. Linville (1992) reported that elderly women were not as

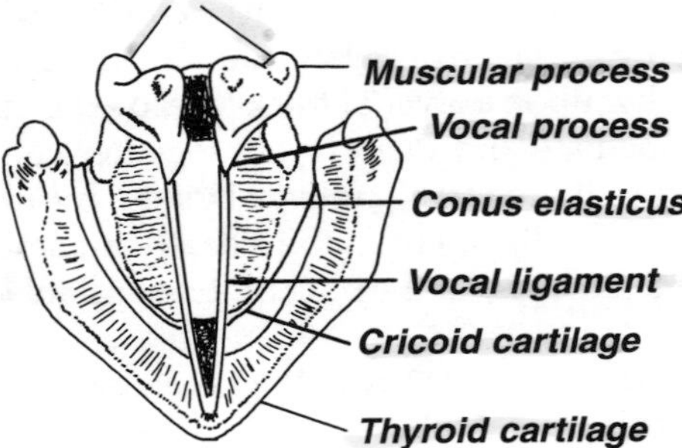

Figure 4–37. Superior view of the larynx illustrating relation of vocal ligament to arytenoid, cricoid, and thyroid cartilages.

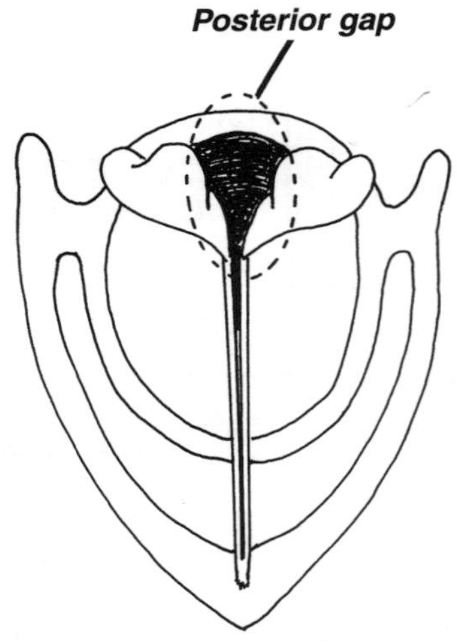

Figure 4–38. The posterior glottal gap.

likely as young women to demonstrate a posterior glottal gap. The elderly subjects in Linville's study were more likely to have an anterior gap or a spindle-shaped gap. Bloedel (1994) reported that both women and prepubescent boys had breathier vowels than men, perhaps because the women and youth have larynges of similar size and a similar ratio of membranous to cartilaginous portions of the vocal folds.

The Intrinsic Muscles of the Larynx

The intrinsic muscles are muscles having both attachments (origin and insertion) within the larynx, itself. They are illustrated in Figure 4–39. Table 4–3 gives details on these muscles, including the origin, insertion, action, and comments. The general function of these muscles is to abduct (open) or adduct (close) the folds, but they also affect vocal fold length and tension. The intrinsic muscles play roles in respiration, swallowing, and vocalization. Although the emphasis in this book is on the last of these, it should be remembered that the intrinsic muscles have functions with critical survival value. As a group, the intrinsic muscles are well adapted to their crucial functions (Malmgren & Gacek, 1992). First, the fibers of these muscles have an abundant supply of **mitochondria**, the energy packets of cells. Second, the muscles are characterized by high rates of oxidative enzyme processes, which reflect their brisk metabolic activity. Third, they possess very high densities of surface capillaries (blood vessels) to support the high metabolic rates. These three properties indicate that the intrinsic muscles have ample capability for high metabolic activity. These muscles are made for quick actions.

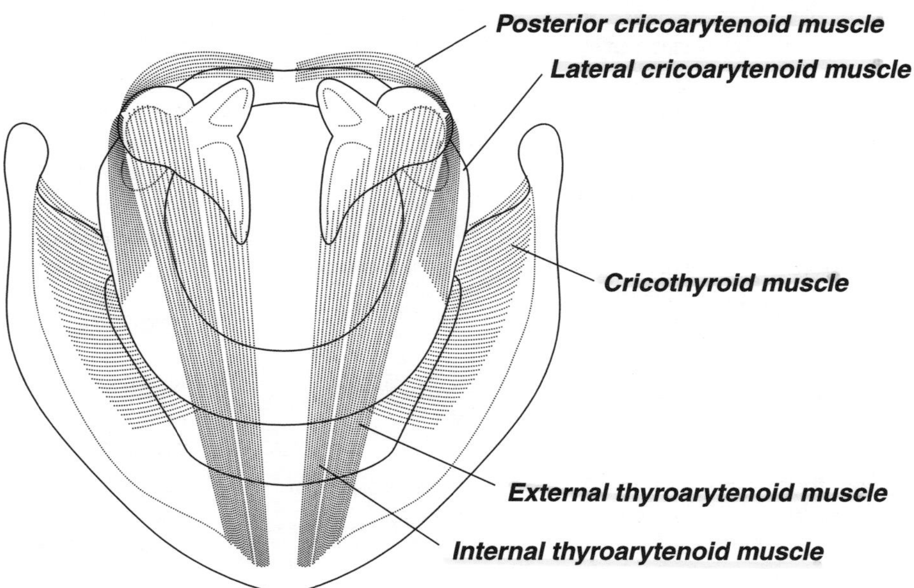

Figure 4–39. Intrinsic muscles of the larynx visible in a superior view.

Table 4–3. Origin, insertion, and primary action of the intrinsic muscles of the larynx.

Muscle	Origin	Insertion	Action
Cricothyroid	Arch of cricoid (antero-lateral aspect)	Inferior cornu and caudal margin of thyroid	Pulls thyroid forward and elevates arch of cricoid; regulates vocal pitch by tensing or lengthening vocal folds
Thyroarytenoid	Angle of thyroid	Vocal processes of arytenoid	Pulls arytenoid forward and rotates it
Vocalis	Angle of thyroid	Vocal processes of arytenoid	Regulates contraction of vocal folds; tensor of folds
Thyroepiglottic	Angle of thyroid	Aryepiglottic fold	Depresses epiglottis and closes entrance to larynx
Posterior crico-arytenoid	Posterior surface of cricoid	Muscular process of arytenoid	Opens and tenses vocal folds; only abductor in larynx
Lateral crico-arytenoid	Superior border of arch of cricoid	Muscular process of arytenoid	Closes, tenses vocal folds; adductor
Transverse arytenoid	Postero-lateral margin of arytenoid	Same region on contralateral member	Approximates arytenoids; adductor
Oblique arytenoid	Posterior surface and lateral margin of arytenoid	Apex of contra-lateral member	Draws apices of arytenoids together; adductor
Aryepiglottic	Apex of arytenoid	Aryepiglottic fold	Assists in closure of epiglottis
Superior thyro-arytenoid	Angle of thyroid	Vocal process of arytenoid	Assists in shortening and reducing tension on vocal folds

Selected muscle actions are shown schematically in Figure 4–40. The principal abductor is the **posterior cricoarytenoid** muscle (also shown in Figure 4–41), which opens the airway for ventilation. This muscle has a moderately fast contraction time of about 30 ms and is the only intrinsic muscle innervated by the **superior laryngeal nerve**, a branch of cranial nerve X (to be discussed in Chapter 7). The **lateral cricoarytenoid** muscle is a major adductor and as such is the antagonist of the posterior cricoarytenoid. It has two primary functions: It adducts the vocal folds and creates a **medial compression force**. In other words, this muscle not only approximates the folds, but it also helps to keep the folds tightly squeezed together. This muscle has a fast contraction time of about 15 ms. Its speed is important in reflexive adduction

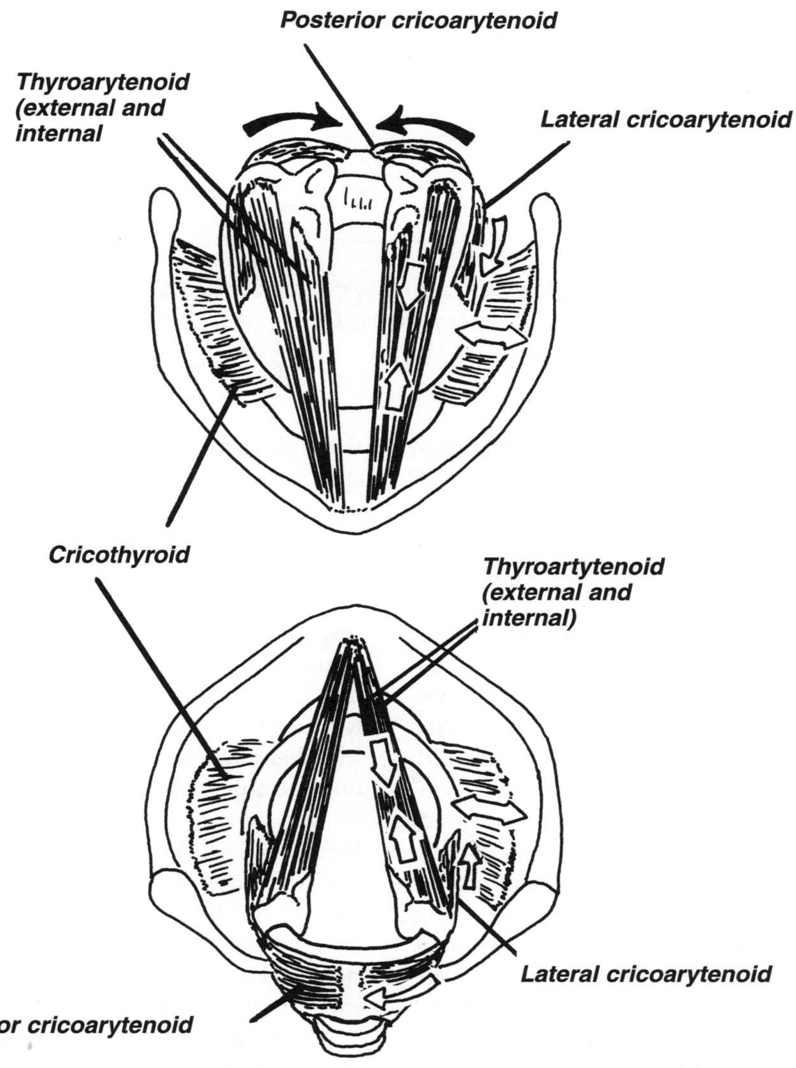

Figure 4–40. The actions of selected intrinsic muscles of the larynx. The arrows indicate muscle actions.

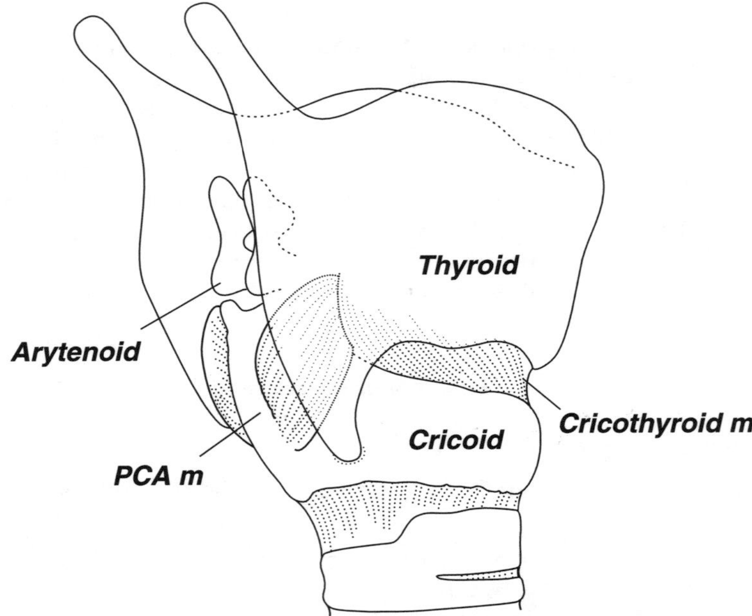

Figure 4–41. Posterolateral view of larynx, showing cricothyroid and posterior cricoarytenoid (PCA) muscles.

of the larynx to prevent entry of foreign particles. The **thyroarytenoid** muscle runs from the angle of the thyroid cartilage to the vocal processes of the arytenoid cartilage. Its course parallels that of the true vocal fold, ventricle, and false vocal fold. This muscle can be divided into two parts, the thyroarytenoid proper (lateral part) and the **vocalis** (also called the **thyrovocalis**) muscle (medial part). The vocalis muscle forms the bulk of the vocal fold. The **cricothyroid** muscle adjusts the relationship between the cricoid and thyroid cartilage and, in so doing, affects the foundation of the arytenoids and therefore the length and tension of the vocal folds. This muscle is used in speech and song to adjust vocal pitch. The cricothyroid has two primary divisions: the pars recta and the pars oblique. These are shown in the photograph of Figure 4–42, which is is an anterior view of the larynx and the trachea. Other structures that can be seen in this figure are the thyroid cartilage, cricoid cartilage, and epiglottis. The **oblique line** of the thyroid cartilage is the point of attachment for two muscles discussed in a following section.

The two **interarytenoid muscles** are the **transverse arytenoid** and the **oblique arytenoid** muscles (Figure 4–43). They adjust the relationship between the two arytenoids, with the transverse muscle drawing them together near midline and the oblique muscle tipping the arytenoid apexes toward one another. The transverse arytenoid muscle helps to adduct the vocal folds. The oblique arytenoid serves both to adduct the folds and to promote medial compression. The **aryepiglottic** muscle helps to close the epiglottis and is therefore important in airway protection during swallowing and other activities. The cuneiform cartilage mentioned briefly earlier in the chapter is embedded in tissues associated with this muscle.

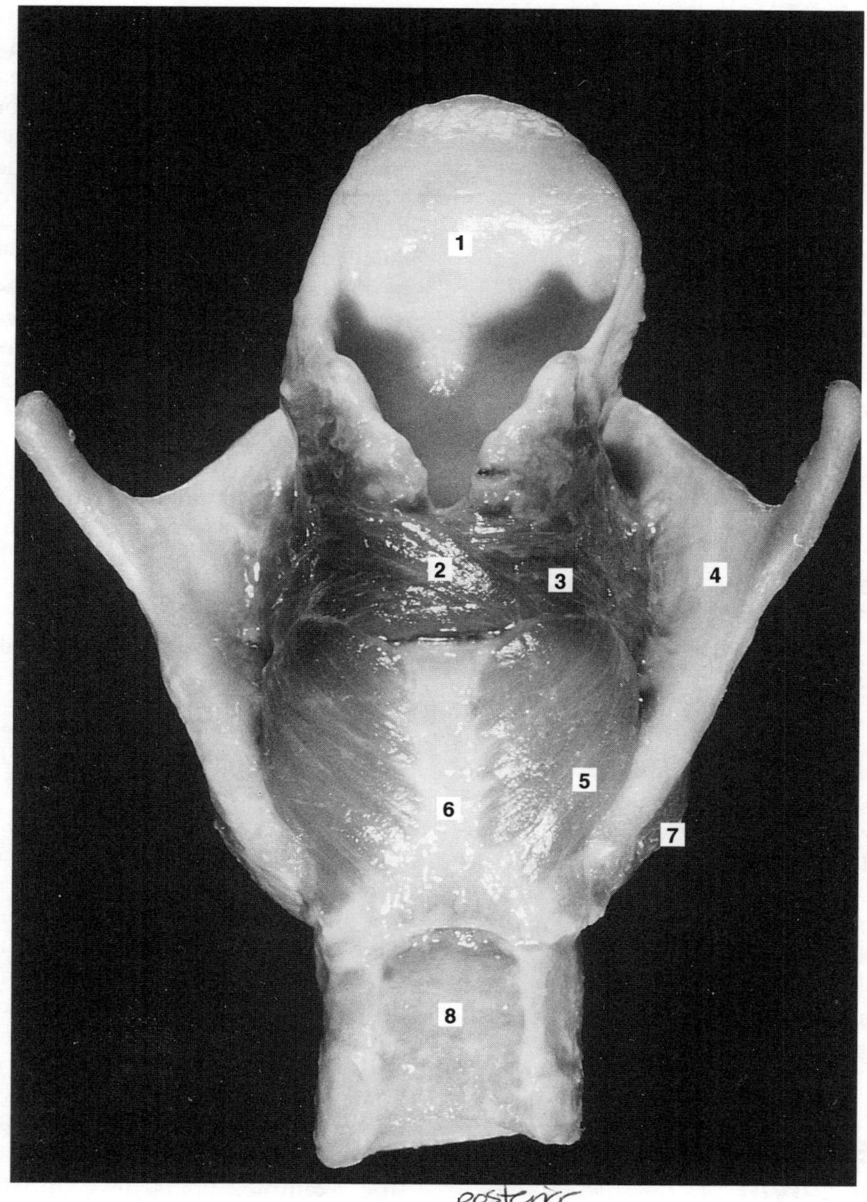

Figure 4–42. A photograph of an anterior view of the larynx and cricothyroid muscle. 1 = epiglottis, 2 = thyroid cartilage, 3 = oblique line, 4 = portion of median cricothyroid ligament, 5 = arch of cricoid cartilage, 6 = pars recta of cricothyroid muscle, 7 = pars oblique of cricothyroid muscle, and 8 = trachea. (Dissection by Joel C. Kahane; photograph courtesy of Joel C. Kahane.)

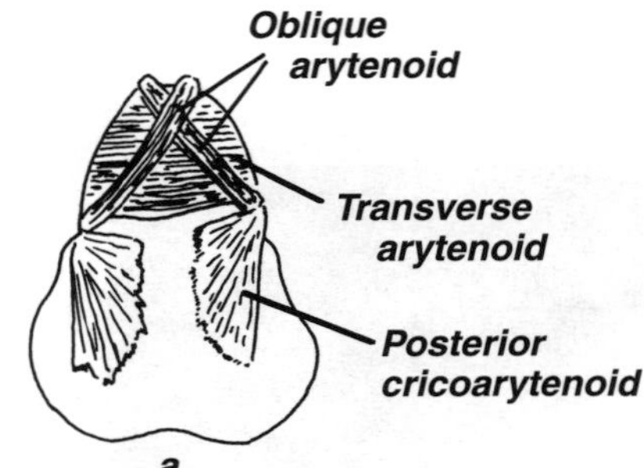

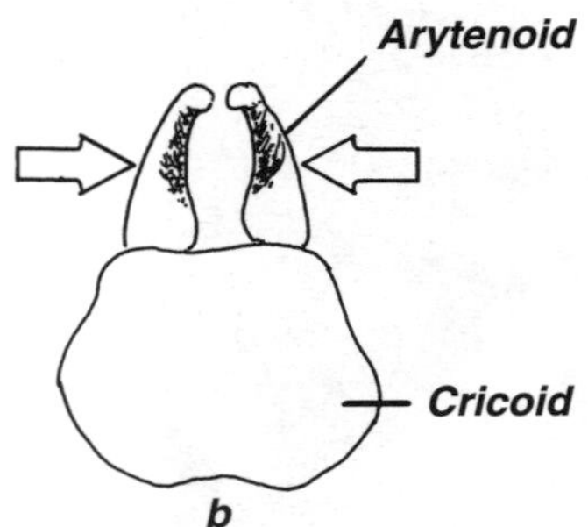

Figure 4-43. a. The interarytenoid muscles; **b.** arytenoid and cricoid cartilages, with arrows showing adduction of the arytenoids.

Several of the intrinsic muscles of the larynx are shown in the photograph of Figure 4–44, which is a posterior view of the larynx. Muscles visible in this photograph are the oblique arytenoid, transverse arytenoid, posterior cricoarytenoid, and the pars oblique portion of the cricothyroid. This photograph also shows the relationship among the epiglottis, thryoid cartilage, cricoid cartilage, and trachea.

The Extrinsic Muscles of the Larynx

The extrinsic muscles are muscles having one attachment on laryngeal structures and the other attachment on another structure external to the larynx. Table 4–4 summarizes the extrinsic muscles with respect to attachments, origin, and specific comments. The extrinsic muscles can be divided into **suprahyoid** and **infrahyoid** sets, depending on whether their external attachment is superior or inferior to the hyoid (Figure 4–45). The suprahyoid muscles are the **stylohyoid, digastric, mylohyoid,** and **geniohyoid**. Because these muscles have an origin that is superior or antero-superior to the hyoid and insert on the hyoid bone, their contraction has the general consequence of elevating the laryngeal framework or drawing it forward. These muscles are detailed in Chapter 5, because they participate in movements of the tongue and jaw. The infrahyoid muscles are the **sternohyoid, sternothyroid, thyrohyoid,** and **omohyoid**. These muscles have an origin that is inferior to the hyoid and insert on the hyoid bone or the thyroid cartilage. Their contraction generally depresses the laryngeal framework. Within its attachments, the larynx, then, can move up and down, and forward and backward.

A more detailed description of the suprahyoid and infrahyoid muscles is in Table 4–4.

Laryngeal Function in Speech and Song

A simple but useful introduction to the control of phonation is to recognize two dimensions of laryngeal regulation (Kitzing & Lofqvist, 1982). The first is the longitudinal tension of the vocal folds. Adjustment of this dimension relates to regulation of fundamental frequency. The second is the abduction and adduction of the vocal folds. This dimension relates to the regulation of voicing (such as voiced-voiceless contrasts), aspiration (turbulence noise generated at the glottis), and voice quality (for example, hoarseness, breathiness, creakiness). Different languages make different uses of these regulatory mechanisms. Some languages use voice quality variations as a linguistic function. English does not. The following sections discuss these two dimensions of phonatory control in more detail, beginning with the question: How do the vocal folds vibrate?

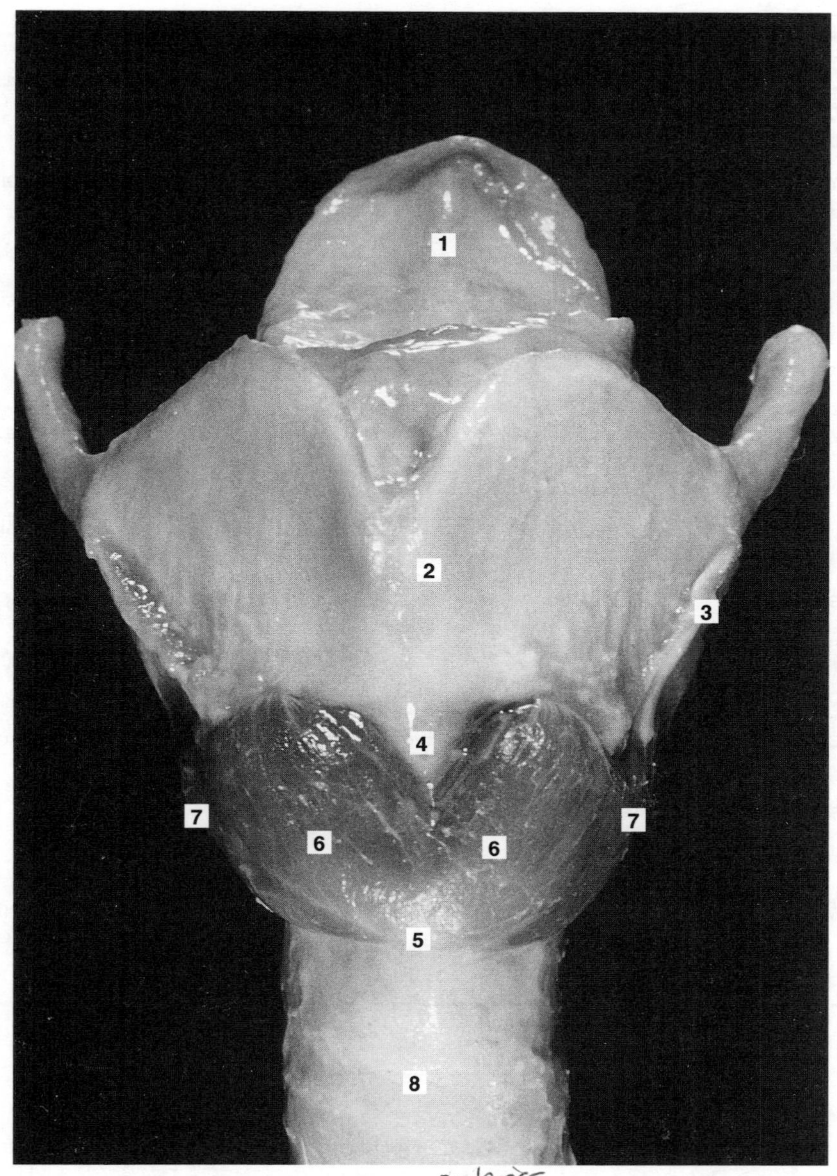

Figure 4–44. A photograph of a posterior view of the larynx and intrinsic laryngeal muscles. 1 = epiglottis, 2 = oblique arytenoid muscle, 3 = transverse arytenoid muscle, 4 = lamina of thyroid cartilage, 5 = posterior cricoarytenoid muscle, 6 = lamina of cricoid cartilage, 7 = pars oblique portion of cricothyroid muscle, and 8 = trachea. (Dissection by Joel C. Kahane; photograph courtesy of Joel C. Kahane.)

Table 4–4. Origin, insertion, and primary action of the intrinsic muscles of the larynx.

Muscle	Origin	Insertion	Action
Suprahyoid muscles			
Anterior belly of digastric	Temporal bone and mandible	Attaches to hyoid by means of a central tendon	Elevates hyoid or assists in depressing mandible
Posterior belly of digastric	Temporal bone and mandible	Attaches to hyoid by means of a central tendon	Elevates hyoid or assists in depressing mandible
Stylohyoid	Styloid process of temporal bone	Body of hyoid	Pulls hyoid up and back
Mylohyoid	Mandible	Body of hyoid	Elevates hyoid and tongue
Geniohyoid	Mandible	Body of hyoid	Pulls hyoid up and back
Infrahyoid muscles			
Sternohyoid	Clavicle and sternum	Hyoid bone	Pulls hyoid down
Sternothyroid	Sternum and cartilages of first two ribs	Thyroid cartilage	Depresses thyroid
Thyrohyoid	Thyroid cartilage	Hyoid bone	Pulls hyoid down draws thyroid up
Omohyoid	Scapula	Hyoid bone	Draws hyoid down

"The ability to look at the voice in action was a mystery first solved by Manuel Garcia in 1854. At Place de l'Odeon in Paris, in a cottage that belonged to his sister, a Diva,

Manuel Garcia had the idea to look at the vocal folds by a complex mirror system using sunlight. It was the birth of laryngology [the medical specialty that deals with diseases of the larynx]."

(J. Abitbol, *Atlas of Laser Voice Surgery*. San Diego: Singular Publishing Group, 1995, p. 78.)

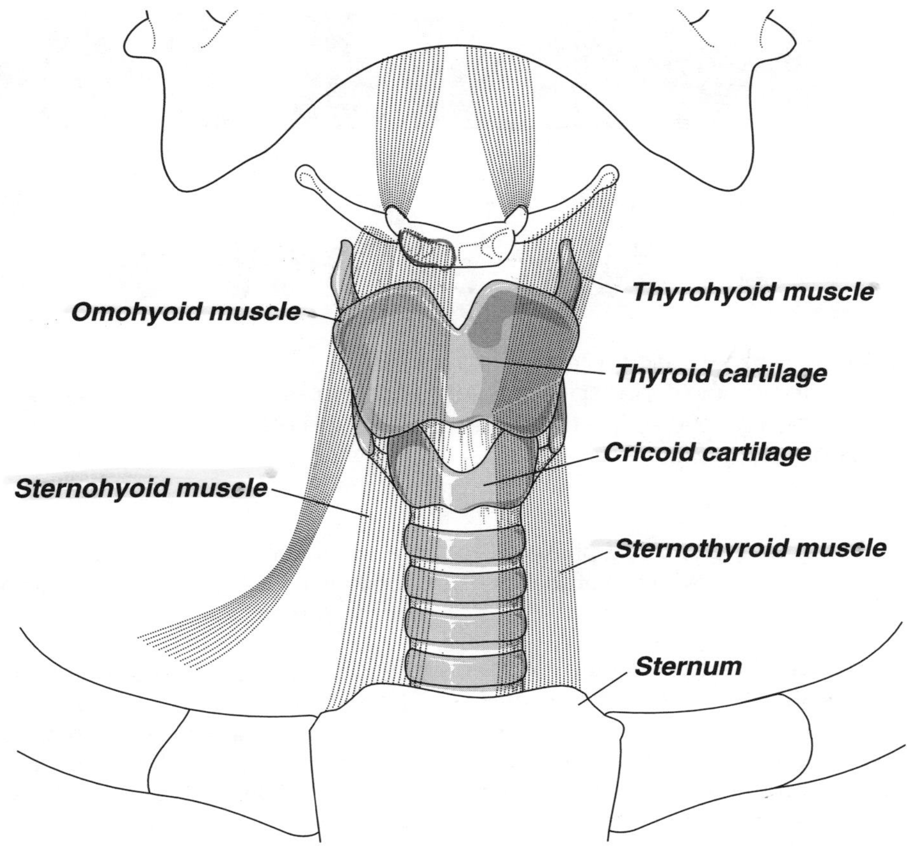

Figure 4–45. The extrinsic (infrahyoid) muscles of the larynx.

Vocal Fold Vibration

Vocal fold vibration is essentially a self-sustaining oscillation with two major factors. The first factor is the development of a mucosal traveling wave and its interaction with the airflow through the glottis (Berke & Gerratt, 1993; Scherer, 1995; Titze, 1994). This traveling wave, or **surface wave**, is evident as an inferior-to-superior movement of the mucosa. It is depicted in Figure 4–46, which shows two ways of viewing one cycle of vocal fold vibration. Because it is difficult to represent the complexity of vocal fold motion in a single illustration, one approach is to show the vocal folds in both coronal and superior perspectives (Childers & Krishnamurthy, 1985; Hirano, 1981; Schonharl, 1960). This kind of illustration captures at least some of the three-dimensional character of the action of the vocal folds. The upper part of Figure 4–46 shows a coronal section, and the lower part shows a superior view. In the lower part of the figure, the folds are represented schematically as two bands, one above the other. The upper band represents the superior margin of the fold, and the lower band represents the inferior margin. Notice that the superior and inferior margins of the folds move in a somewhat different manner. This is called the **vertical phase difference.** When the vocal folds are blown apart, the inferior margins separate before the superior margins. When the folds come together, the inferior margins precede the

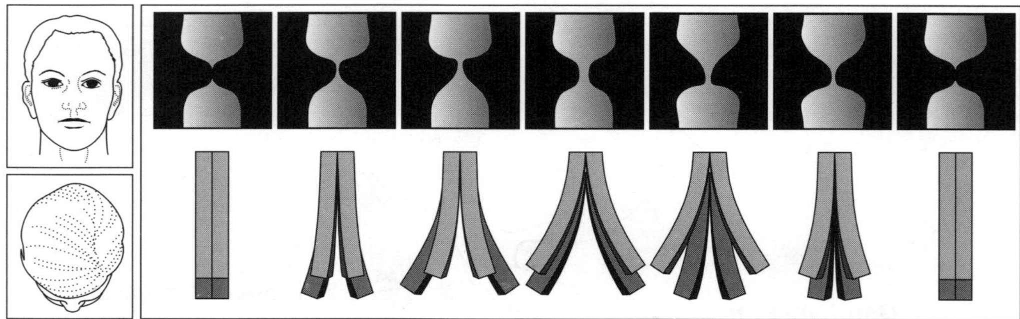

Figure 4–46. A schematic representation of the traveling wave seen during vocal fold motion. The series at the top represents a coronal section through the folds. The series at the bottom shows the relative motions of the upper and lower margins of the folds, from a superior view.

superior margins. This vertical phase difference is the primary evidence of the surface wave of vocal fold vibration.

The second factor in self-sustaining oscillation is the creation of alternating pressures within the glottis that separate the folds and then bring them together again. These pressures are ordinarily developed by the respiratory system. As a person begins to phonate, the following events occur:

1. Subglottal air pressure of suitable magnitude is developed. A minimum subglottal pressure, called the **phonatory threshold pressure** or **oscillation threshold pressure** is needed to set the vocal folds into vibration. Once the folds begin to vibrate, a slightly lower subglottal pressure will maintain the vibration. The phonatory threshold pressure varies somewhat with fundamental frequency, given that the tension of the vocal fold cover increases with increases in frequency. The threshold pressure ranges from about 3 cm H_2O (0.3 kPa) at low fundamental frequencies to about 6 cm H_2O (0.6 kPa) at high fundamental frequencies. (See Exercise 4–2). For lung pressures higher than the threshold pressure, energy transferred from the airflow to the vocal folds exceeds the energy lost by dissipation, helping to maintain oscillation. Excessive subglottal pressure can fail to initiate phonation or will cause an irregular phonatory pattern.

2. The vocal folds are placed in an appropriate adductory position and a suitable medial compression force is achieved. The adductory position of the vocal folds is illustrated in Color plate 2 at the back of this book. If the vocal folds are very tightly adducted, phonation is not likely because a very large subglottal pressure would be required to force them apart. Also, if the vocal folds are insufficiently adducted, phonation is not likely because the air from the trachea simply will escape through the glottis. The intrinsic muscles are particularly important in regulating vocal fold adduction and the appropriate medial compression force.

3. The subglottal air pressure pushes the vocal folds laterally and superiorly to initiate the first cycle of vibration. This event will occur following appropriate regulation of the events described in (1) and (2) above. To put it simply, the air pressure blows the folds apart.

4. Continuing cycles of vibration are sustained by the recoil forces of the vocal folds and aerodynamic forces developed below and within the glottis. It is in this sense that vocal fold vibration is self-sustaining. As noted, energy transfer between airflow and the vocal folds contributes to the self-sustaining oscillation.

A barn-door analogy is helpful in understanding these phenomena. Imagine a barn door connected by a spring to the door frame. A strong wind blows the door open, but the stretched spring then pulls it shut again. As this process is repeated, the door will swing open and closed, as the aerodynamic force provided by the wind is succeeded by the restoring force from the spring. Of course, the barn door is a rigid structure and therefore would not exhibit the vertical phase difference described earlier. Vocal fold vibration has a complexity that reflects the biomechanical properties of vocal fold tissue.

The Cover-Body Theory of Phonation

This theory posits that the vocal adjustments in speaking and singing are regulated by changing the mechanical properties of the different layers of tissue in the vocal folds (Hirano, 1974; Hirano & Kakita, 1985). As mentioned earlier, the vocal fold can be viewed from a mechanical perspective as having two primary layers, a cover layer near the surface of the fold and a body layer deeper in the fold. By contracting different laryngeal muscles, the talker or singer can change the relative stiffness of these two layers and thereby bring about different patterns of vocal fold vibration. For example, weak contractions of both the vocalis and cricothyroid muscles will cause a slackness of both the cover and body. The resulting phonation will be soft, with a low fundamental frequency. But if the vocalis muscle contracts vigorously while the cricothyroid activity is relatively weak, the body will become stiffer than the cover. This adjustment will result in a louder phonatory pattern produced at a medium fundamental frequency.

A simple but fairly effective model of the vocal folds is shown in Figure 4–47. The vocal folds are represented by two masses connected by a spring. The upper mass

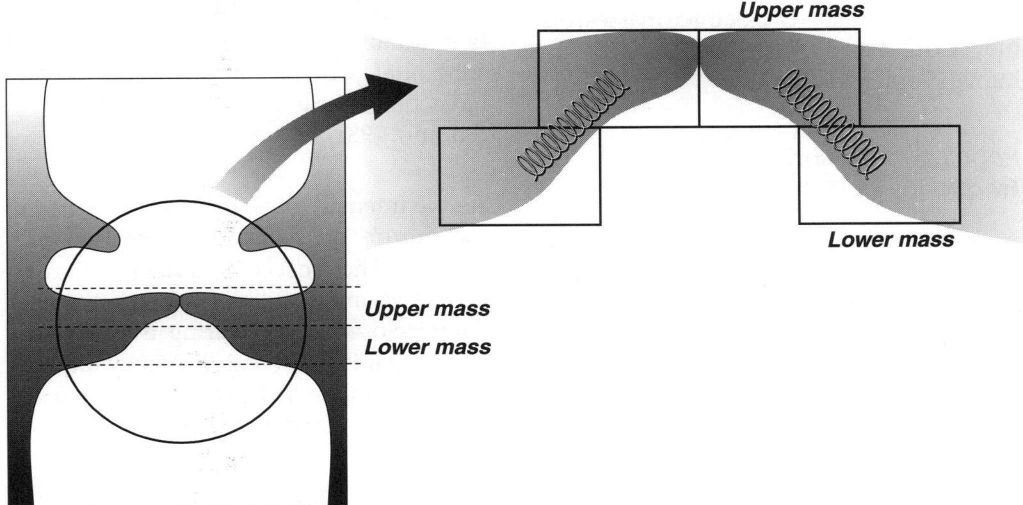

Figure 4–47. A simple two-mass model of the vocal folds. The upper and lower masses are connected by a spring.

corresponds to the portion of the vocal folds and the lower mass to the inferior portion. During vocal fold vibration, the two masses interact to produce a vibratory pattern that has both horizontal and vertical components. This two-mass model (Ishizaka & Flanagan, 1972; Ishizaka & Matsudaira, 1972) was introduced to show how aerodynamic forces generated by subglottal pressure and the flow of air through the glottis (Bernoulli forces) are sequenced with elastic forces in the vocal fold tissues to produce the continuous vibrations of the vocal folds. The two-mass model shown in Figure 4–47 can be compared with the schematic representation of vocal fold motion in Figure 4–46. A general property of the model is that one mass (the body) participates primarily in lateral motion, whereas the other mass (the cover) is responsible for the surface-wave behavior (the vertical phase difference described earlier). Storey and Titze (1995) modified this model by using two "cover" masses coupled laterally to a "body" mass. The behavior of their three-mass model resembled that of the actual vocal folds in several important respects. The work on two and three-mass models of the vocal folds is a good example of the design of models that are simple but effective. The models have low dimensionality (two or three masses) but they exhibit properties like those of the human vocal folds.

Regulation of Fundamental Frequency of Phonation

As noted earlier, longitudinal tension is regulated to control fundamental frequency. Adjustments of the laryngeal muscles influence the length and tension of the vocal folds. A general equation for a string model for frequency applies to vocal fundamental frequency:

Don't Know

$$f_0 = 1/2L\,(T/\rho)^{0.5}$$

where T is the tension of the vocal fold mucosal cover,

rho (ρ) is the density of the tissue, and

L is the length of the vibrating vocal folds.

An important implication of this equation is that, as vocal fold length increases, the increase in tension is greater than the length increase itself. Therefore, fundamental frequency is determined primarily by the tension of the vocal fold cover and not by vocal length per se.

Regulation of Intensity of Phonation

If fundamental frequency (or its primary perceptual correlate of vocal pitch) is related primarily to the tension of the vocal fold cover, then what determines vocal intensity (and its primary perceptual correlate of loudness)? The major determinant of vocal intensity is the subglottal pressure. As subglottal pressure increases, the nature of the airflow through the glottis changes to produce an increase in acoustic intensity. As noted earlier, the phonatory threshold pressure is about 3–6 kPa. The sound produced at this level of subglottal pressure is about 45–65 dB SPL. With increases in subglottal pressure above this minimum value, the acoustic intensity of the voice increases. Subglottal pressure in conversation usually stays below 10 cm H_20, but subglottal pressures of up to 50 cm H_20 have been measured in loud phonation (Hirano, 1981).

As the intensity of phonation is increased, the nature of vocal fold vibration also changes. The most consistent effects are an increased amplitude of vibration and a longer closed phase during the vibratory cycle. That is, the vocal folds stay together longer and then swing apart more widely. This effect is illustrated in Figure 4–48.

Women's voices, because of their higher harmonics, generally can produce more intense sounds than males' voices. However, the *Guinness Book of World Records* (Russell,

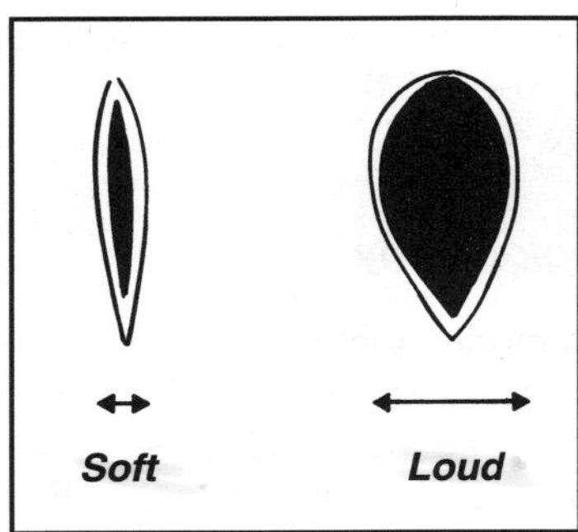

Figure 4–48. Schematic illustration of vocal fold motion during two different levels of vocal intensity.

1987) cites two men for record-breaking accomplishments in vocal intensity. The Annual World Shouting contest was won by Anthony Fieldhouse on September 9, 1984, at Scarborough, England, with a call that was registered at 112.4 dBA. The *Guinness Book* acknowledges Neil Stephenson of Newcastle-upon-Tyne, England, with the "highest scientifically measured emission" of 123.2 dBA for a scream produced on May 18, 1985. The isle of England seems to be the home of stentorian efforts, or perhaps the English are just especially inclined to measure how loud they can shout and scream. For ordinary people who do not set records for intensity, even loud vocal efforts carry little farther than 200 yards or so on a quiet day. This limitation is not entirely unfortunate. If voices were louder, we would overhear more arguments than we do now and would have much greater levels of background noise from other people's conversations. It is often a blessing that voices do not carry further than they do.

Other Laryngeal Functions

The discussion to this point has pertained to phonation, or laryngeal vibration, with a particular emphasis on the frequency of vibration. However, the larynx does more in speech and song than vibrate. At various times, vibrations cease and the vocal folds abduct, as during inspiration, silent pauses, whispering, and voiceless consonants. At other times, the vocal folds join together with considerable medial compression to make a firm aerodynamic seal. This situation happens especially during strenuous exercises or forceful efforts, such as heavy lifting, childbirth, or defecation. To account for these laryngeal actions, additional concepts are needed. In the main, these concepts relate to the second basic dimension of the laryngeal control of phonation, namely, the control of abduction and adduction of the vocal folds.

In the production of voiceless consonants, vibration of the vocal folds is interrupted by an action that has been called the **laryngeal devoicing gesture**. This gesture has a fairly stereotypic appearance across a variety of contexts. First, it has been reported that there is a close temporal relationship between this laryngeal gesture and movements of the articulators of the upper airway. For example, to make a [p] as in *pay*, the talker produces a laryngeal devoicing gesture carefully timed so that the maximum laryngeal abduction coincides with the beginning of the release of the bilabial closure (Lofqvist & Yoshioka, 1981).

When a person lifts a heavy object, he or she is likely to grunt. The grunt is produced with adducted vocal folds. If the folds were not adducted, it would be impossible to make a grunting noise. You might try this simple experiment: Imagine that you are about to lift an extremely heavy object. Bend over and do what you would naturally do just before you expend your effort to make the lift. Can you sense that you take in a deep breath and adduct your vocal folds? Firm adduction of the folds helps to make the thoracic and abdominal cavities rigid, thereby providing support for the action of heavy lifting. A second example of the importance of vocal fold adduction for forceful actions is in childbirth.

Instructors of the **Lamaze** method teach the expectant mother and her "coach" to control pushing and blowing. Pushing is the means by which the baby is forced through the vaginal canal. To push, the mother-to-be closes her vocal folds so that the thoracic-abdominal cavity is rigid. Blowing is used to expend energy without pushing the baby. The right timing of pushing and blowing is a major objective in this approach to childbirth.

This principle has clinical implications for speech and voice. For example, if a person (say a 60-year-old man with Parkinson's disease) has a very weak voice related to insufficient medial compression of the vocal folds, the clinician might ask the man to phonate while using his arms to lift himself up from a chair. The lifting action usually will be accompanied by increased medial compression of the vocal folds. Therefore, it often happens that the voice becomes stronger during the lifting maneuver. With training, this principle can be carried over to routine phonation for speech.

The Glottogram

The study of the voice in both health and disease relies on knowledge of the vibratory pattern. Therefore, it is important to have techniques that permit an analysis of this pattern. The **glottogram** is a graph of the laryngeal (voice source) waveform. The general procedure to produce a glottogram is to record the time-varying area of the glottis, as might be obtained from looking down upon the vocal folds and graphing the area of visible glottal opening over time. As the vocal folds vibrate, the glottis alternately opens and closes. These motions result in a roughly triangular-shaped wave, with the baseline representing closure and the peak representing maximal opening (Figure 4–49). The graph is called an **area glottogram**. There are various laboratory techniques to create this graph or a similar representation of vocal activity. For the purposes of this chapter, five general ways are covered.

Cinematography

This is a motion picture technique in which pictures are taken of the vibrating vocal folds. The rate at which the pictures are taken must be much faster than the usual rate used to make commercial motion pictures, which is 24 frames per second. To capture the events in vocal fold vibration, a high-speed camera is used. The resulting pictures can be analyzed to measure the glottal area. Although this is a relatively direct way to determine vocal fold activity, it is rather expensive and tedious. Cinematography is historically important because it was one of the earliest methods used to understand vocal fold vibration (Moore, 1938). The use of this technique led to significant progress in the first half of the 20th century.

Stroboscopy

The general idea of **stroboscopy** is to take pictures of an event in synchrony with a flashing light. If the pictures are taken at a rate that approximates, but is not identical to, the frequency of vibration of an object, the result is a kind of slow-motion analysis. It is important to note that the pictures are timed so that perhaps only one picture is taken for each cycle of vibration. Practically speaking, this method uses stroboscopic light to obtain sampled images of the vocal folds. If vocal fold vibration is reasonably periodic, the sampled images can be projected to show a slow-motion picture of the vocal folds. What appears to be a single cycle of vibration is in fact a product of many cycles. Successful stroboscopy usually requires that the subject being examined opens the mouth widely, extends the tongue, and tolerates a laryngeal mirror (or

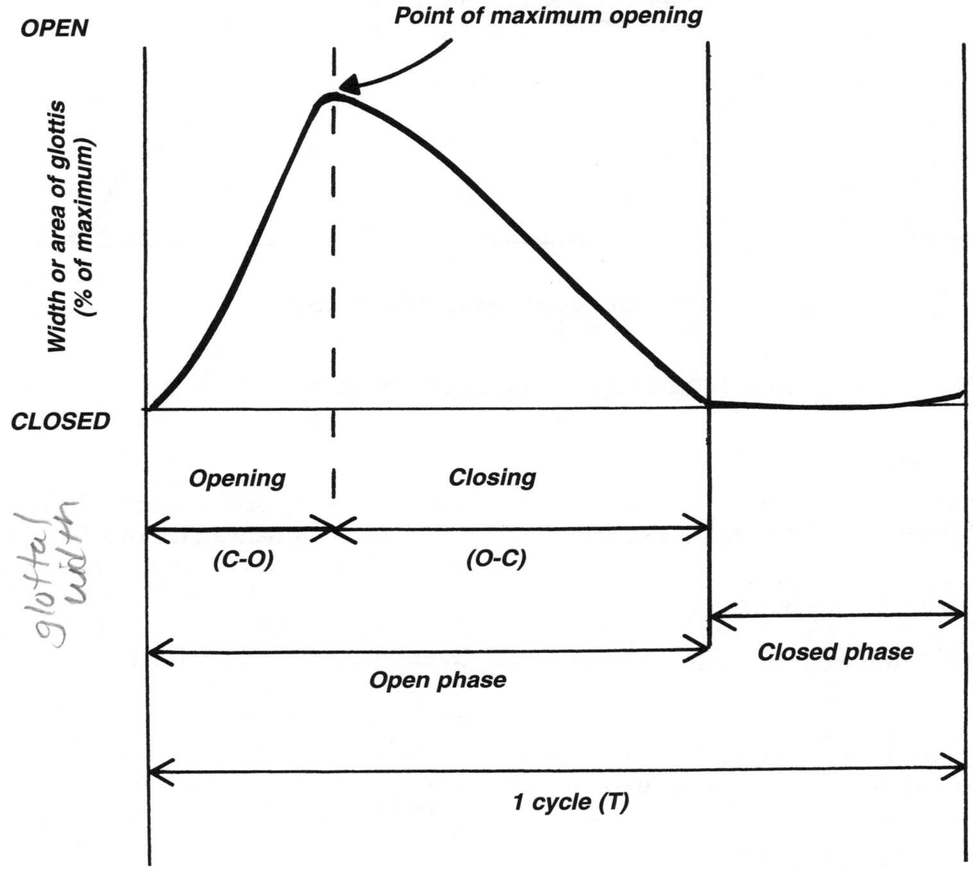

Figure 4–49. The glottal area waveform, or glottogram. Commonly used measurement intervals are shown.

fiberoptic device) positioned for viewing of the vocal folds. Not every subject finds this a comfortable position. Analysis can be tedious, although methods are being developed to reduce the labor involved. An example of stroboscopic images of vocal fold vibration is shown in a color photograph at the end of the book (Color plate 5).

Electroglottography (EEG)

The third way of obtaining the glottogram is to record the signal from two electrodes placed on either side of the neck, overlying the wings of the thyroid cartilage. As the vocal folds open and close during vibration, the signal recorded from the electrodes changes in intensity. The signal reflects changes in the contact area of the vocal folds. This technique, called **electroglottography** (EGG), is noninvasive, so there is little problem with intolerance by the subject. A schematic example of an EGG waveform is shown in Figure 4–50. The technique has some limitations in how well it records vocal fold movements. It is quite good at registering the closure of the vocal folds, but not so good an an index of other features of vibration. A par-

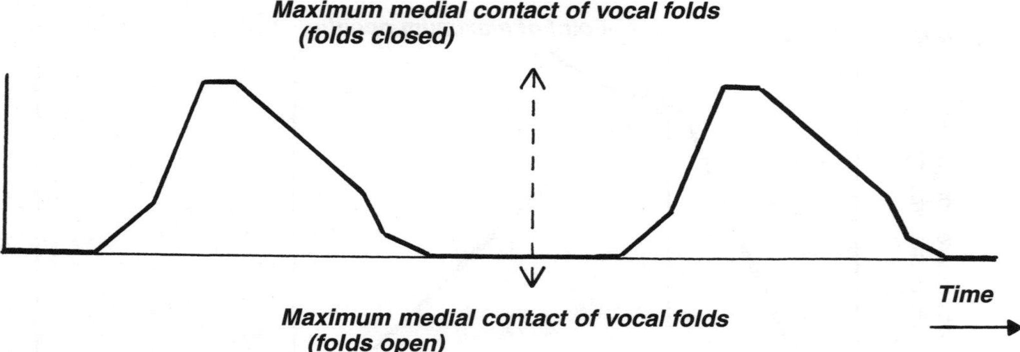

Figure 4–50. The electroglottogram (EGG) signal representing vocal fold motion.

ticularly good discussion of the EGG is found in Childers and Krishnamurthy (1985).

Photoglottography (PGG)

In the fourth method, variations in light intensity are used to monitor vocal fold activity. **Photoglottography** uses a light source on one side of the vocal folds and a **photosensor** on the opposite side. As the folds vibrate, the intensity of the light picked up by the photosensor varies as the vocal folds open and close.

Inverse Filtering 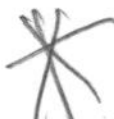

An *inverse* operation is one that is opposite in order or effect. Basically, **inverse filtering** is the opposite of the way in which speech is normally produced. The normal process is conceptualized as the **source-filter** theory of speech production. This theory states that the acoustic energy produced by the vibrating vocal folds is filtered by the pharyngeal, oral, and nasal cavities (which comprise the vocal tract). Speech production therefore has two major components, the source (vibrating vocal folds) and the filter (the supralaryngeal cavities, or vocal tract). The acoustic output is a combination of source and filter. This theory is discussed in more detail in Chapter 9. If the filter characteristics are known, then it should be possible to obtain the source function by an inverse operation, namely, remove the effects of the filtering. This is the basic idea of inverse filtering. For best results, it is usually accomplished with the use of a special mask (Rothenberg, 1973). The airflow recorded in this procedure is proportional to glottal opening. The larger the glottal opening, the greater the airflow. Of course, when the glottis is closed, there is no airflow. Therefore, the flow glottogram resembles the area glottogram obtained from the other methods previously described.

It is possible to use two or more techniques to study vocal fold motion. Figure 4–51 shows the relations among stroboscopy, EEG, and PGG in the study of vocal fold motion in a dog. The points labeled on the EEG and PGG waveforms correspond to the labeled stroboscope photographs.

Features of the Glottogram

The glottogram is a particularly useful graph to understand vocal fold vibration in relation to different voice types. Certain measurements derived from the glottogram serve this purpose (Figure 4–50). One such measure is the **duty cycle** or **open quotient**, which is the proportion of a vibratory cycle that the vocal folds are open. It is during the open phase that the folds are "on duty," that is, producing sound. Duty cycle tends

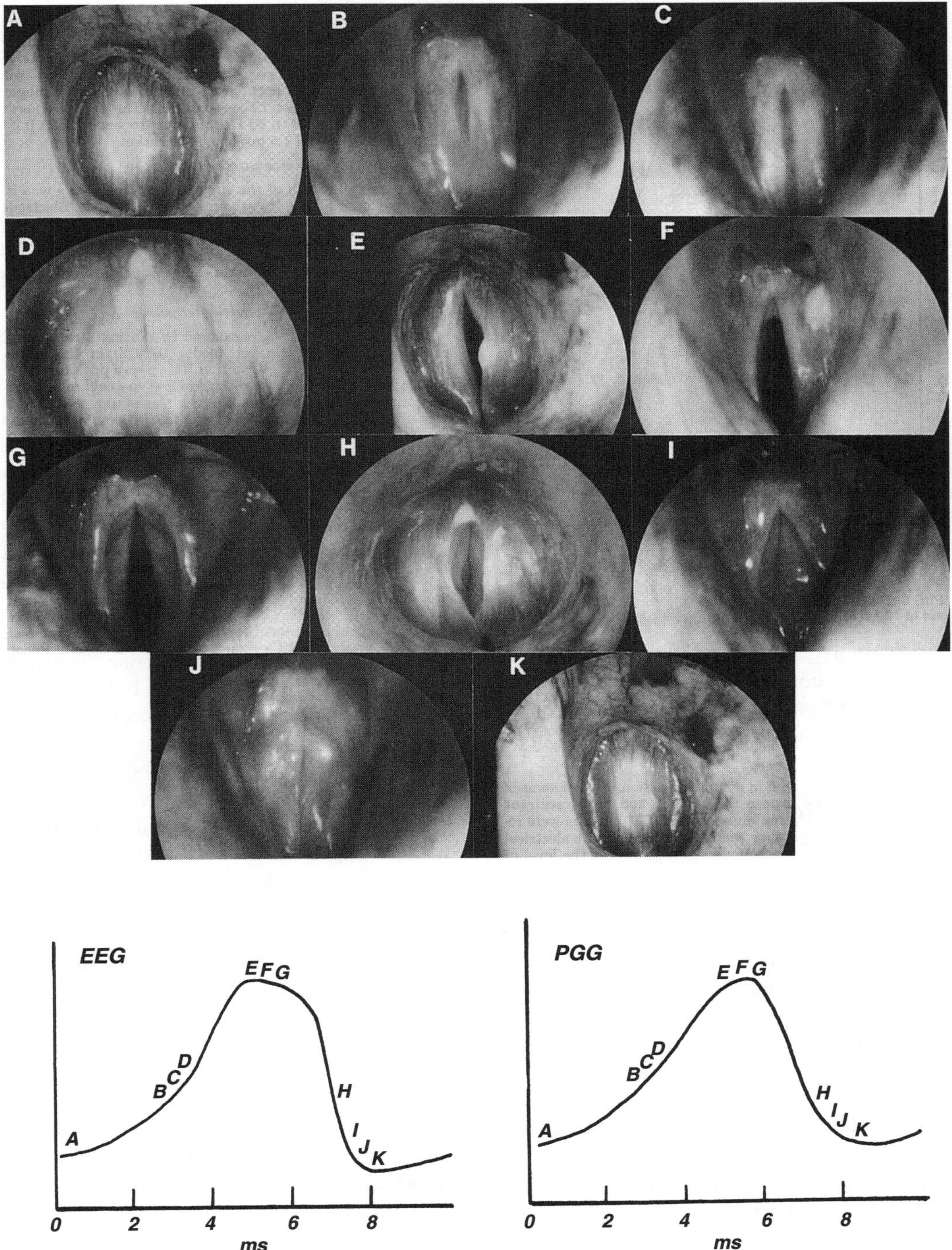

Figure 4–51. Combined stroboscopic, EEG, and PGG recordings of vocal fold motion in a dog. (Reprinted from "Laryngeal modeling: Theoretical, in vitro, in vivo." by G. S. Berke, D. M. Moore, D. G. Hanson, D. R. Hantke, B. R. Gerratt, & F. Burstein, 1987, *Laryngoscope, 97*, 1987, p. 875. Copyright 1987 by *Laryngoscope*. Reprinted with permission.)

to decrease with increases in vocal intensity, meaning that the folds stay closed for a longer time during the vibratory cycle. The **speed quotient** is a measure of the symmetry of the opening and closing portions of the open phase. It is calculated as

Speed quotient = (C – O) / (O – C),

where (C – O) and (O – C) are measured as in Figure 4–44.

The **speed index** is another measure of symmetry of the opening and closing phases. It is calculated as

Speed index = ([(C – O) – (O – C)] / [(C – O) + (O – C)].

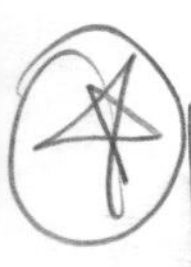

Another important measure that can be derived from the glottogram is the slope of the closing phase. This phase is particularly important in determining acoustic characteristics of the voice. The greater the slope of the closing phase, the greater the energy in the higher harmonics of the voice.

briefly look over

A Brief Review of the History of Voice Science

The following is a capsule of voice science history. It summarizes major progress in the understanding of laryngeal function in speech and song.

Claudius Galen, the famous Greek anatomist of the second and third century, first identified the larynx as the instrument of voice. He also described the three major cartilages and the paired muscles. The great Leonardo Da Vinci turned his attention to the vocal organ and included several drawings of the larynx in his textbook *Quaderni d'Anatomica* published in 1500. A few years later, Andreas Vesalius corrected some errors in Galen's work, noting, for example, that there are two arytenoids rather than one. At about the same time, Gabrielle Fallopio introduced the term "cricoid" for the cartilage now known by that name, and Caspar Bauhinus provided an accurate description of the three pairs of extrinsic muscles and the five pairs of intrinsic muscles, which he also named. In the 18th century, Giovanni Battista Morgagni described laryngeal anatomy in greater detail and also noted pathologic changes in the larynx related to voice disorders. The ventricle of Morgagni is named after him. In 1839, Johannes Muller introduced the **myoelastic** (or **myoelastic-aerodynamic**) theory of phonation, based on the concept that air from the lungs is the active element in voice production, causing vibration of the essentially passive vocal folds. Modifications to this theory were offered by a number of scientists, but one of the most influential descriptions was published in 1958 by van den Berg (who is sometimes credited as the originator of the myoelastic-aerodynamic theory). In 1950, Raoul Husson proposed an alternative theory, the **neurochronaxic theory**. Husson believed that a nerve impulse from the brain initiated each cycle of vocal fold vibration. Therefore, faster impulses would be required as vocal fundamental frequency increased. Husson's theory was not confirmed by experiments, leaving the myoelastic-aerodynamic theory as the most generally accepted account of vocal fold vibration. This theory has been validated by experiments on human vocal folds and by work with models such as the two- and three-mass models discussed earlier in this chapter. One major direction of current work is on the fluid mechanics of vocal fold vibration.

Contemporary issues in the study of laryngeal function include fractal and chaotic models (the concepts of fractals and chaos are introduced in Chapter 2). Baken (1990) used fractal analysis to model the irregularities in the period and amplitude of the glottal waveform. Chaos models were used by Steinecke and Herzel (1995) and by Herzel, Berry, Titze, and Saleh (1994). In the Herzel et al. paper, voice qualities such as hoarseness, creaky voice, and vocal fry were associated with patterns of chaotic behavior. Specific mechanisms were proposed for some vocal pathologies:

1. A desynchronized motion of the left and right vocal folds was hypothesized for localized lesions (e.g., a nodule or small mass on the vocal folds) and unilateral paralysis (a paralysis of the vocal fold on one side). The two folds fail to move in a comparable time relationship.

2. A desynchronization of both the horizontal and vertical modes of vibration was associated with vocal fry (a low-pitched, irregular voice quality).

3. Interaction between the true and false vocal folds was suspected for a voice quality known as pressed voice. Typically, the false folds are not approximated in voice production.

4. An interaction of vocal fold oscillations with vortices and resonances generated in the glottal region also was considered as a factor in some pathologies. That is, the pattern of vocal fold vibration can be affected by conditions surrounding the vocal folds.

A detailed discussion of these new concepts of vocal function is outside the scope of this introductory text. But it is important to note that the understanding of vocal fold vibration is being influenced by the new science of chaos theory. This is an example of how progress in physics and applied mathematics can have far-reaching implications in the study of physiology and behavior.

Life Course Issues 

In the newborn and the infant, for the first few months of life, the larynx is situated relatively high in the neck close to the hyoid bone (Figure 4–52). This high position protects the airway and enables the infant to take food and to breathe virtually simultaneously. This anatomic arrangement can be life-preserving, because it reduces the risk of choking. The larynx descends at around 4 to 6 months and grows rapidly during the first 18 months of life. Also during this interval, the laryngeal cartilages and related tissues become softer and less pliable (Tucker & Tucker, 1979). According to descriptions by Kahane (1978, 1982), the laryngeal cartilages increase in size while retaining their basic shape, with the exception of the anterior aspect of the male thyroid cartilage.

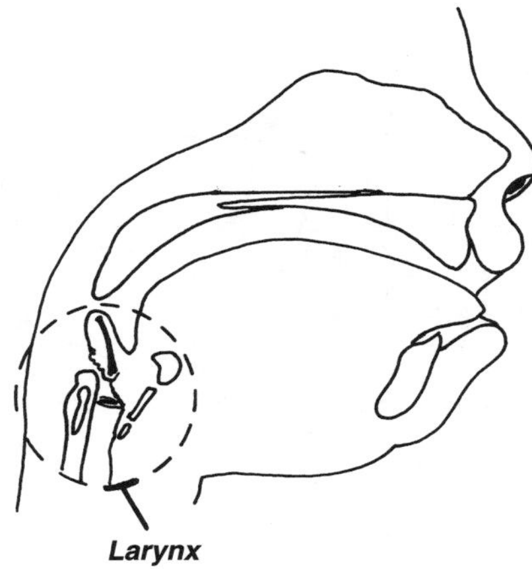

Figure 4–52. Position of the larynx in a newborn.

The thickness of both the vocal folds and the membranous portion of the glottis (the space between the vocal folds) is proportionately larger in the infant than the adult, as shown in Figure 4–53. As Verhulst (1987) commented, the neonate's vocal fold is very wide in proportion to its length. Because the arytenoid is relatively large in the newborn, one half of the infant glottal length is cartilaginous, compared to only one third in the adult.

The length of the vocal folds in newborns is on the order of 4–6 mm. The length increases to about 8 or 9 mm at the age of 6 years. At some point between 6 and 12 years of age, vocal fold length begins to show a sex-related difference. The length of

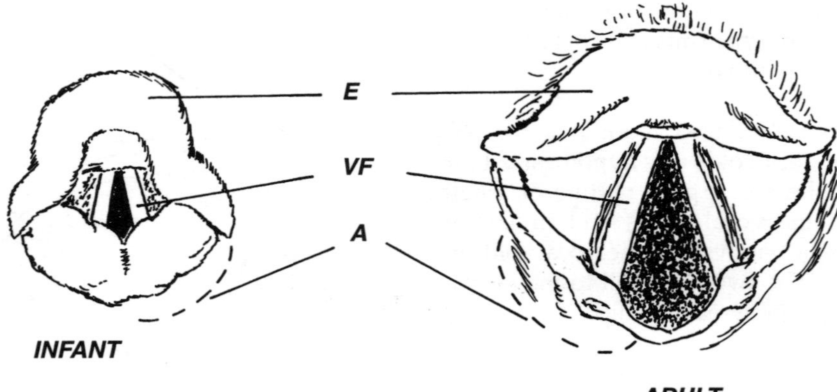

Figure 4–53. Comparison of the vocal folds of neonate and adult. E = epiglottis; VF = vocal folds; A = arytenoid cartilage. Note that in the newborn, the vocal fold is thick relative to its length, and the arytenoid is relatively large compared to the overall vocal fold length.

the folds increases to about 12–17 mm in a girl at puberty, compared to about 15–25 mm in a boy. The average length of a woman's vocal fold is about 21 mm and the average for a man is about 29 mm. The increase in vocal fold length is graphed in Figure 4–54. A growth spurt is especially evident for adolescent males. The developmental variations in vocal fold length are related to changes in mean fundamental frequency. As the length of the folds increases, the fundamental frequency decreases. Some acoustic studies of fundamental frequency show a male-female difference by the age of about 5 to 8 years (Glaze, Bless, & Milenkovic, 1988; Hasek, Singh, & Murray, 1980). These early sex differences may not necessarily reflect differences in vocal fold length, but could be attributable to differences in height or weight, changes in the vocal tract, or to cultural factors (Glaze et al., 1988).

The entire lamina propria in the newborn is uniform, so that distinct layers within this region cannot be identified (Color plate 4 in the Appendix). The three layers seen in the adult lamina propria emerge with development. Between the ages of 1 to 4 years, the vocal ligament (intermediate and deep layers of the lamina propria) appears. Between the ages of 6 to 15 years, differentiation occurs between the two layers of the ligament. Adultlike structure of the vocal folds is present by the age of about 16 years. It is important to note that development of the laryngeal tissues continues well after the ages by which children typically have mastered the sounds of their language. According to Kahane's (1988) measurements of the weights of the intrinsic muscles of the larynx in infants and adults, the values for infants are proportionate to those for adults. Apparently, then, development of the larynx preserves the relationship among the muscles, at least as far as weight is concerned. Growth of the major laryngeal cartilages is graphed in Figure 4–55, which shows the weight increases of the thyroid, cricoid, and arytenoid cartilages in males and females in two age comparisons: prepuberty to puberty and puberty to adult. Some major events in laryngeal development are listed in Table 4–5. As noted in the table, males typically undergo the adolescent voice change be-

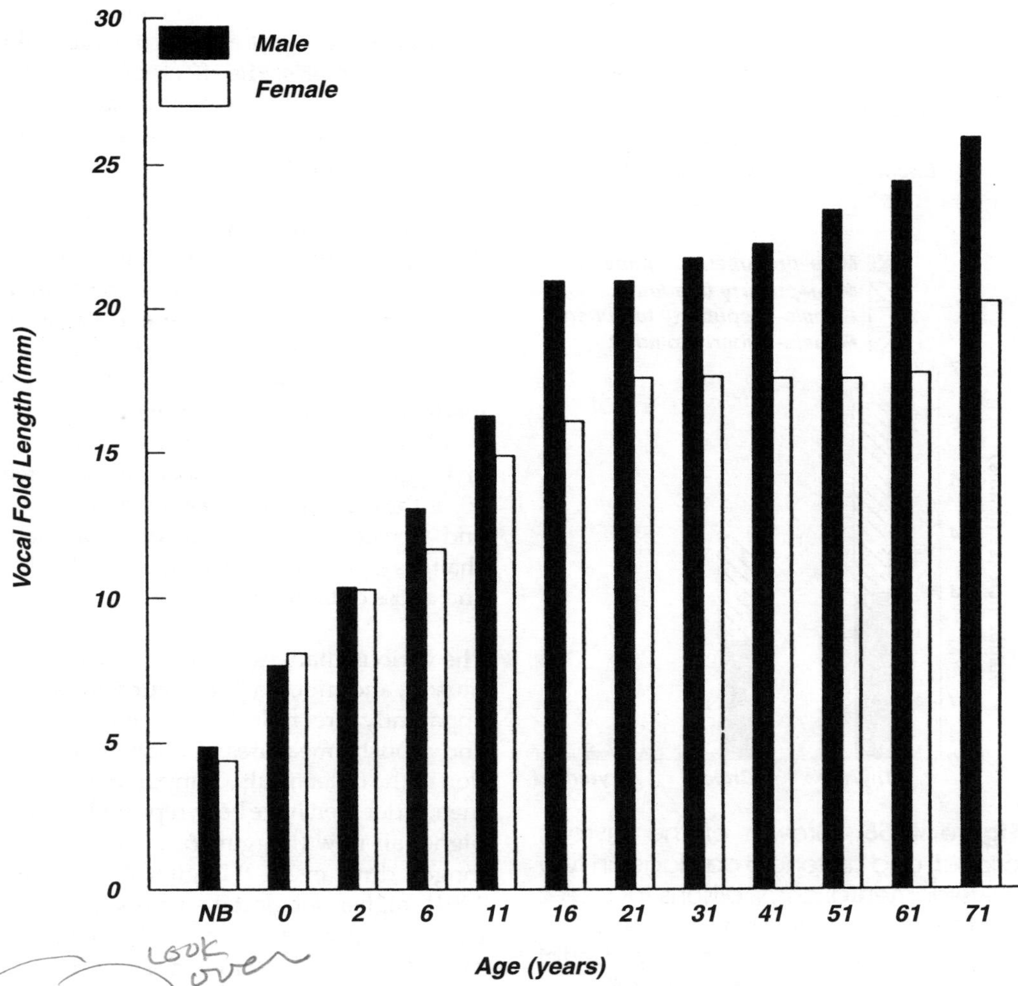

Figure 4–54. Vocal fold length as a function of age in male and female subjects. NB = newborn, *18*, pp. 105–109. (Based on data in "Length of the Human Vocal Folds by Age," by A. G. Kazarian, L. S. Sarkissian, & D. G. Isaakian, *Zhurnal Eksperimentalnoi I Klinicheskoi Meditsiny*, 1978.

tween 12.5 to 14.5 years of age (Hollien, Green, & Massey, 1994). The voice change corresponds to a growth spurt of the laryngeal structures.

The development of laryngeal form and function is a subject of continuing and much-needed investigation. The details are beyond the scope of this text, but the interested reader is referred to Kent and Vorperian (1996) and Netsell, Lotz, Peters, and Schulte (1994).

With aging in the adult, the laryngeal tissues undergo a number of changes that can affect phonatory function (Benjamin, 1988; Kahane & Beckford, 1991; Linville, 1995; Mueller, Sweeney, & Baribeau, 1985). In particular, changes are observed in the histologic structure of the laryngeal cartilages and vocal folds. As mentioned earlier, the thyroid and cricoid are composed of hyaline cartilage, which ossifies with age so that the cartilage eventually becomes bone.

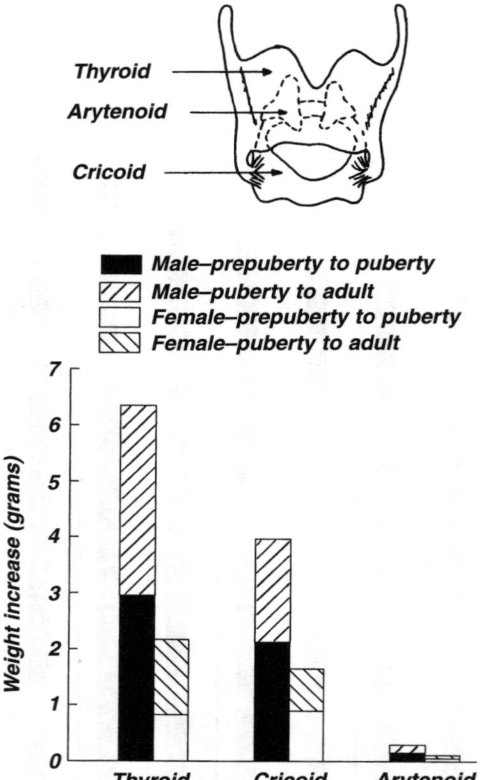

Figure 4–55. Growth of the thyroid, cricoid, and arytenoid cartilages in two developmental comparisons for males and females. (Based on data reported in "Growth of the Human Prepubertal and Pubertal Larynx," by J. S. Kahane, 1978, *American Journal of Anatomy, 151*, pp. 14–17; "Growth of the human prepubertal and pubertal larynx," by J. S. Kahane, 1982, *Journal of Speech and Hearing Research*, 1982, *25*, p. 449; and "Development of the craniofacial-oral-laryngeal anatomy: A review," by R. D. Kent and H. K. Vorperian, 1995, *Journal of Medical Speech-Language Pathology, 3*, p. 172.)

However, the elastic cartilages never ossify. Ossification appears to commence by the third decade for males and by the fourth decade for females. It has been reported that the female larynx never completely ossifies, at least not to the extent that has been observed in males. The effects of age on the larynx may be most evident in singing, in areas such as reduced vocal range or limited vocal dynamics.

Age-related changes in the vocal folds alter their appearance and biomechanical properties. The superficial layer of the lamina propria thickens with aging and becomes **edematous** (swollen with fluid), and the density of the fibers decreases. The intermediate layer becomes thinner as the elastic fibers atrophy and decrease. The deep layer thickens in males, especially after age 50, as the collagenous fibers increase in size and density. A likely outcome of these changes is a stiffening of the vocal folds and a loss of flexibility.

The various changes in laryngeal cartilage, muscle, and mucosa that occur with aging apparently are reflected in aerodynamic and acoustic measures of phonatory function in the older adult. Compared to young men, older men have been reported to have higher air flow (Higgins & Saxman, 1991), longer duty cycle (Higgins & Saxman, 1991), higher subglottal air pressure (Higgins & Saxman, 1991), and higher fundamental frequencies (Hollien & Shipp, 1972; Honjo & Isshiki, 1980; Mueller et al., 1985). Studies have not shown similar airflow changes in aging women (Biever & Bless, 1989; Higgins & Saxman, 1991; Morris & Brown, 1987; Sapienza & Dutka, 1996), but several reports have indicated a decreased fundamental frequency as women age (Benjamin, 1981; Honjo & Isshiki, 1980; Linville, 1987; Mueller et al., 1985; Russell, Penny, & Pemberton, 1995; Stoicheff, 1981). In one of the very few longitudinal studies, Russell et al. (1995) reported that speaking fundamental frequency decreased by nearly 50 Hz in six women studied between 1945 and 1993. This is a substantial drop in frequency and may account for listeners' ability to distinguish younger and older

Table 4–5. Developmental milestones in the laryngeal system.

Age	Typical Event or Pattern
Birth	Laryngeal position is high in neck, similar to nonhuman primate anatomy. Vocal folds are 5 to 7 mm long. Entire lamina propria is uniform, i.e., there is no lamination corresponding to adult histology. About one-half of the infant glottal length is cartilaginous.
4 yrs	Vocal ligament appears between 1 to 4 yrs.
6 yrs	Vocal fold length is about 8 mm in both sexes. The two layers of vocal ligament become differentiated between 6 to 15 yrs.
8 yrs	Sex differences begin to emerge in laryngeal tissues.
12 yrs	Differentiation of lamina propria nearly complete. Adolescent voice change begins in males between 12.5 to 14.5 yrs. Length of vocal folds is about 12–17 mm in pubescent girls and about 15–25 mm in pubescent boys.
16 yrs	Adult morphology of vocal folds achieved.
Adult	Vocal length is about 21 mm in women and about 29 mm in men. About one-third of vocal fold length is cartilaginous.

women by their voices. A study by Linville and Fisher (1985) indicated that fundamental frequency alone is an effective cue for age estimation of women's voices.

It appears that some measures of phonation become more similar between men and women as they age. One of the most notable is the tendency for men to show an increased fundamental frequency and for women to show a decreased fundamental frequency. Hollien, Green, & Massey (1984) proposed a male-female coalescence model of aging in which hormonal changes associated with menopause in the female undo some of the hormone-related differences between males and females that occur at puberty. Menopause, in particular, appears to influence women's fundamental frequency. Stoicheff (1981) found that women who reported having completed menopause had a lower f_0 (by an average of about 20 Hz) than women of similar ages who had not completed menopause. This difference should be readily perceptible as a lower pitched voice in the postmenopausal woman.

Figure 4–56 illustrates the general pattern of change in vocal fundamental frequency for the first 10 years of life. Newborns have large variations in their vocal fundamental frequency, but a value in the range of 400 to 500 Hz can be taken as typical. Vocal fundamental frequency then falls to a value of around 200 to 300 Hz during childhood. Mean values of fundamental frequency for vocalizations by males and females from age 10 to 80 years are graphed in Figure 4–57. Marked changes occur during adolescence, especially in males. The pattern of fundamental frequency in older adults is becoming better defined as the result of recent studies. Figure 4–57 lends some support to the conclusion that fundamental frequency tends to increase with advanced age in males, but to decrease somewhat in females. As more people live to advanced ages, it will be interesting to see new data on vocal function. In perhaps the only published study of vocal function in centenarians, Awan and Mueller (1992) reported a mean fundamental frequency of about 177 Hz for nine women with a mean age of 102

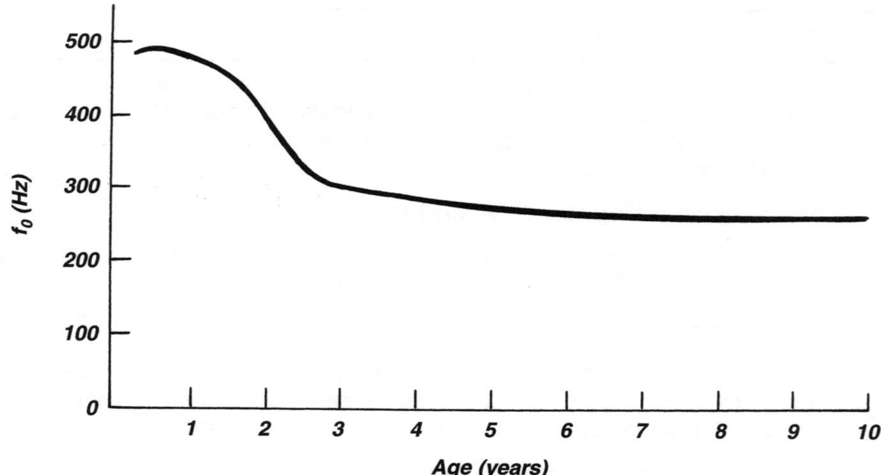

Figure 4–56. Mean f_0 values in males and females for the ages birth to ten years. (Based on data from "Anatomical and neuromuscular maturation of the speech mechanism: Evidence from acoustic studies," by R. D. Kent, 1976, *Journal of Speech and Hearing Research, 19,* 421–447; and *Reference Manual for Communicative Sciences and Disorders: Speech-Language Pathology,* by R. D. Kent, Austin, TX: Pro-Ed.)

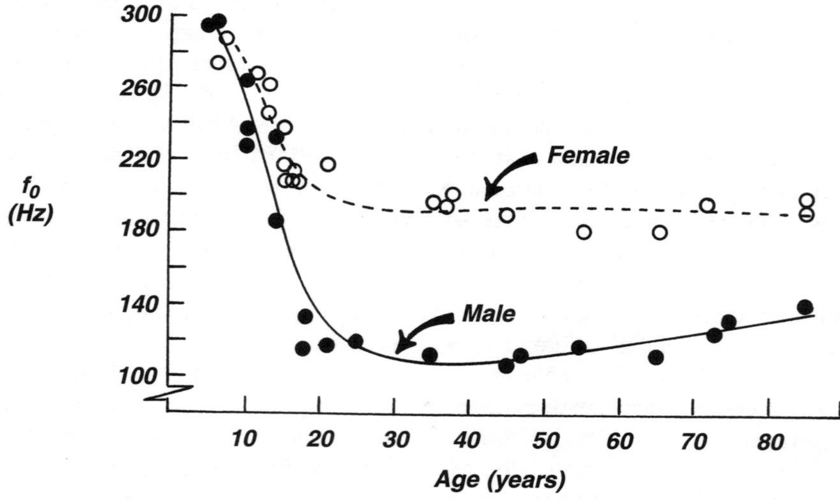

Figure 4–57. Mean f_0 as a function of age for male and female subjects for the period of 10 to 80 years. The data points represent mean or median values from selected published studies (see caption to Figure 4–56).

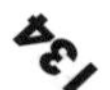

years. When this value is compared with the data in Figure 4–57, it is consistent with the decrease of fundamental frequency in aged women.

Some major conclusions regarding fundamental frequency during the life course are:

1. The newborn has a fundamental frequency of about 400 Hz, which is maintained with little change over the first year of life. However, it should be noted that this is an average value and that vocal fundamental frequency can vary considerably from baby to baby and from time to time in the same baby. Some of a baby's higher pitched shrieks may have a fundamental frequency of 1000 Hz or higher. A general instability in control of fundamental frequency is a characteristic of the infantile voice.
2. Fundamental frequency is fairly stable during childhood, from about age 4 to 10 years.
3. Males and females have roughly similar values until about 12 years of age, although some reports show a subtle male-female difference emerging by 5 to 8 years. It is difficult to disentangle biological and cultural factors that may cause these male-female differences. After age 12, males undergo a relatively large and rapid change in mean fundamental frequency.
4. Young men have a mean fundamental frequency of about 130 Hz, about one octave lower than the mean of 250 Hz for young women. This octave difference is maintained until old age.
5. With advanced age, fundamental frequency tends to increase in men, but decrease in women. Therefore, the sex difference in fundamental frequency tends to narrow with increasing age. A relatively high-pitched older man may be difficult to distinguish from a relatively low-pitched older woman.

Sex Differences in Laryngeal Function

As discussed in the preceding sec. elsewhere in the chapter, males and fe. differ in several aspects of laryngeal fu.c-tion. Besides having a higher fundamental frequency, women tend to have a breathier voice quality. But these are not the only differences. It has been interesting to note the difficulty in trying to model the female voice for computer-generated speech. Valuable sources of information on the differences between the male and female voice are Klatt and Klatt (1990), Morris and Brown (1987), and Titze (1989). Differences between male and female voices also have been described impressionistically, but some of the characteristics that appear in the literature may be hard to reconcile with more quantitative data (Henton, 1989).

Note on Clinical Application

This application note demonstrates the difference between adduction of the vocal folds and medial compression of the folds. Recall that adduction refers to the movement of the folds toward midline, and that medial compression refers to the force created between the folds. The folds can be adducted with varying degrees of medial compression. If the adducted folds have inadequate medial compression, the voice will be weak and ineffective. This situation sometimes occurs in **Parkinson's disease**, a neurological disorder that typically results in tremor, rigidity, and slowness of movement. Many individuals with Parkinson's disease have reduced phonatory ability. Frequently, their voice quality is breathy and weak. Presumably, they can adduct the folds, but lack suitable medial compression. A clinical technique that is used to increase medial compression is to ask the subjects to phonate while lifting themselves up from a chair or while pushing their arms together in an isometric exercise. Recall from earlier comments in this chapter that the vocal folds tend to be closed tightly during lifting or other activities. Activities that increase the medial compression force tend to improve the quality of phonation. This technique can be incorporated as part of a behavioral management to strengthen the voice in Parkinson's disease (Ramig, Bonitati, Lemke, & Horii, 1994).

Voice and Individuality

A recurrent theme in this book is that speech and voice have both a public and an individual aspect. Although all speakers with a suitable anatomy and physiology produce voice and therefore have the capability for spoken language (a public function), individuals often can be recognized by their voices (an individual distinctiveness). Interestingly, the words **person** and **personality** are related to the Latin phrase **per sona**, which means "the sound of the voice passes through." The English words *person* and *personality* are derived from the Latin **persona** which originally was the mouthpiece of a mask worn by actors. Moses (1954) explains these word derivations and writes generally about the relationships between voice and individuality, emotion, and personality. In an important sense, we are our voices.

Summary

The larynx is the instrument of voice. Its role in speech and song is especially evident as the tone produced by vibrations of the vocal folds. But the larynx has other functions as well, and an examination of these functions reveals that the tissues of the larynx enable a number of adjustments of the airway that extends from the respiratory system to the supralaryngeal system. For activities such as rest breathing, the vocal folds are adducted to permit the ready flow of air into and out of the lungs. When a person lifts a heavy object, the vocal folds adduct to make a tight seal that insures rigidity of the chest wall and abdomen. During speech the vocal folds adduct for voiced sounds and abduct for voiceless sounds and pauses. The length and tension of the folds are continuously adjusted to produce changes in prosody. The larynx is capable of refined adjustments that contribute to the intelligibility and quality of speech.

CHAPTER SUMMARY

This chapter has introduced the respiratory and laryngeal systems, with the primary goal of showing how they participate in the process of phonation, or the generation of voice. These systems work closely together, not only for phonation, but for a large number of activities, including coughing, sneezing, heavy lifting, and ordinary breathing. The respiratory and laryngeal systems are composed of a large number of bones, cartilages, tendons, muscles, and other tissues. The anatomy presented here is by no means greatly detailed, as the discussion is directed toward a functional understanding of two systems. Each system is complex in its own right, and the two are coregulated to support basic life processes as well as to produce the basic energy sources of speech. Although phonation typically is a lifelong capability, both the respiratory and laryngeal systems change in conspicuous ways during development and aging. These changes are important to the understanding of speech and song during the life course. They also are important in clinical evaluations as performed in **otolaryngology** (the medical specialty that deals with the ear, nose, and throat) or in speech-language pathology. The air pressures, air flows, and vibratory energy generated by the combined respiratory-laryngeal apparatus are used by the upper airway to produce articulate speech. The next chapter continues the account of how speech is produced. It pertains to the anatomy and physiology of the speech production system that lies above the larynx.

On The Reference Shelf

General references for readers who seek a deeper or extended discussion of selected issues.

Culbertson, W. R., & Tanner, D. C. (1997). *Introductory speech and hearing anatomy and physiology workbook*. Boston: Allyn & Bacon.
Readers who like a workbook format for the study of anatomy might enjoy this recently published book.

Hixon, T. J., and collaborators (1987). *Respiratory function in speech and song*. Boston: College-Hill Press.
This book is a collection of research papers on respiration by Hixon and colleagues over a period of two decades.

Kahane, J. C., & Folkins, J. F. (1984). *Atlas of speech and hearing anatomy*. Columbus, OH: Charles E. Merrill.
Reproductions of drawings and photos of the structures of speech and voice.

Orlikoff, R. F., & Kahane, J. C. (1996). Structure and function of the larynx. In N. J. Lass (Ed.), *Principles of experimental phonetics* (pp. 112–181). St. Louis: Mosby.
A brisk and informative summary of laryngeal anatomy and physiology.

Seikel, J. A., King, D. W., & Drumright, D. G. (1997). *Anatomy and physiology for speech and language*. San Diego: Singular Publishing Group.
This recently published book on anatomy and physiology features clear discussions and illustrations.

Sundberg, J. (1987). *The science of the singing voice*. DeKalb, IL: Northern Illinois Press.
The title is apt: Sundberg, a master of the vocal arts and sciences, discusses how song is produced.

Titze, I. (1994). *Principles of voice production*. Englewood Cliffs, NJ: Prentice Hall.
The author summarizes the state of voice science in a lucid and comprehensive book.

Weismer, G. (1985). Speech breathing. In R. G. Daniloff (Ed.), *Speech science* (pp. 46–72). San Diego: College–Hill Press.
A concise, effective summary of speech breathing research.

West, B. J., & Goldberger, A. L. (1987, July/August). Physiology in fractal dimensions. *American Scientist*, *75*, 354–365.
A concise discussion of fractals in physiology, including the respiratory system.

Chapter References

Abitbol, J. (1995). *Atlas of laser voice surgery*. San Diego: Singular Publishing Group.

Awan, S. N., & Mueller, P. B. (1992). Speaking fundamental frequency characteristics of centenarian females. *Clinical Linguistics and Phonetics*, *6*, 249–254.

Baken, R. (1990). Irregularity of vocal period and amplitude: A first approach to the fractal analysis of voice. *Journal of Voice*, *4*, 185–197.

Benjamin, B. J. (1981). Frequency variability in the aged voice. *Journal of Gerontology*, *36*, 722–736.

Benjamin, B. J. (1988). Changes in speech production and linguistic behaviors with aging. In B. B. Shadden (Ed.), *Communication behavior and aging: A sourcebook for clinicians* (pp. 162–181). Baltimore: Williams & Wilkins.

Berg, J. van den (1958). Myoelastic-aerodynamic theory of voice production. *Journal of Speech and Hearing Research, 1*, 227–244.

Berke, G. S., & Gerratt, B. R. (1993). Laryngeal biomechanics: An overview of mucosal wave mechanics. *Journal of Voice, 7*, 123–128.

Berke, G. S., Moore, D. M., Hantke, D. R., Hanson, D. G., Gerratt, B. R., & Burstein, F. (1987). Laryngeal modeling: Theoretical, in vitro, in vivo. *Laryngoscope, 97*, 871–881.

Biever, D., & Bless, D. (1989). Vibratory characteristics of the vocal folds in young adult and geriatric women. *Journal of Voice, 3*, 120–131.

Bloedel, S. (1994). *An analysis of the acoustic correlates of breathy phonation in the speech of adult men and women and pre-pubescent males.* Unpublished master's thesis, University of Wisconsin-Madison.

Britt, E. J., Shelhamer, J., Menkes, H., Cohen, B., Meyer, M., & Permutt, S. (1981). Sex differences in the decline of pulmonary function with age. *Chest, 1*(Suppl.), 79S–80S.

Childers, D. G., & Krishnamurthy, A. K. (1985). A critical review of electroglottography. *CRC Critical Reviews in Biomedical Engineering, 12*, 131–161.

Comroe, J. H., Forster, R. E., Dubois, A. B., Briscoe, W. A., & Carlsen, E. (1957). *The lung.* Chicago: Year Book Publishers.

Draper, M. H., Ladefoged, P., & Whitteridge, D. (1959). Respiratory muscles in speech. *Journal of Speech and Hearing Research, 2*, 16–27.

Glaze, L. E., Bless, D. M., Milenkovic, P., et al. (1988). Acoustic characteristics of children's voice. *Journal of Voice, 2*, 312–319.

Harden, J. R., & Looney, N. A. (1984). *International Journal of Pediatric Otorhinolaryngology, 7*, 11–19.

Hasek, C., Singh, S., & Murray, T. (1980). Acoustic attributes of children's voices. *Journal of the Acoustical Society of America, 68*, 1252–1265.

Hayflick, L. (1994). *How and why we age.* New York: Ballantine Books.

Henton, C. (1989). Fact or fiction in the description of male and female pitch. *Language and Communication, 9*, 299–311.

Herzel, H., Berry, D., Titze, I, & Saleh, M. (1994). Analysis of vocal disorders with methods from nonlinear dynamics. *Journal of Speech and Hearing Research, 37*, 1008–1019.

Higgins, M. B., & Saxman, J. H. (1991). A comparison of selected phonatory behaviors of healthy aged and young adults. *Journal of Speech and Hearing Research, 34*, 1000–1010.

Hirano, M. (1974). Morphological structure of the vocal cord as a vibrator and its variations. *Folia Phoniatrica (Basel), 26*, 89–94.

Hirano, M., (1981). *Clinical examination of voice.* New York: Springer-Verlag.

Hirano, M., & Kakita, Y. (1985). Cover-body theory of vocal fold vibration. In R. G. Daniloff (Ed.), *Speech science.* San Diego: College-Hill Press.

Hirano, M., Kiyokawa, K., Kurita, S., & Sato, K. (1986). Posterior glottis: Morphological study in excised larynges. *Annals of Otology, Rhinology, and Laryngology, 95*, 576–581.

Hirano, M., Kurita, S., & Nakashima, T. (1981). Growth, development and aging of human vocal folds. In D. M. Bless & J. H. Abbs (Eds.), *Vocal fold physiology: Contemporary research and clinical issues* (pp. 22–43). San Diego: College-Hill Press.

Hirano, M., & Sato, K. (1993). *Histological color atlas of the human larynx.* San Diego: Singular Publishing Group.

Hixon, T. J., & Weismer, G. (1995). Perspectives on the Edinburgh studies of speech breathing. *Journal of Speech and Hearing Research, 38*, 42–60.

Hodge, M. M., & Rochet, A. P. (1989). Characteristics of speech breathing in young women. *Journal of Speech and Hearing Research, 32*, 466–480.

Hoit, J. D., Hixon, T. J., Watson, P. J., & Morgan, W. (1990). Speech breathing in children and adolescents. *Journal of Speech and Hearing Research, 33*, 51–69.

Hoit, J. D., Hixon, T. J., Altman, M. E., & Morgan, W. J. (1989). Speech breathing in women. *Journal of Speech and Hearing Research, 33*, 51–69.

Hollien, H., Green, R., & Massey, K. (1994). Longitudinal research on adolescent voice change in males. *Journal of the Acoustical Society of America, 34*, 80–84.

Hollien, H., & Shipp, T. (1972). Speaking fundamental frequency and chronological age in males. *Journal of Speech and Hearing Research, 15*, 155–159.

Honjo, I., & Isshiki, N. (1980). Laryngoscopic and voice characteristics of aged persons. *Archives of Otolaryngology, 106*, 149–150.

Husson, R. (1950). *Etude de phenomenes physiologiques et acoustiques fondamentaux de la voix chantee*. Unpublished thesis, University of Paris.

Ishizaka, K., & Flanagan, J. L. (1972). Synthesis of voiced sounds from a two-mass model of the vocal cords. *Bell System Technical Journal, 51*, 1233–1268.

Ishizaka, K., & Matsudaira, M. (1972). *Fluid mechanical considerations of vocal cord motion*. (SCRL Monograph No. 8). Santa Barbara, CA: Speech Communication Research Laboratories.

Kahane, J. C. (1978). A morphological study of the human prepubertal and pubertal larynx. *American Journal of Anatomy, 151*, 11–20.

Kahane, J. C. (1982). Growth of the human prepubertal and pubertal larynx. *Journal of Speech and Hearing Research, 25*, 446–455.

Kahane, J. C. (1983). A survey of age-related changes in the connective tissue of the human adult larynx. In D. Bless & J. H. Abbs (Eds.), *Vocal fold physiology: Contemporary research and clinical issues*. San Diego: College-Hill Press.

Kahane, J. C. (1988). Histologic structure and properties of the human vocal folds. *Ear, Nose and Throat Journal, 67*, 322–330.

Kahane, J. C., & Beckford, N. S. (1991). The aging larynx and voice. In D. Ripich (Ed.), *Handbook of geriatric communication disorders* (pp. 165–186). Austin, TX: PRO-ED.

Kahane, J.C., & Kahn, A.R. (1984). Weight measurements of infant and adult intrinsic laryngeal muscles. *Folia Phoniatrica, 36*, 129–133.

Kent, R. D., Kent, J. F., & Rosenbek, J. C. (1987). Maximum performance tests of speech production. *Journal of Speech and Hearing Research, 52*, 367–387.

Kent, R. D., & Vorperian, H. K. (1995). Anatomic development of the craniofacial-oral-laryngeal systems: A review. *Journal of Medical Speech-language Pathology, 3*, 145–190.

Kitzing, P., & Lofqvist, A. (1982). Aeodynamic aspects of phonation. In P. Hurme (Ed.), *Vox humana. Papers in Speech Research* (pp. 103–114). Jyvaskyla, Finland: University of Jyvaskyla.

Klatt, D. H., & Klatt, L. (1990). Analysis, synthesis, and perception of voice quality variations among female and male talkers. *Journal of the Acoustical Society of America, 87*, 820–857.

Leff, A. R., & Schumacker, P. T. (1993). *Respiratory physiology: Basics and applications*. Philadelphia: W. B. Saunders.

Linville, S. E. (1987). Maximum phonational frequency range capabilities of women's voices with advancing age. *Folia Phoniatrica, 39*, 297–301.

Linville, S. E. (1992). Glottal gap configurations in two age groups of women. *Journal of Speech and Hearing Research, 35*, 1209–1215.

Linville, S. E. (1995). Vocal aging. *Current Opinion in Otolaryngology and Head and Neck Surgery, 3*, 183–187.

Linville, S. E., & Fisher, H. B. (1985). Acoustic characteristics of perceived versus actual age in controlled phonation by adult females. *Journal of the Acoustical Society of America, 78*, 40–48.

Lofqvist, A. & Yoshioka, H. (1981). Interarticulator programming in obstruent production. *Phonetica, 38*, 21–34.

Malmgren, L. T., & Gacek, R. R. (1992). In A. Blitzer, M. F. Brin, C. T. Sasaki, S. Fahn, & K. S. Harris (Eds.), *Neurologic disorders of the larynx* (pp. 36–44). New York: Thieme Medical Publishers.

Mitchell, J. L., Hoit, J. C., & Watson, P. J. (1996). Cognitive-linguistic demands and speech breathing. *Journal of Speech and Hearing Research, 39*, 93–104.

Moore, P. (1938). Motion picture studies of the vocal folds and vocal attack. *Journal of Speech and Hearing Disorders, 3*, 235–238.

Morris, R., & Brown, W. (1987). Age-related measures among adult women. *Journal of Voice, 1*, 38–43.

Moses, P. J. (1954). *The voice of neurosis*. New York: Grune & Stratton.

Mueller, P. B., Sweeney, R. J., & Baribeau, L. J. (1985). Acoustic and morphologic study of the senescent voice. *Ear, Nose, and Throat Journal, 63*, 71–75.

Netsell, R., Lotz, W. K., Peters, J. E., & Schulte, L. (1994). Developmental patterns of laryngeal and respiratory function for speech production. *Journal of Voice, 8*, 123–131.

Palmer, J. M. (1993). *Anatomy for speech and hearing* (4th ed.). Baltimore: Williams & Wilkins.

Ramig, L. O., Bonitati, C. M., Lemke, J. H., & Horii, Y. (1994). Voice treatment for patients with Parkinson's disease: Development of an approach and preliminary efficacy data. *Journal of Medical Speech-language Pathology, 2*, 191–209.

Rochet, A. P. (1991). Aging and the respiratory system. In D. Ripich (Ed.), *Handbook of geriatric communication disorders* (pp. 145–163). Austin, TX: Pro-Ed.

Rothenberg, M. (1973). A new inverse-filtering technique for deriviing the glottal airflow waveform during voicing. *Journal of the Acoustical Society of America, 53,* 1632–1645.

Russell, A. (Ed.). (1987). *Guinness book of world records.* Toronto: Bantam Books.

Russell, A., Penny, L., & Pemberton, C. (1995). Speaking fundamental frequency changes over time in women: A longitudinal study. *Journal of Speech and Hearing Research, 38,* 101–109.

Sapienza, C. M., & Dutka, J. (1996). Glottal airflow characteristics of women's voice production along an aging continuum. *Journal of Speech and Hearing Research, 39,* 322–328.

Sato, K., Kurita, S., Hirano, M., & Kiyokawa, K. (1990). Distribution of elastic cartilage in the arytenoids and its physiologic significance. *Annals of Otology, Rhinology and Laryngology, 99,* 363–368.

Scherer, R. C. (1995). Laryngeal function during phonation. In J. S. Rubin, G. Korovin, R. T. Sataloff, & W. J. Gold (Eds.), *Diagnosis and treatment of voice disorders* (pp. 86–104). New York: Igaku-Shoin Medical Publishers.

Schonharl, E. (1960). *Die Stroboskopie in der praktischen Laryngologie.* Stuttgart: Thieme Verlag.

Sodersten, M., & Lindestad, P.-A. (1990). Glottal closure and perceived breathiness during phonation in normally speaking subjects. *Journal of Speech and Hearing Research, 33,* 601–611.

Stathopoulos, E. T., & Sapienza, C. (1993). Respiratory and laryngeal measures of children during vocal intensity variation. *Journal of the Acoustical Society of America, 94,* 2531–2543.

Steinecke, I., & Herzel, H. (1995). Bifurcations in an asymmetric vocal fold model. *Journal of the Acoustical Society of America, 97,* 1874–1884.

Stoicheff, M. L. (1981). Speaking fundamental frequency characteristics of nonsmoking female adults. *Journal of Speech and Hearing Research, 24,* 437–441.

Storey, B. H., & Titze, I. R. (1995). Voice simulation with a body-cover model of the vocal folds. *Journal of the Acoustical Society of America, 97,* 1249–1260.

Titze, I. R. (1989). Physiologic and acoustic differences between male and female voices. *Journal of the Acoustical Society of America, 85,* 1699–1707.

Titze, I. (1994). *Principles of voice production.* Englewood Cliffs, NJ: Prentice-Hall.

Tritten, P. J., & Lleo, A. de S. y (1995). Voice quality analysis of male and female Spanish speakers. *Speech Communication, 16,* 354–368.

Tucker, J. A., & Tucker, G. F. (1979). A clinical perspective on the development and anatomical aspects of the infant larynx and trachea. In G. B. Healy & T. J. I. McGill (Eds.), *Laryngo-tracheal problems in the pediatric patient.* Springfield, IL: Charles C. Thomas.

Verhulst, J. (1987). Development of the larynx from birth to puberty [in French]. *Revue De Laryngologie Otologie Rhinologie, 108*(4), 269–270.

Winkworth, A. L., Davis, P. J., Ellis, E., & Adams, R. D. (1994). Variability and consistency in speech breathing during reading: Lung volumes, speech intensity, and linguistic factors. *Journal of Speech and Hearing Research, 37,* 535–556.

Exercises

4-1. This exercise is suitable for a class or other group of people, preferably a group containing both males and females. Using a stop watch, determine the maximum time that each person can phonate the vowel /ɑ/ (as in *pot*) after a maximal inspiration. Plot the results in a bar graph and evaluate the intersubject variability in maximum phonation times. Compare your data with those in Figure 4–26.

4-2. To get an idea of how much air pressure is used for phonation, conduct this simple experiment. You will need a straw, a centimeter rule, and a tall glass or tube (about 10 cm in height) filled with water. Dip the straw into the glass to a depth of 6 cm. Then take a deep breath of air and blow gently into the straw until you see bubbles forming at the end of the straw. When the bubbles begin to form, you have generated an air pressure of 6 cm H_2O, which is the air pressure typical of conversational speech. Now immerse the straw to a depth of 9 cm H_2O and again blow into the straw until bubbles form. This is an estimate of the subglottal air pressure needed for a loud voice, as in shouting.

4-3. To discover how the understanding of speech breathing has changed, read T. J. Hixon and G. Weismer, "Perspectives on the Edinburgh studies of speech breathing," *Journal of Speech and Hearing Research*, 1995, *38*, 42–60. Prepare a brief summary of how Hixon and Weismer's account of speech breathing differs from the classic description provided by Draper, Ladefoged, and Whitteridge (1959).

4-4. The following exercise is based on the videotape, *Measuring speech production: A video demonstration of speech instrumentation* (available from the Acoustical Society of America). View the following video demonstration: *Physiologically based models of phonation* (by Ingo R. Titze). Then prepare a brief report that discusses what you learned from the video.

4-5. Using modeling clay of different colors, construct the cartilages of the larynx, using the drawings in this chapter (or the reference books) as a guide. Then assemble them into a model of the whole larynx.

4-6. Using a sheet of colored paper, draw and cut out 3 pairs of paper strips with the following dimensions:

Pair 1: 5 mm long and 2 mm wide;

Pair 2: 19 mm long and 4 mm wide;

Pair 3: 25 mm long and 5 mm wide.

Now place the two slips of each pair adjacent to one another lengthwise and place them over a sheet of paper of a different color. The paired slips of paper are approximately the size of the vocal folds of a neonate, an adult woman, and an adult man. When the members of a pair are placed together lengthwise, they resemble the adducted vocal folds. Now draw the slips of paper representing the woman's vocal folds slightly apart (1 or 2 mm) at *one* end to simulate the posterior glottal gap. *Note*: the vocal fold lengths specified in this example are roughly accurate, but the widths are chosen more from illustrative convenience.

4–7. Using Figure 4–35, Figure 4–36, and Color plate 3 as a guide, draw a diagram of the layered structure of the adult vocal fold. Then label this drawing by identifying the epithelium, the layers of the lamina propria, and the vocalis muscle. Using colored pencils, color and label the following divisions: cover, transition, and body.

4–8. As noted earlier in this chapter, Leonardo Da Vinci was one of the first to record a systematic description of the anatomy, physiology, and pathology of the larynx. He also conducted a number of experiments on phonation. Among these experiments was squeezing the lungs of a goose to generate laryngeal tones. Discuss how this experiment relates to the modern understanding of phonation, especially the aerodynamic-myoelastic theory.

CHAPTER

5

The Upper Airway of Speech Production

"The tongue, by its power of manifold motion, moves forward and back, narrows and widens, arches and flattens in its various parts; the lips open and contract; the palate rises and lowers; the nasal passages are closed and unclosed; the teeth approach and separate,—all these movements take place in every varying combination, shaping the column of vibrating breath; and from each separate combination results a sound of distinct and recognizable quality, capable of appropriation as a thought-symbol."

(Albert Salisbury, *Phonology and Orthoepy*. Madison, WI: Wm. J. Park & Sons; 1879; pp. 14–15).

ANATOMY OF THE UPPER AIRWAY

The human head is specialized for executive functions (by virtue of the large brain it contains), for processing sensory information (thanks to the receptors for vision, audition, olfaction, and taste), and for communication by speech (owing to the respiratory airway that has been commandeered for the production of spoken language). The face is a natural focus for our visual attention. We recognize one another largely by facial appearance. We discern emotions partly by noticing facial expressions. And we can see the actions of speaking. It is common practice to use the "head and shoulders" shot in television to give the viewer a good opportunity to gather information from the all-important region of the face. One of the most critical regions is the mouth. As we will see, most of the muscles of facial expression insert into the mouth. But the mouth is also the primary outlet for the sounds of speech. So for both visual and auditory information, the human mouth is the centerpiece of communication.

The upper airway is that part of the speech production system that extends from the vocal folds to the opening of the mouth and nose. This section of airway is a complex anatomic system that comprises the pharynx, tongue, cheeks, jaw, lips, palate, and nasal cavity (Figure 5–1). This system

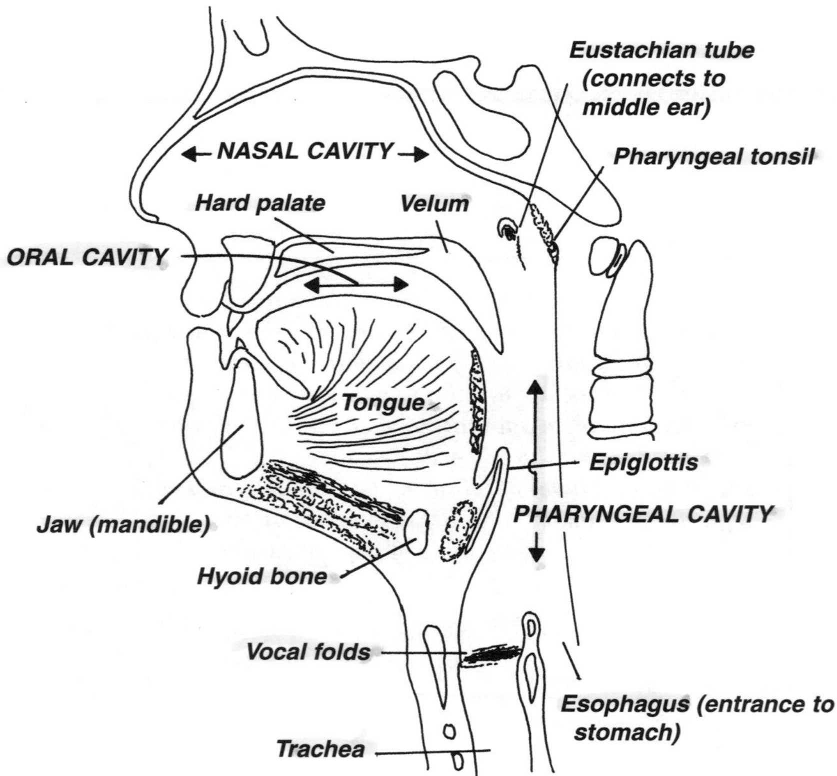

Figure 5–1. Midsagittal section of the vocal tract, with major structures labeled.

is also known as the **vocal tract**, an acoustic concept discussed in Chapter 9. It is responsible for shaping the sound energy provided by the respiratory and laryngeal systems into the distinctive sounds of speech, the phonetic elements of language. The system pictured in Figure 5–1 is not only the speech production system but also the system by which the lungs are ventilated and by which food is chewed and swallowed. Some call this system the **aerodigestive tract** in recognition that it moves both air and food. The same system is host to the functions of talking and singing. It is unwieldly and jarring to refer to this system as the vocal-aerodigestive tract, so the simple term "vocal tract" is used, given this book's focus on speech.

For the present, it should be noted that the vocal tract is the primary region in which speech sounds are formed as recognizable vowels and consonants. The formation of these sounds is accomplished through the actions of **articulation** (*articulate* means to move), **resonance** (*resonate* means to vibrate at a preferred or natural frequency, as discussed in Chapter 2), and **turbulence noise production** (*turbulence noise* is the kind of sound used in the fricatives that occur at the beginning of the words *see* and *she*).

The ultimate goal, then, is to understand how movements of structures such as the tongue or lips can produce acoustic events that a listener recognizes as a speech sound in a particular language. The path to such understanding is: first, to learn some basic anatomy; second, to learn about the physiology of speech; and, third, to learn about acoustics. This chapter primarily addresses the first two of these. Chapter 8 continues the discussion of physiology, and Chapter 9 deals with the acoustics of speech. To study any one of these—anatomy, physiology, acoustics—will lead to some understanding of speech, but it is only by studying all three of them that the power of speech can be appreciated.

We begin our discussion of vocal tract anatomy with two adults, a man and a woman. Men and women differ in their upper airways. First, men have longer airways and this fact has important consequences in the later discussion of speech acoustics. Men and women also differ in the shapes of the speech organs. The total length of a man's vocal tract is approximately 17 cm measured from the vocal folds to the lip opening. The corresponding distance for a woman is about 14 or 15 cm. A major sex difference is that men have a proportionately longer pharynx, the tube that reaches from the vocal folds to the soft palate as shown in Figure 5–2a (adult male) and 5–2b (adult female). We will soon examine the vocal tract of a newborn to learn of other differences in vocal tract configuration.

However, before looking at the newborn's vocal tract, we examine the vocal tract of a chimpanzee (Figure 5–3). This may seem a digression but, in fact, as far as the upper airway of speech is concerned, the chimpanzee may have more relevance to the human newborn than does the human adult. Note the following features of the chimpanzee's upper airway in Figure 5–3 (a comparison with Figures 5–1 and 5–2 may be helpful):

Larynx—positioned high in the neck and close to the tongue;

Epiglottis—touches the velum;

Tongue—most of the tongue mass is oriented horizontally; there is little in the way of a pharynx or vertical dimension.

Shape of vocal tract—basically a gently curved tube (unlike the right-angle configuration evident in Figures 5–1 and 5–2.)

Clearly, the chimpanzee has a different anatomy of the upper airway than does the adult human. How does the chimp's anatomy compare with that of the human newborn? The answer is at hand: Com-

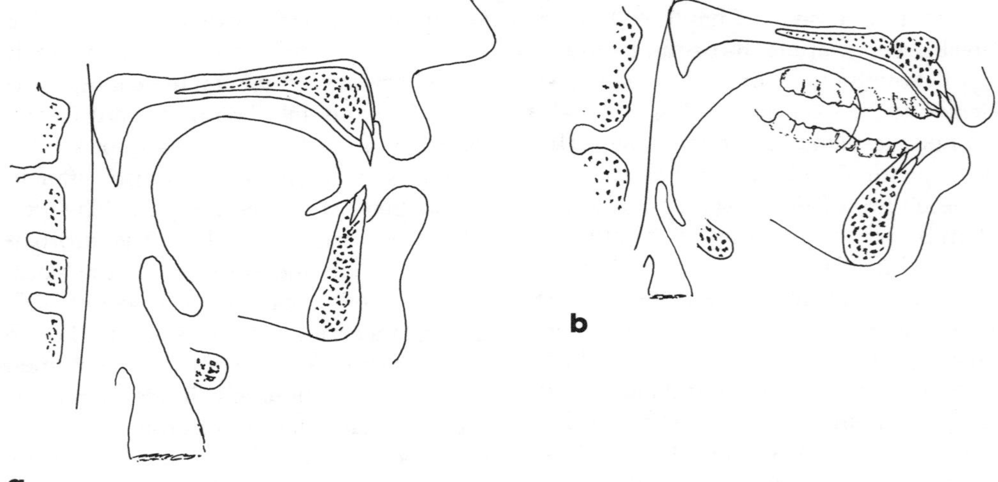

Figure 5–2. Vocal tracts of (**a**) an adult male and (**b**) an adult female.

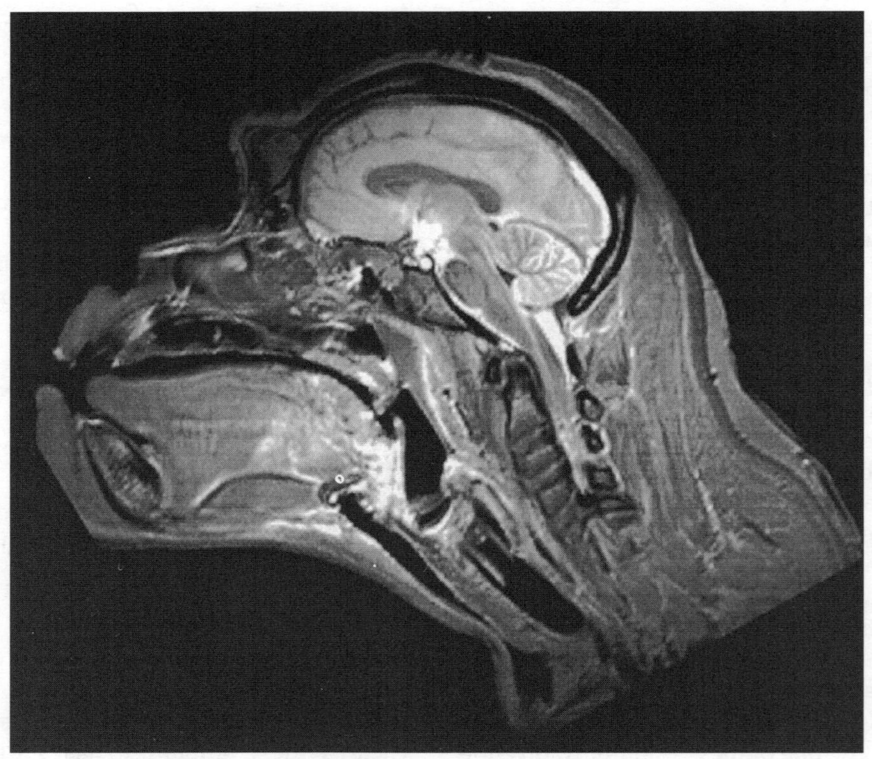

Figure 5–3. Magnetic resonance image (MRI) of the vocal tract of a chimpanzee. (Courtesy of Dr. Sugio Hayama.)

pare the newborn's upper airway (Figure 5–4) with that of the chimp and the human adult. If you decide that the human newborn has an upper airway anatomy that resembles that of the chimp more than the human adult, you are in the company of several speech scientists, anatomists, linguists, and anthropologists. (Chapter 13 has more to say about this.) The vocal tract of the neonate is rather like that of nonhuman primates and rather less like that of the adult human.

Granted (if you will) that human newborns look rather like chimpanzees as far as the upper airway is concerned, then how does the human newborn come to possess an anatomy like that of the human adult? The answer in a word is **remodeling**. The anatomy of the upper airway changes quite remarkably as the human develops in the first few years of life. The system is transfigured as bones grow and change in shape, as soft tissues develop, and as the infantile anatomy is subjected to the forces generated during feeding. These developmental mechanisms are important to the understanding of the shaping of the vocal tract in adults. The following sections pertain primarily to the adult vocal tract, but comments are included on the developmental precedents of the adult morphology—that is, on what happens in infancy and childhood. Because virtually every structure in the upper airway undergoes some kind of developmental change, lifecourse issues are included in the general presentation rather than compiled at the end of the chapter, as was the case in Chapter 4.

The Oral and Nasal Cavities

As seen in Figure 5–1, the oral and nasal cavities form a kind of parallel passageway for the sounds of speech. The boundaries of the oral cavity are formed by the

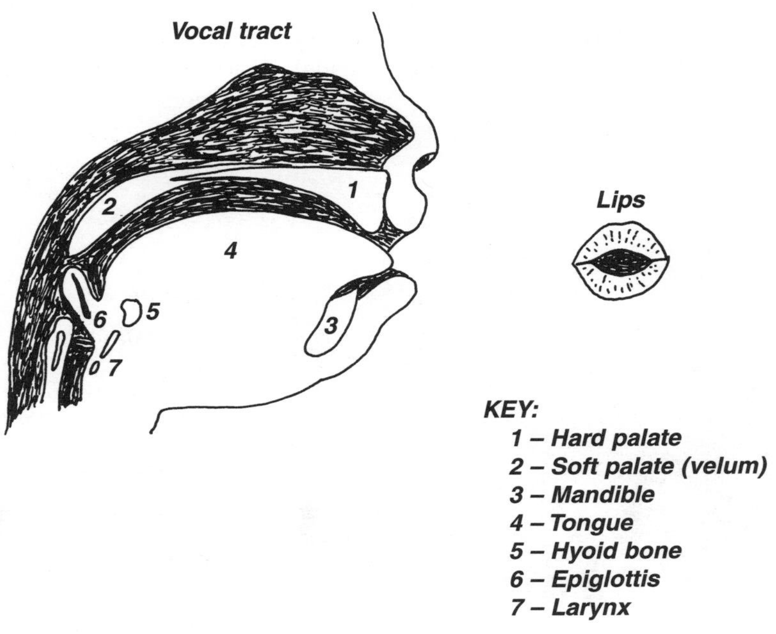

Figure 5–4. Vocal tract of a human neonate (newborn). Compare with Figures 5–2 (a and b) and 5–3.

lips anteriorly and the **anterior** and **posterior faucial pillars** (two muscular arches, as shown in Figure 5–5) posteriorly. Later in this chapter, the pillars are described in terms of the muscles that give them form. For the nasal cavity, the nares form the anterior boundary and the velopharynx is the posterior boundary. The oral and nasal cavities are joined at the velopharynx. Aside from the valving movements of the velopharynx, the nasal cavity has little variation in its shape or length. It is basically a chamber of fixed dimensions, although the soft tissues that line this cavity can swell in disease (such as the common cold) or certain atmospheric conditions. The oral cavity is much more changeable, and its dimensions change continuously in speech production as the consequence of movements of the tongue, lips, jaw, and pharynx. The oral cavity is enclosed by bony and soft tissues, as discussed in following sections. But first, some consideration is given to the oral environment itself.

The oral cavity is usually moist by virtue of the secretion of saliva from glands in the cheek and the floor of the mouth. Saliva is produced at the daily rate of about 750 ml (Provenza & Seibel, 1986). Saliva is obviously important for chewing food and seems to be important even for the mistakenly termed "dry swallow." Few, if any, swallows are really dry, as the **bolus** (material to be swallowed) for non-nutritive swallow is typically a small quantity of saliva. The need for a saliva bolus may be the reason why we eventually find it difficult or impossible to perform repetitive swallows. How many swallows can you perform in a sequence? When the salivary flow is depleted, swallow becomes difficult.

Speakers who talk for long periods often complain of a dry mouth and may seek to replenish their oral moisture with a sip of water. Why does the mouth dry out? The dehydration results partly from evaporation of moisture as the mouth is opened to the typically dryer air of the atmosphere. However, moisture is lost in substantial amounts as water is sprayed from the mouth during speech. Some talkers tend to produce highly visible sprays of saliva, but all talkers release less visible saliva droplets into the air. It has been estimated that about 2.5 droplets are expelled with every word (Bodanis, 1995)—a rather unusual liquid correlate of linguistic output. A 1-hour conversation that proceeds at the

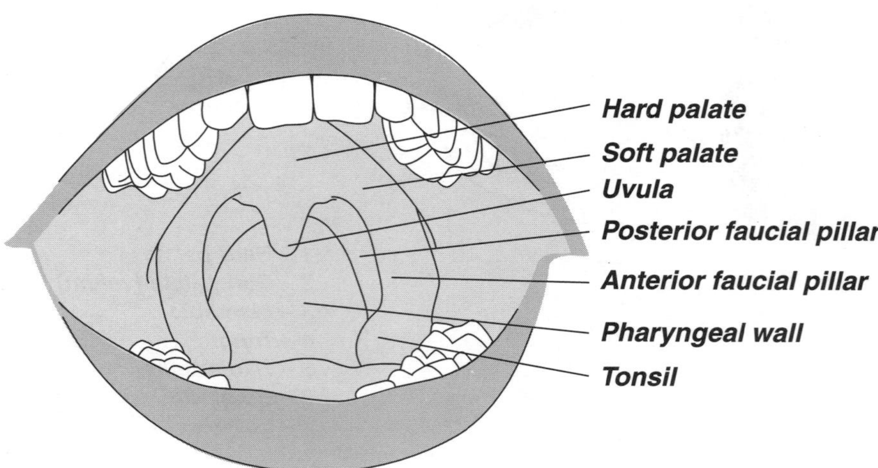

Figure 5–5. The oral cavity as viewed though the open mouth.

rather leisurely pace of 50 words per minute would produce about 7,500 droplets of saliva, which may remain in the air for an hour or more. Little wonder that we are susceptible to airborne infections. Matters become much worse if a talker sneezes into the open air, as a single sneeze may expel about a million high-velocity droplets. Listeners to an ordinary conversation are subject to an incessant, but mostly invisible, cloud of saliva. The highly energetic conversations typical of many social and athletic events generate multiple saliva storms.

The point of this rather unsavory discussion is that speech articulation is lubricated by saliva. Any condition that causes dryness of the mouth can make speech more difficult. The other extreme, excessive saliva, can also be undesirable, especially from an esthetic point of view. Salivary flow should be sufficient during speech to maintain the desired lubrication. The saliva-producing glands that line the oral cavity secrete the fluids that enable mastication and speech. These glands are described in some detail later in the chapter, following a preliminary discussion of oral anatomy.

The functions and health of the oral cavity depend on the mucosa that line all soft tissues. This oral mucosa is formed of two layers: an outer epithelium and a lamina propria (a layer of connective tissue that underlies the epithelium). The mucosal lining of the oral cavity varies regionally according to functional requirements. The three major functional types of oral mucosa are: **lining mucosa, masticatory mucosa**, and **specialized mucosa**. These are distinguished in part by the characteristics of the epithelium, especially whether it is **keratinized, parakeratinized**, or **nonkeratinized**. Keratinized epithelium has surface cells that have lost their nuclei and the cytoplasm has been replaced by keratin filaments. Parakeratinized epithelium has surface cells that retain their nuclei and contain few if any keratin filaments. Nonkeratinized epithelium has surface cells with intact nuclei and no keratin filaments. The lining mucosa is the general lining tissue of the oral cavity and is found on all soft tissues except the **gingiva** (the oral mucosa found around the necks of the teeth), hard palate, and the dorsal surface of the tongue. Lining mucosa has a smooth, shiny appearance. The epithelium is nonkeratinized. The masticatory mucosa is found on the gingiva and hard palate. The epithelium is keratinized or parakeratinized. The lamina propria is well supplied with collagenous fibers that cause the epithelium to adhere tightly to the underlying bone. The masticatory mucosa is designed to withstand the grinding and abrasive forces of chewing. The specialized mucosa covers the superior or dorsal surface of the tongue. The epithelium is mostly composed of modified keratinized cells. The mucosa also contains **papillae** (small pockets or crypts), which may in turn contain taste buds.

A warm, moist environment is often host to large populations of bacteria, and the oral cavity is no exception. Bacteria often are the cause of "bad breath," and oral hygiene is often an effective preventive. In addition, bacteria can promote the development of dental plaque, a hard substance that adheres to the teeth and may contribute to gum (periodontal) disease. Saliva protects the teeth from caries by constantly depositing mucoprotein and sialoprotein on the teeth's surfaces. This deposit eventually forms a nonmineralized protective layer called the **acquired pellicle** (Avery, 1994).

Like the oral cavity, the nasal cavity is normally warm and moist. These attributes enable the nasal passageway to condition the inhaled air, so that it is humidified and reasonably close to body temperature by the time it reaches the lungs. The air conditioning is pushed to its limits in cold, dry weather. In an effort to provide the desired humidification, the mucosa of the nasal passages secrete copious amounts of moisture, causing the nose to run.

In addition to their role in air conduction and air conditioning, the nasal passages also clean the air. This is accomplished in two major ways. First, many inspired particles adhere to the sticky mucous lining of the nasal cavities. If the mucous lining were not refreshed, these particles would accumulate. To avoid this problem, the mucous lining is renewed and the contaminated mucus is transported to the nasopharynx by a process called **mucociliary transport**. *Mucociliary* refers to cilia that move in response to a mucosal load, thereby transporting the mucus posteriorly to the nasopharynx where it is eventually swallowed. The stomach is the eventual destination of most of the nasal mucus. This mechanical cleansing of the air is accompanied by defense mechanisms that inactivate or kill bacteria, viruses, and other undesirable agents. The defensive capabilities use a variety of enzymes and other substances, including lysozyme, lactoferin, proteases, hydrolases, and interferons (Riechelmann, Hinni, Klimek, & Mann, 1995). As a result, the posterior nasopharynx can be nearly sterile in healthy subjects.

Of course, the nose and nasal cavities also are the means of odor detection. The sensitivity of the sense of smell is remarkable. The human nose can detect the presence of vanillin in a concentration of only one part per million. Olfaction is important for many reasons. Fragrances and aromas contribute to the pleasures of eating and drinking, but also are part of our general sensory interactions with different environments. In addition, certain odors alert us to the presence of unpleasant or hazardous substances, such as the odor of something burning.

The oral and nasal cavities are the portals to the alimentary and respiratory tracts. They are the first line of exposure to agents that are taken into the body during eating and breathing. One defensive measure against harmful agents is the presence of a ring of lymphatic tissue that includes the **palatine tonsil**, **lingual tonsil**, and **nasopharyngeal** (or **pharyngeal**) **tonsil**. The tonsils form **lymphocytes** that are part of the body's protection against harmful microorganisms. Additional information on these lymphatic tissues is given later in this chapter.

Cranial and Facial Bones

The bony framework is a good place to begin, especially because the discussion of muscles and other soft tissues often will mention bony attachments and points of reference. This section introduces the major bones of the skull and face. The reader should be forewarned that, in the adult, most of these bones are tightly interlocked. Therefore, it can be difficult to isolate them from adjacent bones.

The bones of the cranium and some of the bones of the face are illustrated in Figure 5–6. The **cranium** is the bony case for the brain. Its topmost part, or skull cap, is sometimes called the **calvarium** (Christ was crucified on a hill called Calvary, or Golgotha, which was named after its skull-like appearance). The face includes the forehead as well as the skeletal framework of the eyes, nose, and mouth (Dickson & Maue-Dickson, 1982).

The classic growth curves for major body tissues were described by Scammon (1930) and are reproduced in Figure 5–7. Different tissues have different patterns of growth and development. The cranium follows the neural growth curve, which ensures that the cranium keeps pace with

Bones of the Skull

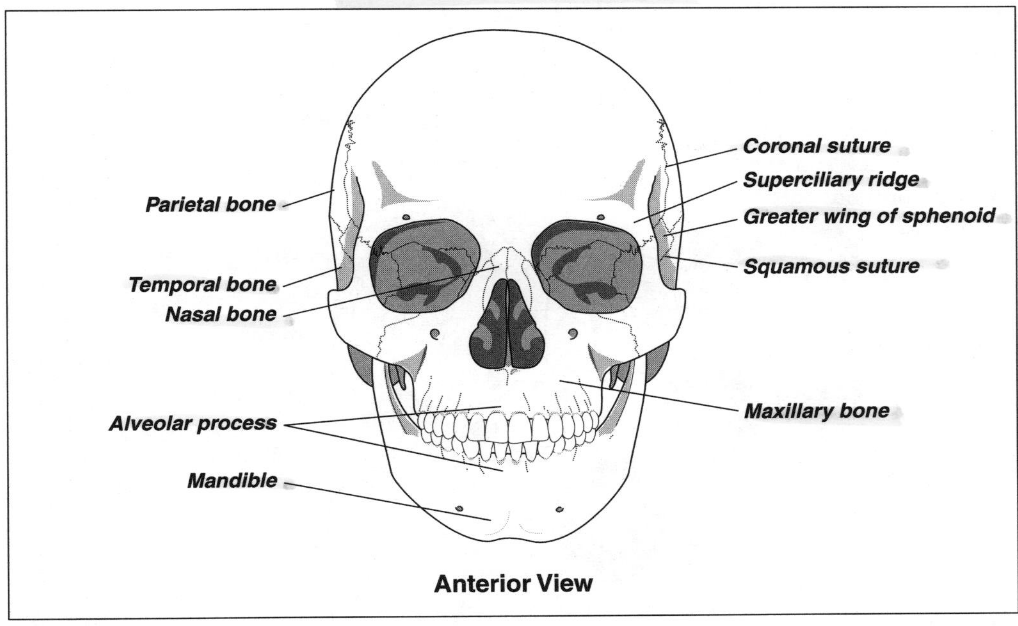

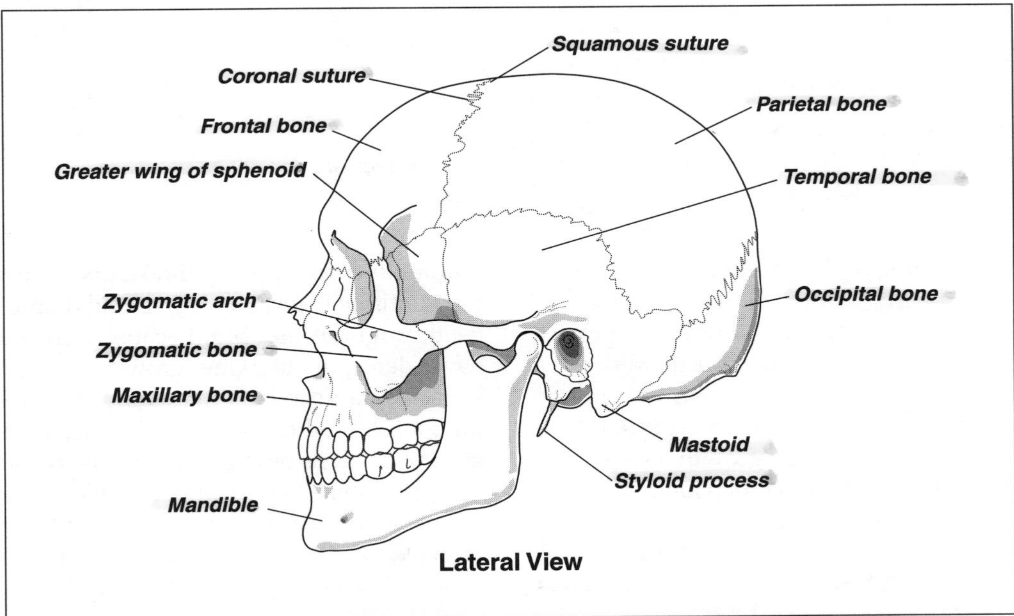

Figure 5-6. The bones of the face and cranium, shown in anterior, lateral, and inferior views. *(continued)*

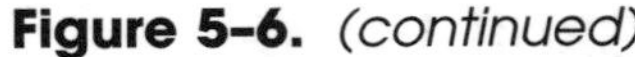
Figure 5–6. *(continued)*

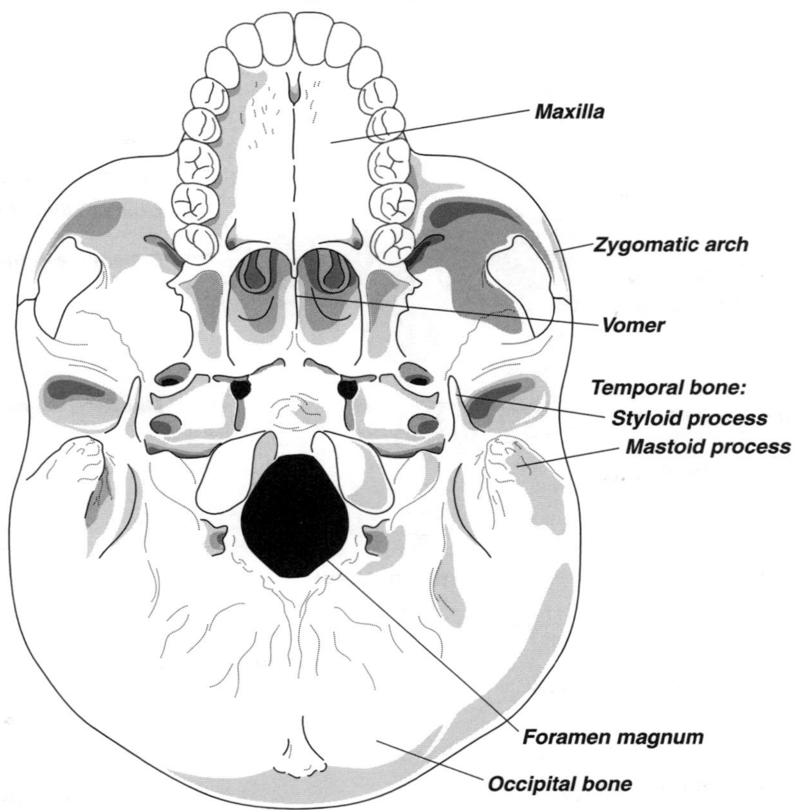

the growing brain. The brain and cranium reach nearly adult size by 6 to 8 years of age. These structures have an early growth acceleration and reach maturity in size at a very young age. In contrast, the middle and lower front regions of the face follow the general somatic growth curve. The growth occurs over a much longer interval than for the cranium, with adultlike size of the lower face reached at about 16 to 18 years. Humans, like mammals and birds generally, have a **determinate bone growth**, meaning that growth of the bones ceases at maturity. Some other species, particularly reptiles, have indeterminate bone growth. Dinosaurs are suspected to have had indeterminate growth, which could explain their often monstrous proportions (Chinsamy & Dodson, 1995). In reptiles and presumably dinosaurs, bones can continue to grow in length and diameter throughout life. But, because humans have determinate bone growth, certain kinds of surgery in humans are delayed until adulthood to avoid interference with growth patterns or to prevent postsurgical complications. For example, rhinoplasty (surgical reconstruction of the nose) for cosmetic or nonurgent medical purposes usually is done in young adulthood rather than childhood.

An important theory of bone growth in the craniofacial complex is the **functional matrix theory** (Moss, 1968), which holds that the growth and development of bone is largely determined by the forces exerted on the bones by muscular actions. That is,

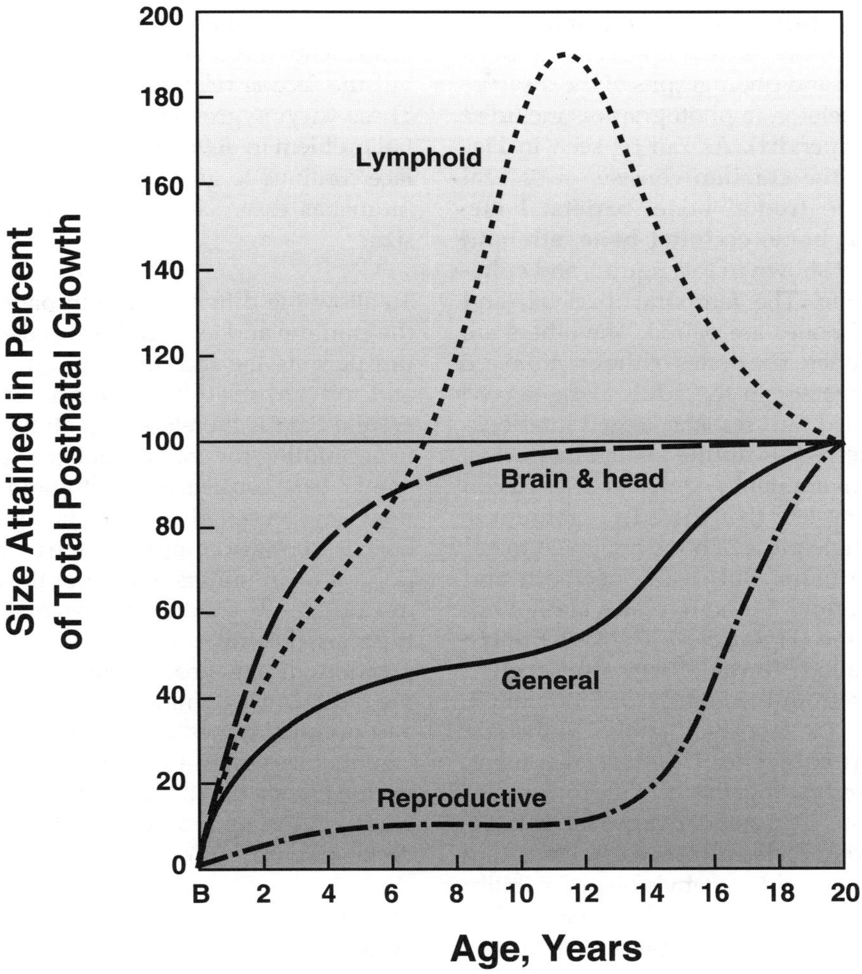

Figure 5–7. The classic growth curves of human tissues.

function determines structure. It is posited that there is no genetic blueprint for bony growth other than a general instruction to ossify (Ranly, 1988). As ossification proceeds, bones assume shapes that reflect the functions of the craniofacial complex. The structures involved in speech are shaped to a large degree by the forces developed during feeding, that is, chewing and swallowing. For this reason, some specialists believe that children with problems in chewing and swallowing may be at risk for maldevelopment of the oral structures that eventually serve speech.

Before turning to study of the individual bones of the skull and face, it is helpful to note that many of these bones become tightly fused in the adult, so that it can be difficult to distinguish them. The neonate's skull contains 45 separate bones, compared to only 22 in the adult (Lowrey, 1973). Pierce, Mainen, and Bosma (1978) is a good source of information on the bones of the neonate. The bones do not disappear with development; rather, they become locked together to form a rigid bony vault. Once they are fused, they can be separated only with considerable force.

The individual bones of the cranium and face are more easily appreciated from drawings and photographs of the disarticulated skeleton (a photograph is included in the appendix). As can be seen in Figure 5–6, the cranium consists of several bones, the **frontal bone, parietal bone, temporal bone, occipital bone, ethmoid bone** (not shown in this figure), and **sphenoid bone**. The temporal, parietal, and ethmoid bones are paired. The others are single bones. The bones of the cranium are fused together in the adult along jagged lines called **sutures** (the jagged interlocking patterns are captured better by fractals than conventional geometry). The fusion is so complete that the adult cranium is like a single piece of bone hollowed to encase the brain. But in the newborn and young infant, the bony plates are not entirely fused (Figure 5–8). The larger openings, called **fontanelles** (also spelled *fontanels*, from the French for "fountain"), are what the layperson knows as the soft spots on a baby's head. With development, the plates fuse together and the fontanelles disappear. One good reason for the unfused bony plates during early life is that that they provide a baby's head flexibility as it passes through the birth canal. The malleability of the infantile skull is further demonstrated in the practices of a Native American group that shaped infant skulls by binding them to swaddling boards. The result of this practice was a flattened ovoid skull thought to be highly desirable. An inadvertent flattening of the infant skull can be produced if the baby is always positioned to lie on the same side of the head.

As Figure 5–6 illustrates, the front of the skull is formed primarily by the frontal bone; the sides by the frontal, parietal, and temporal bones; the back by the parietal and occipital bones; and the base by the occipital, ethmoid and sphenoid bones. The skull base is of particular importance in understanding the growth of the face relative to the cranium. Recall that the cranium reaches adult size early in childhood, but the face is relatively slow to mature. These varying growth rates pose a potential problem in development: How can the face continue to grow even when the cranium has essentially reached its mature size?

To allow the different growth patterns of the cranium and face, the base of the cranium permits the face to grow downward and forward relative to the cranium. The **cranial base** is therefore of central interest in accounting for craniofacial growth. The cranial base consists of the ethmoid, sphenoid, and occipital bones. The sphenoid bone is a bone of complex shape that is important to an understanding of the anatomy of speech production. Its major features are illustrated in Figure 5–9, and its position in the head is shown in Figure 5–10. During childhood, the sphenoid and occipital bones are joined by a cartilage that serves as a major growth center for the cranial base. This union of the two bones is the **spheno-occipital synchondrosis** (Figure 5–11).

The following discussion considers the 14 facial bones (five paired bones and two un-

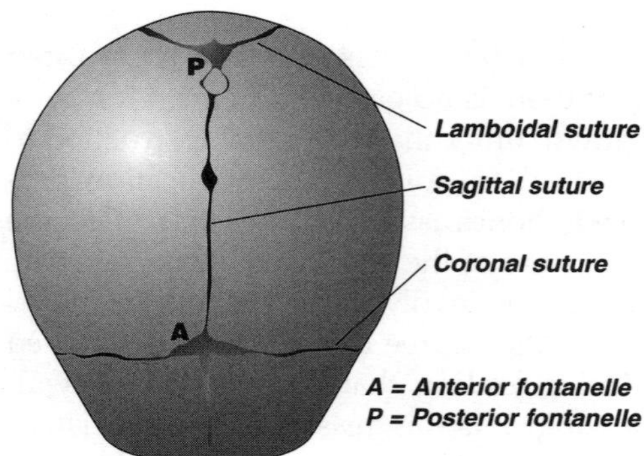

Figure 5–8. The sutures and fontanelles of the cranium.

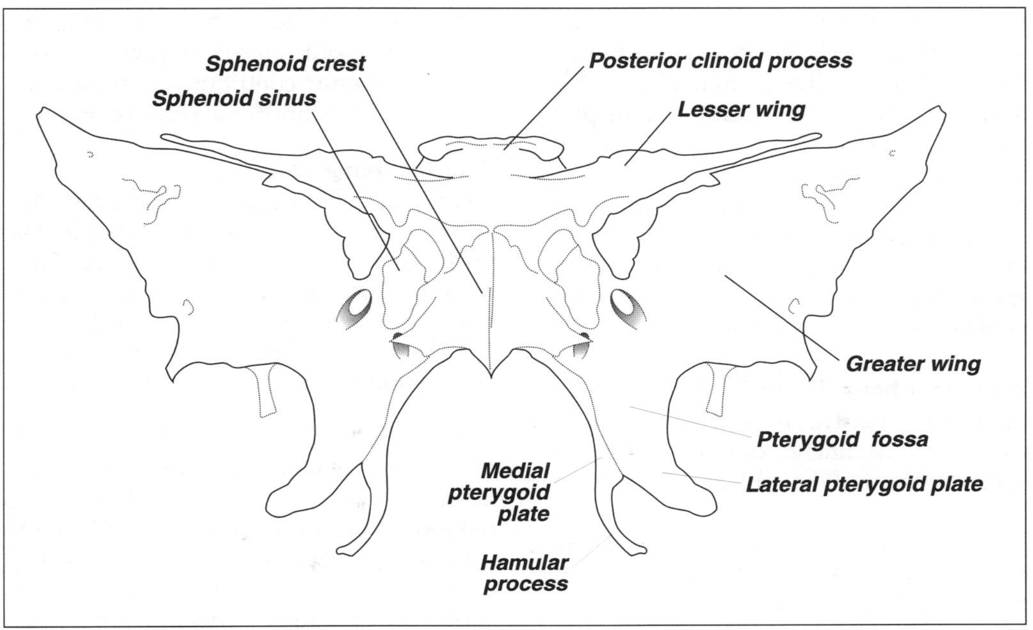

Figure 5-9. The sphenoid bone with major features labeled.

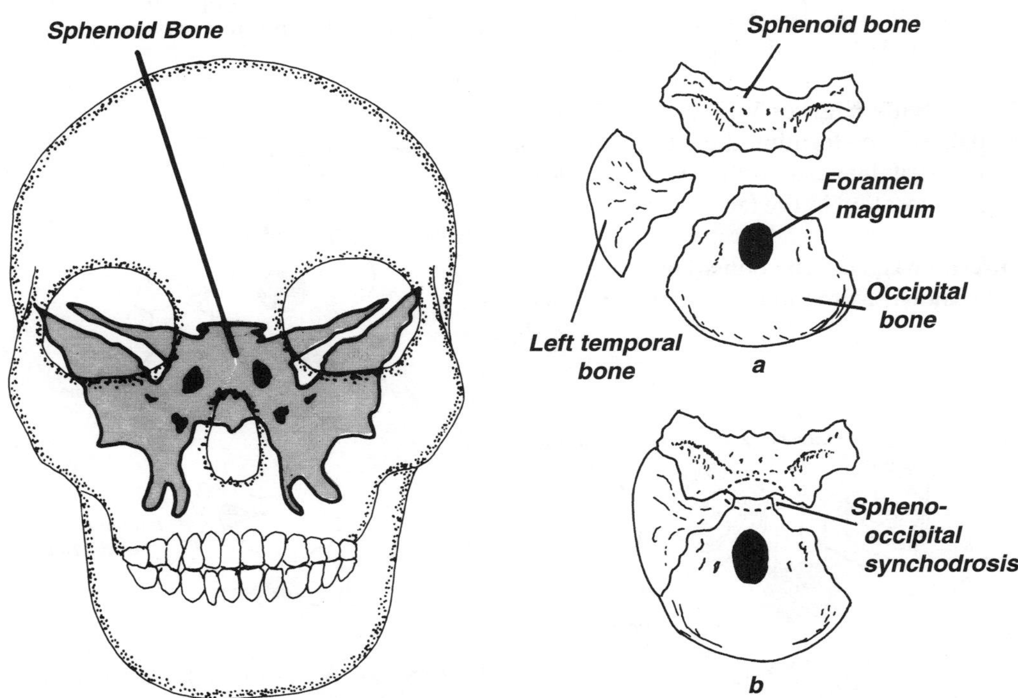

Figure 5-10. The sphenoid bone shown relative to the skull.

Figure 5-11. The spheno-occipital synchondrosis.

paired bones) one at a time. Unless otherwise stated, the listed bones are paired. Most of them are illustrated in Figures 5–6, 5–12, 5–13, and 5–14. In addition, the photograph in Figure 5–15 shows several of the bones discussed in this section. This photograph is especially helpful in understanding the relationships of the bones that form the oral and nasal cavities. It also shows the location of several sinuses (air pockets) to be discussed later.

Zygomatic bone (Figure 5–12) is also called the cheek bone. This bone does in fact give rise to the prominence of the cheek. It also forms the floor of the orbit of the eye.

Nasal bone (Figure 5–12) is a paired bone of oblong shape. The two bones lie adjacent to one another at the bridge of the nose.

Lacrimal bone (Figure 5–13) is a fragile bone that makes up the anteromedial wall of the orbit of the eye. It is associated with the lacrimal gland, which produces tears.

Vomer bone (Figures 5–14 and 5–15) is an unpaired bone forming the inferior-posterior part of the nasal septum. It has a midsagittal location in the face.

Inferior nasal concha bone (Figure 5–13) is also known as the inferior turbinate. This bone is often likened to a scroll positioned at the lateral wall of the nasal cavity. Its convoluted structure contributes to the air conditioning capability of the nasal passages.

Palatine bone (Figures 5–13 and 5–15) takes roughly the shape of the letter "L" (when viewed from front or behind) and is positioned at the posterior boundary of the nasal cavity. The vertical part of the palatine bone forms the posterior nasal cavity, and the horizontal part serves as the posterior section of the floor of the nasal cavity.

Maxilla bone (Figures 5–12, 5–13, 5–14, and 5–15) is sometimes called the maxilla or upper jaw. The maxillae help to form the roof of the mouth, the floor and lateral wall of the nose, one part of the eye orbit, and the maxillary sinus. Figure 5–15 shows how the maxilla bone separates the nasal and oral cavities.

Mandible bone, or simply the mandible, is of particular interest to the study of

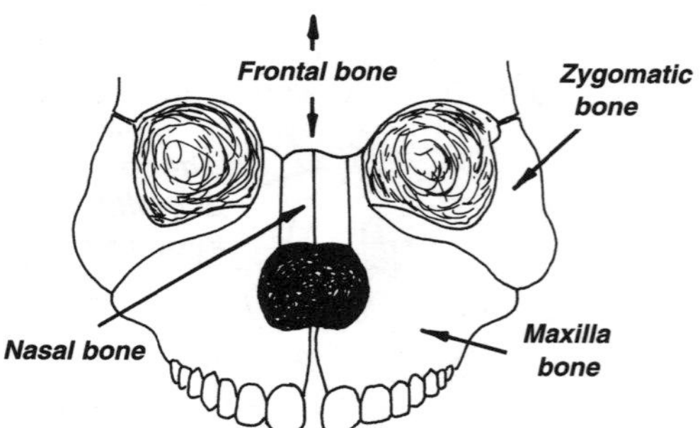

Figure 5–12. Schematic drawing of bones of skull and face, from anterior view.

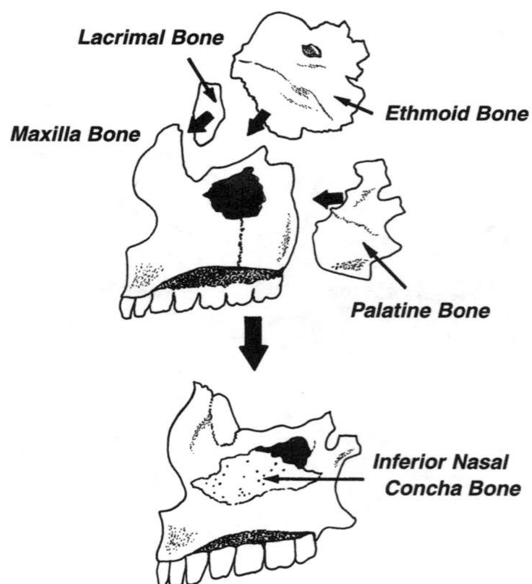

Figure 5–13. Selected facial bones related to the maxilla. The upper part of illustration shows the bones separately; the lower part shows their fused appearance.

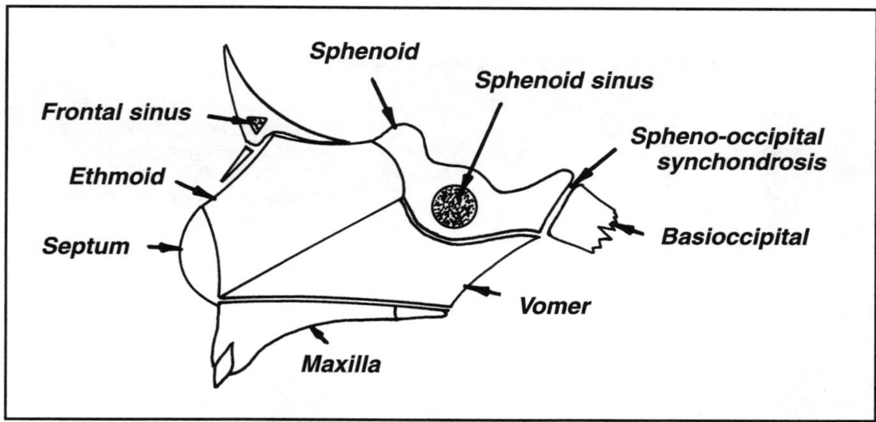

Figure 5–14. Schematic drawing of a midsagittal section to show selected bones of skull and face.

speech and other oral functions and therefore is discussed in some detail. The mandible is shown in Figure 5–16. It is considered an unpaired bone but, in fact, is the result of the fusion of two bones. Because the fusion is accomplished at birth or shortly thereafter, it is considered an unpaired bone.

The mandible is the only movable bone in the craniofacial skeleton. Movement is possible because of the **temporomandibular joint (TMJ)** formed by the insertion of the **condyle** or **condyloid process** into the articular disk of the mandibular fossa of the temporal bone (Figure 5–17). The temporomandibular joint permits a hingelike motion, a sliding motion, and lateral motion of the jaw. The maximum opening of the mandible is about 55–60 mm (33° of angular variation) in men and about 50–55 mm (35° of angular variation) in women (Pullinger, Liu, Low, & Tay, 1987). The normal resting position of the jaw allows a small incisal opening of about 3 mm in adults (Niswonger, 1934). The TMJ is subject to dysfunctions that can result in joint pain, limitations in opening, locking, and an audible click on (jaw) opening movements. Symptomatic TMJ dysfunction may be experienced by as much as one quarter of the adult population (Solberg, Woo, & Houston, 1979).

The mandible grows by two basic means. One is the conversion of growing cartilage to bone. This conversion occurs primarily at the midline symphysis (active until about the end of the first year) and the condyles (active until adulthood). The second means of mandibular growth is the deposition and resorption of bone. That is, bone is deposited in some regions but resorbed in others. Growth of the mandible through bone deposition occurs primarily at the alveolar margin, posterior border of the ramus, and upper edge of the ramus (including the condyle, coronoid process, and mandibular notch). Resorption occurs at the anterior border of the ramus, and the mesial surface of the body and ramus. Growth of the mandible is shown schematically in Figure 5–18.

One of the largest studies of mandibular growth is Walker and Kowalski's (1972) report on 800 typical white American subjects. Their data showed that mandibular growth was slow and steady for females between 8 and 20 years of age. The mandible grew rapidly in males between 12 and 16 years. Moss, Moss-Salentijn, and Ostre-

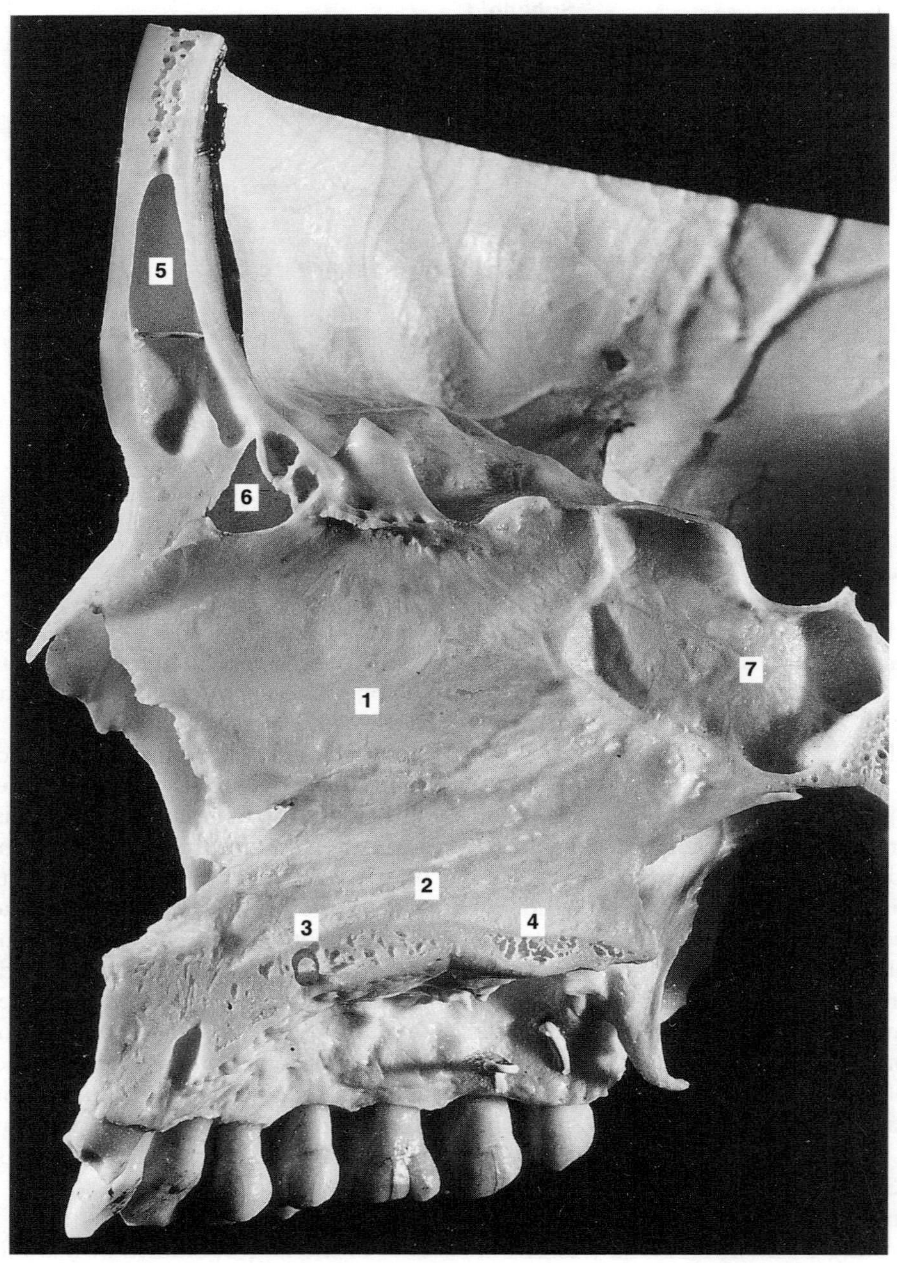

Figure 5–15. Bony nasal septum and related paranasal sinuses. 1 = perpendicular plate of ethmoid bone, 2 = vomer bone, 3 = nasal crest of maxilla bone, 4 = nasal crest of palatine bone, 5 = frontal sinus, 6 = ethmoid sinus, and 7 = sphenoid sinus. (Photograph courtesy of Joel C. Kahane.)

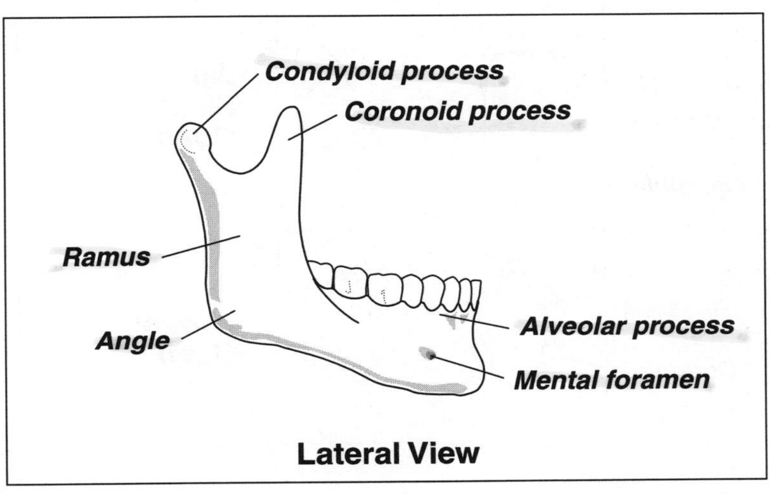

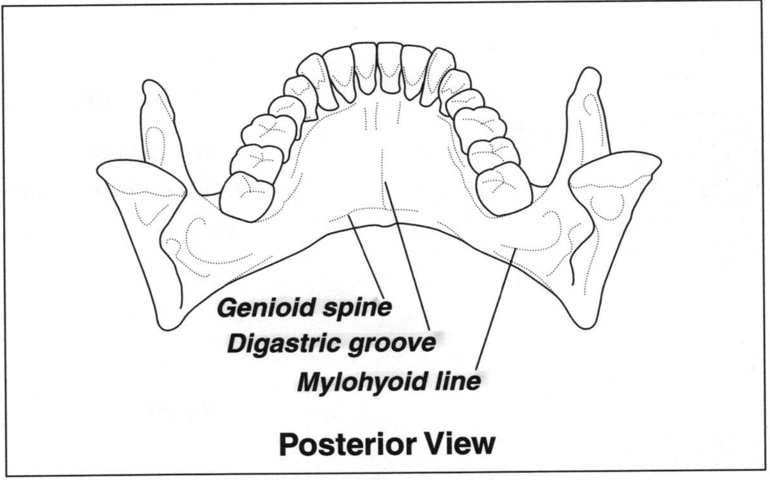

Figure 5–16. Lateral and posterior views of the mandible or jaw bone.

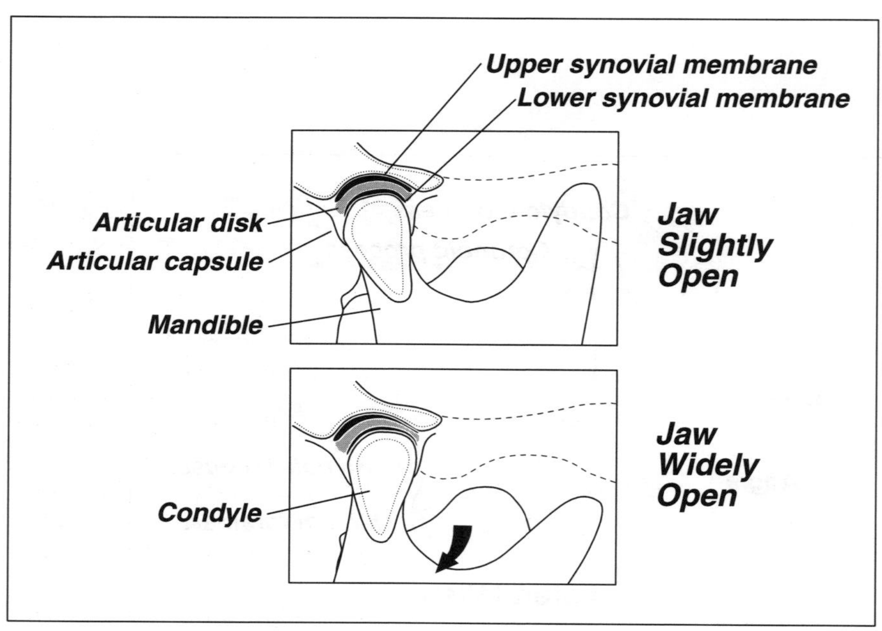

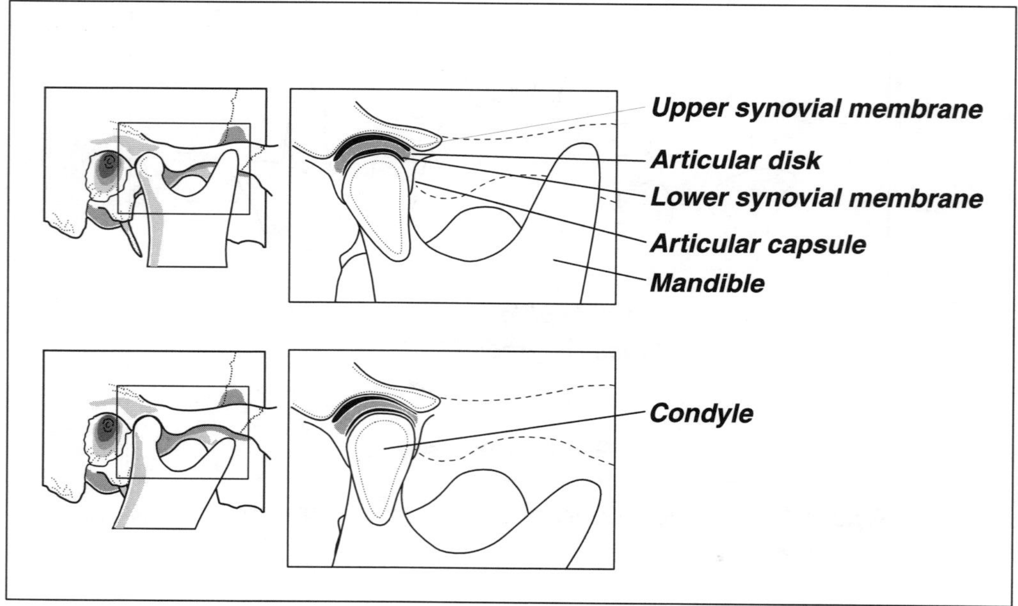

Figure 5-17. The temporomandibular joint.

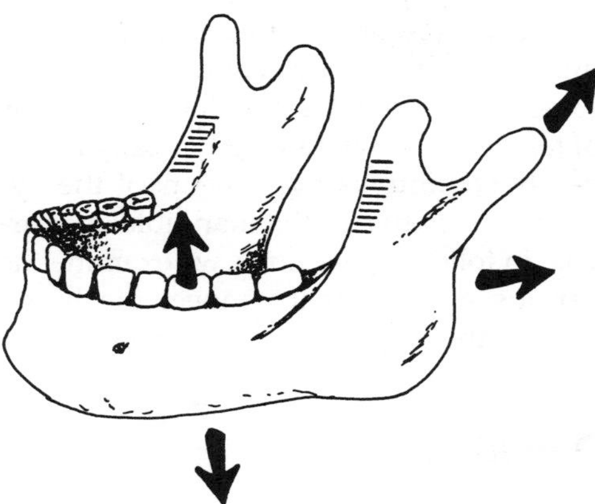

Figure 5–18. Growth of the mandible. The arrows indicate major directions of growth; the dashed lines indicate regions of bone resorption.

icher (1974) described the growth of the mandible as follows:

1. It is **allometric**, that is, it fits the relative growth curve, $y = bx^e$ (the natural number e is discussed in Chapter 2).
2. It can be described by a logarithmic growth curve (similar to the logarithmic spiral discussed in Chapter 2).
3. It is **gnomic**, meaning that it changes only in size and not shape.

The **hyoid bone** is pictured in relation to other structures in Figure 5–19 and individually in Figure 5–20. This bone is shaped like a horseshoe and supports both the tongue and larynx. The hyoid and mandible together can be regarded as the skeletal pedestals for the tongue. The hyoid bone is situated in the neck just above the larynx. It can be palpated quite easily in most people. To locate it, first touch your finger to the superior notch of the thyroid cartilage. Then, move your finger upward slightly until you feel a bony projection. This is the hyoid bone. In most people, it is located roughly parallel to the lower border of the mandible. However, in infants, the hyoid is positioned relatively higher than in the adult. A good anatomic reference for the hyoid position is its level relative to the

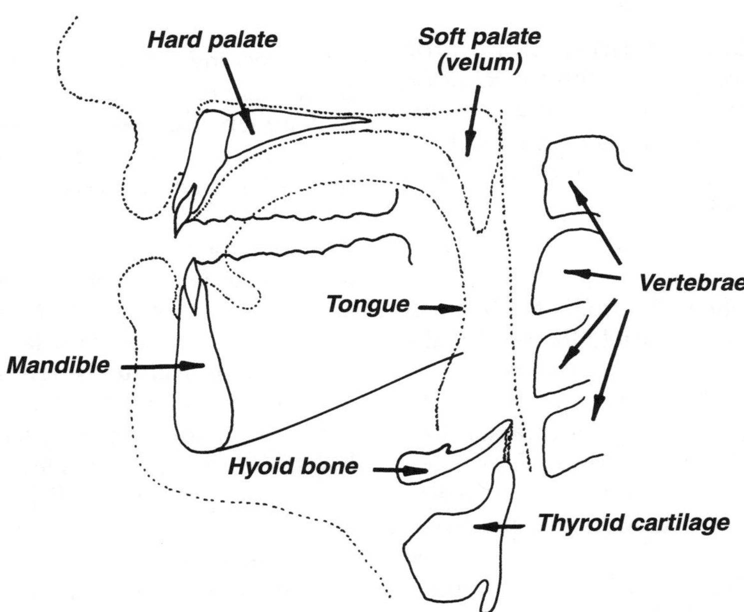

Figure 5–19. The hyoid bone relative to major craniofacial structures.

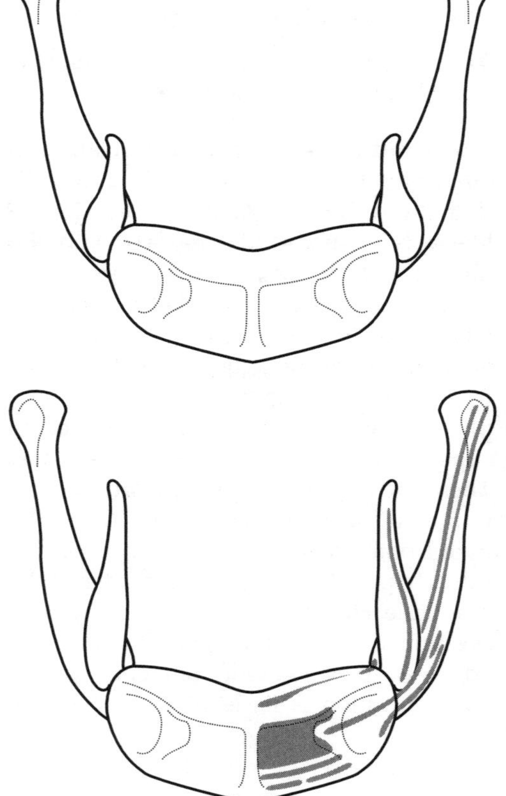

Figure 5–20. The hyoid bone. The upper drawing shows the hyoid bone from a superior view. The lower drawing shows muscle attachments as shaded regions on a superior view of the hyoid bone.

cervical vertebrae. In adults, the hyoid is situated at approximately the level of the body of the fourth cervical vertebra, but in infants it is located near the junction of the second and third cervical vertebrae (Ardran & Kemp, 1972; Bench, 1963). A cephalometric study of children between 6.5 to 17.5 years of age showed that the hyoid bone descended by up to 33 mm in some individuals (Blocquel, Laude, Lafforgue, & Devillers, 1990). The hyoid is the sole floating bone in the human body. It has no direct attachments to other bones, and this freedom from osseous connections is one reason for its variable position. X-ray films of talking and swallowing typically reveal nearly continuous movements of the hyoid bone relative to the mandible and larynx. In following sections, we examine the various muscles that connect the hyoid bone to the tongue, mandible, and larynx.

Dentition

> *"The teeth are very important in many functions of the body. They are essential for protecting the oral cavity and in aquiring and chewing food, as well as in aiding the digestive system in breaking down food. They are necessary for proper speech, and their appearance can be a very positive sexual attraction."*
>
> (R. W. Brand & D. E. Isselhard, *Anatomy of Orofacial Structures*. St. Louis: C. V. Mosby, 1977, p. 3).

The foregoing discussion of the bones of the face is a foundation for a consideration of dentition. The teeth insert into the maxillary and mandibular bones. Like bones, the teeth are a hard structure.

Although the teeth begin to develop in the fetus, their first visible emergence is at about 6 months of age. The first set of teeth is referred to as the **milk teeth**, **primary dentition**, or **deciduous dentition**. Whatever they are called, their basic property is that they are the temporary teeth of childhood. The arrangement of teeth in this first set is illustrated in Figure 5–21. The second set of teeth begin to emerge at about 4 years of age and these teeth are called the **secondary dentition**, or **permanent dentition**. The arrangement of teeth in this second set is shown in Figure 5–22. The teeth

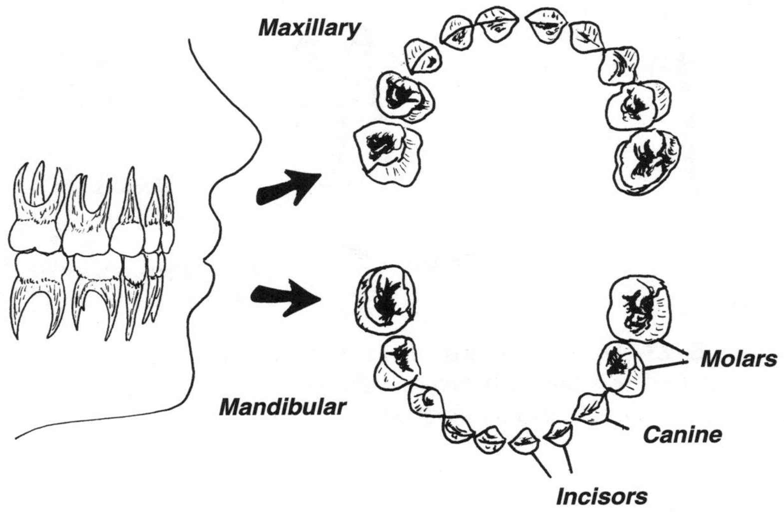

Figure 5–21. The arrangement of teeth in the primary dentition.

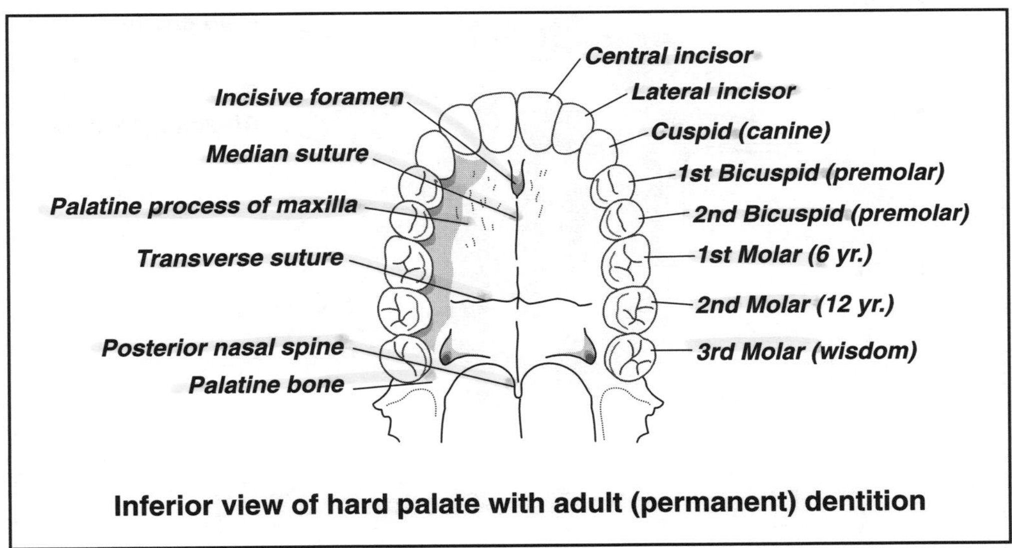

Figure 5–22. The arrangement of teeth in the secondary dentition.

in both the deciduous and permanent dentition can be regarded as units embedded in the alveolar processes of the maxilla and mandible. Each tooth consists of three parts shown in Figure 5–23: **crown, neck,** and **root**. Additional parts of a tooth can be seen in the diagrammatic longitudinal sections of Figures 5–24 and 5–25 (these two figures illustrate different types of teeth). The crown, the exposed portion of the

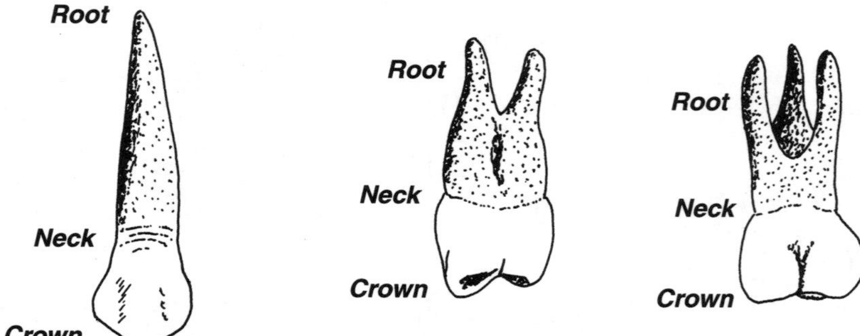

Figure 5–23. Major divisions of a tooth: crown, neck, and root. Three different types of teeth are shown. Note variations in root: single, bifurcated, and trifurcated.

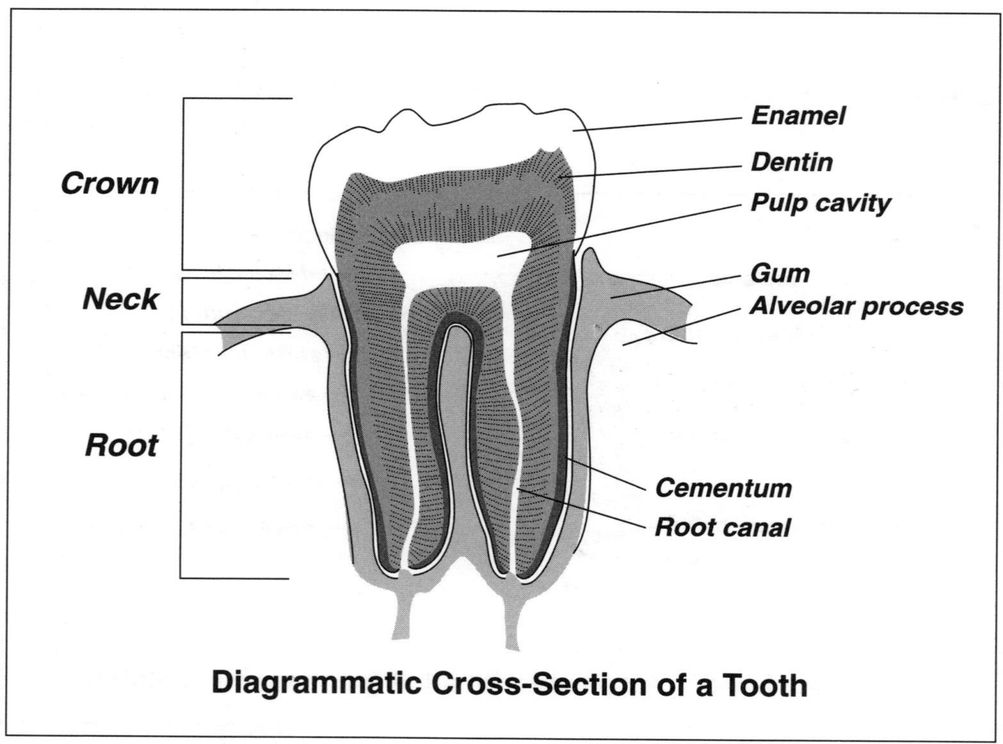

Figure 5–24. The structure of an individual tooth (molar), shown in cross-section. The tooth has a bifurcated root.

tooth, is covered with **enamel**, which is the hardest substance in the body. **Dentin** makes up most of the tooth and encloses a cavity filled with dental pulp, the **pulp chamber**. The **root canal** is the extension of this chamber into the root of the tooth. The root is embedded in the tooth sockets (alveolus) and is secured by fibers of the **periodontal ligament**. These fibers, embedded in a mineral called **cementum**,

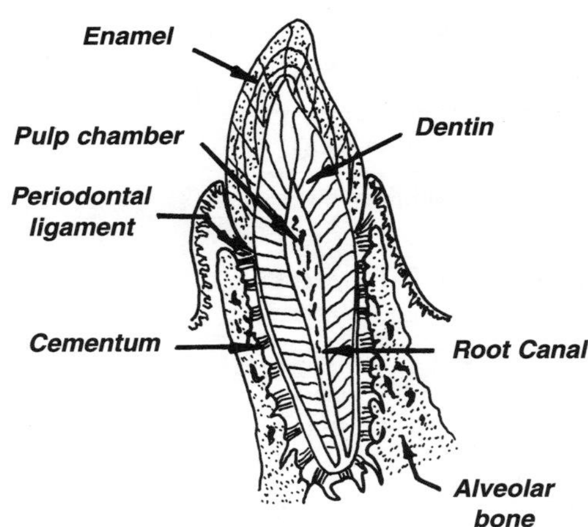

Figure 5-25. The structure of an individual tooth (incisor), shown in cross-section. The tooth has a single root.

connect the teeth in a chainlike fashion to give them a collective unity that is important to the understanding of dental growth and the practice of orthodontia. For example, one reason for orthodontic treatment is crowded teeth. Orthodontia can lead to a rearrangement of the teeth in the periodontal ligament. The essential idea is that the teeth are not simply independent units inserted in the tooth sockets. Rather, they are linked anatomically to serve as a functional unit.

The three important stages in dental development are (1) the initial mineralization or calcification, (2) crown completion, and (3) root completion. Calcification begins in utero for the deciduous teeth and postnatally for the permanent teeth. Careful inspection of the gums of a newborn will reveal tiny indentations. These recesses mark the eventual position of the primary teeth. The emergence of the teeth beyond the gums is called **emergence**. As shown in Table 5–1 the primary teeth begin to emerge at about 6 months and typically require another 20–24 months to complete their emergence by about 2½ years of age. The secondary teeth begin to emerge at about 4 years and require about 14 more years to complete their emergence at about 18 years of age. Wide individual variations are seen in the eruption of both the deciduous and permanent teeth. The normal variation in eruption can be 6 to 12 months on either side of the mean age for the deciduous teeth and 12 to 18 months on either side of the mean age for the permanent teeth. Calcification and emergence of the permanent teeth is earlier in girls than boys by about 1 to 6 months (Demirjian, 1980). But sex differences are not evident in the calcification of the deciduous teeth.

One clinical interest in dentition is that it might be used as one index of maturation. The degree to which dental status can be used as such an index depends on the correlation between dental status and other indexes of maturation, such as skeletal maturation. A number of studies have shown that the correlation between dental maturation and skeletal maturation is quite low (Demirjian, 1980). Lewis (1991) reported that dental ages and left hand-wrist skeletal ages were only moderately associated. For some subjects, the dental and skeletal ages differed by as much as 36 months. Widmer (1992) also concluded that there is only a small correlation between dental eruption time and skeletal maturity, body height, or psychomotor maturity.

The mandible and the dentition form a relationship called **occlusion**. Essentially, occlusion is the relation between the upper (maxillary) and lower (mandibular) dental arcades. One of the most popular systems used to describe occlusion is **Angle's classification**, which consists of three occlusal relationships based on the relative positions of the maxillary and mandibular first permanent molars (Figure 5–26).

Angle's Class I (neutrocclusion)—The first permanent molar of the maxilla is about one-half tooth posterior to the first permanent molar of the mandible. Individual teeth may be misaligned or rotated, but the occlusion is normal.

Table 5-1. Emergence of the primary and secondary dentition.

	Eruption	Shedding
	Primary Dentition	
Central incisors		
Maxillary	6–8 months	7–8 years
Mandibular	5–7 months	6–7 years
Lateral incisors		
Maxillary	8–11 months	8–9 years
Mandibular	7–10 months	7–8 years
Cuspids (canines)		
Maxillary	16–20 months	11–12 years
Mandibular	16–20 months	9–11 years
First Molars		
Maxillary	10–16 months	10–11 years
Mandibular	10–16 months	10–12 years
Second molars		
Maxillary	20–30 months	10–12 years
Mandibular	20–30 months	11–13 years
	Secondary Dentition	
Central incisors		
Maxillary	7–8 years	
Mandibular	6–7 years	
Lateral incisors		
Maxillary	8–9 years	
Mandibular	7–8 years	
Canines (cuspids)		
Maxillary	11–12 years	
Mandibular	9–11 years	
First premolars (bicuspids)		
Maxillary	10–11 years	
Mandibular	10–12 years	
Second premolars (bicuspids)		
Maxillary	10–12 years	
Mandibular	11–13 years	
First molars		
Maxillary	6–7 years	
Mandibular	6–7 years	
Second molars		
Maxillary	12–13 years	
Mandibular	12–13 years	

(continued)

	Eruption	Shedding
Third molars		
Maxillary	17–22 years	
Mandibular	17–22 years	

Source: Adapted from "Developmental Pediatrics" (p. 32) in *Nelson Textbook of Pediatrics* (13th ed.) edited by R. E. Behrman & V. C. Vaughan, 1987, Chicago: W. B. Saunders.

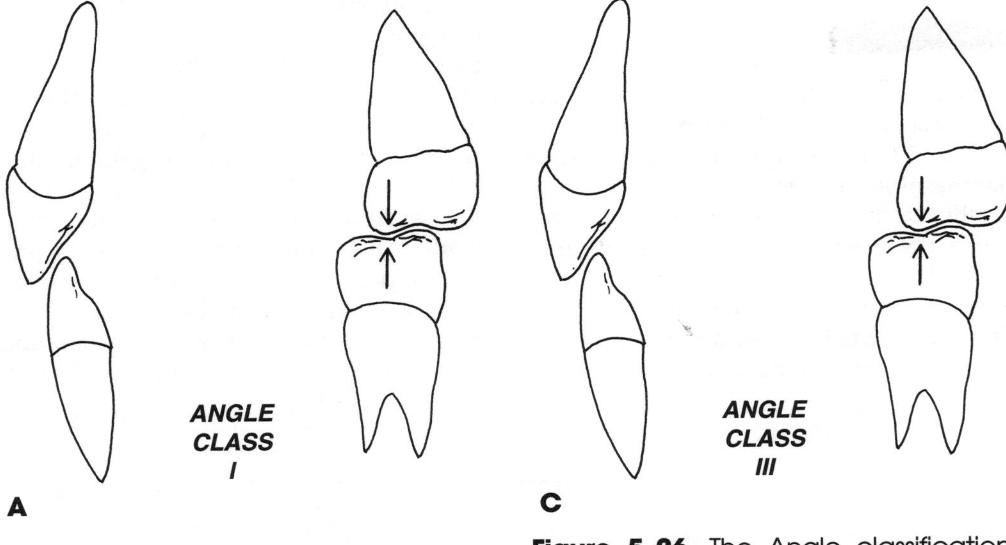

Figure 5-26. The Angle classifications of occlusion: Class I, Class II, and Class III.

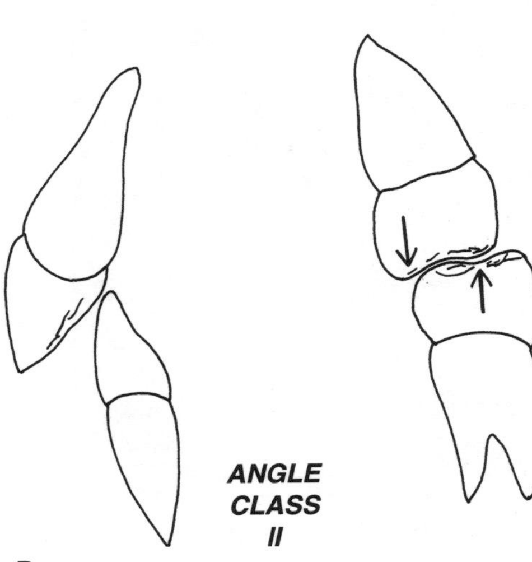

Angle's Class II (distocclusion)—the first mandibular molar is posterior to the normal position defined in Class I.

Angle's Class III (mesiocclusion)—the first mandibular molar is anterior to the normal position defined in Class I.

It has been estimated that only about one-half of young people in the United States have normal jaw and dental relationships, with very severe malocclusions occurring in about 15% of the population (Evans, 1994).

Occlusal patterns are typically established during infancy. The relation of the gum pads to the erupting teeth is stabilized during the first year of life, and occlusal contact for the first primary molars is achieved by the age of 16 months (Widmer, 1992). Once this occlusal contact is established, the jaw typically closes to the same position each time it is closed. Therefore, the age of about 16 months is an important time in the development of muscular control of the jaw.

The Sinuses

Certain of the bones of the face contain hollow spaces called **sinuses** (Figures 5–15 and 5–27). These are sometimes called **paranasal sinuses** in recognition of their location around the nasal structures. Because these cavities are air-filled, they make the head lighter and may contribute to some resonance phenomena in speech. The sinuses are lined with mucus (continuous with the mucous lining of the nasal passages) and drain into the nasal cavities. They are susceptible to infections, which result in a medical condition called **sinusitis** (meaning infection or inflammation of one or more sinuses). The sinuses are named after the bones in which they are found. They are the **frontal sinus, ethmoid sinus, sphenoid sinus,** and **maxillary sinus**. The maxillary sinuses, located directly beneath the eyes, are the largest and can be identified even in infants. One theory of the formation of the sinuses is that they are created as the facial bones grow out and away from the center of the craniofacial skeleton. At birth, the sinuses may be barely evident, but they grow in size, especially when the permanent teeth erupt and also following puberty (Mafee & Carter, 1995). Spaeth, Krugelstein, and Schlondorff (1997), reporting the results of a large study on sinus development, concluded that (1) the ethmoid cells are present in nearly all newborns; (2) the sphenoid sinus has a period of rapid growth extending from birth to about 5 years, and (3) the frontal sinus has a period of accel-

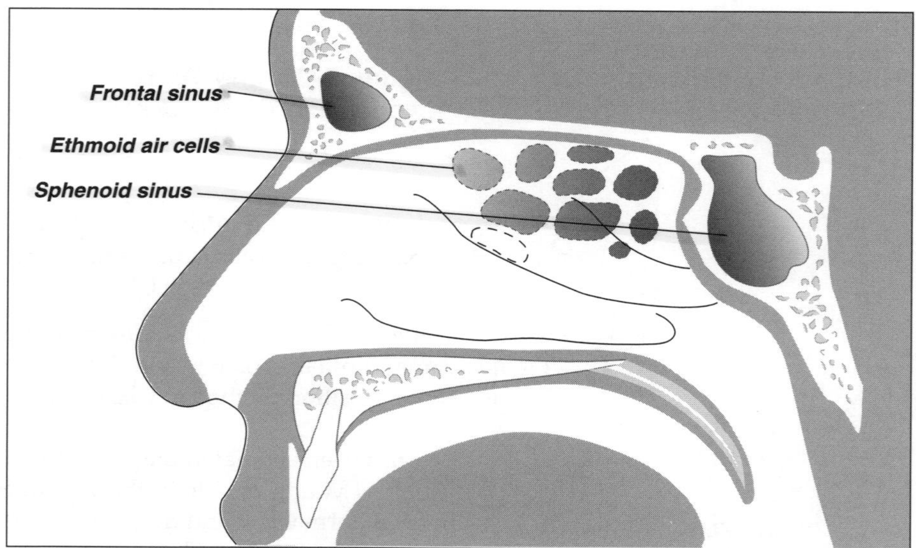

Figure 5–27. Sagittal section of the head showing the frontal, ethmoid, and sphenoid sinuses.

erated growth that begins at about 3 or 4 years and extends to about 12 years.

This completes the examination of the hard tissues of the cranium and face. Our attention now goes to the soft tissues, especially the muscles.

The Oral Cavity, Oropharynx, Nasopharynx, and Laryngopharynx

The oral cavity, as shown in Figure 5–1, connects to the pharynx. The pharynx may be divided into the regions of oropharynx, nasopharynx, and laryngopharynx. The oropharynx is the middle portion of the pharynx. It lies above the laryngopharynx and below the nasopharynx. The oropharynx is posterior to the oral cavity and anterior to the cervical vertebrae. It is shown in Figure 5–28. The oropharynx is important for the production of speech, for mastication, and for the early stages of swallowing. The oropharynx is closely associated with the oral cavity, and this discussion pertains to both.

As commented near the beginning of this chapter, the oral cavity and adjacent oropharynx are equipped with salivary glands that have a dual role of lubrication: first, they lubricate the bolus for swallowing, and, second, they lubricate the movements for speech. Most of the salivary output (about 65% of the 750 ml of daily salivary

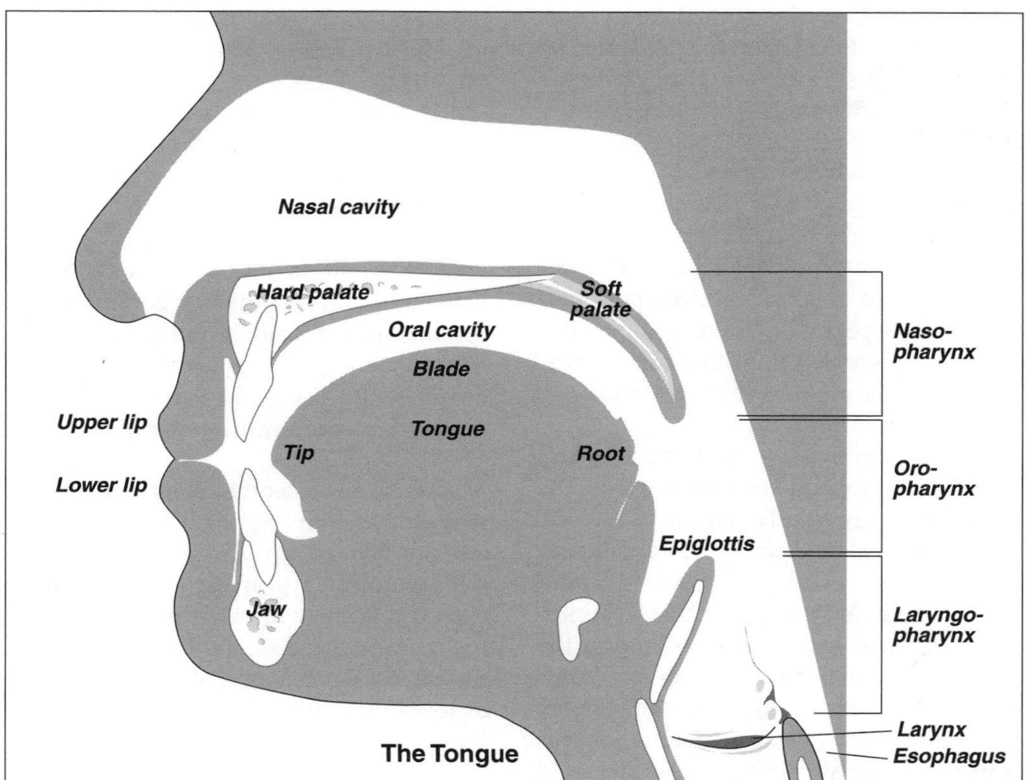

Figure 5–28. Midsagittal section of the head, showing the oropharynx, nasopharynx, and laryngopharynx.

secretion) comes from the **submandibular gland**, which can be palpated: Move your finger along the inferior border of the mandible, beginning just behind the point of the chin. As you move your finger backward, you should detect a small depression or notch on the inferior border. Stop at this point and then move your finger medially. You should feel a lump, which is the submandibular gland.

An additional 25% of salivary volume is produced by the **parotid gland** which is situated on the side of the face near the ear. This is quite a large gland but its salivary secretion is less than half that of the submandibular gland. Next in production of salivary volume at about 15% of the total volume is the **sublingual gland**, which is located near the anterior floor of the mouth, close to the mandibular canines. In addition to these glands, a number of minor salivary glands also produce fluids, but not in sufficient quantity to assist swallowing. They often are more important for tissue lubrication.

Situated immediately below the oropharynx, the laryngopharynx extends down to the entrances of the larynx and the esophagus. This deepest part of the pharynx is closely related to laryngeal structures, particularly the epiglottis. The laryngopharynx is in some respects a transition between the larynx and the supralaryngeal cavities.

The nasopharynx looks down directly into the oropharynx and laryngopharynx. The nasopharynx is closely related to the soft palate and will be discussed in detail later in the chapter. The laryngopharynx and nasopharynx are not easily viewed without the aid of instruments, although the oropharynx can be viewed with the unaided eye if the mouth is sufficiently open. One of the simplest instruments for this purpose is a small mirror such as that used by dentists. A more sophisticated approach is a fiberoptic instrument, which has its own light source.

We turn next to a discussion of the muscles that make up the primary functional components of the upper airway: jaw, tongue, lips and face, and pharynx.

The Jaw Muscles

The jaw muscles are also known as the muscles of mastication, the deep facial muscles, or the craniomandibular muscles. These muscles generally have their origins on the skull or other bony structure and insert on the mandible. Their primary actions are to perform the vertical and horizontal movements of mastication, but they also assist speech by contributing to movements of the lips and tongue. In addition, they stabilize the jaw for actions such as swallowing.

Elevation of the jaw is accomplished primarily by three paired muscles, the **mandibular elevators**, illustrated in Figure 5–29 and described as follows.

Temporalis muscle originates broadly on the temporal fossa of the temporal bone and its overlying fascia. The fanlike fibers converge and pass inferiorly to form a tendon that inserts on the anterior borders of the coronoid process and the ramus of the mandible. As might be imagined from its attachments, contraction of the temporalis muscle can elevate and retract the mandible.

Masseter muscle is actually a muscle with two groups of fibers, one being superficial and one being deep. The origin of the masseter is on the zygomatic arch. The fibers extend inferiorly to insert on the angle of the mandible and on the lateral surface of the ramus. Contraction of the masseter elevates the mandible and therefore closes the mouth opening.

Internal (medial) pterygoid muscle takes its origin from the lateral pterygoid plate. The fibers course inferiorly to insert on the

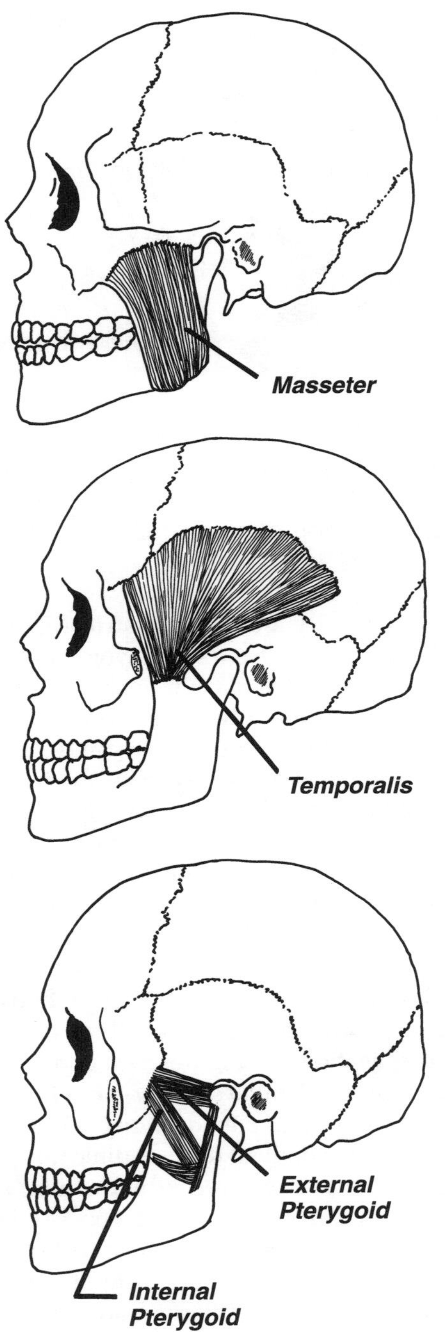

Figure 5–29. Selected jaw muscles including three muscles of mandibular elevation: masseter, temporalis, and internal (medial) pterygoid. One muscle of mandibular depression, the external (lateral) pterygoid also is shown.

ramus and the angle of the medial surface of the mandible. This muscle asists in elevating the mandible. The fibers of the internal pterygoid and masseter form a sling around the angle of the masseter. The pair of muscles is indeed sometimes called the **mandibular sling** (Figure 5–30).

The following muscles serve primarily to depress or lower the mandible. These **mandibular depressors** are illustrated in Figures 5–29, 5–31, and 5–32.

External (lateral) pterygoid muscle (Figures 5–29 and 5–31) is a two-headed muscle, meaning that it has two origins, both on the sphenoid bone. One origin is on the fossa of the great wing of the sphenoid bone; the other is on the lateral surface of the lateral pterygoid plate of the sphenoid bone. The course of the fibers is mostly horizontal as they reach their insertion on the neck of the condyle of the mandible and the articular disk of the temporomandibular joint. This muscle depresses (lowers) the mandible but alternating contraction of each side can produce lateral movements of the mandible. The relative positions of the internal and external pterygoid are most easily appreciated from an inferior view looking up through the mandible (Figure 5–33).

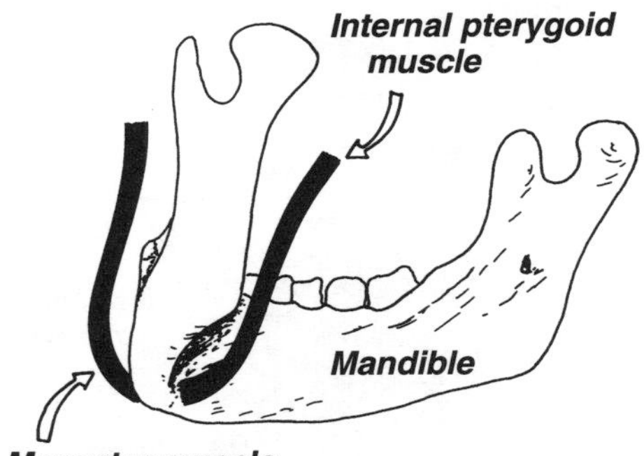

Figure 5–30. Illustration of how the masseter and internal pterygoid muscles form a sling for mandibular elevation.

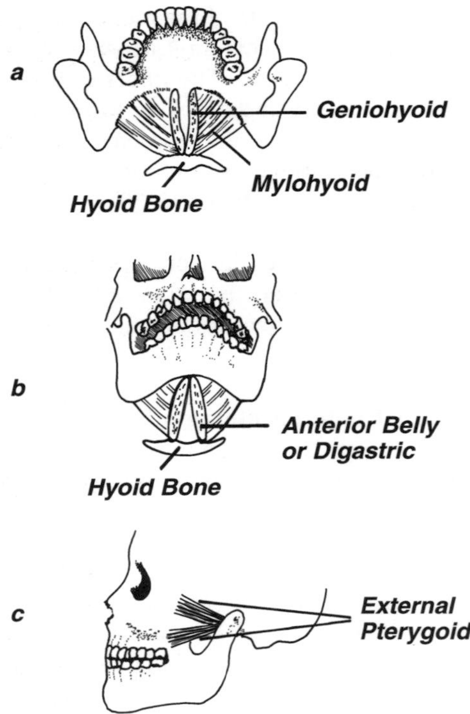

Figure 5–31. The muscles of mandibular depression: external pterygoid, anterior belly of digastric, mylohyoid, and geniohyoid.

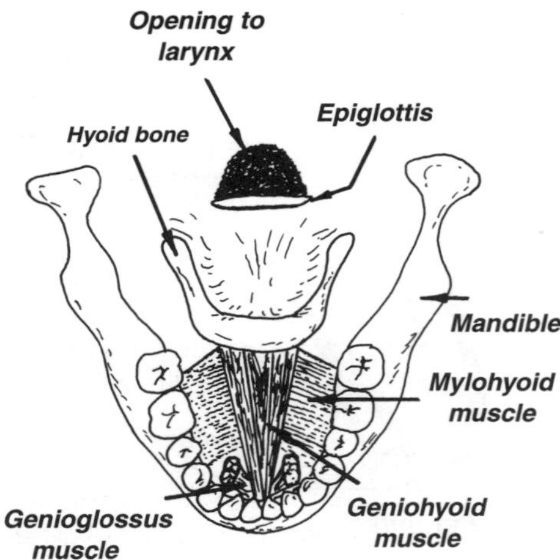

Figure 5–32. Superior view looking into mandible, hyoid bone, and epiglottis, to show the genioglossus, geniohyoid, and mylohyoid muscles.

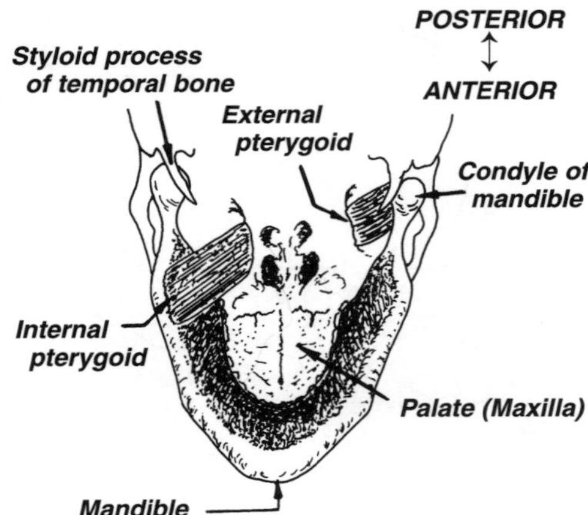

Figure 5–33. Inferior view looking up into mandible to show locations of internal and external pterygoid muscles.

Anterior belly of the digastric (Figure 5–31) is often listed as a suprahyoid muscle. The name *digastric* refers to its two bellies. The digastric muscle has a posterior and anterior belly, the latter of which can depress the mandible. It originates on the deep surface of the jaw and runs posteriorly and inferiorly to insert on a tendon, which in turn attaches to the hyoid bone. If the hyoid bone is fixed, then contraction of the anterior belly of the digastric can lower the jaw.

Mylohyoid muscle, another suprahyoid muscle, forms the muscular floor of the mouth, as shown in Figures 5–31 and 5–32. This muscle originates on the **mylohyoid line**, a ridge that extends along the deep surface of the body of the mandible roughly from the symphysis (midline union) to the region of the third molar. Its fibers then course medially and somewhat posteriorly and inferiorly to meet with the contralateral muscle at the **median raphe**, a line of connective tissue. The mylohyoid muscle can lower the jaw if the hyoid bone is stabilized.

Geniohyoid muscle (Figures 5–31 and 5–32) also is a suprahyoid muscle. It runs from the deep surface of the mandibular symphysis posteriorly to the body of the hyoid bone. This is a paired muscle, with its bellies situated on either side of midline. Its course is roughly parallel with that of the anterior belly of the digrastric, which is inferior to the geniohyoid.

The elevators are particularly strong muscles, given the need for breaking food particles. Jaw closing strength is considerable, great enough to break teeth if not carefully regulated. Jaw closing force is monitored by specialized receptors that enable us to produce sufficient force to break up food particles while not damaging the dentition. The greater strength of the jaw closing muscles as compared to the jaw opening muscles is the trick of the alligator wrestler. Because the alligator has relatively weak muscles for jaw opening, the alligator's jaws can be held shut relatively easily by a human. But beware the open jaws!

> *Note:* See Exercise 5–6 for a discussion of a newly discovered muscle of mastication. If the existence of this muscle is confirmed, then textbook discussions of the muscles of mastication will have to be revised to include a muscle that escaped identification until 1996.

Tongue

> ***"Likewise the tongue is a small part of the body but it makes great boasts."***
>
> (James 3:5)

Here is an anatomy riddle: What do the following have in common: an elephant's trunk, an octopus' tentacle, and a human tongue? The answer (besides the obvious fact that the three words begin with the same letter, *t*) is that each of these organs is an example of a **muscular hydrostat**. This term is applied to muscular organs that do not have a skeleton of cartilage or bone. A muscular hydrostat is defined as a structure that maintains a constant volume as its muscles contract (Kier & Smith, 1985). A water-filled balloon is a crude analogy. Of course, the balloon does not possess muscles, but if the balloon is manipulated by hand, it exhibits some of the properties of the muscular hydrostat, especially the preservation of volume as it undergoes changes in shape. One of the mechanical advantages that a hard skeleton provides for movement is that it gives a rigid support against which muscles can operate. But what is the means by which a muscle devoid of bony or cartilaginous skeletal support can achieve its contractile force? An interesting property of a muscular hydrostat is that it provides its own skeletal support through muscular contraction and the incompressibility of its internal fluids. Without such internally generated skeletal support, the elephant could not lift heavy objects with its trunk, the octopus could not squeeze prey with its tentacles, and the tongue could not press against the insides of the mouth. By selective contraction of certain muscles, the muscular hydrostat can make a rigid support upon which the contraction of other muscle fibers can accomplish selective movements of other parts of the tongue.

The tongue can be functionally divided into five parts as shown in Figure 5–34: **body**, **root**, **dorsum**, **blade**, and **tip**. These divisions are particularly important in describing lingual actions to produce the sounds of speech. The body is the major mass of the tongue. The root is the portion that extends along the pharynx and in fact forms the anterior wall of the pharyngeal tube. The dorsum is the broad dorsal surface of the tongue. The blade is toward the front of the tongue just behind the tip.

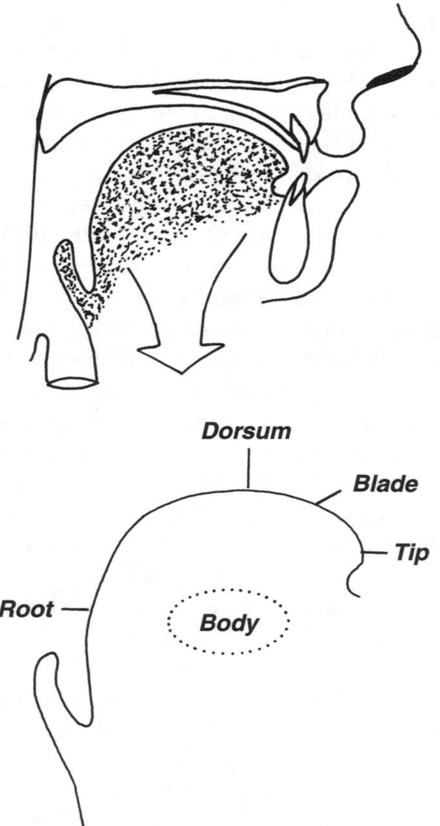

Figure 5–34. The functional divisions of the tongue: body, root, dorsum, blade, and tip.

The tongue is made up primarily of muscle, and the various muscles that form it are divided into two groups, intrinsic and extrinsic. These terms are defined in the same way as for the muscles of the larynx. Intrinsic muscles are muscles that have both attachments (origin and insertion) within the organ, itself. Extrinsic muscles have one attachment in the organ in question and another attachment on another structure. Because the tongue generally is mobile compared to the other structures to which it is connected, the origins of extrinsic muscles are outside the tongue and the insertions are inside the tongue.

The intrinsic muscles form a three-dimensonal matrix of motor fibers within the tongue (Figure 5–35). The intrinsic muscles are called the **superior longitudinal muscle** (running from back to front just under the lingual surface), **inferior longitudinal muscle** (also running from back to front and lying beneath the superior longitudinal muscle), the **transverse muscle** (running from side to side) and the **vertical muscle** (running from the oral surface to the mandibular surface of the tongue and therefore at right angles to both the longitudinal and transverse muscles). The intrinsic tongue muscles are responsible for fine movements of the tongue and are involved in the more delicate adjustments of shape and position.

The extrinsic muscles of the tongue connect the tongue to surrounding structures including the mandible, hyoid bone, palate, styloid process of the temporal bone, and pharynx. Each of these muscles includes the word *glossus*, or *glosso* (meaning "tongue") and another word indicating the external structure of attachment. Descriptions given here are quite general for two reasons: (1) this text is intended as an introduction to anatomy and not as an anatomical atlas, and (2) there are discrepancies and uncertainties in the anatomical literature pertaining to the tongue muscles (DiFoggio, 1984). Anyone who requires precise information on these muscles is advised to consult the literature carefully, taking into account the inconsistencies in muscle description.

The extrinsic muscles of the tongue are illustrated as a group in Figures 5–36, 5–37, and 5–38. Figure 5–36 depicts the general orientation of four of the muscles. Figure 5–37 shows a combination of intrinsic and extrinsic muscles. Figure 5–38 is a schematic drawing that represents the directions of muscle contraction for the extrinsic muscles as well as two of the intrinsics. It may

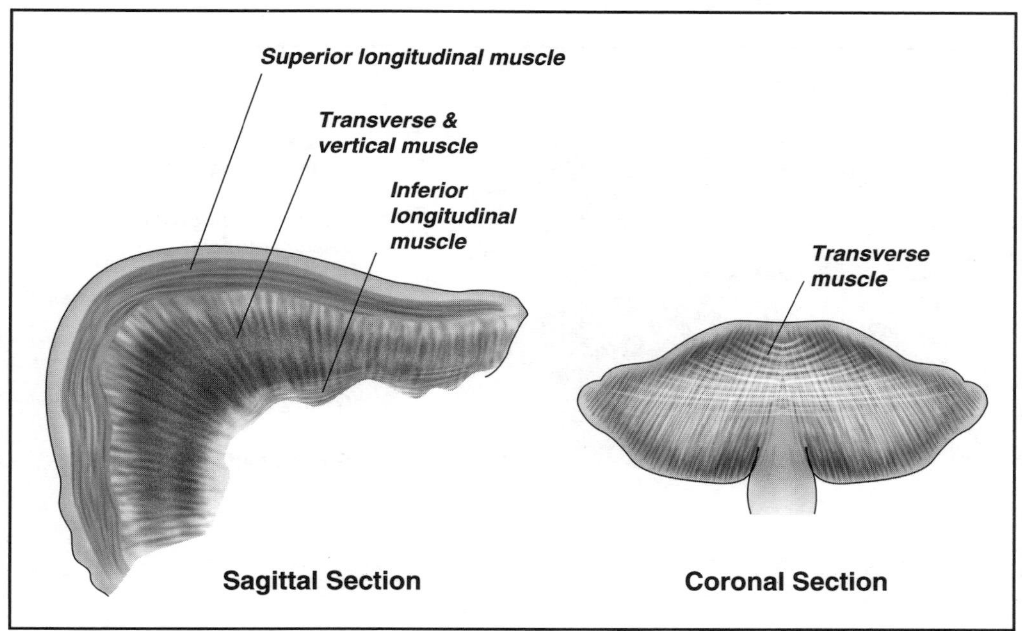

Figure 5–35. The intrinsic muscles of the tongue shown in sagittal and coronal sections: superior longitudinal, inferior longitudinal, vertical, and transverse.

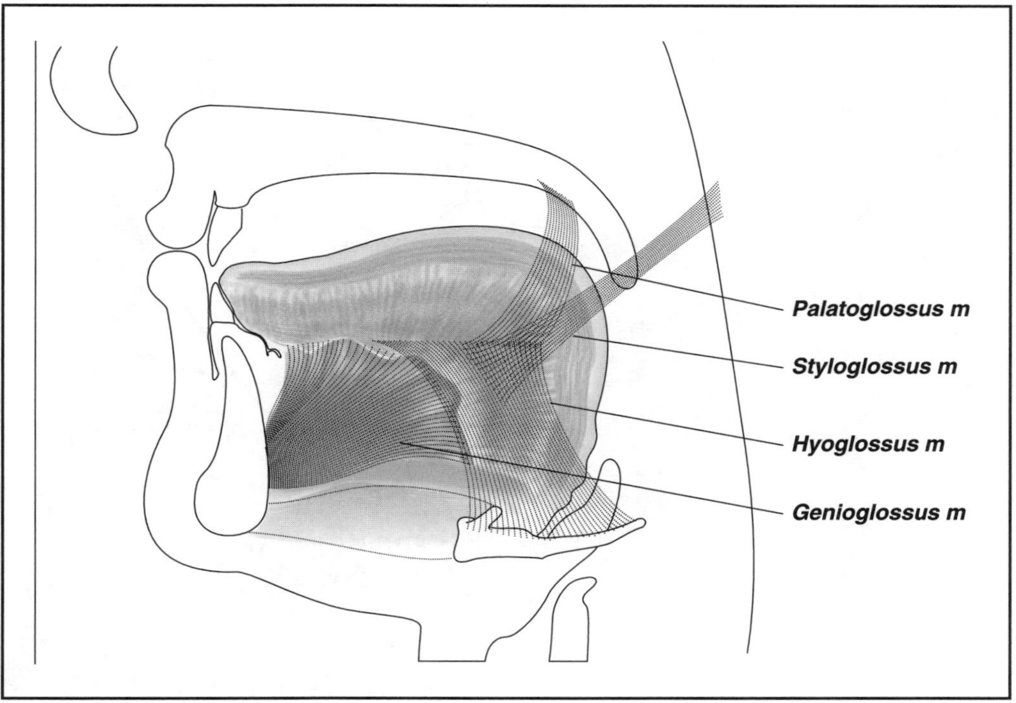

Figure 5–36. The extrinsic muscles of the tongue: palatoglossus, styloglossus, hyoglossus, and genioglossus.

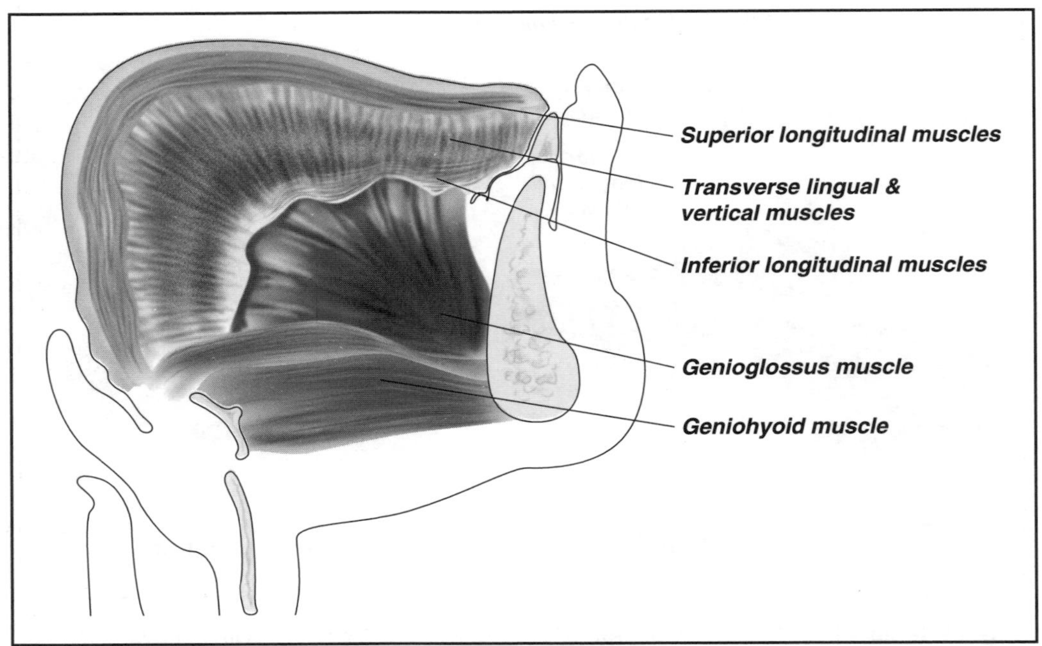

Figure 5–37. The genioglossus and geniohyoid muscles shown along with the intrinsic tongue muscles in a midsagittal section.

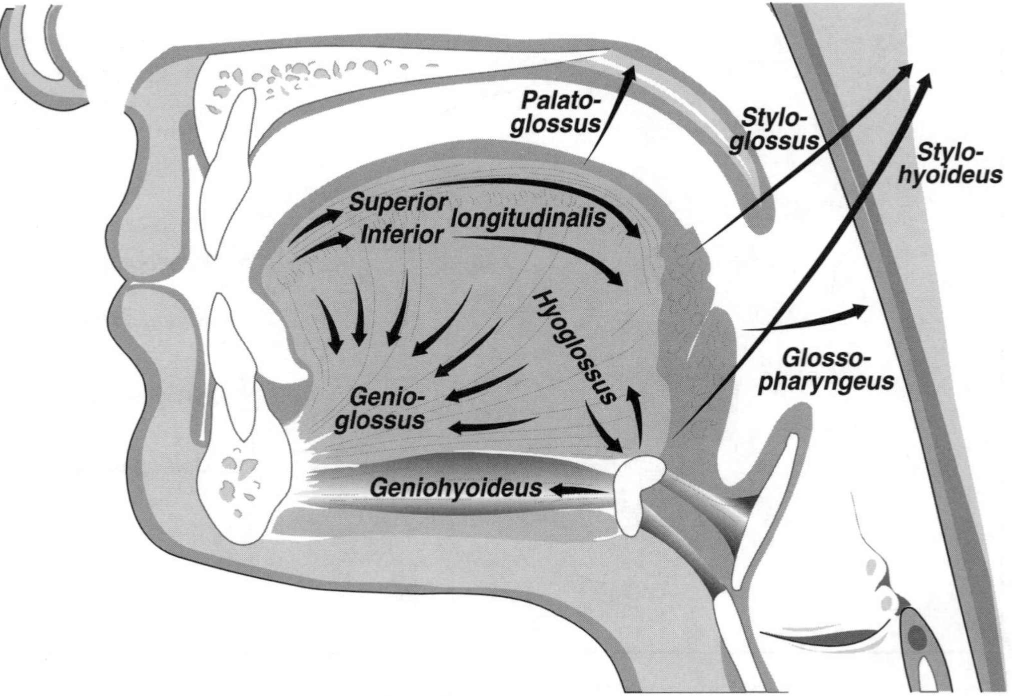

Figure 5–38. The actions of the extrinsic tongue muscles. The superior and inferior longitudinal muscles also are shown.

be helpful to compare the drawings of the individual muscles that follow with these composite illustrations to understand their relationships. The extrinsic muscles follow with brief descriptions:

Genioglossus muscle (Figure 5–39) makes up much of the bulk of the tongue. Its fibers fan outward from its origin on the midline of the lingual surface of the mandible to insert widely over the tongue (from apex to root) and even the hyoid bone. Various authorities recognize different fiber groups of the genioglossus. Depending on which fibers contract, this muscle can protrude the tongue tip, depress the tongue, or form a midline groove.

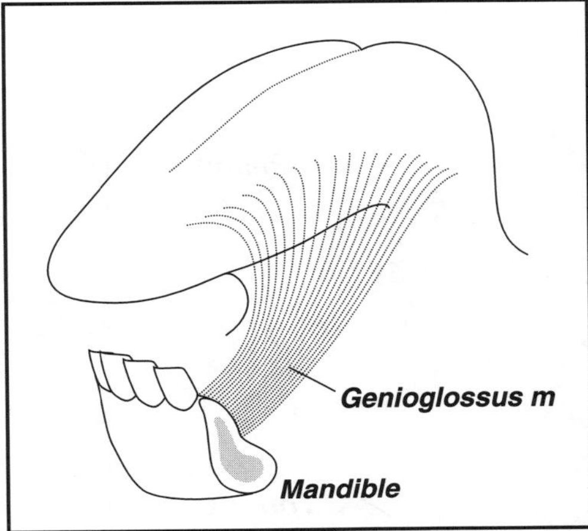

Figure 5–39. The genioglossus muscle.

Hyoglossus muscle (Figure 5–40) originates on the greater cornu of the hyoid bone and inserts on the sides of the posterior part of the tongue. It acts to depress the tongue and pull it backward.

Palatoglossus muscle (Figure 5–41) is also called the **glossopalatine** muscle. Later in this chapter, this muscle will be included in the discussion of the muscles of the palate. That is, this muscle can be regarded as both a tongue muscle and a palatal muscle (DiFoggio, 1984). Furthermore, its origin and insertion can be reversed between tongue and palate, depending on which structure is the more mobile. The term "palatoglossus" suggests that the palate is the origin (hence fixed) and the tongue is the insertion (hence movable). The palatoglossus has its origin in the palatal raphe (the midline of the palate) and inserts on the tongue, primarily the superficial mus-

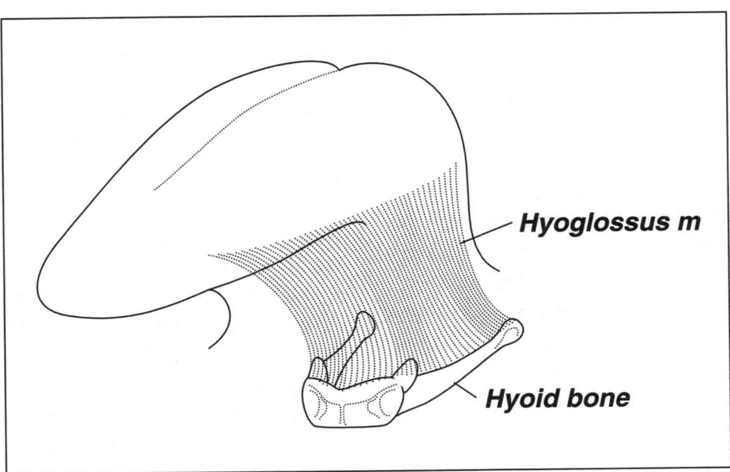

Figure 5–40. The hyoglossus muscle.

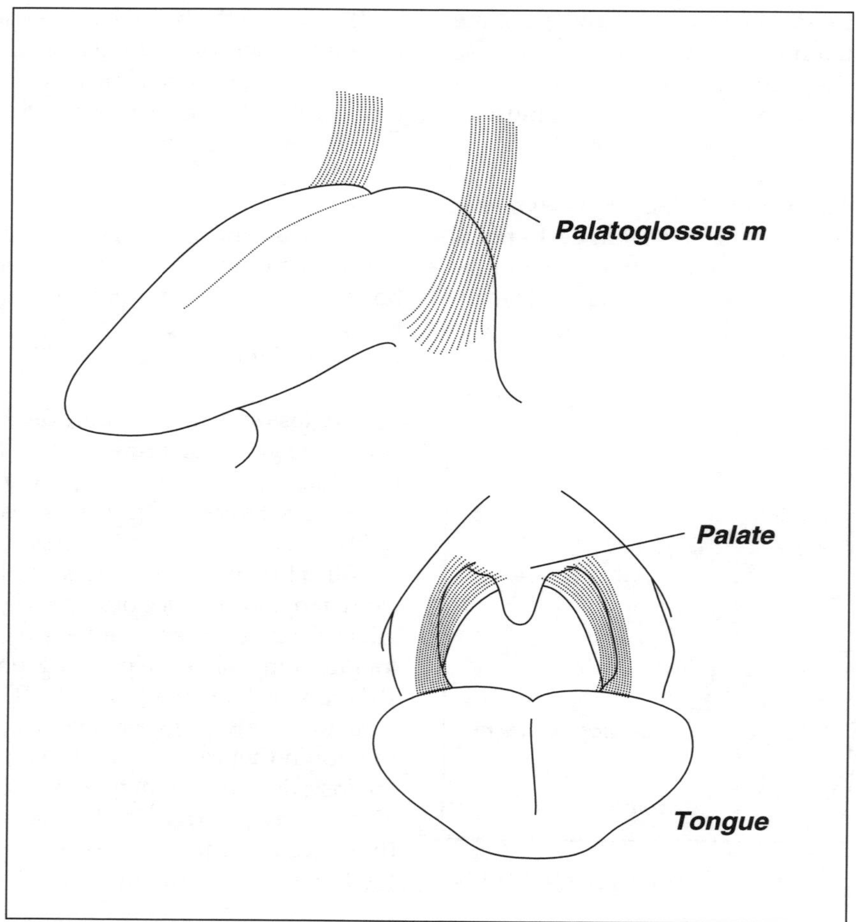

Figure 5–41. The palatoglossus muscle.

cles at the lateral margins and bottom, as well as the transverse muscle. Contraction serves to elevate the tongue.

Styloglossus muscle (Figure 5–42) takes its origin on the spikelike projection of the styloid process of the temporal bone. Its course is anterior, inferior, and somewhat medial to its insertion on the lateral margins of the tongue. Its contraction pulls the tongue upward and backward.

Glossopharyngeus muscle is discussed along with the muscles of the pharynx, but is noted here to indicate its attachment to the tongue.

Tongue Functions

The complex musculature of the tongue endows it with a multitude of movement possibilities. It can bunch, protrude, retract, wag from side to side, curl up its tip, form a midline groove, and explore the oral cavity within which it resides. This able musculature is accompanied by a rich vasculature. Beaven and Brooks (1988), a good source of general information on anatomy, physiology, embryology, and pathology of the tongue, comment that the organ's rich blood supply is "necessary for the rapid and almost continuous use of tongue muscles" and "has also produced an ability for rapid multiplication and turnover of sur-

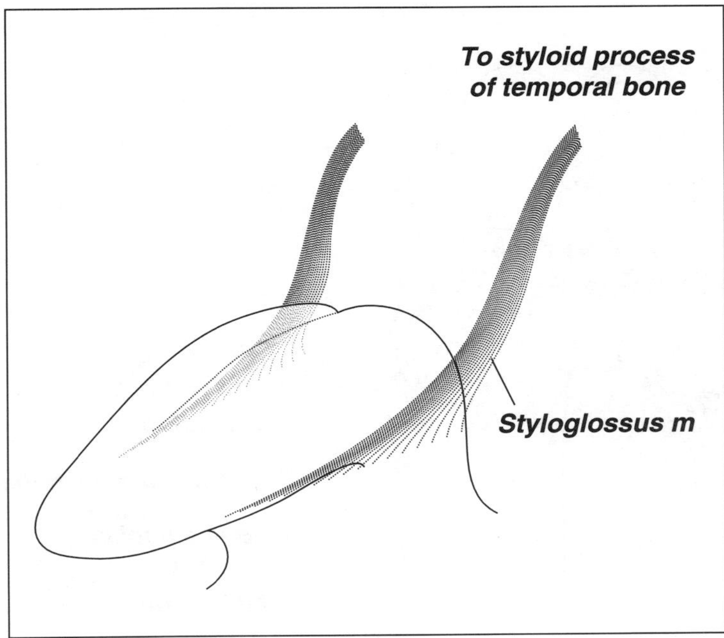

Figure 5–42. The styloglossus muscle.

face cells" (p. 13). The tongue muscles also form major boundaries of the oral cavity. For example, the floor of the mouth is composed especially of the mylohyoid and geniohyoid muscles.

Growth of the Tongue

The tongue of the newborn nearly fills the oral cavity. It is oriented primarily in the horizontal plane and has relatively little pharyngeal extension. The posterior third of the tongue gradually descends into the pharyngeal cavity during the first few years of life. From a review of developmental information, Kent and Vorperian (1995) concluded that the tongue attains its adult size at about age 16, in keeping with the overall maturational schedule of the craniofacial complex. The growth of the tongue is in general harmony with that of the mandible and lips. This synchrony in growth would seem to be an important factor that assists regulation of this multiarticulate apparatus. The size of the tongue correlates well with body weight or height. An enlarged tongue (hypertrophic tongue) is seen in some clinical conditions, including Down syndrome and possibly sudden infant death syndrome (Siebert & Haas, 1988).

Lingual Tonsil

Located on the posterior third of the tongue is a mass of lymphatic tissue called the lingual tonsil (Figure 5–43). It extends from the circumvallate papillae to the base of the epiglottis. The lingual tonsil contains dozens of crypts that are invested in its epithelium. The palatine tonsil is considered along with the nasopharyngeal tonsil in the section on the nasopharynx.

Lingual Papillae. The papillae are cup-shaped depressions that contain the taste buds, the sensory end-organs of taste (gustation). The different types of papillae are arranged on the tongue surface as shown in Figure 5–43.

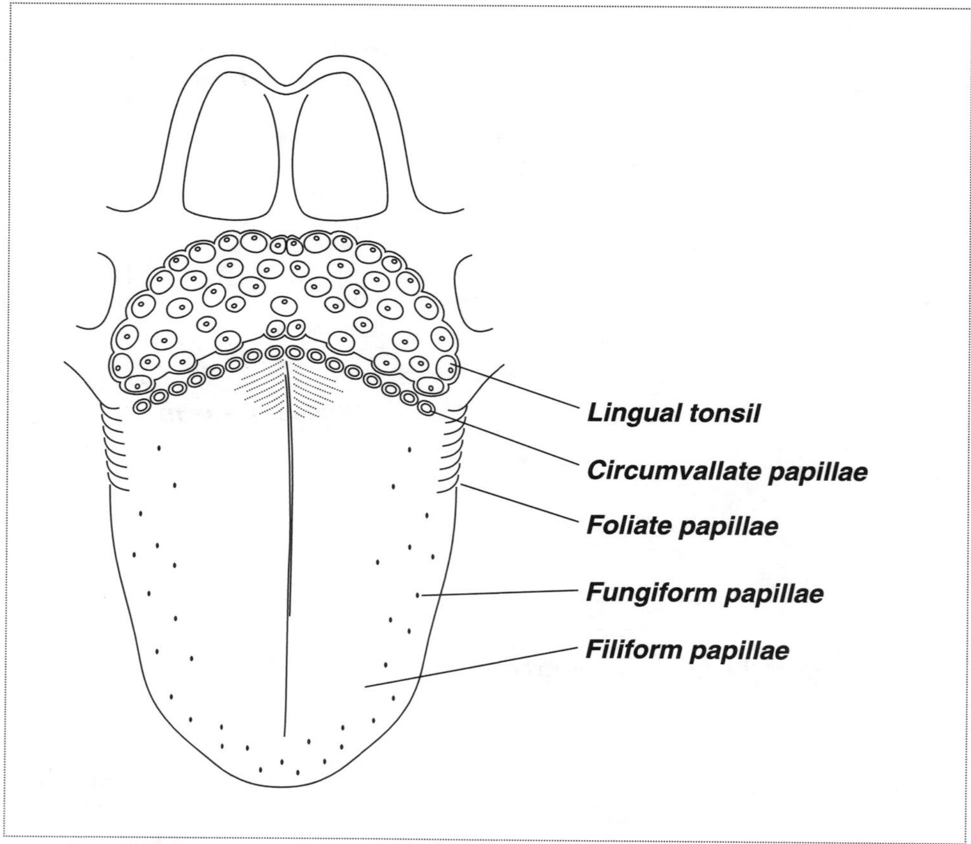

Figure 5–43. Superior aspect of tongue showing lingual tonsil and various papillae.

Lips and Face

Taken together, the facial muscles are often referred to as the muscles of facial expression, because this is their major collective function. Some authors refer to them as the superficial facial muscles, in distinction to the deep facial muscles associated with the mandible. The facial muscles are not as a group involved in speech, and therefore the discussion of these muscles is condensed. However, those facial muscles that act on or make up the lips are very much involved in speech, and these are the focus of this discussion. These are the labial and circumoral (around the mouth) muscles. The muscles of the lips and face are shown in the form of drawings in Figures 5–44 and 5–45. Figure 5–46 is a photograph of a partial dissection that reveals several facial muscles in an older adult.

The lips are a sphincteric muscle, meaning that they form a variable opening. The muscle that constitutes this sphincter is the **orbicularis oris** muscle (a name that basically denotes the orbit of the mouth). The fibers of several facial muscles run from surrounding areas of the face to converge on the oral sphincter and become its fibers. For this reason, the orbicularis oris does not have a definite insertion or origin. Nor does it have fibers distinct from the muscles that converge on the labial region. Lip

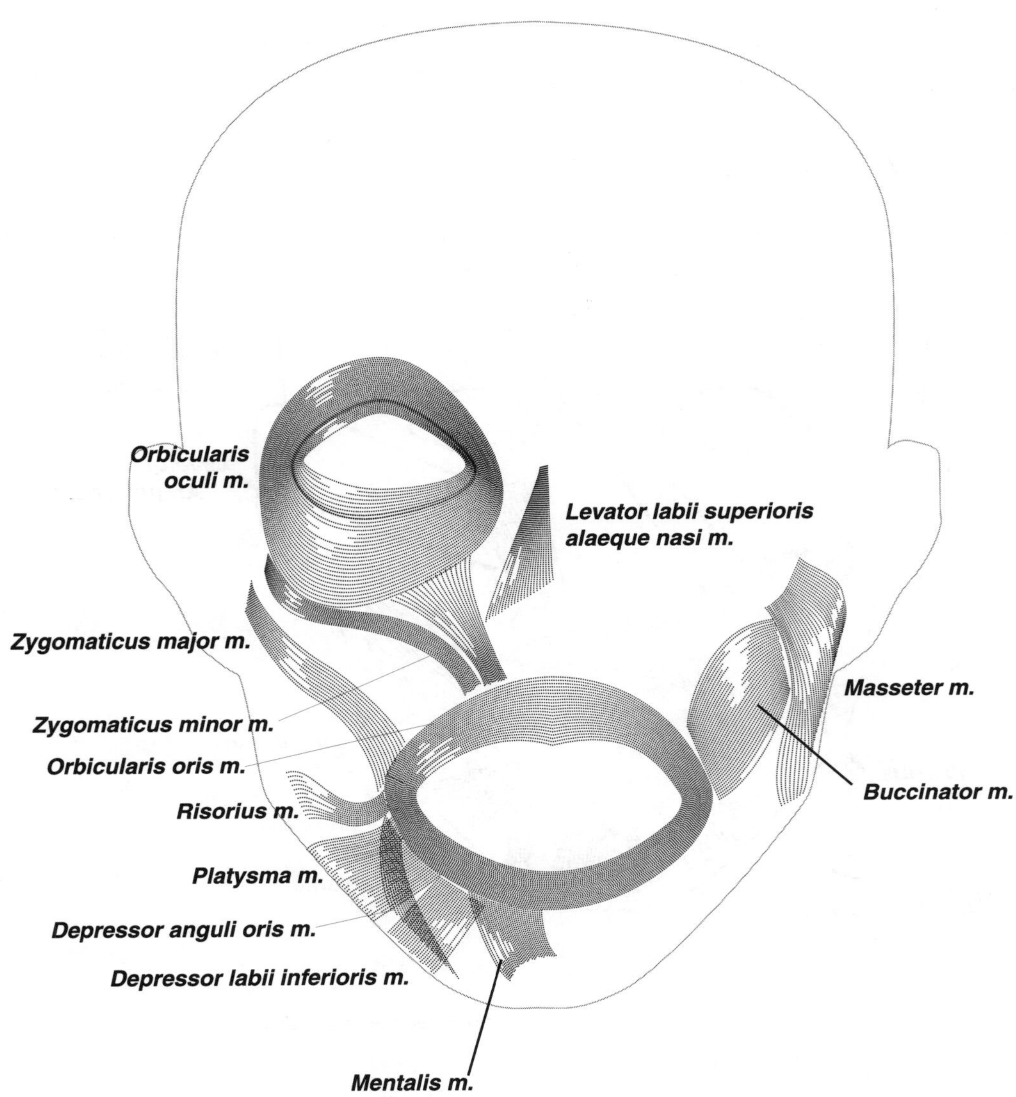

Figure 5–44. The muscles of the lips and face shown in a schematic anterior view.

movements frequently reflect the action of more than one muscle. One labial action that is most characteristic of the contraction of the fibers of the orbicularis oris as a whole is puckering of the lips. For this reason, this muscle is referred to as the "kissing muscle." The facial muscles that attach to the lips but have an origin elsewhere are called extrinsic muscles. These are sometimes grouped into four sets: (1) the transverse muscles, which have an essentially horizontal course; (2) the angular muscles, which run obliquely to the corners of the mouth; (3) the labial, or vertical, muscles, which have a vertical orientation; and (4) the parallel muscles, which run adjacent and parallel to the lip. As the various muscles are discussed individually, they are classified as within one of the four muscle sets.

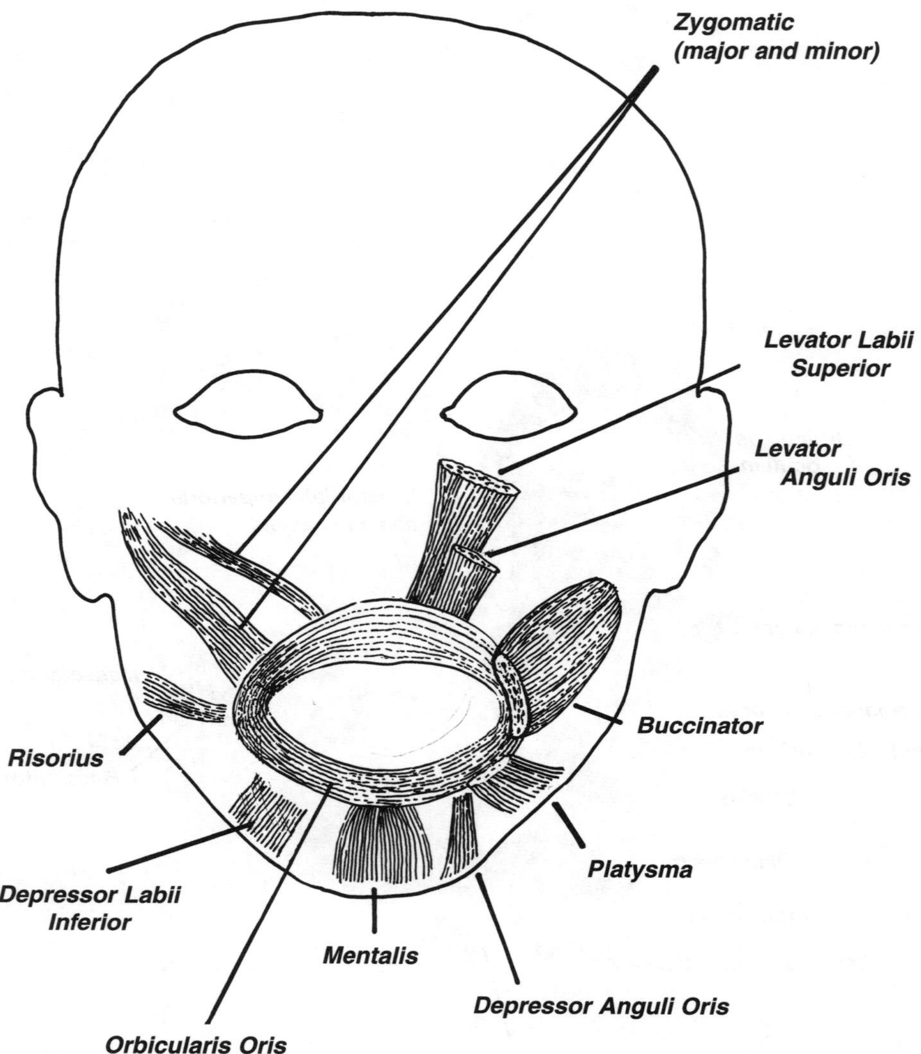

Figure 5–45. The muscles of the lips and face shown in a schematic posterior view, that is, looking out from the facial skeleton.

Transverse Facial Muscles

These work to pull the corners of the mouth laterally and are:

Buccinator muscle, also called the bugler's muscle, is the primary muscle of the cheek. The root *bucca* is Latin for cheek or mouth; therefore, the word *buccal* refers to the cheek. Dentists refer to the buccal surface of teeth when they want to refer to the surfaces adjacent to the cheek tissue. The buccinator has a complex origin but mainly from the pterygomandibular raphe, which is a ligament that connects the pterygoid with the mandible. Being classified as a transverse facial muscle, the buccinator runs horizontally to insert into the upper and lower lips. Contraction of the buccinator serves to pull the corners of the mouth

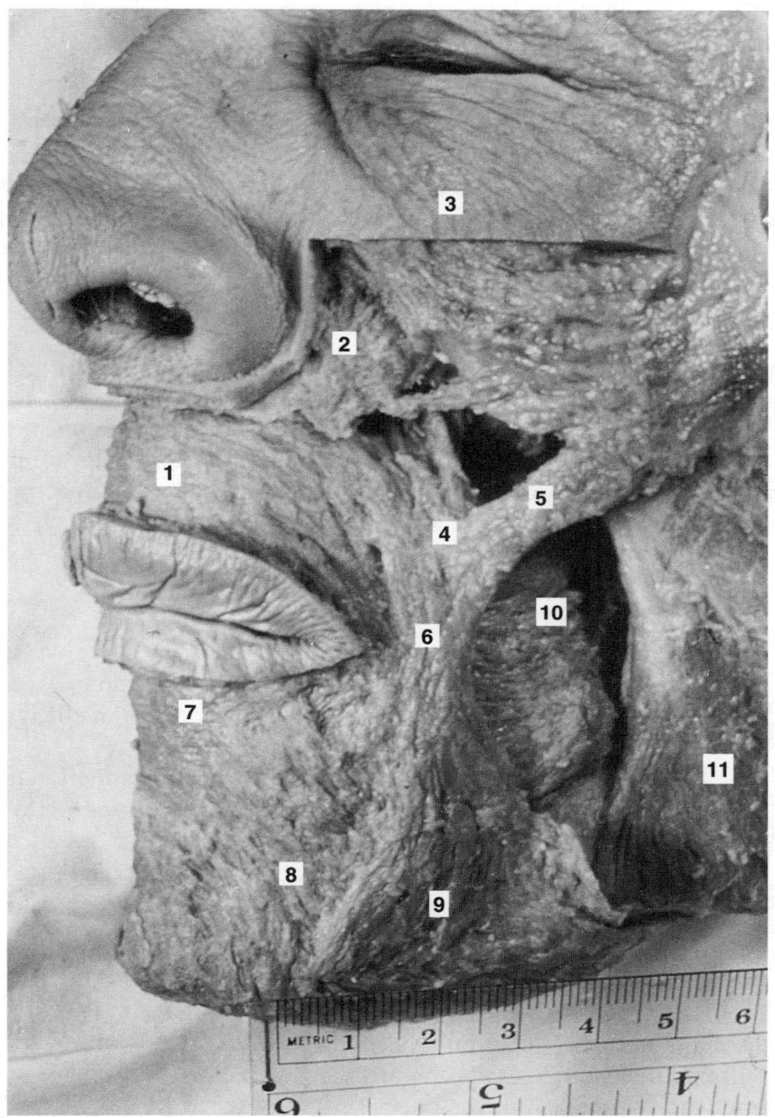

Figure 5–46. Photograph of right facial muscles of an older adult. 1 = orbicularis oris superior muscle, 2 = levator labii superior muscle, 3 = orbicularis oculi muscle (a muscle of the orbit of the eye), 4 = levator anguli oris muscle, 5 = zygomatic (major) muscle, 6 = modiolus, 7 = orbicular oris inferior muscle, 8 = depressor labii inferior muscle, 9 = depressor anguli oris muscle, 10 = buccinator muscle, 11 = masseter muscle. (Courtesy of Joel C. Kahane.)

laterally and to press the lips and cheek against the teeth. The buccinator is partially visible in the dissection of Figure 5–46.

Risorius muscle, also known as the laughing muscle (the Latin *risus* means laughter), takes its origin from a fascia that overlies the masseter muscle, one of the elevators of the mandible. It inserts primarily into the corner of the mouth. The action is to draw the mouth angle laterally.

Angular Facial Muscles

Act to pull the mouth angle up or down, or to elevate the upper lip or depress the lower lip:

Levator labii superior muscle originates broadly from the lower margin of the orbit and surrounding regions and runs inferiorly to insert into the upper lip. It elevates the upper lip and may contribute to eversion (turning inside out) of the lip.

Levator labii superior alaeque nasi muscle originates on the maxilla and courses mostly downward to divide into two portions, one of which inserts into the lateral cartilage of the nose and the other into the orbicularis oris. This muscle can dilate the nostrils or elevate the upper lip.

Zygomatic muscle has an origin on the zygomatic bone and runs inferiorally and medially to insert into the orbicularis oris, especially at the corner of the mouth. Contraction draws the mouth angle upward and lateralward. A broad smile is associated with contraction of the zygomatic.

Depressor labii inferior muscle originates on the mandible and inserts into the lower lip. Its action is to pull the lip downward and lateralward.

Vertical Facial Muscles

Act to depress or evert the lower lip or to elevate the upper or lower lips:

Mentalis muscle arises from the mandible and runs vertically into the orbicularis oris and the integument of the chin. Its contraction can evert (turn outward, as in a curling action) the lip or wrinkle the chin.

Depressor anguli oris muscle originates on the mandible and inserts primarily into the orbicularis oris at the angle of the mouth. Contraction can depress the angle of the lip or help to compress the lips by pulling the upper lip down toward the lower lip.

Levator anguli oris muscle runs downward from the maxilla to insert into the upper and lower lip near the angle of the mouth. It acts to elevate the corner of the mouth or to assist in compressing the lips by pulling the lower lip upward against the upper lip.

Parallel Facial Muscles

Act to draw the corner of the mouth medially and upward or medially and downward:

Incisivus labii superior muscle arises on the maxilla just superior to the canine teeth and runs lateralward to the angle of the mouth. It acts to pull the corner of the mouth medially and upward, as in a pucker.

Incisivus labii inferior muscle arises from the mandible near the lateral incisors and courses horizontally to insert into the orbicularis oris near the angle of the mouth. Contraction causes the corner of the mouth to be pulled medially and downward.

Platysma

Finally, the **platysma** muscle is often discussed with the facial muscles because it covers an extensive region of the lower face. Some writers classify it as a superior cervical muscle. Its origin is somewhat controversial, but seems to be primarily from the fascia overlying the pectoralis major and deltoid muscles. It may include fibers that originate on the mandible. Insertion is to the corner of the mouth. Its action is thought to be to draw the lower lip and corner of the mouth downward and laterally outward. However, it also may contribute to smiling and compressing the lips.

Growth of the Lips

The overall development of the lips can be specified as increases in width, height, and convexity (Burke, 1980). Growth studies generally point to two growth spurts, an early spurt between birth and 2 years and a later acceleration between 10 and 17 years. During the infantile growth spurt, the lips nearly double in width. The second growth spurt coincides with growth acceleration of the mandible, especially in males (Walker & Kowalski, 1972). In addition to changes in size and shape, the lips change in other ways during development. These other changes can be described with respect to the labial epithelium, which has three regions: hairy cutaneous, glabrous, and papillary (Thach, 1973). In infants, the papillary zone is generously supplied with papillae. These apparently give mobility and adhesive properties to the lips. These features would facilitate formation of an oral seal during suckle feeding.

FACIAL EXPRESSION: DEVELOPMENTAL AND UNIVERSALIST CONCEPTS

The infant's lips may be well adapted to nutritional needs, but they also demonstrate a precocious function in another realm. One of the earliest facial expressions to appear in a child, and one of the most universal facial expressions in the world is the smile. Children begin smiling by about 3 months of age, and this is true of children who are congenitally blind and blind-deaf, as well as children who have sight and hearing. The smile is remarkable not only for its early emergence and its universality, but also for the mastery of motor coordination that it represents. As Konner (1986) expressed it, "the facial muscles behind the smile—the risorious, along with zygomaticus major and other, more delicate sheets of tissue—must contract in a precisely orchestrated concatenation to produce a genuine smile, implying the existence of a genetically determined central neural mechanism of great coordination" (p. 4).

Within the last 20 years, some developmental psychologists have argued for a substantial revision of ideas about infant facial expressions. An earlier dominant view was that the child could imitate facial expressions at about 1 year of age, and this ability was a major event in social-cognitive development (Piaget, 1962). But Meltzoff and Moore (1977) reported the startling result that infants only 12 to 21 days old could imitate adult expressions of tongue protrusion, mouth opening, and lip protrusion. This phenomenon has been replicated in several studies in several different countries (Meltzoff & Moore, 1993), but some scientists dispute these observations and believe that general arousal reactions may be involved rather than genuine imitative responses. Assuming that the imitations are genuine, the explanation for this early imitative capacity is also controversial, but one explanation is that infants can relate information from multiple modalities. For present purposes, it is sufficient to draw attention to the phenomenon as an interesting possibility of early orofacial motor abilities of babies. Neonates may possess the ability to make different facial expressions, and can imitate several different facial expressions produced by adults, apparently without the need for previous exposure to these expressions.

Facial Muscles and Aging

We have seen that a large number of muscles attach to various regions of the face and are responsible for a rich repertoire of facial expressions. The same muscles account for many of the wrinkles that appear with aging. Because the facial tissues are continuously being pulled this way or that, they eventually suffer some wear and tear. Another factor that contributes to the wrinkling process is the aging of the facial tissue, such as the loss of collagen. If we never smiled or frowned, our faces might look younger longer. But our social worlds would be much poorer for the loss of animated faces. And perhaps we would feel older while looking younger.

Pharyngeal Muscles

The pharynx is the passage that connects the nasal cavity, oral cavity, and laryngeal cavity. This passage is vital to the movement of air and food. The anatomic boundaries of the pharynx are the cranial base superiorly and the esophageal opening inferiorly. This section emphasizes the oropharynx and laryngopharynx; the following section discusses the nasopharynx.

The primary muscles of the pharynx are shown in Figure 5–47. From an overall perspective, these muscles can be viewed as composing a muscular tube that gradually narrows in diameter in the inferior direction. This muscular tube is formed by

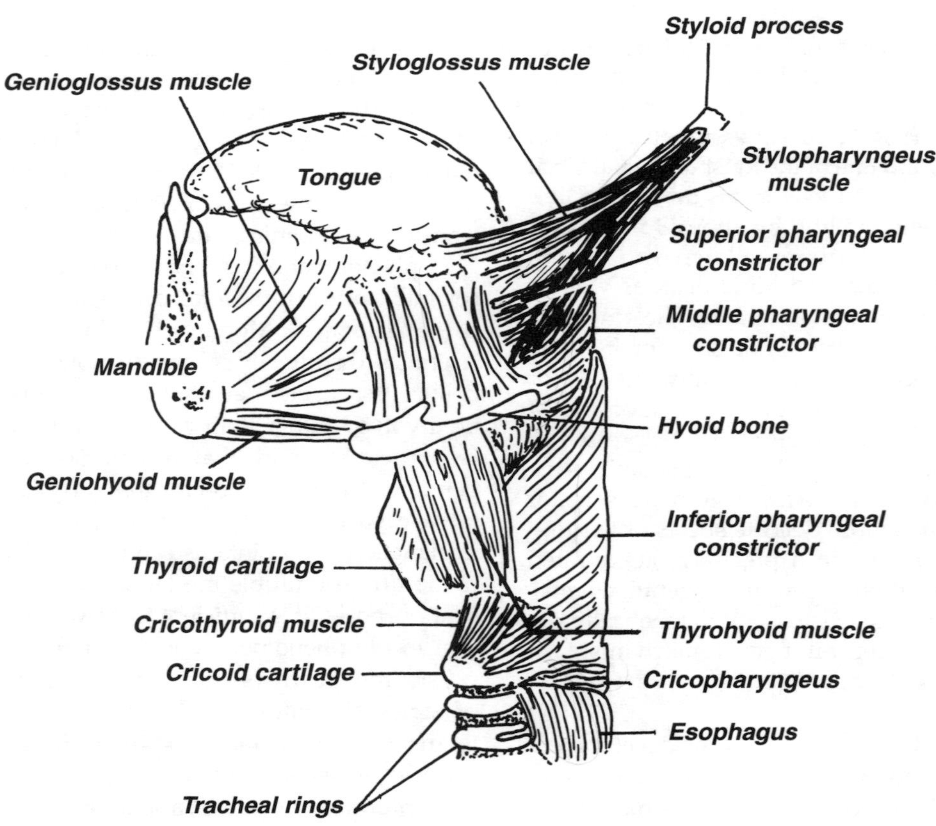

Figure 5–47. The primary muscles of the pharynx, shown in a lateral view of a partly dissected head and neck.

three large, thin muscles, the **pharyngeal constrictors**. These fan-shaped muscles overlap one another rather like shingles. The **inferior constrictor** is the largest and strongest of the pharyngeal constrictors. It takes its origin primarily from the sides of the thyroid cartilage and then wraps around the lower to mid regions of the pharynx. Located at the lower margin of the inferior constrictor is another muscle, the **cricopharyngeus**, which arises from the cricoid cartilage and encircles the superior opening of the esophagus. The cricopharyngeus can be regarded as a muscular valve at the opening of the esophagus.

The **middle constrictor** lies superior to the inferior constrictor and is partly overlapped by it. The middle constrictor extends from the horns of the hyoid bone to encircle the middle pharynx. Proximal to the middle constrictor are two other muscles, the **stylopharyngeus** and the **salpingopharyngeus**. Because these muscles are not particularly important to speech, they are not discussed in detail here. The **superior constrictor** is at once the weakest and most complex of the pharyngeal constrictors. Its origin is primarily from the skeletal framework of the soft palate, including the medial pterygoid plate, the hamulus of the pterygoid, and the pterygomandibular ligament that connects the pterygoid bone with the mandible. The superior constrictor wraps around the upper pharynx.

Nasopharynx

The nasopharynx is situated above the soft palate. When the soft palate is closed, it forms the floor of the nasopharynx. In its shape, the nasopharynx can be likened to an inverted cone with membranomuscular walls. The large dimension of the cone is within the nasal cavity and the narrow dimension is the velopharyngeal port. The anatomy of this system in human adults is unique among mammals. It is shown in Figures 5–48, 5–49, and 5–50. Figure 5–48

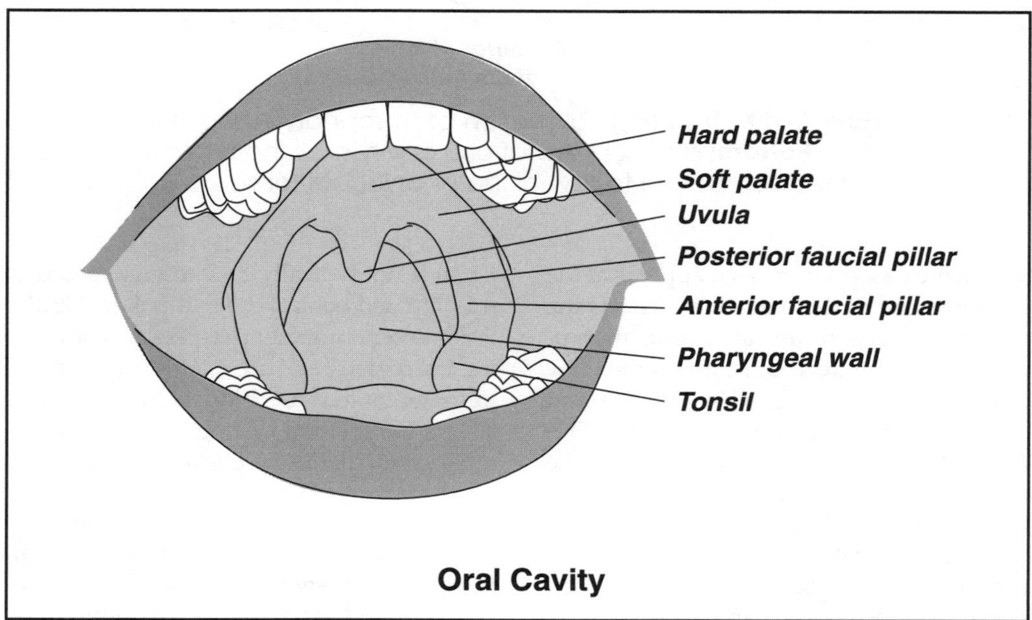

Figure 5–48. The oral cavity as seen through the open mouth. Note position of soft palate and uvula relative to faucial pillars.

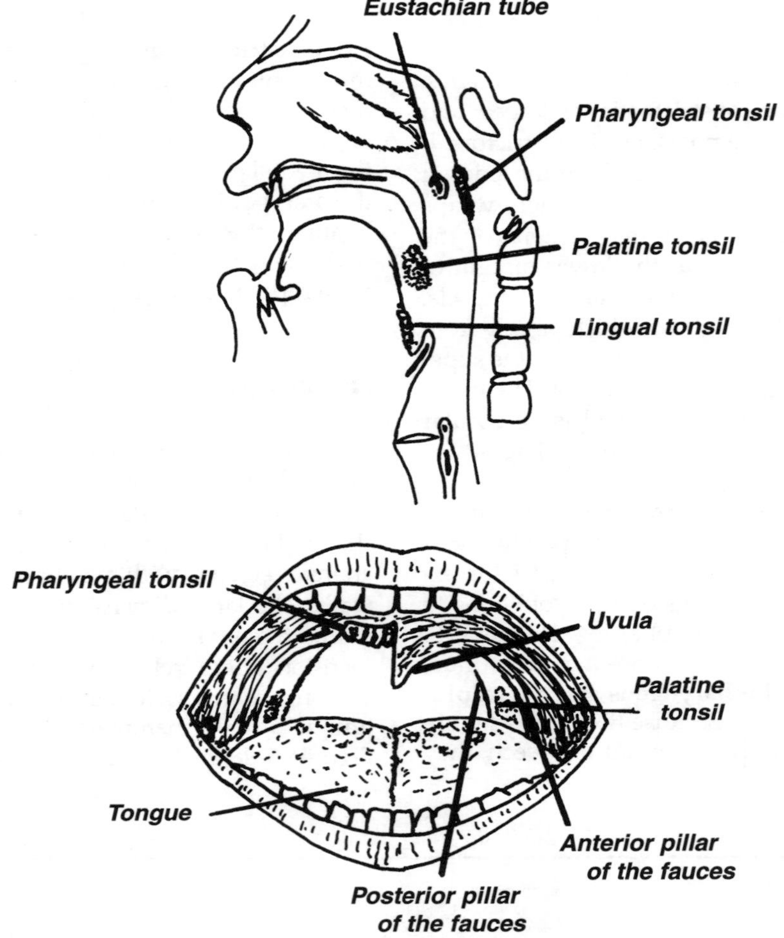

Figure 5-49. Top: sagittal section of nasopharynx showing tonsils. **Bottom:** anterior view of oral cavity showing a partly resected soft palate to reveal the pharyngeal tonsil.

shows the nasopharynx as it appears at the posterior end of the oral cavity. This is the typical oral posture for an examination of the teeth or throat. That is, this is the view that physicians have when the patient opens the mouth and says "ah." Figure 5–49 shows additional detail of the oropharynx and nasopharynx. In particular, it shows the three masses of lymphoid tissue, the lingual, palatine, and pharyngeal tonsils. These tonsils virtually encircle the entrance to the pharynx and are sometimes called **Waldeyer's ring**. The pharyngeal tonsil is not typically easy to view because it is situated behind the soft palate. Figure 5–50 presents another perspective, comparing the regions that are readily visible with the regions that are hidden from view. It shows the relation among the pharyngeal tonsil, soft palate, and eustachian tube.

As mentioned earlier in this chapter, the human infant is like the chimpanzee in having an engagement between the velopharynx and larynx. This anatomic relationship is, in fact, common among mam-

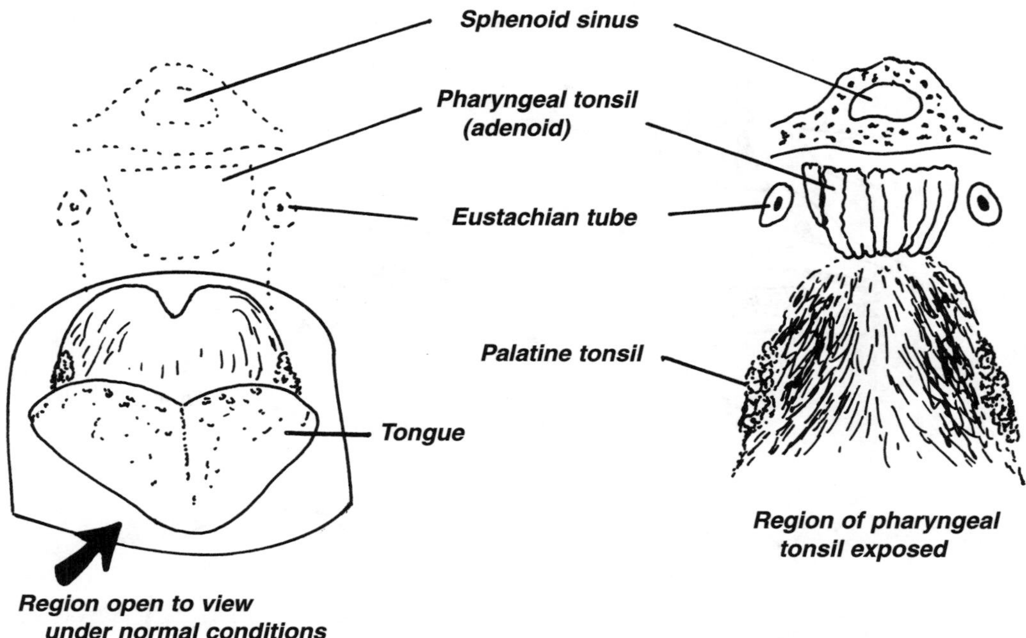

Figure 5–50. Anterior view of oropharynx and nasopharynx, showing locations of structures behind the tongue and soft palate.

mals (Figure 5–51) and is thought to provide an important advantage, in that it enables breathing to continue even during feeding. The close connection of velopharynx and larynx minimizes the risk of choking. The separation of these structures in adult humans is a distinct threat to life, and many people die each year because of choking. Some writers have remarked that such an evolutionary adaptation would seem unlikely unless it were balanced by some special advantage. One possible advantage is speech, because the altered anatomy underlies the manifold sound production capabilities of human speech (Lieberman, 1991). More is said about this issue in Chapter 13. For the moment, we simply pose the question: Is the capability for speech gained at the substantial risk of death through choking?

Located on the lateral wall of the nasopharynx is the **torus tubarius**, the cartilaginous medial portion of the eustachian tube that connects the middle ear with the pharynx. The adenoid, or nasopharyngeal tonsil, is located close to the torus tubarius, near the roof of the nasopharynx. As noted earlier, the eustachian tube is responsible for ventilation of the middle ear.

Some of the sound products of this system are not always welcome. **Snoring** seems to arise in many people as the soft palate relaxes during sleep and falls against the posterior pharyngeal wall. As air moves through the portal, it causes vibration of the flaccid tissues of the palate and pharynx. The sound generation potential of this valve is remarkable. One snorer found his way to the *Guinness Book of World Records* (Russell, 1987, p. 39), for producing an 88 dB snore (equivalent to a motorcycle at full throttle). His wife, now reported to be deaf in one ear, sleeps with her good ear nestled in a pillow.

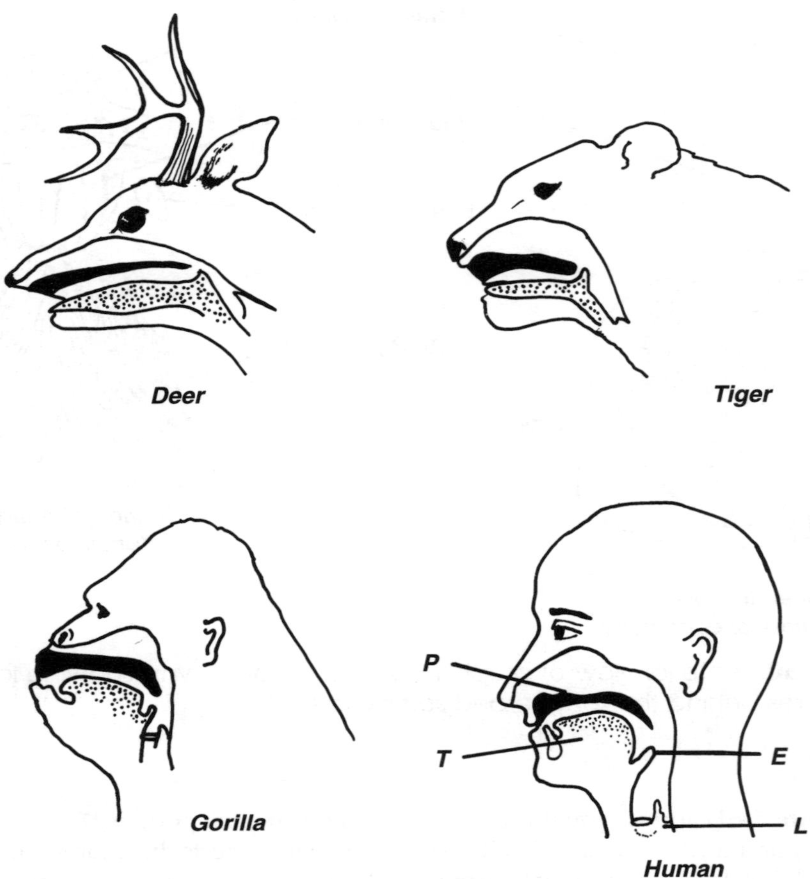

Figure 5–51. Drawings of sagittal sections of the upper airway of selected animals, showing differences from the human anatomy.T = tongue, P = palate, E = epiglottis, L = larynx.

Between infancy and adulthood, the volume of the nasopharynx increases by about 80% (Bergland, 1963). However, the depth dimensions of the nasopharynx are established early in life and change relatively little (Tourne, 1991). The developmental increase in volume of the nasopharynx is attributable largely to increases in the vertical dimension. In other words, the nasopharynx grows long but not wide. Subtelny's (1957) observations show that the nasopharynx grows vertically about 12 mm from the 1st to the 18th year of life, with a relatively uniform rate of growth of slightly less than 1 mm per year. Tourne (1991) noted that the acute angle of the cranial base in the human anatomy produces a more vertical than horizontal direction of pharyngeal growth. Subtelny's (1957) measurements are consistent with this explanation.

A notable feature of the nasopharynx in developmental studies is the lymphoid tissue known as the pharyngeal tonsil or nasopharyngeal tonsil or **adenoids** (although the term *adenoids* is better restricted to enlarged nasopharyngeal tonsils). The pharyngeal tonsil is situated in the midline of the posterior wall of the superior nasopharynx. A closely related tissue is the palatine tonsil, which is typically considered as a structure of the oropharynx, but is more conveniently discussed along with the pharyngeal tonsil. The palatine tonsils project into the oropharynx and are located between the anterior and posterior pillars (for this reason, the palatine tonsils are sometimes called the **faucial tonsils**). They contain numerous branching crypts. These tissues grow in early childhood and then atrophy in mid or late childhood. Hypertrophy of the nasopharyngeal tonsil in childhood may obstruct the passageway for nasal air flow, and hypertrophy of the palatine tonsil can obstruct the oropharynx. Handelman and Osborne (1976) reported that the growth rate of the nasopharyngeal tonsil exceeds that of the bony nasopharynx during the preschool and early school years. Consequently, the lymphoid hypertrophy markedly reduced the nasopharyngeal airway in many of the subjects in this age range. Children of a generation or two ago fairly routinely underwent the surgical removal of the nasopharyngeal tonsil (**adenoidectomy**) and palatine tonsil (**tonsillectomy**). This practice was reconsidered but now appears to be on the rise again, especially for children who have several respiratory infections in a 1-year period.

The Muscles of the Soft Palate

The soft palate, or velum, is a posterior extension of the bony, or hard, palate. The soft palate is composed mainly of muscular fibers and its movements change the volume and shape of the nasal and oral cavities. For speech, the soft palate is critical to the nasal-nonnasal phonetic distinction. For nonnasal sounds, like the consonants in the word "closed," the soft palate is elevated to make a seal with the posterior pharyngeal wall. For nasal sounds, like the consonants in the word "meaning," the soft palate is lowered, so that acoustic energy passes readily through the nasal cavity. These actions are shown in Figure 5–52. The soft palate is also important for swallowing. During the part of swallowing when the bolus passes from the oral cavity into the pharynx, the soft palate closes to prevent the food from entering the nasal cavity. This is discussed in more detail near the end of this chapter. Anyone who tries to murmur the affirmative "hm-hm" (yes) while taking a drink risks the rush of liquid into the nasal cavity.

The soft palate is formed primarily of five muscles (Figure 5–53): the **levator veli palatine**, **tensor veli palatine**, **uvula**, **palatoglossus**, and **palatopharyngeus** muscles. Fibers of a sixth muscle, the **velopharyngeal sphincter**, also extend into the palate, but this muscle is discussed with the pharyngeal muscles. Only one muscle, the uvula (or musculus uvulae), is an intrinsic muscle of the soft palate. The others have one attachment outside the palate.

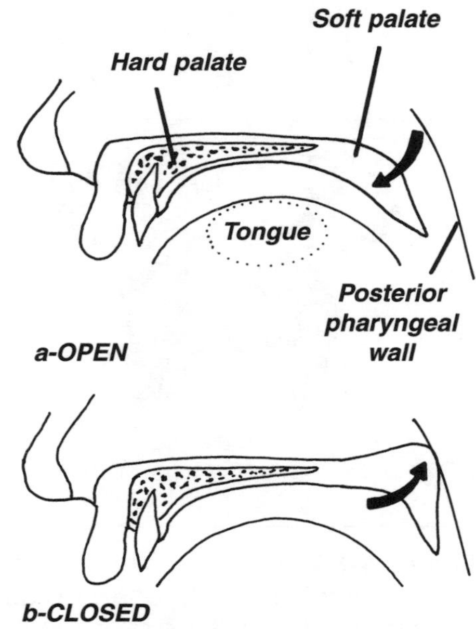

Figure 5–52. Movements of the soft palate.

The levator veli palatine muscle is an elevator of the soft palate. Its fibers originate mainly on the petrous part of the temporal bone and then course downward and medially to insert into the midline of the soft palate (the midline is also called the **palatal raphe**, or **aponeurosis**). Contraction of this muscle pulls the soft palate upward toward the posterior pharyngeal wall. In addition, this muscle may help to dilate the opening of the eustachian tube for ventilation of the middle ear (as discussed in Chapter 6). The levator veli palatini is considered among the velopharyngeal muscles to be the most consistent in size, shape, and location (Moon & Kuehn, in press).

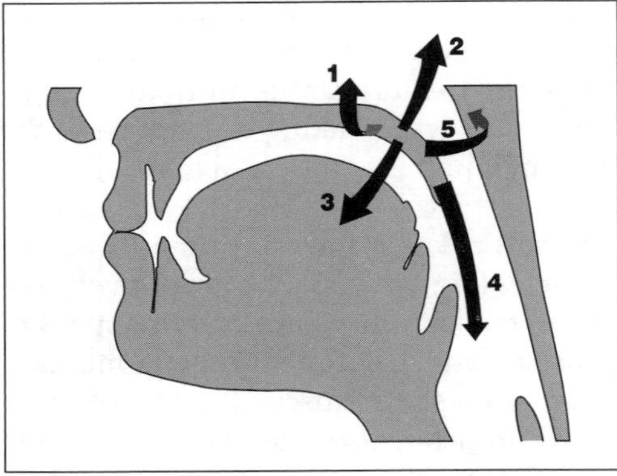

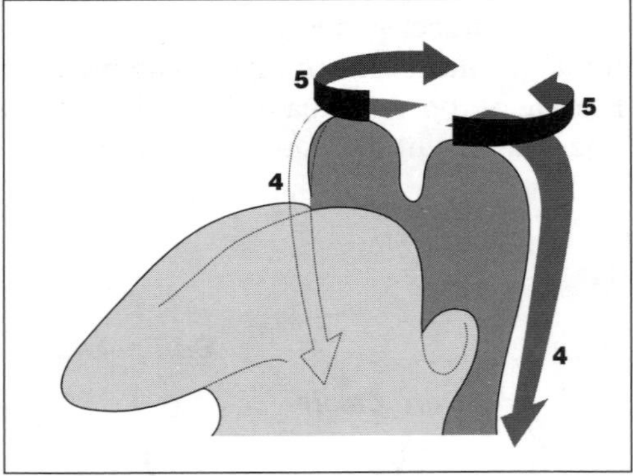

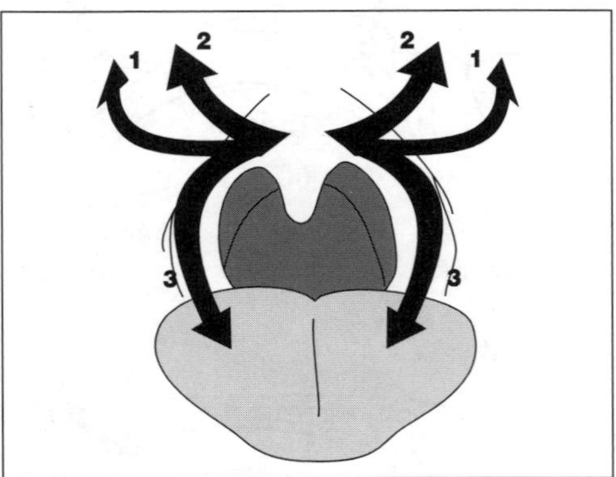

Figure 5–53. Muscles of the soft palate or velopharynx: 1, tensor palatini; 2, levator palatini; 3, palatoglossus; 4, palatopharyngeus, and 5, superior pharyngeal constrictor.

The tensor palatine muscle has a dual origin, the medial pterygoid plate and the lateral walls of the eustachian tube. However, Palmer (1993) suggested that a better description of the second origin would be the scaphoid fossa (cf., Moon & Kuehn, in press). Fibers from the more superior origin run forward and downward to connect to a tendon that goes around the hamulus to insert on the palatal raphe. The primary action of this muscle is to dilate the eustachian tube. It also may serve to tense the palate, which may assist in velopharyngeal closure, but Moon and Kuehn (in press) doubt that any tensing action would be considerable. It has been suggested that one role of the tendon of the tensor palatine muscle is to relieve stress at the junction between the hard and soft palate, rather like the collar at the junction of an electrical cord and its plug (Kuehn & Kahane, 1990).

The uvula muscle is actually two bands of muscle fibers with origins near the posterior nasal spine and the palatal raphe. The two bands continue on either side of midline to insert into the uvula. The uvula muscle is the only truly intrinsic muscle of the velum. The uvula ("little grape") may be a vestigial structure (Palmer, 1993), but it also has been suggested that it can control the stiffness of the nasal aspect of the soft palate and therefore assist in extending the palate (Kuehn, Folkins, & Linville, 1988). However, the uvula per se has very few muscle fibers (Ettema & Kuehn, 1994;

Kuehn & Kahane, 1990). The uvula can be important for clinical examination, because it assumes forms that reflect palatal dysmorphology. For example, a **bifid uvula** is split at the midline and may accompany a cleft of the palate.

The palatoglossus muscle has its origin at the tongue, primarily the superficial muscles at the lateral margins and bottom, as well as the transverse muscle. The fibers pass superiorly to insert into the palatal raphe. The fibers of the palatoglossus form a pair of bundles that are visible as submucosal bulges on either side of the oral cavity. Reference was made to these pillars at the beginning of this chapter. These bulges are called the **anterior pillar of the fauces** (also known as the **palatoglossus pillar**, or the **palatoglossus arch**). See Figure 5–54. Contraction of this muscle can either depress the sides of the soft palate or pull the sides of the tongue upward and backward.

The palatopharyngeus muscle originates at the posterior border of the thyroid cartilage and the fibrous layer of the lower pharynx. Its fibers course superiorly along with the fibers of the stylopharyngeal muscle to form visible bulges on either side of the oral cavity. These bulges are called the **posterior pillar of the fauces** (or the **palatopharyngeus pillar,** or **palatopharyngeus arch**) (Figure 5–54). The bundle of fibers divides into two fasciculi, an inferior one that runs along the posterior aspect of the soft palate and a superior one that enters the palate directly. They insert into the palatal raphe. Contraction of this muscle can have two primary actions, either to depress the soft palate or to elevate the pharynx and larynx. The latter action is a part of the swallowing complex. But it should be noted that the palatopharyngeus muscle is poorly understood, one reflection of which is its designation by two names in the classic anatomic literature, either pharyngopalatine or palatopharyngeus, depending on how its primary action is viewed. Cassell, Moon, & Elkadi (1990) suggested that this muscle actually consists of two well-defined fiber groups, one oriented vertically and the other horizontally.

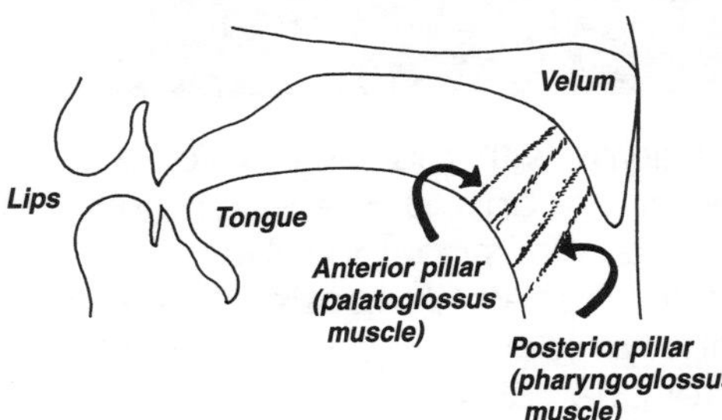

Figure 5–54. The faucial pillars, as seen from a lateral perspective.

Figure 5–55 is a photograph of the nasopharynx with its mucosal surface intact. This photograph shows the relationship between the soft palate (labeled *10*) and various structures of the oral and nasal cavities.

Patterns of Velopharyngeal Action

The basic action of the velopharynx in speech and swallowing is deceptively simple: either close the entry into the nasal cavity or open it. But studies of velopharyngeal function have shown variations with sex plus individual differences in anatomy and stage of development. McKerns and Bzoch (1970) observed three major differences related to sex. First, in males the velum forms an acute angle in its orientation to the posterior pharyngeal wall; but in females, the velum has a right-angle orientation. Second, the extent of the area of the velopharyngeal seal is greater in females. Third, the midpoint of closure in the nasopharynx is superior to the palatal plane in males, but inferior to this plane in females.

Individual differences in the pattern of velopharyngeal valving have been described in several studies (Croft, Shprintzen, & Rakoff, 1981; Shprintzen, 1992; Skol-

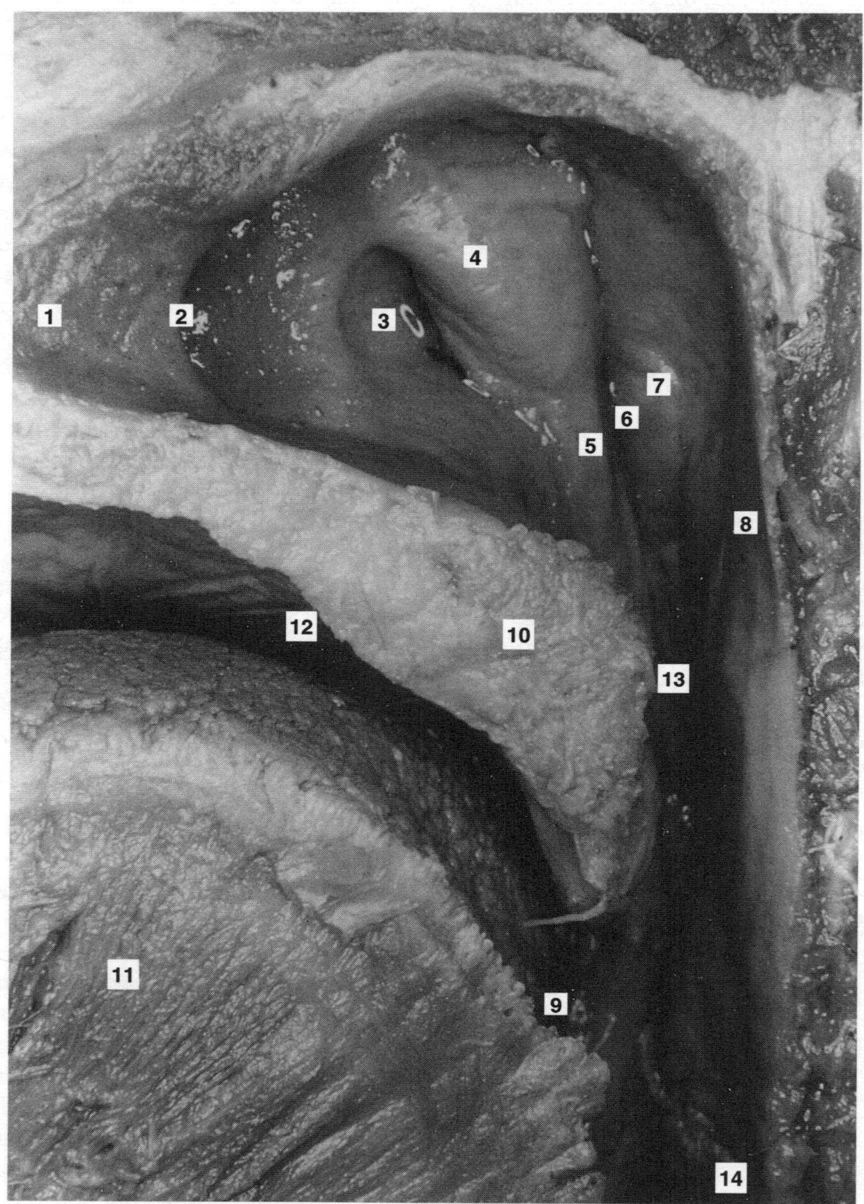

Figure 5–55. Photograph of nasopharynx with mucosal surface intact. 1 = nasal septum, 2 = posterior choana, 3 = eustachian tube orifice, 4 = torus tubarius (cartilage of eustachian tube), 5 = salpingopharyngeal fold, 6 = pharyngeal recess, 7 = posterolateral pharyngeal wall, 8 = posterior pharyngeal wall, 9 = posterior faucial pillar, 10 = soft palate, 11 = tongue, 12 = oral cavity, 13 = nasopharyngeal portal, and 14 = oropharynx. (Courtesy of Joel C. Kahane.)

nick, McCall, & Barnes, 1973). The most frequently observed patterns fall into four categories (Figure 5–56). The coronal pattern (Figure 5–56a) is accomplished mainly by anteroposterior movements of the velum and corresponds to the trap-door analogy of velar motion. The sagittal pattern (Figure 5–56b) relies primarily on movement of the lateral pharyngeal walls. The circular pattern (Figure 5–56c) involves nearly equal movements of the velum and lateral pharyngeal walls. Finally, the circular pattern with **Passavant's ridge** (also called Passavant's pad) (Figure 5–56d) is the combination of the circular pattern just described with the assistance of an anterior movement of a portion of the posterior pharyngeal wall. It is not clear why these different patterns occur,

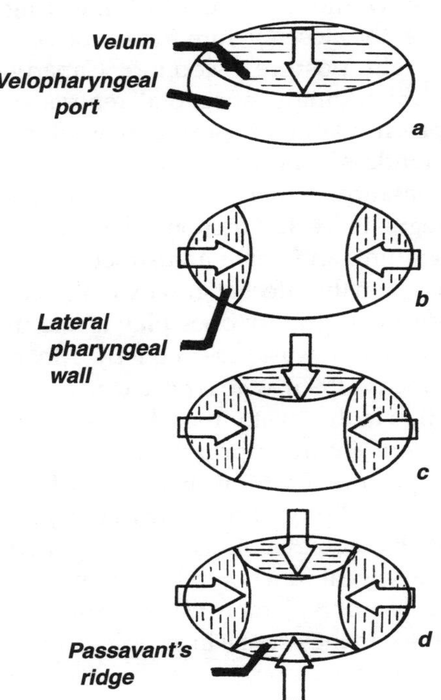

Figure 5–56. Major types of velopharyngeal valving: **a.** Coronal. **b.** Sagittal. **c.** Circular. **d.** Circular with Passavant's ridge. See text for detailed description.

but at least a partial explanation is that they reflect differences in nasopharyngeal anatomy. Finkelstein et al. (1995) studied the relation between pattern of velopharyngeal closure and velopharyngeal anatomy in 60 adults. The coronal pattern of closure was observed especially in subjects who had a wide and "flat" (i.e., a smaller anterior-posterior than left-right dimension) velopharyngeal port in its resting state. Circular and sagittal patterns of closure tended to occur in subjects who had narrower, less flat, and more rounded ports. In addition, it was observed that subjects with coronal patterns of closure tended to have hamulus bones closer to the tubercle of the atlas than did subjects with other closure patterns.

Velopharyngeal function also varies with age and in particular with age-related changes in the proportions of hard and soft tissues. As noted in the beginning of this section, growth of the nasopharyngeal soft tissue is greater than that of the bony structures between 3 to 5 years of age (Jeans, Fernando, Maw, & Leighton, 1981). As would be expected from this disproportionate growth of soft tissue, the nasal airway is narrowest (Fujioka, Young, & Girdany, 1979) and nasal resistance values are at their greatest (Saito & Nishihata, 1981) during this developmental period.

In very young children, velopharyngeal valving is thought to be predominantly velar-adenoidal (Croft, Shprintzen, & Rubin, 1981; Skolnick, Shprintzen, McCall, & Rakoff, 1975). This pattern exploits the typically large adenoidal mass (nasopharyngeal tonsil) in young children (Figure 5–57). But as the adenoid atrophies, a change in velopharyngeal valving occurs. Siegel-Sadewitz and Shprintzen (1986) reported that 60% of their normal subjects changed patterns of velopharyngeal valving between a prepubertal and a postpubertal examination. The size and persistence of the adenoid varies greatly among individu-

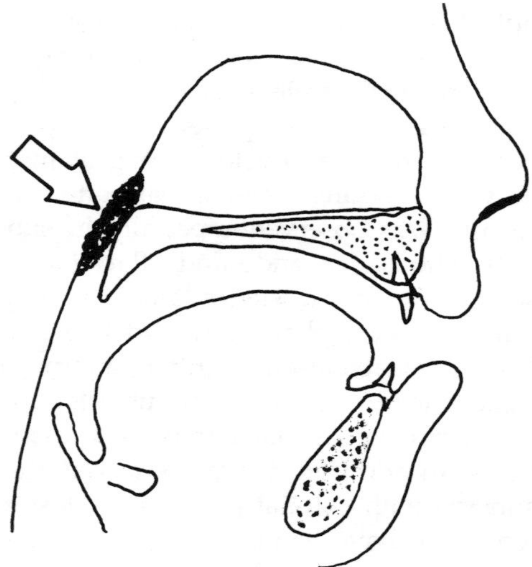

Figure 5–57. Velar–adenoidal form of velopharyngeal valving. Arrow points to adenoid (enlarged pharyngeal tonsil).

als, and it can strongly influence velopharyngeal functions for speech and breathing (Finkelstein, Berger, Nachimani, & Ophir, 1996; Rodenstein & Stanesco, 1986).

With these functional variations in mind, we turn to some general principles of velopharyngeal articulation. First, the velum is elevated primarily by the levator veli palatini muscle, but it appears that at least three different muscles may be involved in velar positioning: levator veli palatini, palatoglossus, and palatopharyngeus (Kuehn, Folkins, & Cutting, 1982). Lowering of the velum may involve three factors: muscle contraction (especially the palatoglossus and palatopharyngeus muscles), gravity, and tissue elasticity (Moon & Kuehn, in press). Classic descriptions of velopharyngeal actions may underestimate the complexity and variability of the forces involved. In particular, the analogy of the soft palate as a trap-door mechanism may be simplistic. Possibly, the velopharyngeal mechanism should be viewed as a muscular hydrostat, as the tongue was described earlier. This suggestion was made by Moon and Jones (1991) and Ettema and Kuehn (1994). Hydrostatic considerations can lead to an understanding of velopharyngeal actions that are different from more classic concepts. For example, Ettema and Kuehn (1994) proposed that the palatopharyngeus muscle could contribute to velopharyngeal closure by "squeezing the contents of the more posterior aspects of the velum and forcing the posterior nasal surface of the velum to conform to the concavity of the surrounding pharyngeal walls, much like forcing a water balloon to conform to the walls of a cylindrical container" (p. 311). For a more detailed discussion of different concepts of velopharyngeal function, the reader is referred to Moon and Kuehn (in press).

Gravity may influence velar function, because it would tend to exert lowering forces on the closed velum for a subject in an upright posture (Moon & Canady, 1995). Interestingly, anecdotal reports of the speech quality of astronauts working in weightless conditions mention an altered nasality. Perhaps the muscle forces that regulate velar function take gravity into account, and some adjustment is required when the effect of gravity is altered. Evidence that gravity does play a role in velar function was presented by Moon and Canady (1995), who reported a greater activation in the levator muscle when subjects were in the upright rather than supine posture. Postural change may be a useful clinical procedure. Duffy (1995) reported that some subjects with impaired velopharyngeal function related to neurological disorders demonstrated improved speech when they spoke in a supine rather than upright position.

Summary

The upper airway of speech production, also called the vocal tract, consists essentially of three interconnected cavities: the oral, nasal, and pharyngeal cavities. It is in these cavities that most speech sounds are formed. The muscles of this system are complex and specialized. At least two muscle groups are sphincters, the oral sphincter of the lips and the velopharyngeal sphincter that separates the oral and nasal cavities. The oral sphincter, composed mostly of fibers of the orbicularis oris muscles, is a converging point of attachment for most of the facial muscles. These muscles, which originate on various parts of the face and skull, insert on or near the mouth opening. Among the muscles of the upper airway, the jaw muscles are most similar to the skeletal muscles of the body that regulate movement about joints and are arranged in agonist-antagonist groups. The jaw rotates about the temporomandibular joint and its actions can be described through the actions of jaw closing and opening muscles. However, the jaw is capable of movement in three dimensions, owing largely to the muscular sling formed by the masseter and pterygoid muscles and to the flexibility of the temporomandibular joint. The tongue and perhaps the soft palate are unique among the muscles of the body in acting like muscular hydrostats, muscular organs devoid of bony or cartilaginous skeleton. The soft palate and the pharyngeal walls form the sphincter of the velopharyngeal port. But the pattern of velopharyngeal closure varies among subjects, apparently in relation to individual differences in the anatomy of soft and hard tissues.

Generalizations are important as a economical approach to knowledge, but they also can obscure exceptions to the general pattern. The structures discussed in this chapter are not fashioned after an invariant blueprint. Most of them are sexually dimorphic in some respect; that is, they do not have the same appearance in males and females. Most of the structures undergo changes in size *and* shape during their development in infancy, childhood, and adolescence. Furthermore, they can vary somewhat from individual to individual, even in the same age-sex group. These individual variations have not been sufficiently studied, so their full consequence is unknown. But it is well to remember that the upper airway has many individual configurations, and some of these may be important in understanding oral functions. For further discussion, see Buck (1997) and Kent and Vorperian (1995).

SWALLOWING

Swallowing, or deglutition, is a major function of many of the structures discussed in this chapter. Swallowing is a relevant topic for this book for several reasons. First, the forces developed during mastication and deglutition help to shape the oral and pharyngeal structures during childhood. Bosma (1975) described the anatomy of speech production as a "performance anatomy," or an anatomy shaped by function. Chewing and swallowing are relatively forceful activities. In contrast, speech usually develops small forces and therefore probably does not contribute greatly to the developmental anatomy. Second, because deglutition uses many of the same muscles that are used to produce speech, clinicians often compare swallowing and speech behaviors to determine the degree of involvement of oral, pharyngeal, and laryngeal muscles in various disease conditions. Third, many speech-language therapists participate in the evaluation and management of swallowing disorders (known as **dysphagias**).

Like speech, swallowing involves a large number of structures in the head and neck. The major purpose of a swallow is to transport a bolus (the mass of masticated food that is ready to be swallowed or simply a volume of liquid) from the oral cavity to the stomach without admitting any of the swallowed substance into the nasal cavity (which could cause nasal reflux) or the larynx (which can cause choking or aspiration of food particles). As noted previously, swallowing in humans is a relatively risky behavior compared to swallowing in nonhuman animals, because humans are more prone to choke when food lodges in the respiratory airway. Swallowing involves a sequence of muscular actions that serve to accomplish the following steps: (1) trap the bolus in the anterior region of the oral cavity, (2) move the bolus from the mouth to the entrance to the pharynx, (3) admit the bolus into the esophagus while the entrance to the larynx is closed, and (4) transport the bolus through the esophagus to the stomach. The performance of a single swallow, therefore, requires muscular actions of the lips, tongue, soft palate, pharynx, larynx, and esophagus. It also is accompanied by a brief interruption of respiration, called an **apneic interval**.

The sequential nature of swallowing often has been recognized by describing the swallow in terms of stages. Figure 5–58 shows several of these stage descriptions, proceeding from the *orad* (oral cavity) direction to the *aboral* (away from the oral cavity) direction. For purposes of discussion, only one stage description is reviewed, based on a summary given in Kennedy and Kent (1985). Most other stage descriptions of swallowing can be understood as modifications of the one discussed here. The stages described below are illustrated in Figure 5–59.

Containment Stage

An anterior seal is formed by the lips and also by the tip or blade of the tongue. The bolus is held in a depression at the front of the tongue. The dorsum of the tongue often arches upward to assist in bolus containment. In effect, the tongue performs a spooning or pooling action to contain the bolus. An additional posterior seal may be effected by the soft palate, which descends to make contact with the tongue. The bolus is also contained laterally by the sides of the tongue. Stabilization of the tongue and lips may be assisted by a partially closed position of the jaw.

Midpalatal Stage

The bolus is squeezed aborally by a progressive wavelike elevation of the anterior tongue, rather like squeezing a toothpaste tube to push the paste toward the opening. At the same time, the dorsum of the tongue is lowered to receive the bolus. The soft palate elevates in advance of the bolus to open the oropharyngeal channel and also to close the velopharyngeal port.

Pharyngeal Compression Stage

This stage begins as the bolus reaches the faucial pillars and soft palate. The passage between the oral cavity and pharynx is called the **isthmus of fauces**. Many authorities believe that this stage is the onset of reflexive control of deglutition, with the preceding stages being more under voluntary control (however, a strict dichotomy of voluntary versus reflexive control may not be justifiable). One feature of this control is cessation of respiratory activity (the apneic interval). The name *compression* derives from the action of the tongue, which flexes backward on the hyoid bone to thrust the bolus posteriorly into the pharynx. Vigorous tongue motion is essential to this stage of the swallow.

Pharyngeal Engulfing Stage

The larynx moves in a superior-anterior direction to tuck under the root of the tongue. The epiglottis tips downward and back-

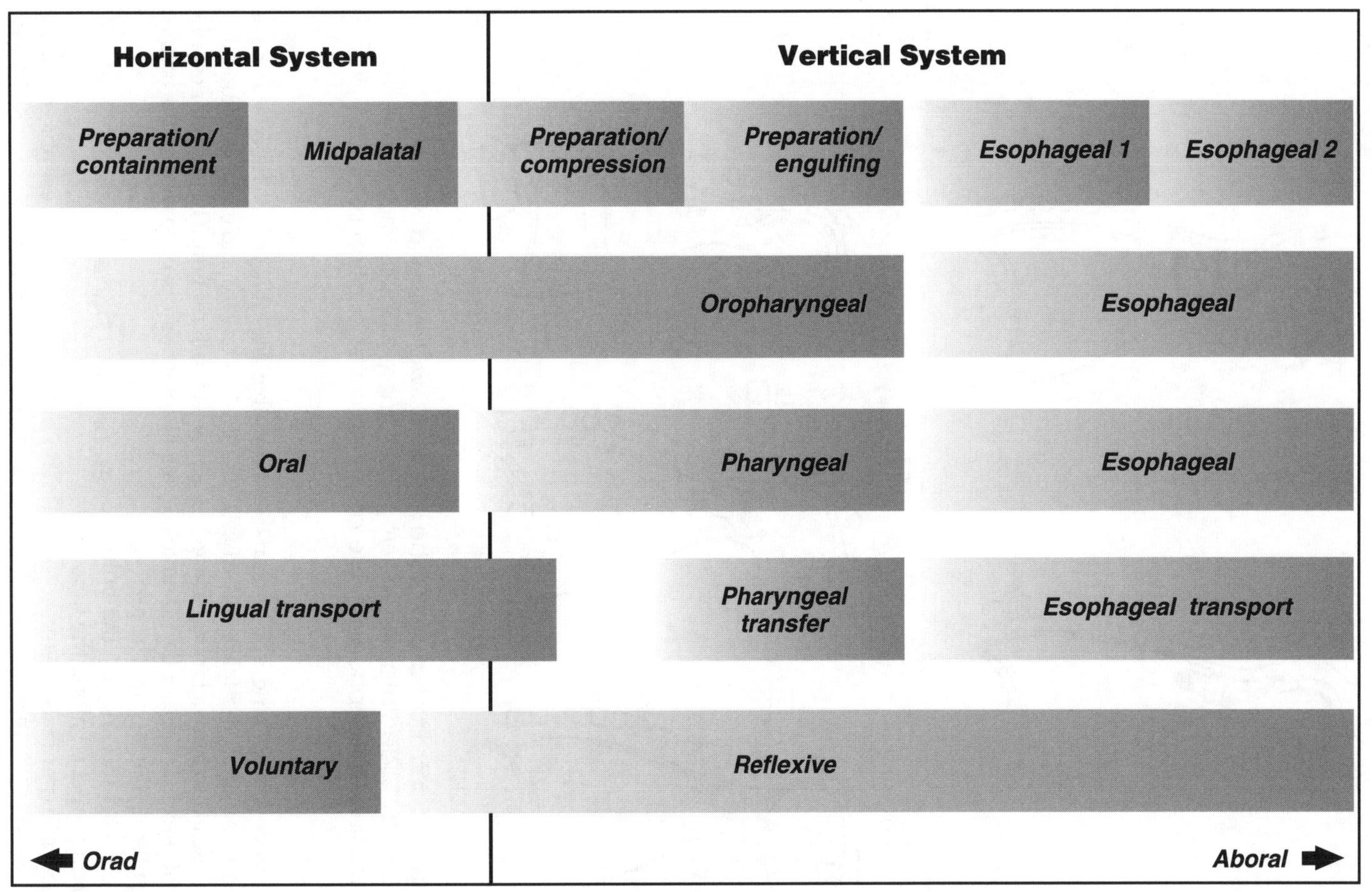

Figure 5–58. Selected stage descriptions of swallowing, shown relative to a horizontal and vertical reference. The oral cavity comprises the horizontal system, and the pharyngeal cavity comprises the vertical system.

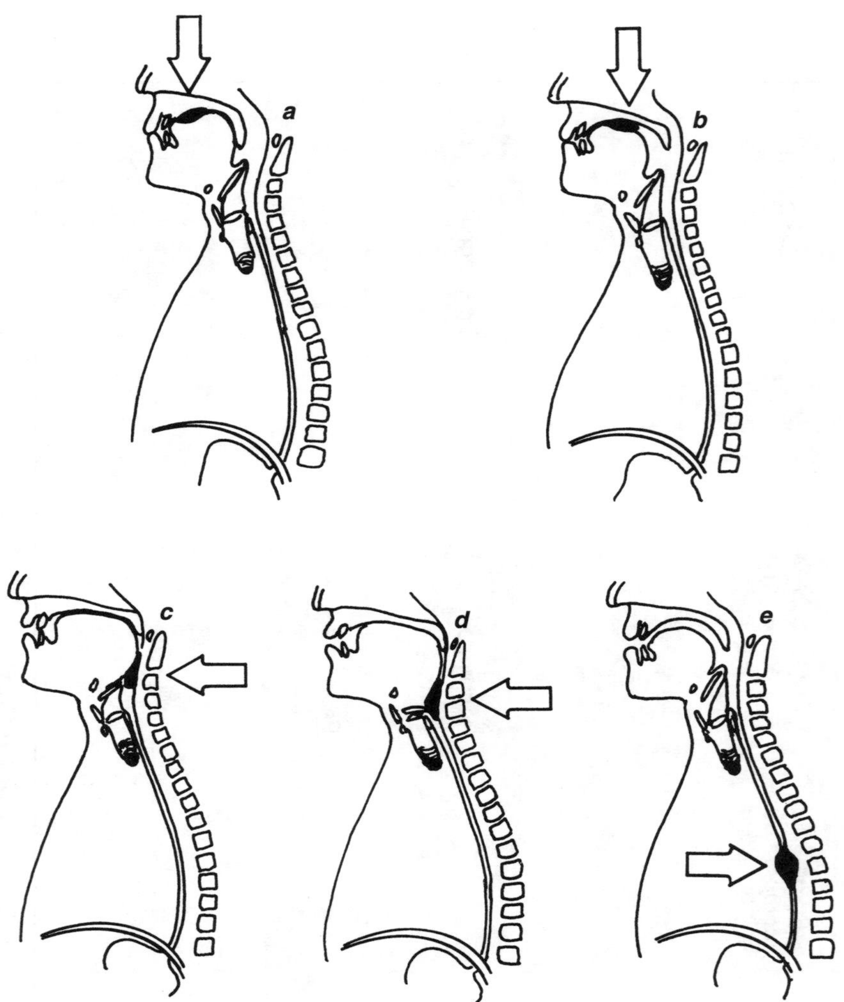

Figure 5–59. Illustrations of the stages of swallowing: **a.** Containment. **b.** Midpalatal. **c.** Pharyngeal compression. **d.** Pharyngeal engulfing. **e.** Esophageal. The arrow indicates position of bolus.

ward to protect the opening into the larynx. At the same time, the false and true vocal folds adduct to form a laryngeal constriction that prevents solid or liquid materials from entering the larynx. The pharyngeal tube elevates to "engulf" the bolus, which is then propelled along the tube by a peristaltic wave (**peristalsis** refers to successive waves of involuntary contraction). The analogy of a snake capturing its prey is sometimes used to describe this stage. Imagine that the pharyngeal tube is a snake that moves toward and engulfs its food in a single smooth motion. The superior esophageal sphincter opens to receive the bolus.

Esophageal Stage

The bolus is moved by esophageal peristaltic contractions until it reaches the gastroesophageal sphincter, the entrance to the stomach. Respiration resumes and the soft palate descends to its rest position to permit nasal breathing. (Some authorities recognize two esophageal substages.)

Bolus transport time is the time required for passage of the bolus for a given stage or for movement between two specified points. Once a solid bolus has been prepared for swallow, the oropharyngeal transport time averages about 2 sec in young adults but about 3–4 sec in older adults (Sonies, Parent, Morrish, & Baum, 1988). There is substantial individual variation in these times. Esophageal transport time ranges from about 0.5 to 1 sec. Generally, liquid boluses have shorter transport times than solid boluses.

Swallowing can be conceptualized as a wave of muscular activity that proceeds from oral cavity to pharyngeal cavity to esophagus. The participation of major structures in the act of swallowing is summarized in Table 5–2. The activation of the various structures is effected in a smooth overlapping fashion. The initial activity in the lips and tongue (with stabilization from the jaw) is followed by activity in the pharynx, soft palate, and larynx. The final stages are associated with the peristaltic muscular activity in the esophagus. Knowledge about swallowing has increased substantially within the last decade. Additional sources of information are listed under **On the Reference Shelf** and in the chapter references. Arvedson and Rogers (1993) discuss swallowing and its disorders in children—their paper is a good source of information on developmental issues in swallowing.

Table 5–2. Participation of various oral and laryngeal structures in swallowing.

	Stages of Swallowing				
Structure	**Preparation and Containment**	**Midpalatal**	**Pharyngeal Compression**	**Pharyngeal Engulfing**	**Esophageal 1 and 2**
Lips	Anterior seal ——————>				
Tongue tip	Anterior seal ——————>				
Tongue dorsum	Bolus retention	Bolus transport			
Tongue root			Bolus transport ——————>		
Jaw	Stabilization ——————>				
Soft palate velopharynx		Closes velopharynx ——————>			Opens
Pharynx			Opens for bolus	Bolus transport	
Epiglottis			Closes entry to larynx		Opens
Esophagus		Superior sphincter opens	Peristaltic transport of bolus		

CONCLUSION

Chapters 4 and 5 summarize the anatomy of the respiratory, laryngeal, and upper airway subsystems of speech production. Although these subsystems figure prominently in speech, they serve many other functions, especially ventilation and food intake. Many writers describe speech as an overlaid function, one that is imposed on physiological systems designed to serve more basic functions that support life. If so, speech is a remarkable opportunist. Drawing on the capabilites of a diverse set of organs, humans have come to rely on the faculty of speech as the primary system of communication. As discussed in Chapter 1, virtually every group of people throughout the world, with the exception of those with a serious hearing impairment, use speech. The anatomy of speech production is complex. Chapters 4 and 5 highlight the major components of the overall system of speech production and should prepare the reader for further study of the anatomy and physiology of this system, of pathologies that impair its function (Chapter 12), or of specialized issues such as inquiry into its evolutionary origins (Chapter 13) or embryology (Chapter 14). The next chapter considers the auditory system, which is a major sensory partner in spoken language.

On The Reference Shelf

Recommended for readers who seek additional information or a different perspective on the material covered in this chapter.

Avery, J. K. (Ed.). (1994). *Oral development and histology* (2nd ed.). New York: Thieme Medical Publishers.
A valuable source on developmental aspects of the oral structures, and their histologic properties.

Brand, R. W., & Isselhard, D. E. (1977). *Anatomy of orofacial structures*. St. Louis: Mosby.
An older, but excellent, book directed toward dentistry.

Seikel, J. A., King, D. W., & Drumright, D. G. (1997). *Anatomy and physiology for speech and language*. San Diego: Singular Publishing Group.
A recent basic text on the anatomy and physiology of speech; accompanied by computer disks and video materials.

Zemlin, W. R. (1988). *Speech and hearing science: Anatomy and physiology*. Englewood Cliffs, NJ: Prentice-Hall.
A classic text, rich in anatomic detail.

Chapter References

Ardran, G. M. & Kemp, F. H. (1972). A functional assessment of relative tongue size. *American Journal of Roentgenology, 114*, 282–288.

Arvedson, J. C., & Rogers, B. T. (1993). Pediatric swallowing and feeding disorders. *Journal of Medical Speech-Language Pathology, 1*, 203–221.

Avery, J. K. (1994). Histology of saliva, pellicle, plaque, and calculus. In J. K. Avery (Ed.), *Oral development and histology* (2nd ed., pp. 382–393). New York: Thieme Medical Publishers.

Beaven, D. W., & Brooks, S. E. (1988). *Color atlas of the tongue in clinical diagnosis*. Chicago: Year Book Medical Publishers.

Bench, R. W. (1963). Growth of the cervical vertebrae as related to tongue, face and denture behavior. *American Journal of Orthodontics, 49*, 183–214.

Bergland, O. (1963). The bony nasopharynx. *Acta Odontologica Scandinavia, 21*(Suppl. 35), 1–137.

Blocquel, H., Laude, M., Lafforgue, P., & Devillers, A. (1990). A cephalometric study of the cervical and palatal movements during growth. *Bulletin Du Groupement International Pour La Recherche Scientifique En Stomatologie Et Odontologie, 33*, 9–18.

Bodanis, D. (1995, April). Pulling *what* out of thin air. *Smithsonian, 26*(1), 76–81.

Bosma, J. (1975). Anatomic and physiologic development of the speech apparatus. In D. B. Tower (Ed.), *The nervous system: Human communication and its disorders* (Vol. 3, pp. 469–481). New York: Raven Press.

Buck, J. M. (1997). Organic variation of the vocal apparatus. In W. J. Hardcastle & J. Laver (Eds.), *The handbook of phonetic sciences* (pp. 256–297). Cambridge, MA: Blackwell.

Burke, P. H. (1980). Serial growth changes in the lips. *British Journal of Orthodontics, 7*, 17–30.

Cassell, M. D., Moon, J. B., & Elkadi, H. (1990). Anatomy and physiology of the velopharynx. In J. Bardach & H. Morris (Eds.), *Multidisciplinary management of cleft lip and palate*. Philadelphia: Saunders.

Chinsamy, A., & Dodson, P. (1995, March/April). Inside a dinosaur bone. *American Scientist, 83*, 174–180.

Croft, C. B., Shprintzen, R. J., & Rakoff, S. J. (1981). Patterns of velopharyngeal valving in normal and cleft palate subjects: A multiview videofluoroscopic and nasendoscopic study. *Laryngoscope, 91*, 265–271.

Demirjian, A. (1980). Dental development: A measure of physical maturity. In F. E. Johnston, A. F. Roche, & C. Susanne (Eds.), *Human physical growth and maturation: Methodologies and factors* (pp. 83–100). NATO Advanced Study Institute Series A: Life Sciences, Vol. 30. New York: Plenum Publishing Corp.

Dickson, D., & Maue-Dickson, W. (1982). *Anatomical and physiological bases of speech*. Boston: Little, Brown.

DiFoggio, J. J. (1984). *An anatomical investigation of the extrinsic lingual musculature*. Unpublished master's thesis, University of Wisconsin-Madison.

Duffy, J. R. (1995). *Motor speech disorders: Substrates, differential diagnosis, and management*. St. Louis: Mosby.

Ettema, S. L., & Kuehn, D. P. (1994). A quantitative histologic study of the normal human adult soft palate. *Journal of Speech and Hearing Research, 37*, 303–313.

Evans, C. A. (1994). Postnatal facial growth, birth through postadolescence. In J. K. Avery (Ed.), *Oral development and histology* (2nd ed., pp. 58–67). New York: Thieme Medical Publishers.

Finkelstein, Y., Berger, G., Nachimani, A., & Ophir, D. (1996). The functional role of the adenoids in speech. *International Journal of Pediatric Otorhinolaryngology, 34*, 61–74.

Finkelstein, Y., Shapiro-Feinberg, M., Talmi, Y. P., Nachmani, A., DeRowe, A., & Ophir, D. (1995). Axial configuration of the velopharyngeal valve and its valving mechanism. *Cleft Palate and Craniofacial Journal, 32*, 299–305.

Fujioka, M., Young, L. W., & Girdany, B. R. (1979). Radiographic evaluation of adenoidal size in children: Adenoidal-nasopharyngeal ratio. *American Journal of Roentgenology, 133*, 401–404.

Handelman, C. S. & Osborne, G. (1976). Growth of the nasopharynx and adenoid development from one to eighteen years. *Angle Orthodontist, 46*, 243–259.

Jeans, W. D., Fernando, D. C., Maw, A. R., & Leighton, B. C. (1981). A longitudinal study of the nasopharynx and its contents in normal children. *British Journal of Radiology, 54*, 117–121.

Kennedy, J. G., III, & Kent, R. D. (1985). Anatomy and physiology of deglutiton and related functions. *Seminars in Speech and Language, 6*, 257–273.

Kent, R. D., & Vorperian, H. K. (1995). *Development of the craniofacial-oral-laryngeal anatomy*. San Diego: Singular Publishing Group.

Kier, W. M., & Smith, K. K. (1985). Tongues, tentacles, and trunks: The biomechanics of movement in muscular hydrostats. *Zoological Journal of the Linnean Society*, *83*, 307–324.

Konner, M. (1986, September/October). The riddle of the smile. *The Sciences*, *26*, 4–6.

Kuehn, D. P., Folkins, J. W., & Cutting, C. (1982). Relationships between muscle activity and velar position. *Cleft Palate Journal*, *19*, 25–35.

Kuehn, D. P., Folkins, J. W., & Linville, R. N. (1988). An electromyographic study of the musculus uvulae. *Cleft Palate Journal*, *25*, 348–355.

Kuehn, D. P., & Kahane, J. C. (1990). Histologic study of the normal human adult soft palate. *Cleft Palate Journal*, *27*, 26–34.

Lewis, A. B. (1991). Comparisons between dental and skeletal ages. *The Angle Orthodontist*, *61*, 87–92.

Lieberman, P. (1991). *Uniquely human*. Cambridge, MA: Harvard University Press.

Lowrey, G. H. (1973). *Growth and development of children* (6th ed.). Chicago: Year Book Medical Publishers.

Mafee, M. F., & Carter, B. L. (1995). Nasal cavity and paranasal sinuses. In G. E. Valvassori, M. F. Mafee, & B. L. Carter (Eds.), *Imaging of the head and neck* (pp. 248–331). New York: Thieme Medical Publishers.

McKerns, D., & Bzoch, K. (1970). Variations in velopharyngeal valving: The factor of sex. *Cleft Palate Journal*, *7*, 652–662.

Meltzoff, A. N., & Moore, M. K. (1977). Imitation of facial and manual gestures by human neonates. *Science*, *198*, 75–78.

Meltzoff, A. N., & Moore, M. K. (1993). Why faces are special to infants—On connecting the attraction of faces and infants' ability for imitation and cross-modal processing. In B. de Boysson-Bardies, S. de Schonen, P. Jusczyk, P. MacNeilage, & J. Morton (Eds.), *Developmental neurocognition: Speech and face processing in the first year of life* (pp. 211–225). Dordrecht, the Netherlands: Kluwer Academic Publishers.

Moon J. B., & Canady, J. W. (1995). Effects of gravity on velopharyngeal muscle activity during speech. *Cleft Palate and Craniofacial Journal*, *32*, 371–375.

Moon, J. B., & Kuehn, D. P. (in press). Anatomy and physiology of normal and disordered velopharyngeal function for speech. To appear in K. Bzoch (Ed.), *Communicative disorders related to cleft lip and palate* (4th ed.).

Moss, M. L. (1968). The primacy of functional matrices on orofacial growth. *Dental Practice*, *19*, 65–74.

Moss, M. L., Moss-Salentijn, L., & Ostreicher, H. P. (1974). The logarithmic properties of active and passive mandibular growth. *American Journal of Orthodontics*, *66*, 645–664.

Niswonger, M. E. (1934). The rest position of the mandible and the centric relation. *Journal of the American Dental Association*, *21*, 1572–1581.

Norton, P. G., & Dunn, E. V. (1986). Night noise. *The Sciences*, *26(4)*, 54–57.

Palmer, J. M. (1993). *Anatomy for speech and hearing* (4th ed.). Baltimore: Williams & Wilkins.

Piaget, J. (1962). *Play, dreams and imitation in childhood*. New York: Norton.

Pierce, R. H., Mainen, M. W., & Bosma, J. F. (1978). *The cranium of the newborn infant*. Bethesda, MD: National Institutes of Health, National Institute of Dental Research.

Provenza, D. V., & Seibel, W. (1986). *Oral histology: Inheritance and development* (2nd ed., p. 407). Philadelphia: Lea and Febiger.

Pullinger, A. G., Liu, S.-P., Low, G., & Tay, D. (1987). Differences between sexes in maximum jaw opening when corrected to body size. *Archives of Oral Rehabilitation*, *14*, 291–299.

Ranly, D. M. (1988). *A synopsis of craniofacial growth*. Norwalk, CT: Appleton & Lange.

Riechelmann, H., Hinni, M., Klimek, L., & Mann, W. J. (1995). Objective measures of nasal function. *Current Opinion in Otolaryngology & Head and Neck Surgery*, *3*, 207–212.

Rodenstein, D. O., & Stanesco, D. C. (1986). The soft palate and breathing. *American Review of Respiratory Disease*, *134*, 311–325.

Russell, A. (Editor-in-Chief) (1987). *Guinness book of world records*. Toronto: Bantam Books.

Saito, A., & Nishihata, S. (1981). Nasal airway resistance in children. *Rhinology*, *19*, 149–154.

Scammon, R. E. (1930). The measurement of the body in childhood. In J. A. Harris, C. M. Jackson, D. G. Patterson, & R. E. Scammon (Eds.), *The measurement of man* (pp. 173–215). Minneapolis, MN: University of Minnesota Press.

Shprintzen, R. J. (1992). Assessment of velopharyngeal function: Nasopharyngoscopy and multiview videofluoroscopy. In L. Brodsky, L. Holt, & D. H. Ritter-Schmidt (Eds.), *Craniofacial anomalies: An interdisciplinary approach* (pp. 196–207). St. Louis: Mosby-Year Book.

Siebert, J. R., & Haas, J. E. (1988). Size of the tongue in sudden infant death syndrome. In P. J. Schwartz, D. P. Southall, & M. Valdes-Dapena (Eds.), *The sudden infant death syndrome. Annals of the New York Academy of Sciences, 533*, 467–468.

Siegel-Sadewitz, V. L., & Shprintzen, R. J. (1986). Changes in velopharyngeal valving with age. *International Journal of Pediatric Otorhinolaryngology, 11*, 171–182.

Skolnick, M. L., McCall, G. N., & Barnes, M. (1973). The sphincteric mechanism of velopharyngeal closure. *Cleft Palate Journal, 10*, 286–305.

Skolnick, M. L., Shprintzen, R. J., McCall, G. N., & Rakoff, S. J. (1975). Patterns of velopharyngeal closure in subjects with repaired cleft palate and normal speech: A multi–view videofluoroscopic analysis. *Cleft Palate Journal, 12*, 369–376.

Solberg, W. K., Woo, M. W., & Houston, J. B. (1979). Prevalence of mandibular dysfunction in young adults. *Journal of the American Dental Association, 98*, 25–34.

Sonies, B. C., Parent, L. J., Morrish, K., & Baum, B. J. (1988). Durational aspects of the oral-pharyngeal phase of swallow. *Dysphagia, 3*, 1–10.

Spaeth, J., Krugelstein, U., & Schlondorff, G. (1997). The paranasal sinuses in CT-imaging: Development from birth to age 25. *International Journal of Pediatric Otorhinolaryngology, 39*, 25–40.

Subtelny, J. D. (1957). A cephalometric study of the growth of the soft palate. *Plastic and Reconstructive Surgery, 19*, 49–62.

Thach, B. T. (1973). Morphologic zones of the human fetal lip margin. In J. F. Bosma (Ed.) *Fourth symposium on oral sensation and perception: Development in the fetus and infant* (pp. 96–117). Bethesda, MD: DHEW Publication NIH 73–546.

Tourne, L. P. (1991). Growth of the pharynx and its physiologic implications. *American Journal of Orthodontics and Dentofacial Orthopedics, 99*, 129–139.

Walker, G. F., & Kowalski, C. J. (1972). On the growth of the mandible. *American Journal of Physical Anthropology, 36*, 111–118.

Widmer, R. P. (1992). The normal development of teeth. *Australian Family Physician, 21*, 1251–1261.

Exercises

5–1. Using the unlabeled drawing in Figure 5–60, identify the bones of the skull.

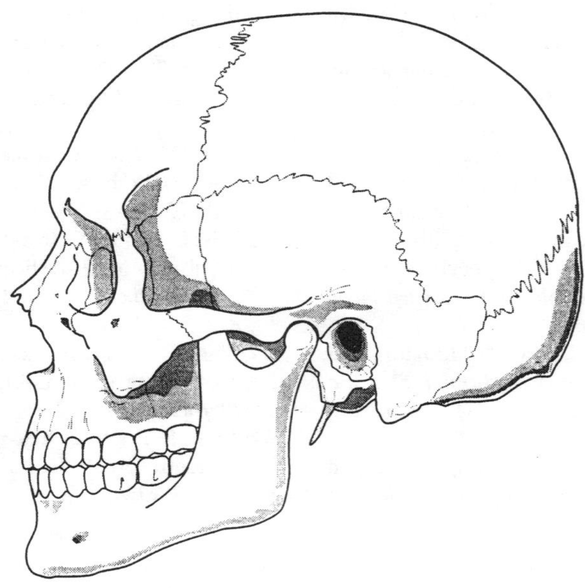

5–2. Describe how the tongue, lips, mandible, and velopharynx change in anatomy across the following ages: 2 years, 6 years, 18 years. Using the illustrations in this chapter as a guide, draw these structures at each of the specified ages.

5–3. Draw the general outline of a frontal view of the human face, sketching in the eyes, mouth, and nose. Then, use different colored pencils to draw in the approximate locations of the muscles of facial expression.

5–4. Discuss the properties of a muscular hydrostat. Why might this model be suitable for the tongue and soft palate, but not for the muscles of the jaw?

5–5. Using modeling clay of different colors, make a model of the tongue as follows. Use one color to make up the genioglossus, which is the bulk of the tongue. With another color, attach clay to the sides of the tongue and shape it to extend upward to form the palatoglossus. A third color will form the hyoglossus. To form this muscle, attach clay to the sides of the tongue and extend it downward. Finally, the fourth color will represent the styloglossus, which runs backward from the sides of the tongue at its posterior region.

5–6. Although refinements in anatomic description continue to be made with respect to issues such as origin and insertion of muscles, it is not often that a new muscle is described. Drs. Gary Hack and Gwendolyn Dunn announced at the 1996 annual meeting of the American Association for the Advancement of Science that they discovered a new muscle, named the **sphenomandibularis**. The muscle was found in 25 cadavers and in living individuals who were studied with magnetic resonance imaging (MRI) scans. The newly discovered muscle has its origin on the sphenoid process behind the eye socket and its insertion on the mandible. Apparently, its fibers have been confused with those of the medial pterygoid, which has a similar insertion. The muscle may have clinical importance in that it could explain certain pains behind the eye that are associated with chewing. To demonstrate that this is, in fact, a new muscle, it needs to be shown that it has an independent innervation and insertions distinct from those of other muscles. Using a model of the skull and mandible or drawings of these structures, try to imagine the location of this muscle and to describe its action.

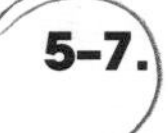

5–7. The bones of the skull and face serve as places of attachment for the muscles of the face, mandible, and neck. The numbers 1–13 on Figure 5–61 represent the points of attachment of several different muscles. Match each number with one of the muscles listed below. (Answers are in appendix.)

Levator labii superioris alaeque nasi
Levator labii superioris
Levator anguli oris
Buccinator
Mentalis
Depressor labii inferioris

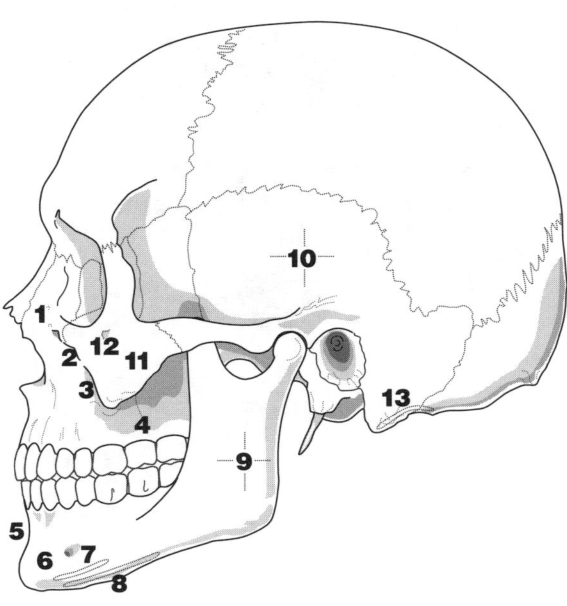

Depressor anguli oris
Platysma
Masseter
Temporalis
Zygomaticus major
Zygomaticus minor
Sternocleidomastoid

5–8. This exercise is like Exercise 1 except that the points of muscle attachment are listed on the basal surface of the skull (Figure 5–62). Match each of the numbers in the drawing with one of the muscles listed below. (Answers are in appendix.)

Musculus uvulae
Palatopharyngeus
Internal pterygoid (deep head)
Internal pterygoid (superficial head)
External pterygoid (upper head)
Masseter
Styloglossus
Stylohyoid
Stylopharyngeus
Posterior belly of digastric
Sternocleidomastoid

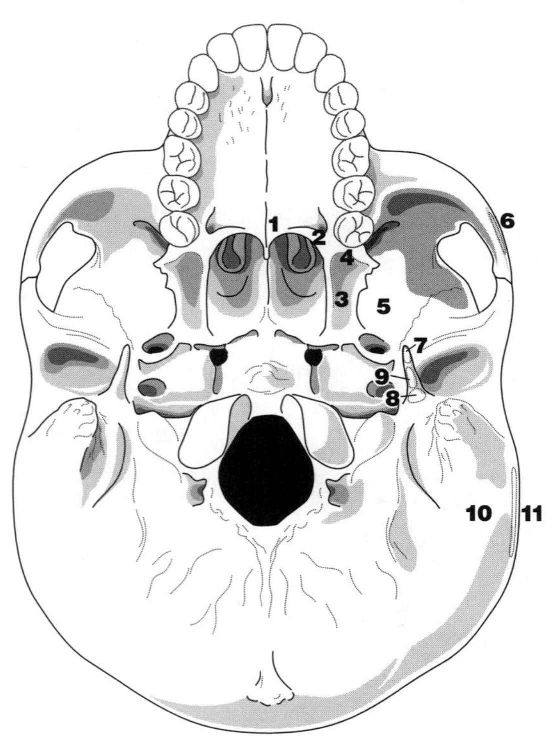

5–9. The following exercises are based on the videotape, *Measuring Speech Production: A Video Demonstration of Speech Instrumentation* (available from the Acoustical Society of America). View one of the following and prepare a brief review of the video demonstration. Your review should include: the name of the technique, a short description of how it works, and an example of its application to the study of speech. Both video demonstrations are contained in "Part Two: Indirect Articulatory Measurements."

Choose either:

Magnetic resonance imaging (MRI) in speech research.

Imaging the tongue with ultrasound.

C H A P T E R

6

The Auditory System

"According to the saga, Heimdal was able to hear the grass grow. Our hearing ability is perhaps not of that kind, but our ear is anyhow almost sensitive enough to record the bounce of an air molecule against the eardrum, while, on the other hand, it can withstand the pounding of sound waves strong enough to set the body vibrating. Moreover, the ear is capable of a selectivity which permits a close analysis of sounds, the various qualities of which determine the characteristics of the spoken word and of instrumental and vocal expressions in the universe of music."

(From C. G. Bernhard's comments concerning the awarding of the Nobel Prize for Physiology or Medicine in 1961 to Georg von Bekesy; reprinted in the *Journal of the Acoustical Society of America, Supplement, The Bekesy Commemorative Issue,* no page number given (1962).)

Audition, the sense of hearing, depends on sensitivity to mechanical vibrations that are ordinarily transmitted through the air. Mechanical sensitivity depends on receptors called **mechanoreceptors**. These are specialized cells that monitor mechanical stimuli such as pressure, position, and movement. There are a variety of mechanoreceptors in the body that provide essential information for a number of different functions. The millions of mechanoreceptors in the skin are the basis of the sensations of touch. The hollow organs of the body, such as the blood vessels and bladder, are equipped with mechanoreceptors that monitor pressure. The skeletal muscles contain mechanoreceptors that provide information on tension and extension.

But the most sensitive mechanoreceptors are the **hair cells** of hearing and balance. Hair cells in one part of the ear are the sensory receptors for audition. Other hair cells serve the sense of balance by responding to linear acceleration (change in motion in a linear direction) or angular acceleration (change in motion in a rotatory direction). The hair cells that serve the senses of audition and balance are the site of mechanoelectrical transduction, or the transformation of mechanical to electrical energy. These cells are encased in the hard temporal bone of the skull (discussed in Chapter 5) in a compartment called the **otic capsule**. The hair cells are subject to stimulation that reaches this hidden area. The understanding of how hair cells work, although far from complete, has advanced remarkably within the last decade. A discussion of current knowledge about the process of hearing begins with a brief look at the gross anatomy of the ear and then continues with a consideration of its microscopic anatomy. The emphasis of this chapter is on anatomy, but a few general comments are made on auditory physiology and the perception of sounds. The perception of speech is considered in some detail in Chapter 10.

GROSS ANATOMY OF THE EAR

The ear is conveniently divided into three parts as shown in overview in Figure 6–1 and a more detailed illustration in Figure 6–2. The first part is the **outer ear**, including the visible appendages on each side of the head. The outer ear captures airborne vibrations and funnels them into a canal called the **external auditory meatus** (or **external auditory canal**). The meatus terminates with the **ear drum**, or **tympanic membrane**. The **middle ear** is a small chamber that contains three tiny bones, the **ossicles**. The **inner ear** is the site of the sensory end organ of hearing, the **cochlea** (Latin for "snail"). Unlike the outer and middle ear, the inner ear is filled with fluid, and it is the motion of this fluid that stimulates the hair cells. The thousands of hair cells that convert mechanical energy to neural impulses are housed in the spiral-shaped and fluid-filled cochlea. The following sections provide additional information on each of the ear's major divisions.

The Outer Ear

The convoluted flap of cartilage and skin that is the most visible manifestation of the ear is referred to technically as the **pinna** or **auricle**. Ironically, this most visible and largest part of the ear is the least important in human auditory function. We can hear fairly well without the pinna, although it serves as a convenient structure to hold eyeglasses in place. It also serves a decorative function for those who wear earrings. The pinna does help somewhat to direct

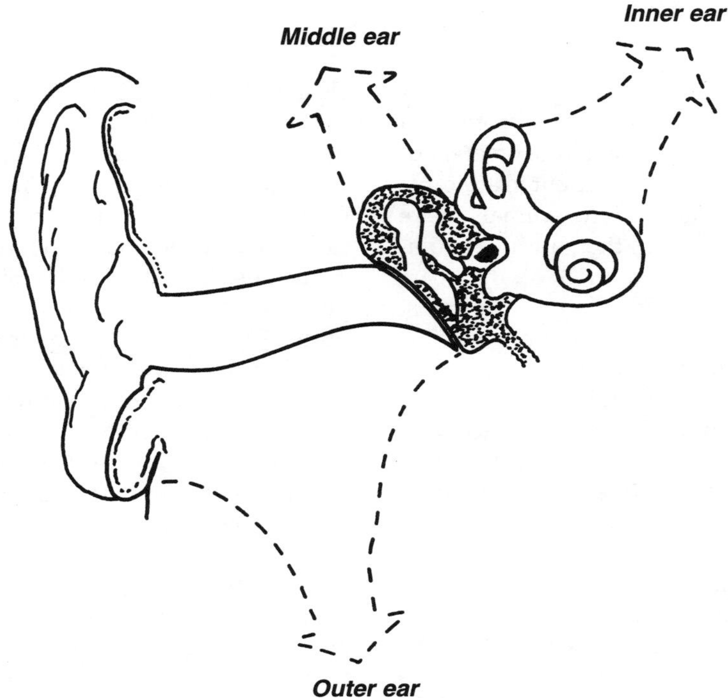

Figure 6–1. The three parts of the ear: outer, middle, and inner.

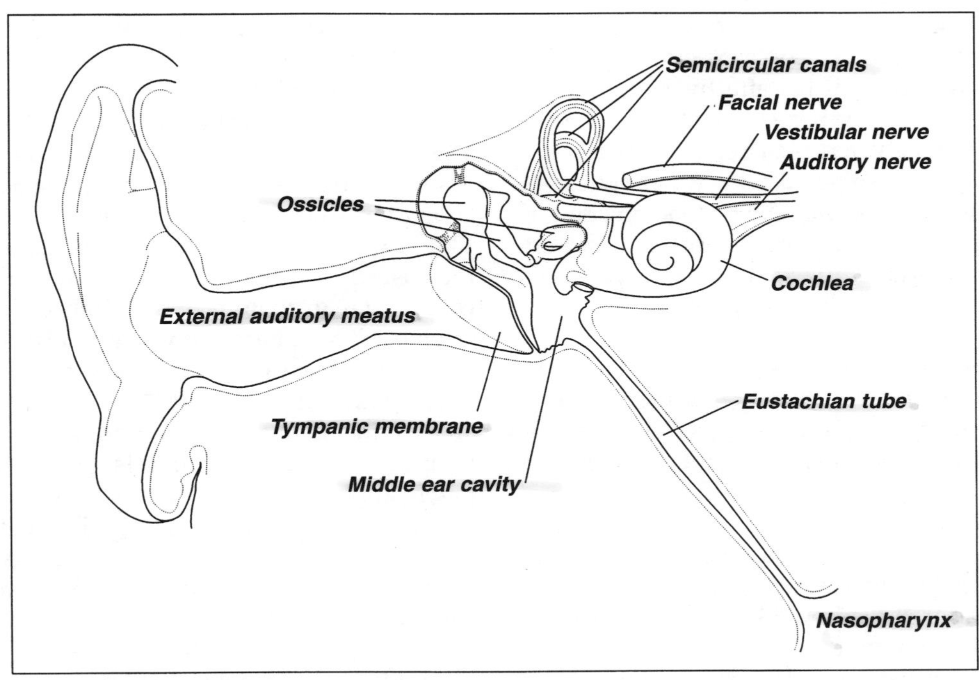

Figure 6–2. Basic anatomy of the ear: structures of the outer, middle, and inner ear.

sound waves into the rest of the ear. But, as most humans have little or no motility of the pinna, head movement is of greater advantage than pinna movement in attempts to capture sound. Many animals have movable pinnas to aid their auditory abilities. Cats and dogs can prick up their ears in response to a sound of interest. For most humans, the term "prick up your ears" is more figurative than literal. Because the pinna is thin-skinned and has virtually no subcutaneous fat, it is susceptible to frostbite. Residents of northern climes need to take precautions to protect the pinna during cold periods.

The pinna funnels sound into the external auditory meatus, sometimes called the **auditory canal**. This tube, S-shaped in the adult, is about 0.6 cm (a quarter inch) in diameter and about 2.5 to 3.0 cm (an inch or so) in length. It is bounded by cartilage in its outer third and by the temporal bone in its inner two-thirds. The cartilage-bounded portion is lined with hair follicles and mucous glands that secrete a wax called **cerumen**. Some people experience a buildup of cerumen that effectively blocks the canal and must be removed by a specialist. Fortunately, cerumen deposits usually are effectively softened with water (Lucente, Lawson, & Novick, 1995). One function of the external auditory meatus is to protect the delicate structures of the middle and inner ear, which lie deeply recessed.

The external auditory meatus terminates at the ear drum, or tympanic membrane, a thin diaphragm that marks the boundary between the outer and middle ear. The ear drum is aptly named if one imagines sound as beating on the drum of the ear. The tympanic membrane can be punctured by physical injury, which is one reason for the admonition that one should never put anything larger than the elbow into the ear canal. The point of this admonition, of course, is that it is risky to put anything into the ear canal. A specialist can clean the canal should this become necessary, but many people have unwittingly damaged their ears in the attempt to clean the canal. The tympanic membrane is fragile and can be ruptured by instruments that probe deeply into the external auditory meatus. As mentioned earlier, one purpose of the external auditory canal is to protect the middle and inner ear. The external auditory canal also warms the air that enters the external ear, which helps to keep the air temperature fairly equal on either side of the tympanic membrane. Unequal air temperatures can result in unequal Brownian (random) motion of air particles, which can be heard as noise (Harris, 1968). (Recall the quotation at the beginning of the chapter, which states that human hearing is just insensitive enough that we do not hear the random movements of air particles.)

The Middle Ear

This (AA) cavity of the ear is about 0.6 cm (a third of an inch) wide and only about 0.4 cm (one-sixth of an inch) deep. This tiny chamber is filled with air and with an arrangement of three tiny bones and their associated tissues. It connects with the nasopharynx (the upper, or nasal, part of the pharynx) by means of a slender tube called the **eustachian tube**, named after the 16th century Italian anatomist, Bartolomeo Eustachio. The name **auditory tube** also is used for this passage, which is about 3 or 4 cm long in adults. The part of the eustachian tube that connects to the middle ear is bounded by cartilage and is normally patent (open). The part of the tube that connects with the nasopharynx is a bellows-like structure that is actively opened by the tensor palatini muscle, which is discussed in Chapter 5.

The middle ear is a biologic gas pocket ventilated by the eustachian tube. We become conscious of the air in the middle ear when atmospheric pressure changes around us, as in scuba diving or flying in a plane. The air is trapped in the middle ear, except when the eustachian tube opens to equalize air pressures between the middle ear and nasopharynx. The uncomfortable sensation one experiences in the ear when scuba diving or changing altitudes in a plane arises because of unequal air pressures within and outside the middle ear. Air pressure pushes against the tympanic membrane, and the direction of the force depends on whether air pressure is greater or lesser within the middle ear than it is outside. The eustachian tube opens during activities such as chewing, swallowing, or yawning. The airplane passenger who experiences middle-ear discomfort is well advised to chew gum vigorously or to yawn.

Both the middle ear and the eustachian tube are lined with a mucociliary system similar to that found in the respiratory airways of the bronchi and trachea. Basically, this system consists of a thin layer of mucus that overlies a bed of cilia. The continuous beating of the cilia transports the mucous blanket along with anything trapped in it, rather like a conveyer belt. Mucus originating in the middle ear is transported through the eustachian tube to the nasopharynx, where it is swallowed. Therefore, the eustachian tube has the twofold purpose of ventilating the middle ear and ridding it of mucus. Mucous blockage is a condition that may lead to infections of the middle ear (Sade & Ar, 1997).

If the eustachian tube is blocked by an ear infection, it can be very difficult to correct an imbalance of air pressures. Rubbing the ears can be a symptom of ear infection in children who are too young to verbalize their discomfort. Young children are more prone to middle ear infections than adults, partly because their eustachian tubes run nearly horizontally when the head is in the upright position. The adult's eustachian tubes have a more diagonal orientation and therefore fluids drain from the middle ear more readily (Figure 6–3). Infections of the middle ear are known medically as **otitis media** (meaning infection of the middle ear). The cumulative incidence for acute otitis media during the period of birth to 24 months has been reported to be more than 40% (Casselbrant, Mandel, Kurs-Lasky, Rockette, & Bluestone, 1995). That is, at least 40% of the infants studied acquired an ear infection during the first 2 years of life. The period of greatest risk was between 6 and 12 months. About 10% of adults also are susceptible to repeated ear infections, possibly because they lack pneumatic (air-filled) cells in the mastoid process of the temporal bone (Sade & Ar, 1997). The mastoid air cells appear to compensate for fluctuations in the gas content of the middle ear. Individuals who lack these cells are at risk for otitis media. It appears that the mastoid air cells, the middle ear, and the eustachian tube form a ventilatory complex that normally resists mucous blockage and disease.

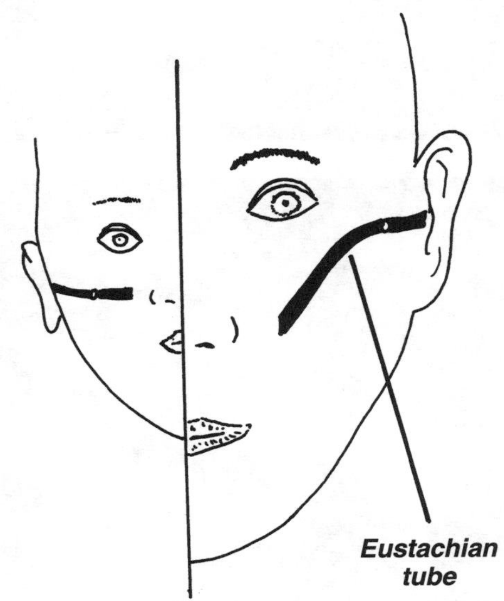

Figure 6–3. Orientation of the eustachian tube in infant and adult.

Recurrent otitis media in children has been proposed as a contributing factor to language and phonological defects. Several studies have supported this relationship (Abraham, Wallace, & Gravel, 1996; Friel-Patti, 1990; Harsten, Nettlebladt, Schalen, Kalm, & Prellner, 1993), but other studies have not (Roberts et al., 1986; Roberts et al., 1989). Perhaps the effect of recurrent otitis media on language and phonological development is not to be found in a simple relationship. This topic continues to attract considerable research interest. We return to this issue in Chapter 10, where it is discussed in relation to the auditory perception of language.

The bones in the ear, the ossicles, are the smallest bones in the human body. They form a small chain of articulated bones, the **ossicular chain** (Figure 6–4). These bones are named, from outermost to innermost, the **hammer** (or **malleus**), **anvil** (or **incus**), and **stirrup** (or **stapes**). The second name given in parentheses is the Latin designation. This tiny chain of bones connects the tympanic membrane with the cochlea. Ligaments within the cavity of the middle ear help to hold the ossicular chain in place. The membrane and bone apparatus of the middle ear converts the vibrations of airborne sound energy to mechanical vibrations. The mechanical energy is transmitted

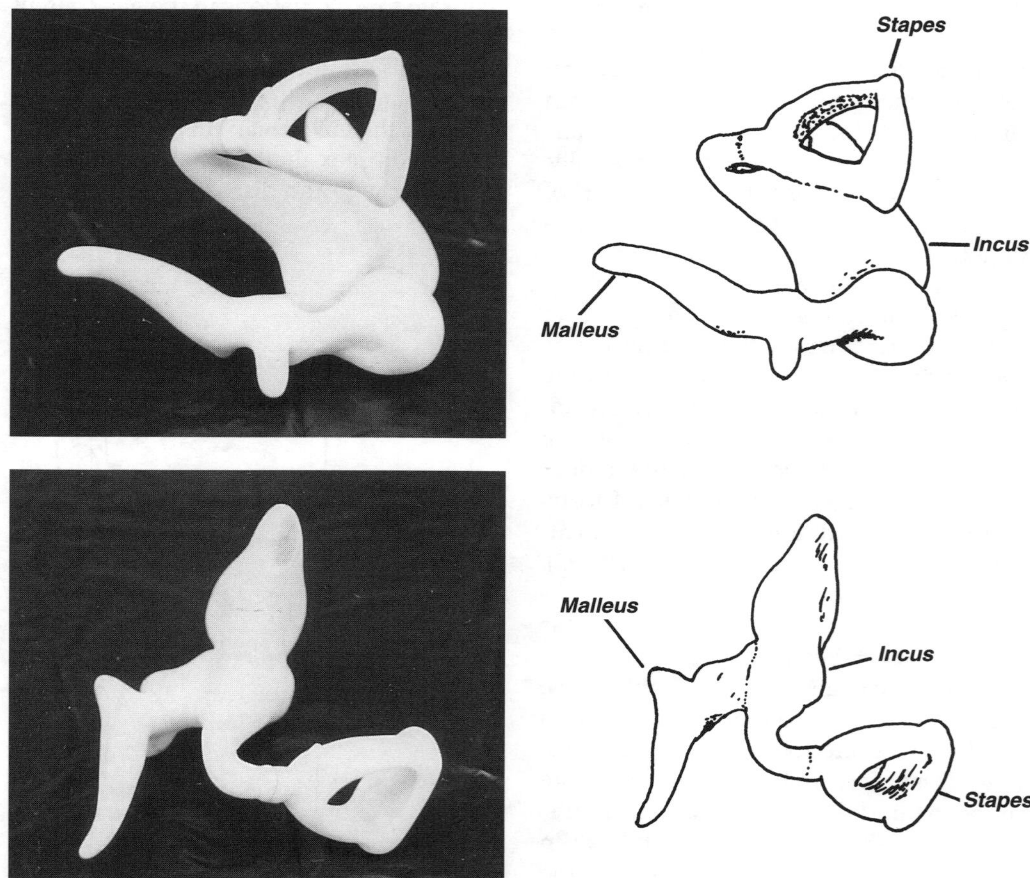

Figure 6–4. Views of the ossicular chain, the three-bone assembly of the middle ear.

from tympanic membrane to malleus to incus to stapes. A convenient way to remember the sequence using the English terms is the mnemonic *has* (**h**ammer to **a**nvil to **s**tirrup). However, the Latin terms are used more frequently by specialists in hearing, so the mnemonic *mis* is an alternative. The last of these bones (stirrup, or stapes) embeds in a window (to be precise, the **oval window**) of the cochlea. Therefore, the mnemonic for the Latin terms might be *misc* (**m**alleus to **i**ncus to **s**tapes to **c**ochlea). And so it is that vibrations from the stapes are delivered to the fluid-filled tubes of the inner ear, which are discussed later.

But this miniature assembly of membrane and bone does more than conduct vibration. It also provides a kind of mechanical advantage in which force is amplified from tympanic membrane to the footplate of the stapes. This amplification happens because of three factors (Yost, 1994):

1. The effective area of the tympanic membrane is about 17 times larger than that of the stapes footplate, which gives rise to a 15 dB increase in pressure going from tympanic membrane to footplate.
2. The ossicles provide a mechanical advantage in the form of a lever action that increases the force at the stapes by about 1.3 relative to the tympanic membrane.
3. Because of its conical shape, the tympanic membrane buckles during its motion to cause a doubling of force between the membrane and the adjacent malleus.

The combination of these three factors yields a maximum pressure increase of about 44:1, which is equivalent to about 33 dB. This increase is important in transferring energy from air, which has little density and high compressibility, to the inner ear fluids, which have high density and little compressibility. Were it not for the middle ear mechanics, the force delivered to the inner ear would be largely reflected (bounced back) because the inner ear would act like a rigid wall compared to the vibrations in the external air. Reflection can occur whenever force is transmitted from a less dense to a more dense medium.

The tiny bones of the middle ear are equipped with two tiny muscles (Figure 6–5). The **stapedius muscle**, which has the

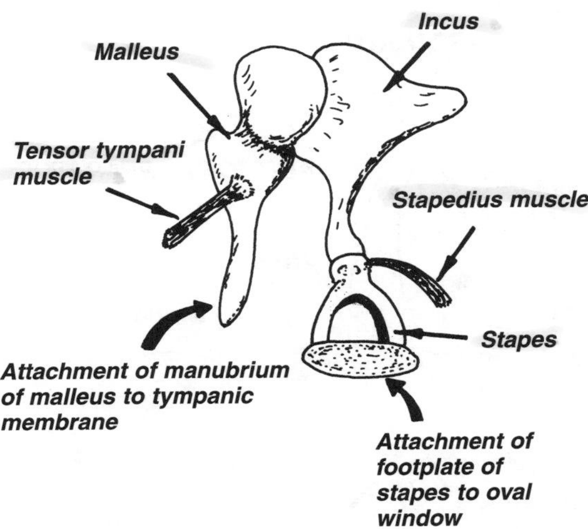

Figure 6–5. The attachments of the tensor tympani and stapedius muscles.

distinction of being the body's smallest, is about 6 mm long. It runs from a bony canal in the middle ear to the head of the stapes. The **tensor tympani muscle** also has an origin in a bony canal, but connects with the manubrium of the malleus. This muscle runs parallel to the eustachian tube and is about 25 mm long. The two muscles have a normal state of tension that helps the operation of the ossicular chain. The stapedius muscle contracts vigorously in response to intense sound, usually 80 dB sensation level (SL) or more. This reflex contraction, the **acoustic,** or **stapedial, reflex,** reduces the transmission of sound energy by 10 to 30 dB and therefore functions as a protective mechanism. This reflex also is part of a general startle reflex.

The footplate of the stapes inserts into the oval window, which looks into the sensory end organ of hearing that is contained in the inner ear. The middle ear's apparatus, built of some of the body's tiniest bone and muscle components, significantly increases the force available to set the fluids of the inner ear into motion. Sound energy enters the external auditory meatus as vibrations of air particles; this energy is converted to mechanical energy by the tympanic membrane and the ossicular chain.

The three-bone ossicular chain is common to mammals. Birds and reptiles have a single middle ear bone, the stapes, which has a cartilaginous extension called the extrastapes. Interestingly, in the development of the mammalian embryo, the malleus has its origin as part of the lower jaw or mandible. During fetal development, the malleus separates from the jaw and becomes a structure of the middle ear. Therefore, ear bones are related to the jaw bone. In fact, from an evolutionary perspective, the middle ear and the jaw were a functional unit in the mammalian ancestors (Crompton & Parker, 1978). Chapter 14 considers this issue from an embryological perspective.

The Inner Ear

The cochlea and the vestibular organ are a closely connected system that sits within the bony case of the temporal bone. Figure 6–6 is a sketch of this apparatus. Basic functions are as follows.

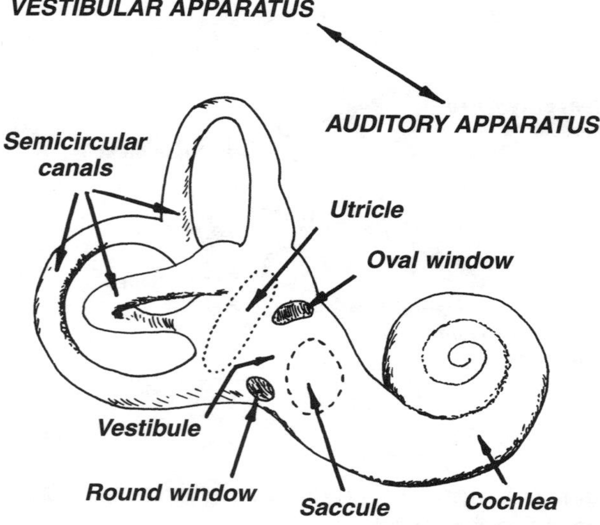

Figure 6–6. The cochlea and vestibular system.

The cochlea is the organ of hearing. As noted earlier, the word "cochlea" is derived from the Latin for "snail." This derivation aptly describes the coiled structure, which bears an interesting resemblance to the shell of the pearly nautilus. The geometry of this spiral has a mathematical simplicity and an esthetic appeal. Descartes called this pattern an equiangular spiral and Jakob Bernoulli termed it the logarithmic spiral. Bernoulli's fascination with this spiral is discussed in Chapter 2. An important characteristic of this spiral is that it retains its original proportions as its size increases. Its mathematical blueprint applies across all sizes. Both the snail and the sense of audition have exploited a geometric relation. On the cosmologic scale, so do the spiral galaxies. The human cochlea has 2⅝ turns. If the cochlea of the adult male is uncoiled and straightened, it reaches to a length of about 35 mm (slightly less than 1½ inches). The number of turns and length of the cochlea vary among mammals.

The vestibular apparatus includes the **vestibule**, **utricle**, **saccule**, and **semicircular canals**. These are essentially fluid-filled sacs and tubes. The vestibule is an oval-shaped cavity that contains the utricle and saccule. The vestibule is filled with a fluid called **perilymph**. The utricle and saccule respond to linear acceleration, as is experienced by a passenger when a car is smoothly accelerated from a stop. The semicircular canals respond to angular acceleration, as experienced when a person is spun in a rotating chair. Each of these does, in fact, have a semicircular appearance and they are arranged at right angles to one another in geometric symmetry. The design is remarkable: three miniature arches arranged in the three dimensions of space.

These parts share a reliance on hydromechanics, or the mechanics of liquids, as discussed in Chapter 2. The cochlea and the vestibular organ are filled with fluids. The hair cells that ultimately generate the neural signals of audition and balance are awash in these fluids. For this reason, the cochlea and the vestibular organ can be considered as hydrodynamic systems. The conversion from mechanical to neural energy relies on the streaming of fluids past the sensitive hair cells of the auditory and vestibular systems.

> ***"Of all the senses, hearing most resembles a contraption some ingenious plumber has put together from spare parts."***
>
> (Diane Ackerman, *A Natural History of the Senses*, New York, Random House, 1990, p. 178.)

The hydrodynamics of the cochlea can be understood more easily by using simplified illustrations of cochlear action. In Figure 6–7, the spiral turns of the cochlea are straightened so that it now appears as a straight tube with a basal end (near the oval window) and an apical end. In fact, some species, such as birds, have a nearly straight tube for a cochlea. The straightened tube of Figure 6–7 would have a length of about 3.5 cm and a width of about 0.4 cm at its thickest region. In Figure 6–8, the interior of the cochlea is exposed to reveal that it is divided by a triangular-shaped duct (the **cochlear partition**) into two fluid-filled passages that run lengthwise together from base to apex. These passages are called the **scala tympani** and the **scala vestibuli**. Both are filled with a fluid called perilymph, which, as noted previously, is also found in the vestibule. The oval window opens into the scala vestibuli (AA), and another opening, the **round window**, opens into the scala tympani (Figure 6–7). A closer look at the cochlear partition (enlargement in Figure 6–8) reveals that it is formed by two membranes that enclose a space filled with another fluid called **endolymph**. These two membranes are **Reissner's membrane** and the **basilar membrane**. The scala tympani, scala vestibuli, and the cochlear partition (also called the **scala media**) thus constitute three divisions that run nearly the en-

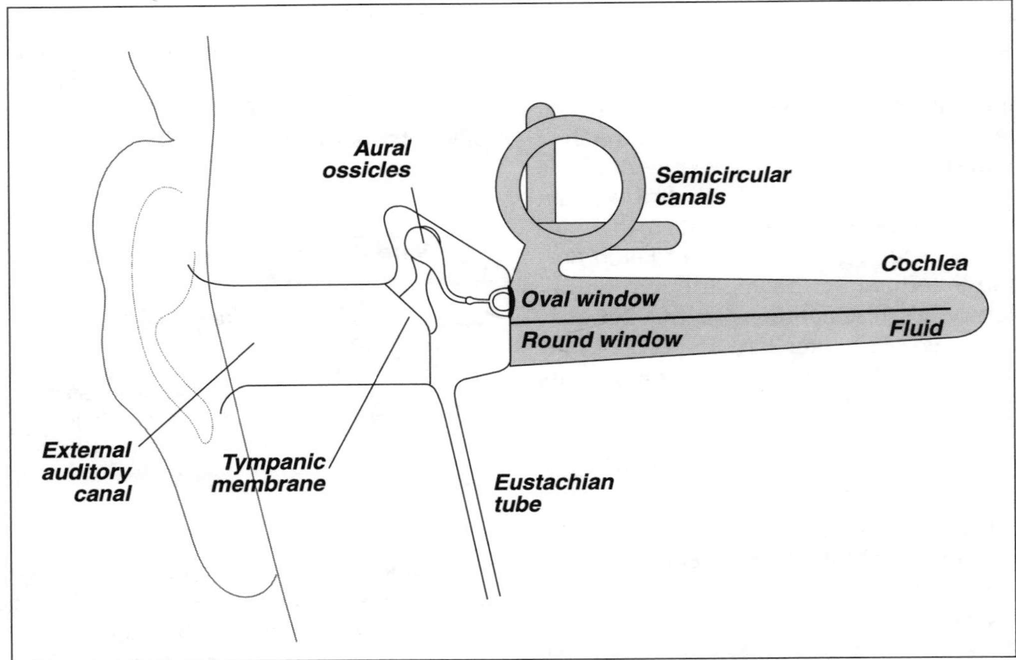

Figure 6–7. Schematic representation of the cochlea, which has been straightened.

tire length of the cochlea. In other words, the cochlea is really three tubes gathered into an elegant spiral. Figure 6–9 is a diagrammatic summary of the structures discussed to this point. It shows how sound waves propagated in the air are converted into mechanical vibrations in the middle ear and then converted into fluid motion in the inner ear.

The structures of interest become smaller and smaller as we proceed deeper into the otic capsule, and our inquiry requires a higher stage of magnification as we examine the details of the cochlear partition. Figure 6–10 shows an enlargement of the cochlear partition. Much of the attention in this chapter is on the **organ of Corti** (Figures 6–8 and 6–10), which is the sensory end-organ of hearing. This organ is located on the side of the basilar membrane that faces the scala media. If the basilar membrane is considered to be the floor of the organ of Corti, then the **reticular lamina** can be regarded as its roof. Covering the roof is another structure, the **tectorial membrane**, which is a collagenous gel. The organ of Corti contains support cells and two types of hair cells, **outer hair cells** and **inner hair cells**, located on either side of the tunnel shown in Figure 6–10. **Deiter's cells** help to support the hair cells. The human cochlea has about 12,000 outer hair cells and about 3,500 inner hair cells. The less numerous inner hair cells are really the sensory receptors for hearing. The role of the outer hair cells is the subject of considerable research and some interesting possibilities are reviewed later in this chapter. First, a further consideration of cochlear hydrodynamics is in order.

As noted in the beginning of this chapter, Georg von Bekesy received the Nobel prize for his work on audition. One of his scientific discoveries was the **traveling wave** within the cochlea. This wave is a fundamental aspect of cochlear hydrody-

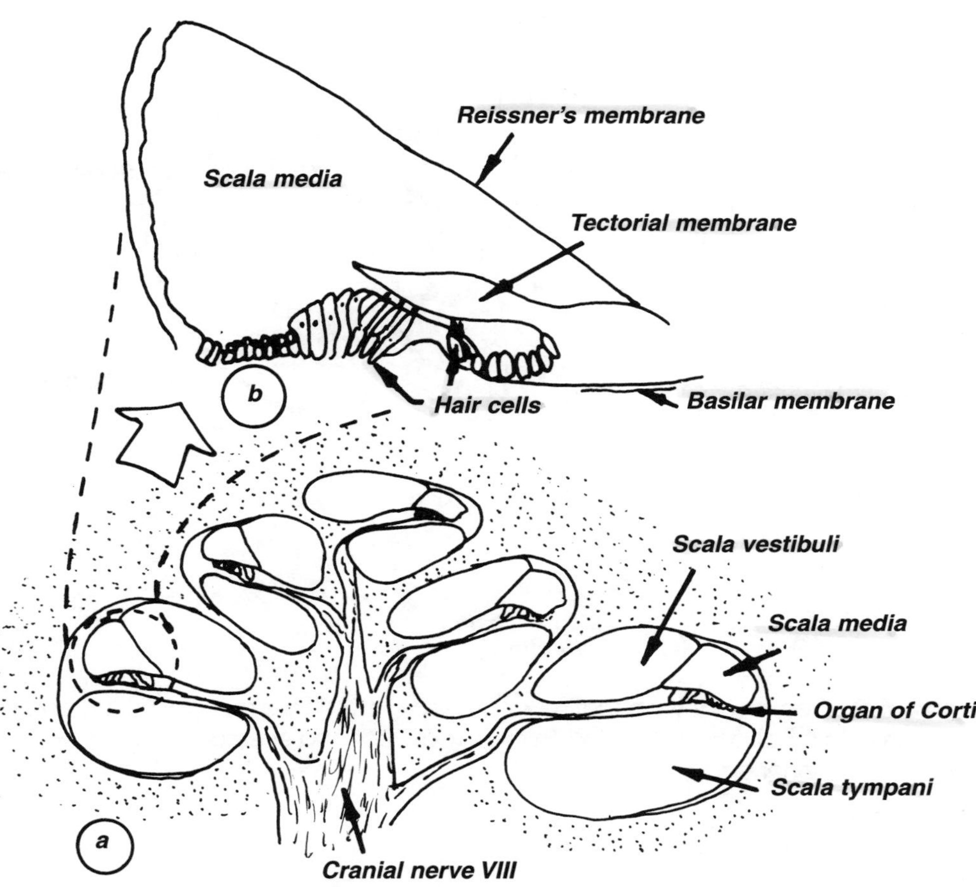

Figure 6–8. a. Drawing of a cross-section of the cochlea. **b.** An enlargement of the organ of Corti.

namics. It arises as follows. In response to sound, the footplate of the stapes pushes in and out against the round window, causing pressure changes within the fluids of the cochlea. As was described by Bekesy, these pressure changes produce a traveling wave that moves along the cochlear partition. Essentially, this is a deformation that proceeds from the oval-window end of the cochlea to its apical end. It is illustrated in a highly schematic way in Figure 6–11. Because the stiffness of the basilar membrane decreases from its base to apex, the speed of wave travel also decreases. For a given frequency of sound vibration, a particular region of the partition undergoes a maximal deformation. Therefore, sounds of different frequencies are associated with maximal displacements at different regions along the basilar membrane. High-frequency sounds are represented at the basal end, and low-frequency sounds are represented at the apical end. The traveling wave accomplishes a kind of mechanical frequency representation.

The maximal displacement of the basilar membrane generally indicates the frequency of stimulation. However, it was recognized several years ago that this mechanical frequency analysis did not account for the exquisite frequency resolu-

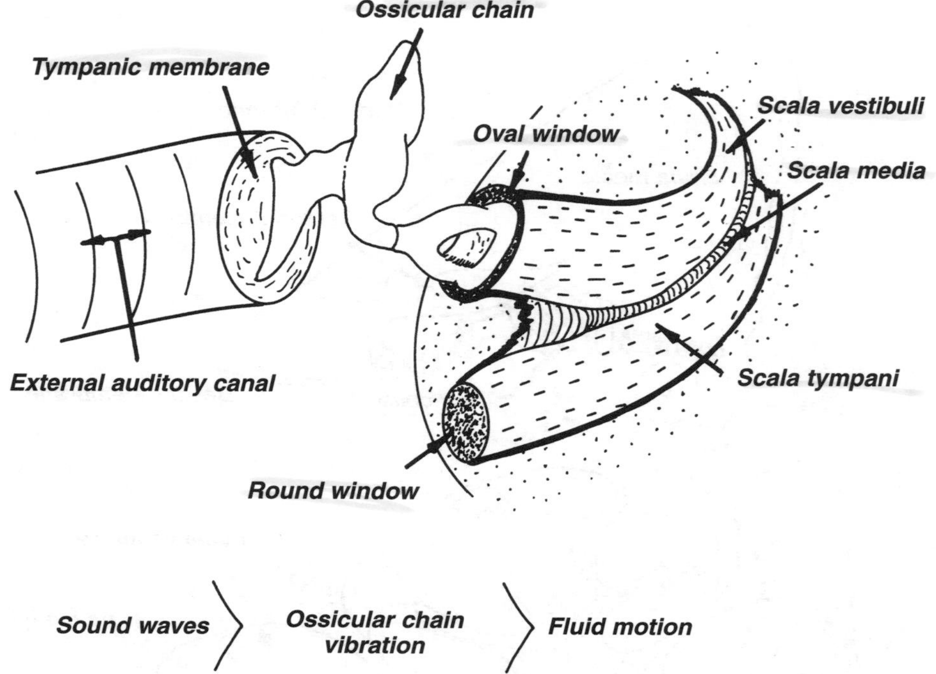

Figure 6–9. Diagram showing that sound waves in the air are received in the outer ear, converted to mechanical vibrations in the middle ear, and eventually converted to fluid motion in the inner ear.

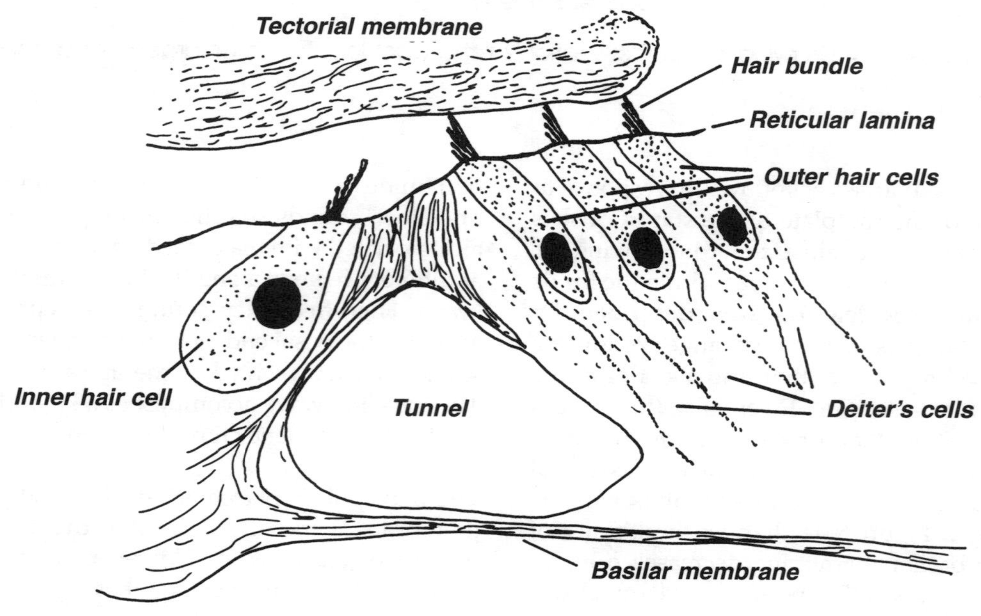

Figure 6–10. The cochlear partition and organ of Corti.

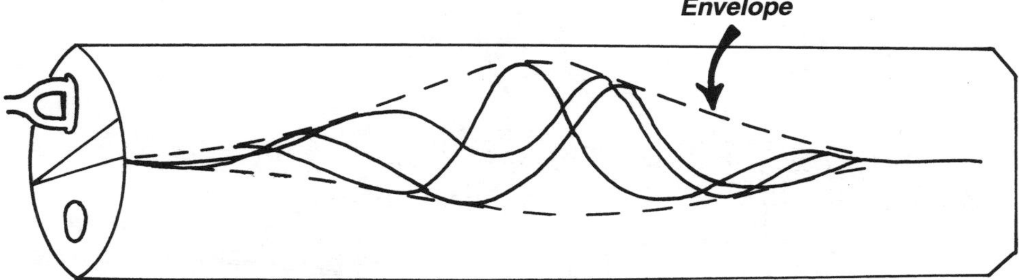

Figure 6–11. Schematic drawing of the traveling wave in the cochlear partition of a straightened cochlea.

tion of the ear. That is, our ability to analyze frequency is better than could be produced by the traveling-wave peak itself. What apparently happens to improve on the mechanical analysis performed by the traveling wave is that, at the region of maximum vibration of the partition, a local source of metabolic energy creates additional vibratory energy. To understand this local source of energy, we need more information about the hair cells of the organ of Corti.

We now turn to a more detailed examination of the inner and outer hair cells. A tuft of slender hairs called a **hair bundle** is located on the hair cell's upper surface (Figures 6–10 and 6–12). This bundle contains two types of "hairs." One has the characteristics of a true cilium and is called the **kinocilium**. The others are rather like the microvilli (tiny projections) of the intestinal wall and are called **stereocilia** (Figure 6–13). The stereocilia are connected by fine extracellular filaments called **tip links**. These filaments provide a functional integrity to the stereocilia, so that they tend to bend corporately rather than individually. By way of analogy, imagine the bristles on a brush that are glued together at their ends. The purpose of the tip links seems to be to focus the tension produced by bundle deformation on tiny mechanosensitive channels in the membrane of the stereocilia. Bending of the hair bundle is the proximal physical stimulus that causes the inner hair cells to generate a neural impulse.

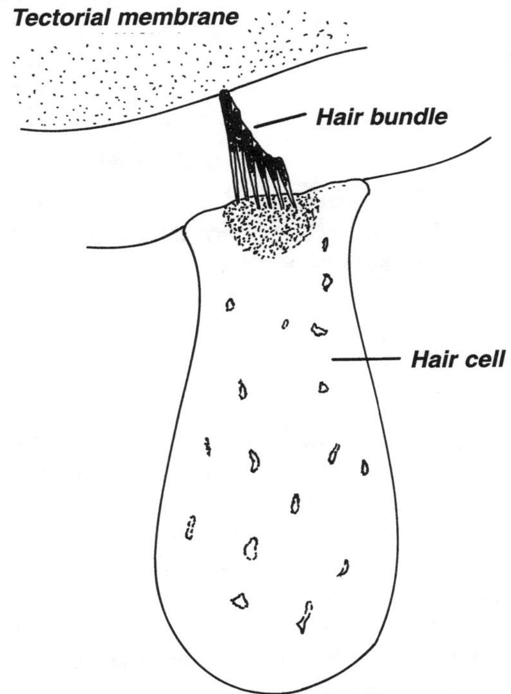

Figure 6–12. Hair cell and hair bundle.

What, then, does the relatively large population of outer hair cells do? Apparently, a major role is to modify the relationship be-

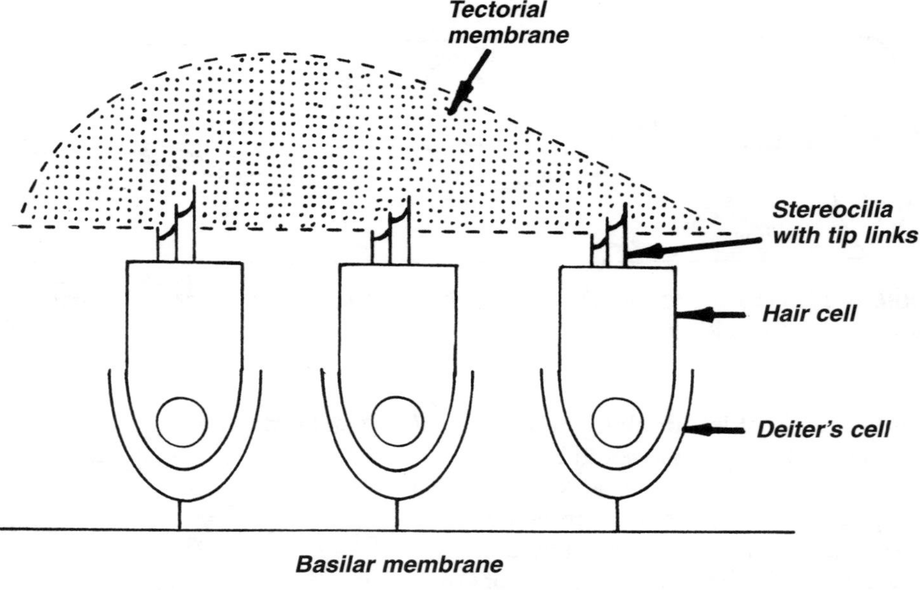

Figure 6–13. Schematic diagram of the organ of Corti, showing hair cells and related elements.

tween the tectorial membrane and the reticular lamina (Figure 6–10). The outer hair cells can cause this modification through a stiffening of their hair bundles. This stiffening changes the physical relationship between the two membranes. In addition, it was recently discovered that these hair cells are capable of something quite unusual—**electromotility**, or changes in shape that occur with electrical stimulation. When voltages pass through these cells, they shorten and lengthen. These movements, though tiny, may serve to amplify and sharpen the traveling wave, or wavelike motion that moves along the cochlear partition in response to sound. The outer hair cells may give a refinement to this wave that enhances our perception of sound. We might say that the outer hair cells provide a fine tuning, or selective amplification, to the traveling wave and in so doing enhance our auditory sensitivity. As explained earlier, some local source of energy, in addition to the traveling wave, is needed to explain the ear's frequency analysis. This local energy is found in the outer hair cell.

Because the cilia of the outer hair cells are attached to the tectorial membrane, these cells can influence the flow of fluids between the tectorial membrane and the organ of Corti. In fact, the streaming of the fluid results from the relative movement between these tissues. A helpful analogy is that the tectorial membrane and the organ of Corti have a relative motion somewhat like the pages of a book that is hung from its spine as its covers are moved back and forth. This motion often is called a shearing motion. The fluid flow, in turn, causes stimulation of the inner hair cells.

ELECTRICAL EVENTS AND RELATED PHENOMENA

It was observed earlier that the bending of the hair bundle is responsible for the generation of a neural impulse. This transduction of mechanical energy to electrical energy is the fundamental event by which the auditory system can transmit signals to the brain. The electrical events can be recorded with electrodes placed in or near the auditory system. One of these signals is briefly considered here; others are discussed in Chapter 7. The electrical signal of primary and immediate interest is the **cochlear microphonic**. This signal is produced only during the presentation of an auditory stimulus. It generally mirrors the intensity and frequency components of the stimulus. For example, if a 1000 Hz tone is presented to the ear, then a cochlear microphonic of the same frequency will be generated. It is believed that the cochlear microphonic is generated at the cilia-bearing end of the hair cells.

A recently discovered phenomenon is the **otoacoustic emission** (OAE). These emissions, first discovered by Kemp in 1978 (but predicted by Gold three decades earlier), are faint sounds produced by the cochlea as it responds to acoustic stimuli. These otoacoustic emissions can be recorded in the human ear canal. Their discovery is an interesting story. Kemp turned to the study of the ear following an earlier career in petroleum engineering. Part of his work in geology involved seismic waves, the echoes that pass through the earth's crust in response to underground explosions. Kemp decided to use the seismic technique on a smaller scale—on the ear. He recorded faint sounds that were generated in response to acoustic stimulation. In some people, the otoacoustic emissions are sufficiently intense that they can be heard by a listener who stands close. The listener might be inclined to say, "I can hear you hearing."

Otoacoustic emissions have attracted great attention from hearing scientists because they provide a new and valuable way to study auditory function. Hundreds of scientific papers have been published on this phenomenon and it is likely that hundreds more will be written. The basic procedure used to record otoacoustic emissions is fairly simple. A miniature probe that contains a sound source is placed in the external canal, along with a sensitive microphone to record the emissions. The emissions are of two types. **Spontaneous otoacoustic emissions** are weak tonal signals that occur naturally, without acoustic stimulation, in a majority of people with normal hearing. These signals may be a sign of good hearing. They are generally inaudible to the people who have them. **Evoked otoacoustic emissions** occur in almost everyone and are elicited with low- to moderate-level test sounds. This type of emission is of great interest because of its potential clinical application. Otoacoustic emissions are particularly appealing, because they appear to reflect the biomechanical activity of the outer hair cells, which are susceptible to various types of disease and other damage (including exposure to loud sounds). Among other applications, otoacoustic emissions may provide a means of testing hearing in infants and subjects who cannot participate in conventional behavioral tests of auditory function. Otoacoustic emissions are reduced or absent in some disorders of the cochlea, and this fact is of great interest in the diagnosis of hearing problems. In addition, because otoacoustic emissions are related to hearing sensitivity, they may provide a means of assessing auditory function.

ENERGY AND INFORMATION FLOW IN THE AUDITORY SYSTEM

Dallos (1988) conceptualized the flow of energy and information within the auditory system as shown by the block diagram of Figure 6–14. Energy is represented by the dark arrows and information by the light arrows. Notice that both energy and information have two-way paths of travel. Acoustic stimulation in the environment

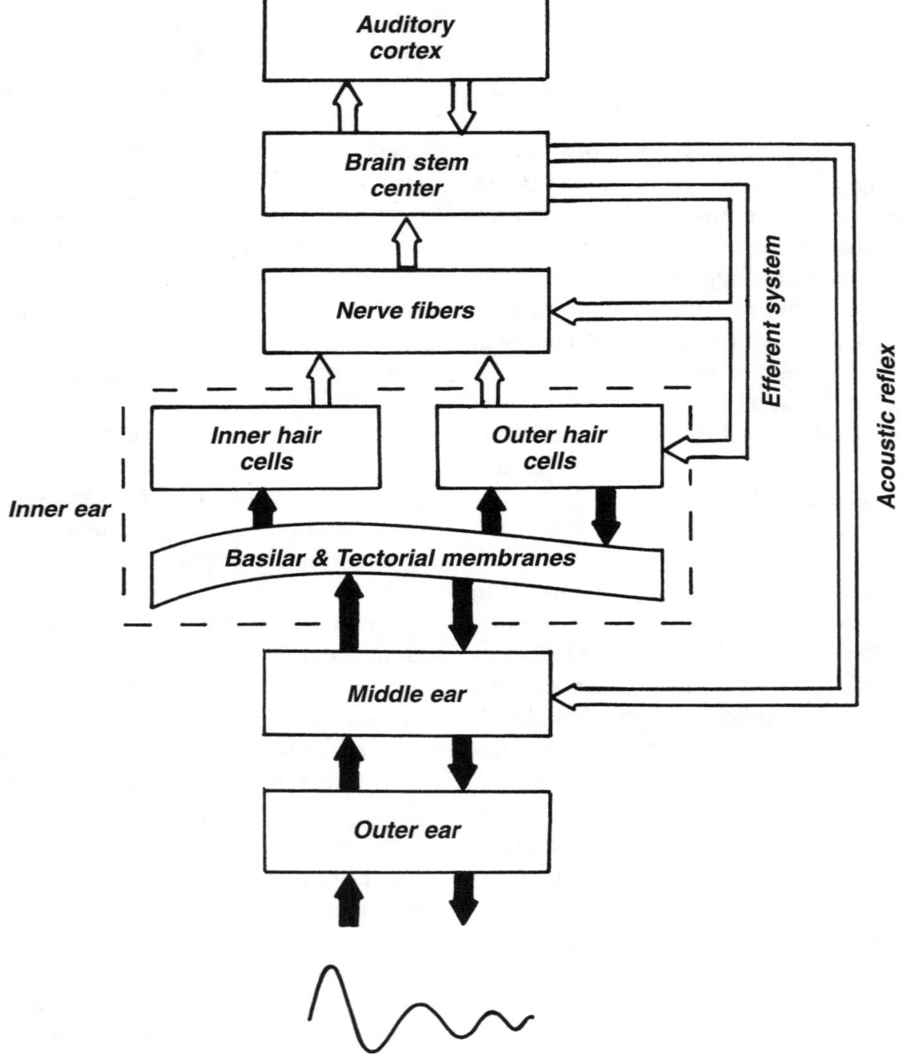

Figure 6–14. Flow of energy and information in the auditory system. The blackened arrows represent energy flow, and the unfilled arrows indicate information flow. (Redrawn from "Cochlear Neurobiology: Revolutionary Developments," by P. Dallos, 1988, *Asha, 30,* p. 55. Redrawn with the permission of the American Speech-Language-Hearing Association.)

causes a flow of energy that proceeds from the outer ear to the middle ear to the inner ear. But a reverse energy flow also is shown. This reverse flow is evidenced by the presence of otoacoustic emissions. Information flow begins in the inner ear with the generation of neural impulses. This information is transmitted along a neural pathway that includes the brainstem and cerebral cortex (which is discussed in more detail in Chapter 7). But a reverse direction of information flow allows the brainstem to influence actions in the inner ear (by means of the efferent system), and the acoustic reflex mediated by brainstem structures can influence the middle ear and the transmission of signals through it. In short, although it seems intuitive to think of energy and information as traveling in only one direction in the auditory system, the evidence indicates that both have bidirectional paths.

SUMMARY OF THE AUDITORY SYSTEM

Given the complexity of this system, it may be helpful to give a brief summary of the major events in audition.

Speech and other acoustic stimuli create vibrations in the air. These vibrations are a form of mechanical energy. The pinna funnels this energy into the external auditory meatus. These are structures of the outer ear. At the termination of the meatus, the tympanic membrane (ear drum) marks the entrance to the middle ear. The primary structures within the middle ear are the three tiny bones (the ossicles: malleus, incus, and stapes) and associated muscles (stapedius and tensor tympani). The stapes has a footplate that inserts into the round window of the cochlea, or inner ear. Within the cochlea, three fluid-filled tubes extend from the basal end nearly to the extreme apical end. The smallest of these tubes is the cochlear partition that contains the organ of Corti, the sensory end-organ of hearing. Mechanical vibrations transmitted through the outer and middle ear produce a traveling wave along the cochlear partition. This displacement causes a bending of the inner hair cells and the generation of neural impulses that are sent to the brain. The traveling wave does not account for the full capability of the ear's frequency analysis. A supplemental factor is a local energy source created by the outer hair cells. This local source enhances the frequency analysis performed by the ear. The result is an acoustic analysis so remarkable that it has challenged the imagination of scientists to explain it and to design models of comparable capability.

COMPARATIVE AUDITORY FUNCTION

Human hearing is not remarkable for its frequency range. Compared to dogs and a number of other mammals, humans have limited hearing for high-frequency sounds. The range of human hearing is usually given as 20–20,000 Hz, with the frequency region of greatest sensitivity around 1000 Hz. A dog's hearing can extend to frequencies of 60,000 Hz or higher, which is why dogs can hear whistles that are inaudible to humans. Some other animals have better hearing than humans for low-frequency sounds (sometimes called **infrasonic** frequencies). For example, elephants produce calls with fundamental frequencies as low as 12 Hz (Payne, Langbauer, & Thomas, 1986). Different animals have varying auditory experience with the world. Sounds that may be very important to dogs and elephants may be completely outside the range of human auditory experience. We may be deaf to sounds that are very important to dogs and cats.

Of course, the auditory frequencies most important to humans are those for speech. As discussed in Chapter 9, most of the energy in speech is contained in a range of frequencies that extends from about 100 Hz to 5000 Hz. Under most conditions, speech is readily recognizable if energy in this range is transmitted. In fact, telephone transmission affords an even smaller range of frequencies, from about 300 to 3500 Hz. This frequency range is quite modest compared to the total range of human hearing and decidedly limited compared to the frequency range for a number of other animal species. However, humans seem to excel in the auditory function of discrimination for frequency, intensity, and duration. That is, we can hear subtle changes in the frequency, intensity, and durations of acoustic stimuli. Therefore, we are well equipped to hear *patterns* of sound. This refined discrimination probably underlies our ability to hear rapid sequences of auditory stimuli such as those that comprise speech. Humans are not alone in the ability to hear complex sound patterns. Research has shown that many animals can detect at least some of the acoustic patterns in the speech signal. This research is considered briefly in Chapter 10.

PSYCHOACOUSTICS

Psychoacoustics, the science that deals with the psychological response to sound, has been highly focused on the auditory system's analysis of frequency. As mentioned in Chapter 2, a Fourier analysis is a form of analysis that decomposes a complex sound into its sinusoidal components. In fact, pure sinusoids seldom occur in the natural world. Sinusoids have been a useful laboratory tool to discover how the ear analyzes frequency. However, other properties of acoustic signals may be just as important, if not more important, in our understanding of audition in the ordinary course of events. An example comes from attempts at synthesizing (producing by computer) the sounds generated by various musical instruments.

Fourier analysis (discussed in Chapter 2) enabled scientists and engineers to determine the composition of sounds created by different horns and stringed instruments. But when attempts were made to synthesize these instrumental sounds from the lessons learned from Fourier analysis, the result was disappointing. The sound quality simply was not convincing. Further study revealed the reason for the deficiency. It turns out that different instruments have different **attacks** (onsets of sound), and these attacks are particularly important in creating the desired instrumental effect. When the synthesized instrumental sounds were given a suitable attack, the signal quality was judged to be much more like the natural instrument. Apparently, the human ear gives special weight to the onset of sounds, even if they are very brief. The ecological advantage of this strategy may be that quick decisions sometimes need to be made about an acoustic event. If an acoustic signal represents a potential danger, then it hardly behooves the listener to perform an extended Fourier analysis of the signal in the hope of gaining maximal information about the sinusoidal components of the sound. Rather, a threatening signal needs to be processed as rapidly as possible, especially if the sound is not accompanied by other sensory information (such as the sound produced in the dark). Hearing is designed in part to provide a rapid analysis of environmental events. The human ear attends especially to sound onsets. This strategy has obvious survival value, but it also has been carried over to the appreciation of music. We see in the chapter on speech perception (Chapter 10) that attending to onsets also is a characteristic of listening to speech.

LIFE COURSE CONSIDERATIONS

Humans are precocious as far as mammalian hearing is concerned. Human auditory function is effective months before birth, but mammals such as the rat and cat only have a postnatal onset of hearing. The adult dimensions and ossification of the human cochlea are achieved before birth (Clopton, 1981), and there are indications of fetal responsiveness to sound (Clopton, 1981; Eggermont, 1989; Lecanuet & Granier-Deferre, 1993). It is estimated that human hearing begins about 5½ months after conception. The cochlea seems to be the limiting factor in onset of hearing because it is the last structure to reach functional maturity. More precisely, the hair cells are the final elements to mature. The hair cells initially begin to differentiate in the first half of the basal turn and the differentiation then spreads basally and apically. The inner hair cells mature before the outer hair cells.

Auditory function in the fetus was tested in an interesting study conducted by Hepper and Shahidullah (1994). They examined fetuses of 19–35 weeks gestational age. Pure-tone stimuli of 100, 250, 500, 1000, and 3000 Hz were presented to a fetus by placing a loudspeaker on the maternal abdomen. Fetal response to sound was movement recorded by ultrasound. At 19 weeks, a response to the 500 Hz tone was noted. With maturation, the response first spread to the lower frequencies of 100 and 250 Hz, and then to the higher frequencies of 1000 and 3000 Hz. At 27 weeks gestational age, almost all the fetuses responded to pure tones of 250 and 500 Hz, but none to the tones of 1000 or 3000 Hz. All fetuses responded to these higher frequencies at 33–35 weeks. The authors believed that these results point to a low-frequency auditory function that may promote language acquisition. Chapter 9 discusses the speech information that may be present in this region of low frequencies. For the present, it can be noted that information about the prosody of speech (e.g., intonation, stress patterns, syllable rhythms) is likely available to the fetus at the earliest stages of auditory development.

Therefore, we enter the world ready to hear and in fact have already been receiving some auditory signals while in the womb. Until 1882, it was generally believed that the fetus had no sensory information about the outside world. In that year, Preyer suggested that the human fetus might respond to sensory stimulation. Both mothers and scientists have proved Preyer to be correct. The supporting evidence from pregnant women was their impression that the fetus moved in response to an intense environmental sound. Scientists have confirmed their report and also have suggested that the fetus can detect the human voice. The mother's voice is particularly likely to be heard by the fetus, but other voices also can be heard in the watery world of the womb. This point is reconsidered in Chapter 10 (Speech Perception) in regard to the question, "When does speech perception begin?" One aspect of this question is to determine why newborns express a preference for the mother's voice and maybe even the mother tongue. To steal some thunder from Chapter 10, it probably reflects the fetus's auditory experience with a particular natural language spoken by a particularly important woman, the mother. Humans are not alone in this respect: It has been shown that bird embryos respond to the calls of the parent birds (Lecanuet & Granier-Deferre, 1993). Humans respond to sound **in utero** and birds **in ovo**. Interestingly, it is in these two species that sound learning is most evident. It appears that the developmental design wastes little time before auditory learning begins. More is said about this in Chapter 7, which pertains to the neural structures of speech and hearing.

Unfortunately, it also may not be very long before some people begin to lose auditory function. In a summary of the effects of aging on audition, Steinberg (1995) noted that:

1. Hearing for high frequencies may decline after the age of 20 years.
2. After the age of about 30 years, hearing in men declines twice as rapidly as hearing in women.
3. Hearing loss for tones of low frequency typically begins in the seventh decade of life.
4. Older women have more sensitive hearing than older men.

Whether because of accumulated damage or because of aging itself, human audition wanes with age. The hypothesis of accumulated damage suggests that long-term exposure of some kind—to too much sound or to toxins, for example—results in a deterioration of the auditory system. The aging hypothesis asserts that normal aging, itself, is a risk factor, for reasons that are not entirely understood. Research has shown that people who live in industrialized societies have poorer hearing than people who live in more noise-free societies (Kryter, 1983). Gordon-Salant (1991) concluded from studies of individuals living in a relatively noise-free environment that aging itself produced only a slight hearing loss, and that this age-related loss was similar for men and women. She explained the differences in hearing between persons in industrialized versus nonindustrialized societies as a combination of risk factors, including noise exposure, diet, medications, cardiovascular disease, and atherosclerosis. Her conclusion was that aging by itself does not greatly impair hearing in most people. Rather, environments and behaviors account for most differences in hearing loss across individuals. However, the results of a large study reported in 1996 indicate that hearing in men declines more rapidly than in women, especially for high frequencies (Morrell, Gordon-Salant, Pearson, Brant, & Fozard, 1996). Perhaps gender interacts with environment and behavior to account for this difference. Given the same exposure to potentially damaging agents, men may suffer greater auditory damage than women because of a greater frailty of their ears. However, more research with adequate controls for factors such as noise exposure is needed to provide a definitive answer to the question of gender differences.

Preservation of hearing may be, in large part, a matter of good behaviors and overall good health. People living in industrialized societies are at risk for a hearing loss beyond their years. For those who wish to preserve their hearing, the implication is clear: Take steps to protect hearing by good nutrition, healthy living, and avoiding excessive noise exposure. The last of these deserves special emphasis, especially because many social events and musical performances expose those in attendance to potentially damaging levels of sound. In addition, many workers in factories and assembly plants are exposed to several hours of intense noise. Some chemical agents, called **ototoxic drugs**, carry a special risk of damaging hearing. Among these agents are aspirin, aminoglycoside antibiotics (such as streptomycin), alcohol, lead, and tobacco.

Elderly listeners may have hearing difficulties especially for auditory stimuli that occur with a competing background message or stimuli that have been multiply degraded, that is, altered in time, frequency, and intensity. One of the most damaging types of degradation is **time compression**, in which the rate of speech is increased without producing spectral distortion (Gordon-Salant & Fitzgibbons, 1995). Time compression speeds up the rate of information in the acoustic signal, and it appears that elderly listeners cannot cope as readily as younger listeners with this increased information rate. The elderly are not the only ones who may be at a disadvantage in the rapid processing of auditory stimuli. Some young people may have a similar difficulty, and it has been proposed that a deficiency in rapid temporal processing contributes to certain disorders of language and reading. This issue is taken up in later chapters. An interesting new technology permits the speech signal to be extended in duration by a selective lengthening of segments such as vowels and silences. This kind of temporal alteration, combined with amplification, may benefit many people with hearing impairments.

Speech and hearing are like hand and glove. Because we speak to be heard, our vocal efforts are closely tied to the sense of audition. The roots of this association reach back to the fetal stage and, barring injury or disease to our vocal and auditory systems, we speak and hear to our dying day.

On The Reference Shelf

Recommended sources for more detailed discussion of the topics in this chapter.

Dallos, P. (1988, July/August). Cochlear neurobiology: Revolutionary developments. *Asha, 30*, 50–56.
A concise review of changing concepts of cochlear functions.

Pickles, J. O. (1988). *An introduction to the physiology of hearing* (2nd ed.). London: Academic Press.
An excellent resource for information on auditory physiology.

Willott, J. F. (1991). *Aging and the auditory system: Anatomy, physiology, and psychoacoustics.* San Diego: Singular Publishing Group.

Yost, W. A. (1994). *Fundamentals of hearing* (3rd ed.). San Diego: Academic Press.
A fine introductory text that covers basic issues in audition.

Chapter References

Abraham, S. S., Wallace, I. F., & Gravel, J. S. (1996). Early otitis media and phonological development at age 2 years. *Laryngoscope, 106*, 727–732.

Casselbrant, M. L., Mandel, E. M., Kurs-Lasky, M., Rockette, H. E., & Bluestone, C. D. (1995). Otitis media in a population of black American and white American infants, 0–2 years of age. *International Journal of Pediatric Otorhinolaryngology, 33*, 1–16.

Clopton, B. M. (1981). Neurophysiological and anatomical aspects of auditory development. In R. N. Aslin, J. R. Alberts, & M. R. Petersen (Eds.), *Development of perception: Psychobiological perspectives* (*Vol. 1*, pp. 111–137). New York: Academic Press.

Crompton, A. W., & Parker, P. (1978, March/April). Evolution of the mammalian masticatory apparatus. *American Scientist, 66,* 192–201.

Dallos, P. (1988, July). Cochlear neurobiology: Revolutionary developments. *Asha, 30,* 50–56.

Eggermont, J. J. (1989). The onset and development of auditory function: Contributions of evoked potential studies. *Journal of Speech-Language Pathology and Audiology, 13,* 5–16.

Friel-Patti, S. (1990). Otitis media with effusion and the development of language: A review of the evidence. *Topics in Language Disorders, 11,* 11–22.

Gold, T. (1948). Hearing II. The physical basis of the action of the cochlea. *Proceedings of the Royal Society of London, Biological Sciences, 135,* 492–498.

Gordon-Salant, S. M. (1991). The audiologic assessment. In D. Ripich (Ed.), *Geriatric communication disorders* (pp. 367–393). Austin, TX: PRO-ED.

Gordon-Salant, S., & Fitzgibbons, P. J. (1995). Recognition of multiply degraded speech by young and elderly listeners. *Journal of Speech and Hearing Research, 38,* 1150–1156.

Hamill, O. P., & McBride, D. W., Jr. (1994). Mechanoreceptive membrane channels. *American Scientist, 83,* 30–37.

Harris, T. T. (1968). Brownian motion in the cochlear partition. *Journal of the Acoustical Society of America, 44,* 176–181.

Harsten, G., Nettlebladt, U., Schalen, L., Kalm, O., & Prellner, K. (1993). Language development in children with recurrent otitis media during the first three years of life. Follow-up study from birth to seven years of age. *Journal of Laryngology & Otology, 107,* 407–412.

Hepper, P. G., & Shahidullah, B. S. (1994). Development of fetal hearing. *Archives of Disorders in Children, 71*(Suppl.), F81–F87.

Hudspeth, A. J. (1989). How the ear's works work. *Nature, 341,* 397–404.

Kemp, D. T. (1978). Stimulated acoustic emissions from within the human auditory system. *Journal of the Acoustical Society of America, 64,* 1386–1391.

Kryter, K. D. (1983). Presbycusis, sociocusis, and nosocusis. *Journal of the Acoustical Society of America, 73,* 1897–1917.

Lecanuet, J.-P., & Granier-Deferre, C. (1993). Speech stimuli in the fetal environment. In B. de Boysson-Bardies, S. de Schonen, P. Jusczyk, P. MacNeilage, & J. Morton (Eds.), *Developmental neurocognition: Speech and face processing in the first year of life* (pp. 237–248). Dordrecht, The Netherlands: Kluwer Academic Publishers.

Lowen, S., & Teich, M. (1992). Auditory-nerve action potentials form a nonrenewal point process over short as well as long time scales. *Journal of the Acoustical Society of America, 92,* 803–805.

Luce, R. D. (1993). *Sound and hearing: A conceptual introduction.* Hillsdale, NJ: Erlbaum.

Lucente, F. E., Lawson, W., & Novick, N. L. (1995). *The external ear.* Philadelphia: W. B. Saunders.

Morrell, C. H., Gordon-Salant, S., Pearson, J. D., Brant, L. J., & Fozard, J. L. (1996). Age- and gender-specific reference ranges for hearing level and longitudinal changes in hearing level. *Journal of the Acoustical Society of America, 100,* 1949–1967.

Payne, K. B., Langbauer, W. R., & Thomas, E. M. (1986). Infrasonic calls of the Asian elephant (Elephas maximus). *Behavioral Ecology and Sociobiology, 18,* 297–301.

Preyer, W. (1982). *Dies seel des kinder.* Leipzig: Fernau.

Pujo, R., & Lavigne-Rebillard, M. (1995). Sensory and neural structures in the developing human cochlea. *International Journal of Pediatric Otolaryngology, 32,* S177–S182.

Roberts, J. E., Burchinal, M. R., Collier, A. M., Ramey, C. T., Koch, M.A., & Henderson, F. W. (1989). Otitis media in early childhood, and cognitive, academic, and classroom performance of the school-aged child. *Pediatrics, 83,* 477–485.

Roberts, J. E., Sanyal, M. A., Burchinal, M. R., Collier, A. M., Ramey, C. T., & Henderson, F. W. (1986). Otitis media in early childhood and its relationship to later verbal and academic performance. *Pediatrics, 78,* 423–430.

Sade, J., & Ar, A. (1997). Middle ear and auditory tube: Middle ear clearance, gas exchange, and pressure regulation. *Otolaryngology—Head and Neck Surgery, 116,* 499–524.

Steinberg, J. (1995, April). The graying of the senses. *The Journal of NIH Research, 7,* 32–33.

Yost, W. A. (1994). *Fundamentals of hearing* (3rd ed.). San Diego: Academic Press.

Exercises

6–1. Starting with a sound in space, such as a note played on a piano, discuss the sequence of events by which the sound energy is transmitted through the external ear, middle ear, and inner ear. In your discussion, describe the role of the major structures listed in an arbitrary order below.

oval window	stapes
tympanic membrane	organ of Corti
external auditory meatus	incus
malleus	pinna

6–2. Using the dimensions given in the text, draw an approximately life-sized illustration of the external auditory meatus, middle ear, and eustachian tube. Alternatively, construct a model of these structures with modeling clay.

6–3. Draw a cross-sectional diagram of the cochlear partition and label the following structures: basilar membrane, tectorial membrane, organ of Corti, inner hair cells, and outer hair cells. Then briefly explain the function of each structure.

6–4. Consult an encyclopedia or textbook on audition to determine the frequency range of hearing for different animals. Make a comparative graph to show the differences in frequency range.

CHAPTER

7

The Neural Basis of Speech

One way of gauging progress in the understanding of the brain is to look at the models and metaphors that have been used in the history of brain study. The early Romans considered the brain to work in terms of the flow of body fluids. Perhaps their innovations with aqueducts to supply water to their communities shaped their views on how bodily functions work. René Descartes in the 17th century, possibly reflecting the enthusiasm for mechanical inventions of the era, likened the brain to a mechanical apparatus with gears, cogs, and cams. A popular model of the 19th century was to view the brain like a system of railway networks. With the 20th century, computing machines became a favored model or metaphor. One variant of this idea was to consider the brain as a system composed of separate specialized modules that compute certain kinds of information in parallel, making their results available nearly simultaneously to some executive structure. Another 20th century approach was to think of the brain as a chemical engine based on the metabolism of oxygen and glucose and the regulation of activities through chemical messengers called neurotransmitters. In a sense, modern thinking about the brain revives the ancient idea of fluids, except that the contemporary notion pertains to tiny amounts of chemicals that form functional watersheds in the complex circuitry of the brain. The models of modern brain chemistry are based on transmitter molecules and their specialized receptors.

> *"The stuff of thought is not caged in the brain but is scattered all over the body . . . There is little doubt now that the brain is a gland; it produces hormones, it has hormone receptors, it is bathed in hormones, hormones run up and down the fibers on individual nerves, and every activity that the brain is engaged in involves hormones."*
>
> (Richard M. Bergland in *The Fabric of Mind*)

THE CELLS OF THE NERVOUS SYSTEM

The Neuron

The cell is the basic unit of all body systems. In the nervous system, the neuron is the primary cell of interest. Like other cells, it has a nucleus that contains the genetic material. Unlike other cells, the neuron rarely can be replaced. The usual dictum is that neurons cannot regenerate. If a neuron dies, it is gone forever. There are some interesting exceptions. Neuronal regeneration has been observed in some nonhuman species, and even in humans, a neuron in the olfactory system is routinely replaced (which is why some people recover from a temporary loss of the sense of smell caused by exposure to toxic chemicals).

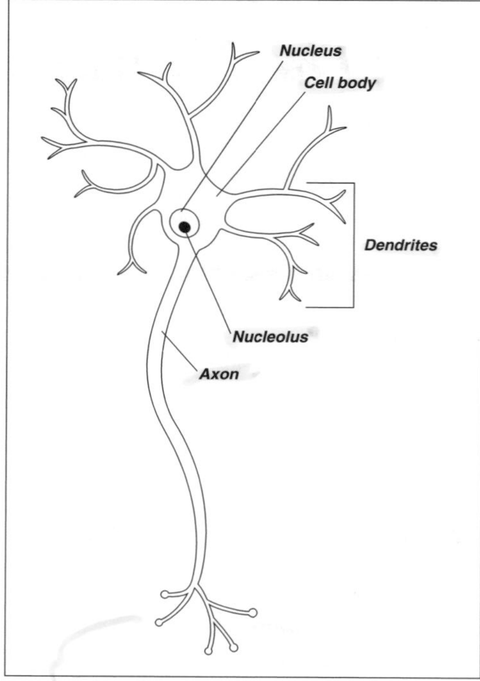

Figure 7–1. Structure of a neuron, showing nucleus, cell body, dendrites, and axon. The dark spot in the nucleus is the nucleolus.

Neurons have varying shapes and sizes, but a typical neuron is illustrated in Figure 7–1. The **neuron cell body** contains the **nucleus** with its dark central **nucleolus**. A number of projections, or **processes**, extend from the cell body. These are the primary means by which one neuron communicates with other neurons and other tissues, such as muscles or glands. The **dendrites** are the numerous short projections that conduct nerve impulses in the direction of the cell body. The **axon** is the single long process that conducts the nerve impulse to other neurons, to muscles, or to glands. The dendrites and axons are sometimes called **nerve fibers**. They appear under microscopy as threadlike structures. Apparently, Rudolf Albert von Kolliker in 1849 was the first to recognize that these fibers were the extensions of nerve cells. This was an important discovery that opened the way for the understanding of neurons as functional units of the nervous system.

The neurons are remarkable for their sheer numbers. Estimates of the number of neurons in the brain generally run in the billions, but may be as high as 20 trillion. The large population of neurons is comforting, especially because all of us lose neurons at a daily pace (one estimate puts the daily loss at 1,000 neurons), beginning before we are born and continuing throughout life. In a sense, the human nervous system is shaped largely by loss. Thousands of irreplaceable cells are shed as a routine matter. But much of the loss is never felt, for the surviving neurons carry out the important business of the nervous system. In fact, loss of neurons is a major factor in the development of the brain. The natural plan seems to be to begin with more neurons than are needed. As some have said, "Nature is profligate." Neurons that make functional contacts with other neurons and receive stimulation associated with behavioral activities are preserved. It is these functional contacts, or connectivities, that make all the difference. Rat brains actually have a higher neuronal density (neurons per unit of area) than human brains, but the brain of the human has a greater number of neurons overall and they are much more richly interconnected than the neurons of the rat brain.

Neurons are specialized. Three basic types are **sensory neurons**, **motor neurons** (or motoneurons), and **interneurons**. Sensory neurons conduct nerve impulses from a sensory receptor at a site, such as the eye or ear. They deliver the sensory information to the brain and spinal cord for processing and interpretation. In general, then, *sensory* impulses travel from the periphery to the more central structures of the nervous system. This direction of travel is called **afferent**. There are about five million sensory neurons in the human body. Motor neurons carry neural instructions from the brain to the muscles or glands. Therefore, *motor* impulses travel from the central nervous system to the periphery (muscles and glands). This direction is called **efferent**. All human actions rely on the nerve impulses sent to the muscles of the body. The motor neurons number in the few hundred thousands. This relatively small number is an important consideration in diseases that attack motor neurons. The interneurons are by far the most numerous and they greatly outnumber the sensory and motor neurons combined. Estimates of the number of interneurons run to the billions or even trillions. The interneurons are the neurons that constitute the neural tissues of the brain and spinal cord. Combined, these structures constitute the **central nervous system** (CNS). The sensory and motor neurons are part of the **peripheral nervous system** (PNS).

Neurons also can be classified by their structure as one of three primary types: **monopolar**, **bipolar**, and **multipolar** (Figure 7–2). The monopolar neuron has its cell body located in a collateral section that connects to the transmitting zone of dendrite and axon. This is the typical neuron of the general somatic sense, that is, the sense of touch and pressure over the surface of the body. The bipolar neuron has its cell body along the main structure of the neuron, with the dendrite extending in one direction from the cell body and the axon in the other. This neuron is found in the special senses, that is, vision, audition, and olfaction. Finally, the multipolar neuron is a Medusalike structure in which multiple dendrites project from a region containing the cell body. The complex branching pattern of the dendrites is another example of a possible fractal design in nature. This neuron is the typical neuron of the CNS and is also the structure of the motor neuron that innervates muscle.

Neuronal Connections

A neuron by itself can accomplish nothing of behavioral interest. But if the neuron

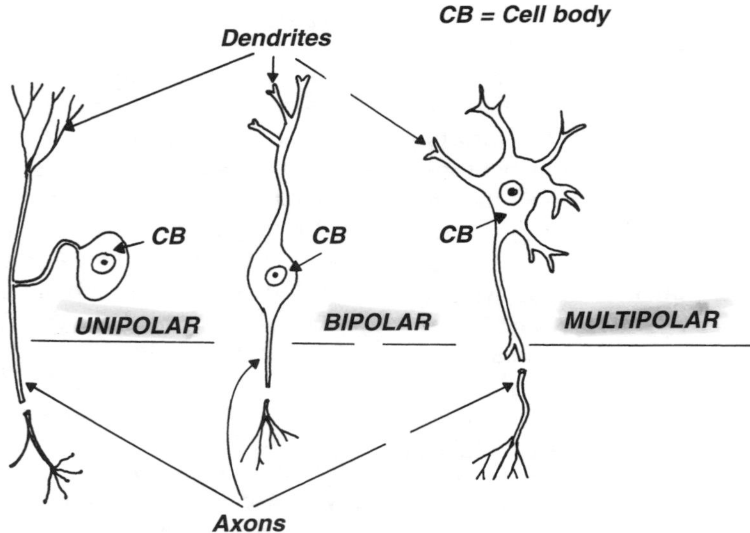

Figure 7-2. Three types of neurons: unipolar (monopolar), bipolar, and multipolar.

communicates with other cells, it can help to shape behavior. Communication between neurons is achieved by the release of small packets of chemicals into the **synapse**, the tiny gap between two neurons. The synapse is illustrated in Figure 7–3. The neuron transmitting the impulse is the **presynaptic neuron**, and the neuron receiving the impulse is the **postsynaptic neuron**. The chemicals involved in the neuronal communication are called **neurotransmitters**. A neurotransmitter is a chemical substance released from the terminal boutons ("buttons") of one neuron into the cleft of a synaptic junction, where it can exercise excitatory or inhibitory influence on the adjacent postsynaptic neuron by interacting with receptor molecules of that neuron. Neurotransmitters are the chemical messengers of the nervous system. The chemicals are contained in the presynaptic terminal in tiny structures called **synaptic vesicles**. Under certain conditions, the vesicles migrate to the **synaptic cleft**, the microscopic space that defines the synapse, and release their contents. In this way, the neurotransmitter substance enters the synaptic cleft. Certain other chemicals released into the cleft take up the substance and can therefore regulate its effects. Receptors in the dendrite of the postsynaptic neuron are specialized to respond to neurotransmitters through a kind of lock and key relationship. The right neurotransmitter can "open" the lock into the receptor and thereby spread neural activity to another neuron. Two kinds of action on the postsynaptic neuron are possible: **excitation** (promoting spread of the neural activity), and **inhibition** (reducing the likelihood of neural activation).

The nervous system may employ as many as 100 different neurotransmitters. But the major ones are glutamate, aspartate, gamma-aminobutyric acid (GABA), and glycine. These neurotransmitters are characterized by having relatively simple and fast actions. They may be central to basic life processes. Glutamate and aspartate are excitatory. It has been discovered that nicotine in tobacco facilitates glutamate, which is perhaps why some smokers get an invigorating lift from tobacco. GABA and glycine are inhibitory. Various other neurotransmitters have slower actions and

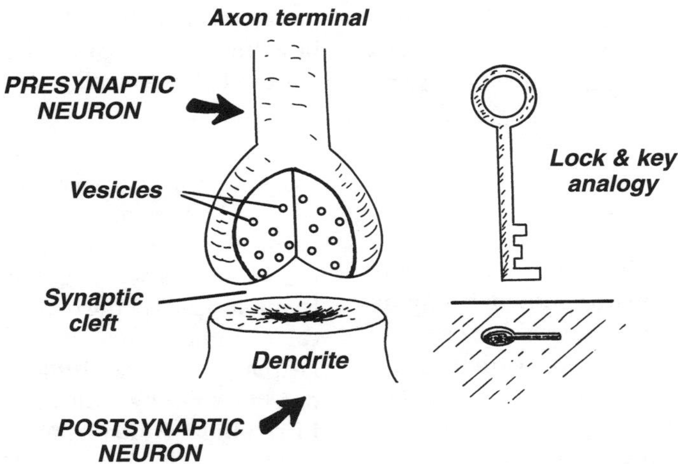

Figure 7–3. Diagram of a synapse showing synaptic vesicles, synaptic cleft, and dendritic surface of postsynaptic neuron. A neurotransmitter released into the synaptic cleft can excite or inhibit the receptor in the postsynaptic neuron, analogous to the mechanism of a key opening a lock.

tend to work with the four major chemicals just listed. Some of these slower acting neurotransmitters relevant to topics in this book are serotonin, norepinephrine, and dopamine. These are also called **neuromodulators** because they modulate or regulate neural activity. The neuromodulators appear to be involved in common psychiatric or neurologic disorders, such as schizophrenia, depression, and Parkinson disease, all of which can affect speech and language. Drugs such as Prozac and Zoloft, among the most frequently prescribed pharmaceuticals in modern medicine, exert an influence on the serotonin system of the brain. In contrast, glutamate, aspartate, GABA, and glycine generally do not seem to be critically involved in psychiatric or neurologic disorders even though they regulate various aspects of behavior.

A single neuron can be influenced by hundreds and even thousands of other neurons. Figure 7–4 is an understated example of neuronal connectivity. In this drawing, the neurons labeled B and C have synaps-

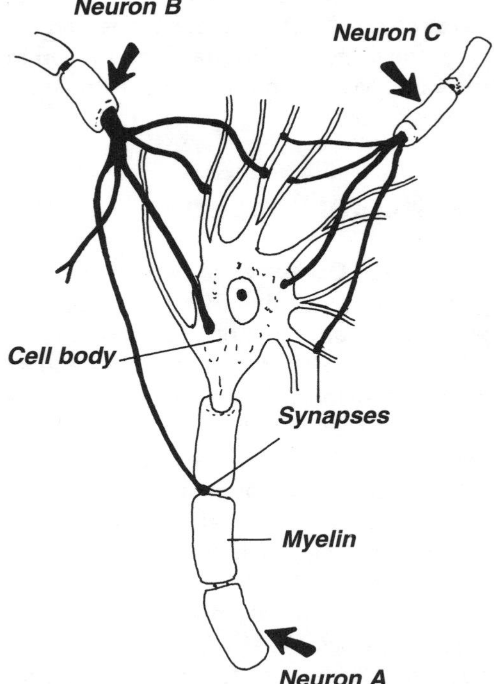

Figure 7–4. Three neurons, A, B, and C, showing the synaptic connections that neurons B and C make with neuron A.

es with the neuron labeled A. The synapses are located widely over the neuron's membrane, including its dendritic branches, its cell body, and even its axon.

Myelin and Glia

Larger axons are insulated with a fatty coating called **myelin**, shown in Figure 7–4. This insulation increases the speed of neural transmission and also reduces interference with the neural message. Demyelinating diseases, such as multiple sclerosis, damage the myelin wrapping around large axons, which leads to impaired functioning of the nervous system.

For all their numbers, neurons are a relatively small population within the nervous system. They are greatly outnumbered by other kinds of cells, especially the **glial cells** (*glia* means glue). Glial cells, also called **glia**, hold neurons in place and also provide nutrients. One of the types of glial cells, the **oligodendroglia**, form myelin in the CNS. Myelin in the PNS is formed by **Schwann cells**.

The Neural Impulse

The ancient Greeks were perhaps off to a good start in believing that fluids were important in brain function. But communication within the brain is not simply a matter of fluid transport. Neurons generate electrical impulses that travel the lengths of nerve fibers. The existence of these electrical impulses as the brain's means of controlling the body was first demonstrated in 1843 by Emil Heinrich Du Bois-Reymond. It was not until 1921 that Otto Loewi discovered that chemicals can stimulate nerves to fire impulses. What this series of discoveries revealed was that neuronal function is a combination of chemical processes and electrical events. The following section summarizes the basic information on how neurons generate an electrical impulse and how this impulse can cause a neighboring neuron to fire as well.

Each neuron can be considered as a tiny biological battery. In general, batteries store electrical potential (or voltage) by accumulating excess positive charges in one terminal and excess negative charges in the other terminal. Cells of the body create an electrical potential across their membranes by keeping the **extracellular fluid** (the fluid outside the cell) positive compared to the **intracellular fluid** (the fluid inside the cell), as illustrated in Figure 7–5. The means to this electrical potential is an electrically charged molecule or atom called an **ion**. Some ions carry a positive charge. Included in this group are sodium (Na^+, where Na is the chemical symbol for sodium and the superscript + indicates the positive charge of the sodium ion) and potassium (K^+). Other ions carry a negative charge. One of these is chlorine (Cl^-). An excess of positively charged sodium ions is typically maintained *outside* a cell and an excess of negatively charged ions is maintained *inside* a cell. The excess of sodium ions is so great in the extracellular fluid that a potential difference (voltage) is created. This imbalance of ions creates the electrical potential, which is realized as a **resting membrane potential** of about –70 millivolts (mV). In comparison, the standard flashlight battery (D cell) has a voltage of 1.5 V. But how is this membane potential maintained? The primary mechanism is the **sodium potassium pump**. Millions of these pumps are in each cell. They act to exchange sodium ions found inside in a cell with potassium ions found outside a cell. As a result, the extracellular fluid is rich in sodium (about tenfold richer than the intracellular fluid) and the intracellular fluid is rich in potassium.

The membrane of a neuron in its resting state is said to be **polarized**. The electrical signal of neuronal transmission is generated by **depolarizing** the membrane, that is,

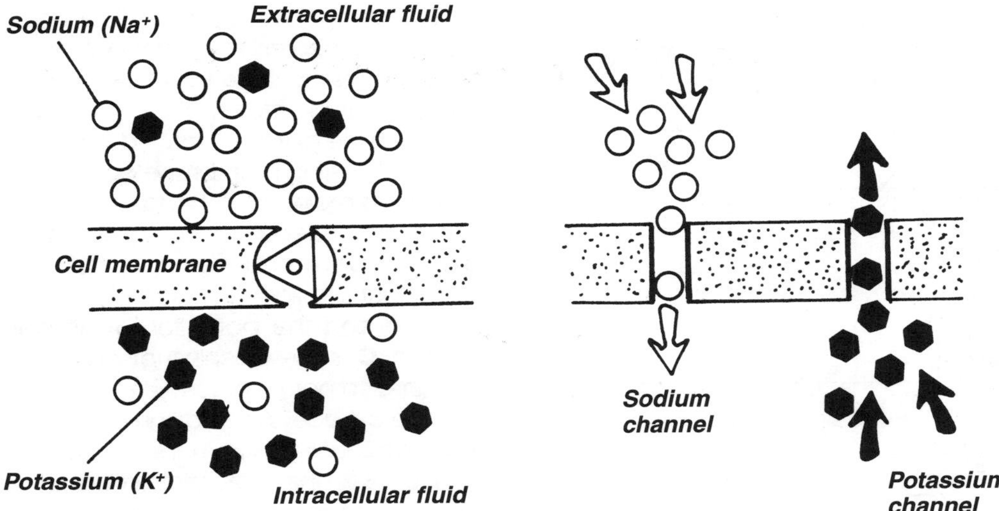

Figure 7–5. Diagram of the sodium-potassium pump *(left)* and membrane channels for sodium and potassium *(right)*.

causing it to lose its polarity (Figure 7–6). The **wave of depolarization** is called an **action potential**. The depolarization begins because some event (typically action in another neuron) momentarily lowers the voltage of a region of the membrane below some threshold. This causes the opening of **voltage-controlled gates** (or channels) that regulate sodium ions. As these channels open, sodium ions flood into the intracellular fluid, causing the membrane potential to reverse its polarity from –70 mV to about +30 mV. This abrupt reversal of polarity is called the **action spike**. Very shortly after the sodium channels are opened to allow sodium ions into a cell, potassium channels are opened so that potassium ions escape into the extracellular fluid. This discharge of the positively charged potassium ions begins to return the cell membrane back to a negative potential. Then the sodium potassium pumps begin their work of maintaining the resting membrane potential.

This depolarization influences only a tiny portion of the cell membrane (about a millimeter of its length), but it causes voltage-controlled gates to open in the adjacent portion of the membrane, which produces another depolarization event. In this way, the wave of depolarization spreads along a nerve fiber. This neural impulse is transmitted in one direction only and is an *all or none* phenomenon (meaning that the impulse is fully present or it is absent; there is no gradation of the electrical event in the neuron). The fuse is sometimes used as an analogy to the firing of a neuron. The fuse is all or none, and, assuming that it is lit at one end, it burns in one direction.

The nerve impulse is conducted along a neuron until it reaches its axon terminals. Here it synapses with other neurons (or in some cases, with muscles or glands) and, assuming that synaptic activation occurs, the nerve impulse is then transmitted along the next neuron. The continuous and widespread activity in the nervous system is a chemoelectrical process involving depolarization of a neuron membrane and synaptic transmission to other neurons.

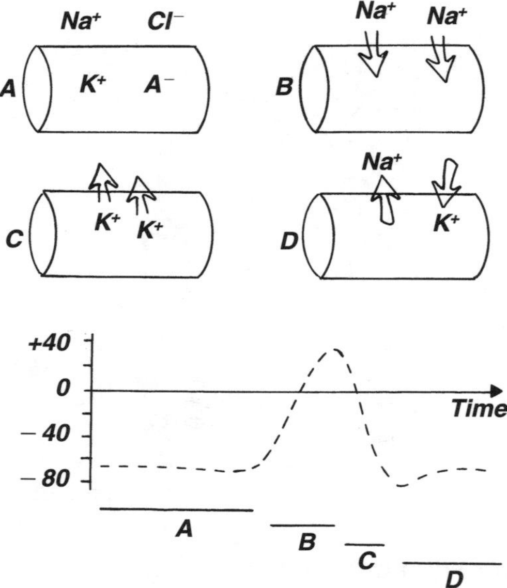

Figure 7–6. Polarization and depolarization of a neuron membrane. **A** represents the resting state in which the sodium pump creates ionic imbalances between the extracellular and intracellular fluid. A resting membrane potential of −70 mV is maintained. **B** marks the neural impulse, or depolarization of the membrane; sodium channels open to allow sodium ions to flood into the intracellular fluid, causing the potential to swing to positive. **C** is the opening of potassium channels to permit potassium to escape into the extracellular fluid. This loss of positive potassium ions from the intracellular fluid causes the potential to begin to return to negative. **D** is the return to the resting membrane potential as the sodium-potassium pump resumes its ionic transport across the cell membrane.

In 1966, the French Academy of Medicine defined clinical death as the cessation of brain activity, rather than stoppage of the heart. It was the first medical group to do so. Others followed suit. One means of ascertaining the presence of brain activity is to record electrical activity from the brain. Such a recording is called an **electroencephalogram** (*electro- + encephalo- + gram;* encephalon refers to the brain), abbreviated EEG. In case of clinical brain death, normal activity patterns are not observed. The EEG in brain death is a "flat line."

Summary

The neuron is the basic unit of the nervous system. An understanding of the neuron and its connections is fundamental to the broader understanding of the nervous system and its operations. Neurons are classified according to their function and structure. The functional classifications are sensory neurons, motor neurons, and interneurons. Sensory and motor neurons are found exclusively in the peripheral nervous system. Interneurons are the primary type of neuron in the central nervous system. The major structural types of neurons are: monopolar, bipolar, and multipolar. Each of these has a cell body, a dendrite, and an axon. The nerve impulse is a wave of depolarization that spreads along the processes of a neuron and can be likened to a burning of a fuse in its all-or-none, one-directional character. Neurons communicate with one another through junctions called synapses. Neurotransmitters are chemical messengers that account for important aspects of synaptic communication. Large populations of neurons share a given transmitter and it is therefore possible to describe the nervous system in terms of transmitter systems.

ANATOMY OF THE NERVOUS SYSTEM

As noted earlier, the human nervous system can be divided into two major systems, the central nervous system or CNS and the peripheral nervous system or PNS, as schematized in Figure 7–7. The CNS is made up of the **brain** and **spinal cord**. We already have noted that the huge population of interneurons is found in the CNS. The peripheral nervous system consists of the 31 pairs of **spinal nerves** that emerge from the spinal cord and the 12 pairs of **cranial nerves** that emerge from the base of the brain. These **peripheral nerves** carry out the sensory and motor functions of the nervous system. The CNS is the site of central operations including the interpretation of sensory stimuli, the preparation of motor responses, storage of memories, thought, and language. The PNS is the system of nerves that carries information to and from the CNS. All sensory information that the brain receives comes by way of the PNS and all actions that the CNS wants to perform depend on PNS transmission of neural instructions to muscles and glands. Figure 7–8 is a general outline of the nervous system and related tissues. The various divisions seen in the outline are discussed in this chapter.

Central Nervous System

> ***The brain is just the weight of God.***
> ***For, heft them, pound for pound,***
> ***and they will differ, if they do,***
> ***as syllable from sound.***
>
> (Emily Dickinson, from Poem No. 632 in *The Poems of Emily Dickinson*, edited by Thomas H. Johnson, ed. Cambridge, MA: The Belnap Press of Harvard University)

Figure 7–9 illustrates in a highly diagrammatic way the major CNS divisions listed in Figure 7–8. The discussion in this chapter refers to these divisions repeatedly. Another diagrammatic representation of the CNS is shown in Figure 7–10, which shows a simplified view of the major stuctures of the CNS, labeled with names that might be less intimidating than those used in Figures 7–8 and 7–9.

The CNS is also called the **neuraxis**. The divisions of the neuraxis are given various names, but one common system uses the base form *encephalon* (meaning brain, as noted earlier) modified by a prefix *tel-* ("far"), *di-* ("between or through"), *mes-* ("middle"), *met-* ("bridge"), and *myel-* ("marrow"). Thus, the divisions are the **telencephalon** (far brain), **diencephalon** (interbrain), **mesen-**

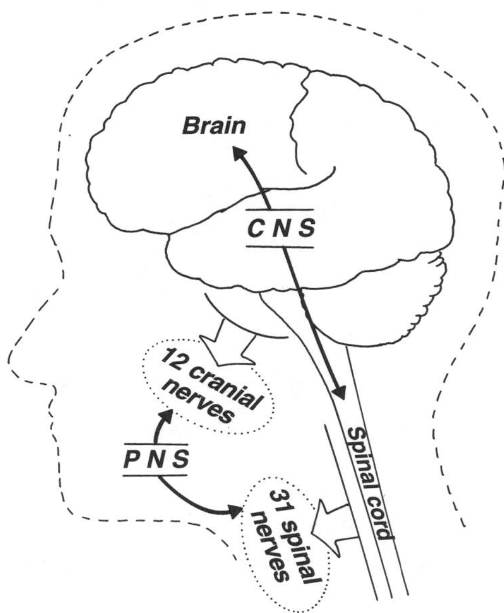

Figure 7–7. Diagram of the central nervous system (CNS) and peripheral nervous system (PNS).

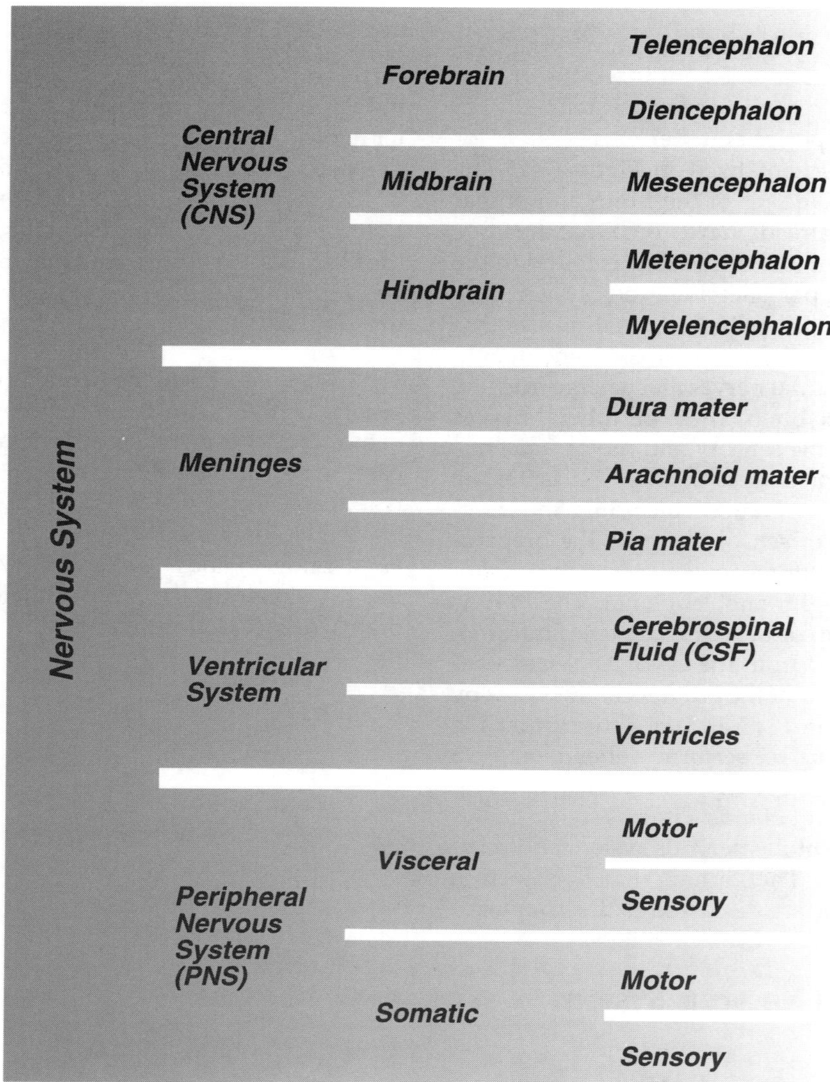

Figure 7–8. General outline of the nervous system.

cephalon (midbrain), **metencephalon** (bridging brain), and **myelencephalon** (marrow brain). The metencephalon and myelencephalon together form a structure called the **hindbrain**. In the following discussion, these divisions are associated with the brain structures listed in Table 7–1.

Cerebral Hemispheres

The **cerebral hemispheres** are the right and left halves of the largest part of the brain. When most people think of the brain, they visualize the cerebral hemispheres (or **cerebrum**). The cerebrum, along with the basal

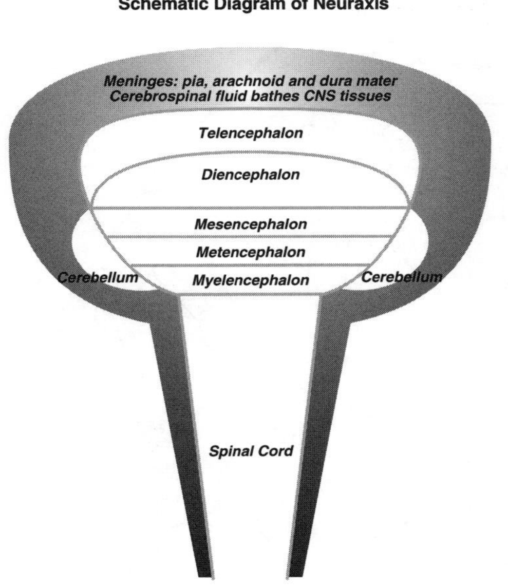

Figure 7–9. Schematic diagram of major parts of the CNS.

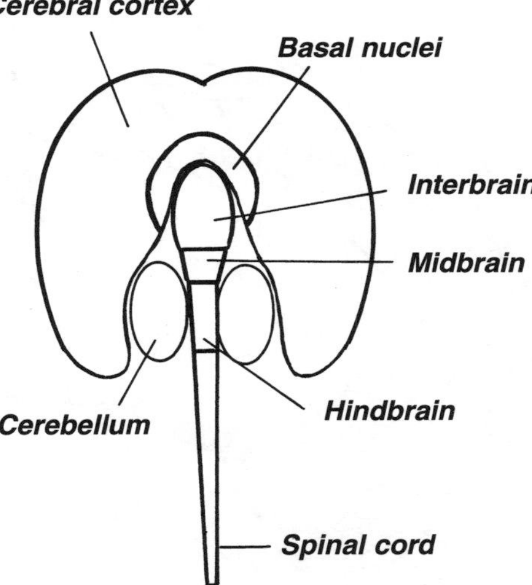

Figure 7–10. Schematic diagram of the CNS (neuraxis), showing major divisions.

Table 7–1. Divisions of the CNS.

Division	Related Structures
Telencephalon	Cerebral hemispheres, basal nuclei
Diencephalon	Thalamus, hypothalamus
Mesencephalon	Midbrain
Metencephalon	Pons
Myelencephalon	Medulla

nuclei, is also known as the telencephalon. The cerebrum is, by far, the largest part of the brain by volume, weight, and surface area. It has a deeply wrinkled surface, as seen in Figure 7–11. The wrinkles are important because they increase the total surface area that can be accommodated within the skull. If the wrinkled cortex is straightened out to form a flat sheet, we would discover that about two thirds of its surface area is hidden in its recesses. The increased area provides for an expansion of the **cerebral cortex**. This cortex is the thin (2–3 mm) bark that envelopes the hemispheres. It consists of six layers of neurons. This bark is part of the brain's **gray matter**. Regions that are gray in color have a high concentration of neuronal cell bodies. That is, gray matter indicates the presence of large numbers of cell bodies of interneurons. The tissue underlying the cortex has a white or pale color derived from the mye-

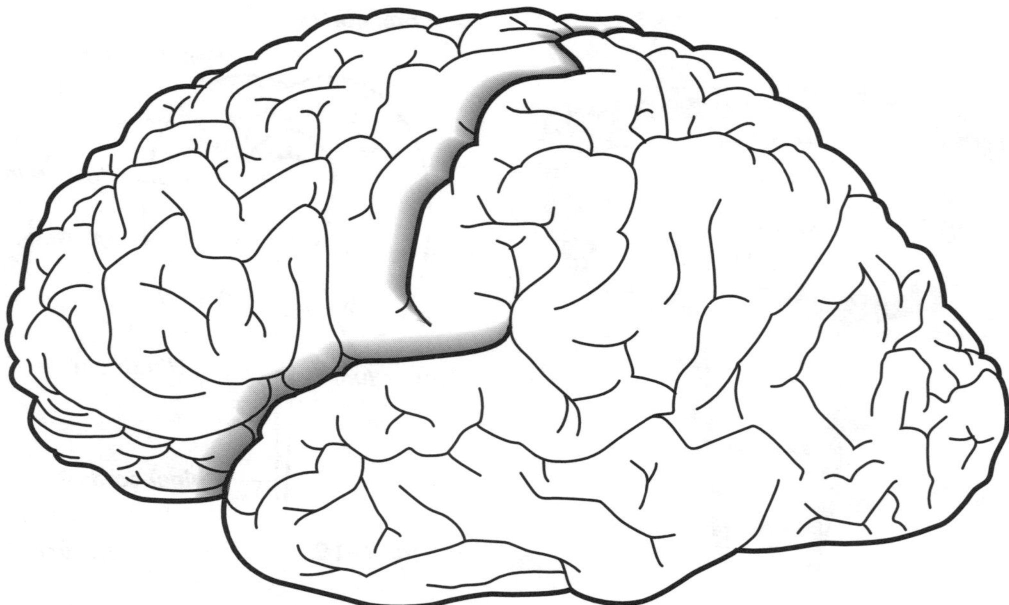

Figure 7–11. Drawing of the surface of the brain, showing its wrinkled surface. Two deep fissures are shaded.

lin coating of the axonic processes. The **white matter** of the CNS therefore reflects the presence of interneuron axons. The gray and white matter distribution is shown in a coronal section of the brain in Figure 7–12.

The outfoldings of the cortical surface are called **gyri** (singular form, *gyrus*) and the infoldings, or grooves, are called **fissures** or **sulci** (singular form, *sulcus*). In this text, the term *fissures* refers to the deepest of the valleys. The convolutions as a whole vary from one brain to the next, but some of the largest convolutions are fairly uniform (Ono, Kubik, & Abernathy, 1990). The most prominent and consistent of the gyri and sulci are frequently used as landmarks for anatomic descriptions. There are three deep fissures: the **longitudinal fissure** that divides the two cerebral hemispheres, the **central fissure** (or **fissure of Rolando**) that divides each cerebral hemisphere into anterior and posterior regions, and the **lateral fissure** (or the **fissure of Sylvius**) that courses along the side of the cerebrum.

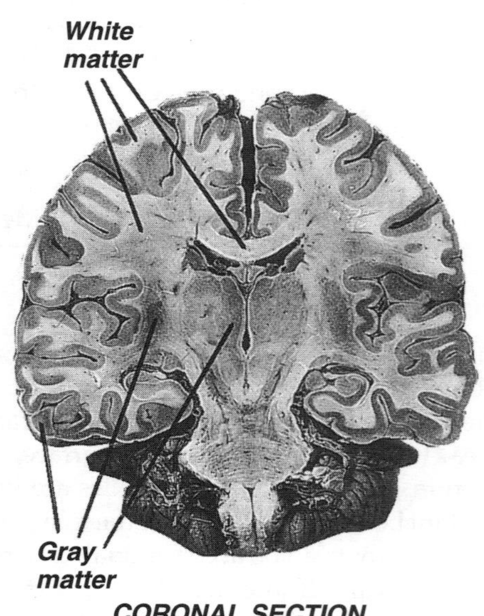

Figure 7–12. A coronal section of the brain to illustrate distribution of white and gray matter.

These fissures are useful boundaries to identify divisions of the brain. The central and lateral fissures, along with smaller gyri and an additional sulcus, are illustrated in Figure 7–13.

The major divisions are called **lobes**. There are five lobes, but only four of them are visible from the outside, as shown in Figure 7–14. The **frontal lobe** is separated from the **parietal lobe** by the central fissure. The **temporal lobe** is separated from both the frontal lobe and parietal lobe by the lateral fissure. The **occipital lobe** lies near the back of the brain. An internal lobe that is not visible without cutting into the brain is the **limbic lobe**.

A visual inspection of the surfaces of the cerebral hemispheres does not reveal any conspicuous differences from region to region, aside from the sulci and gyri. However, microscopic studies show regional differences that give the cortical surface a patchwork-quilt appearance. These differences were mapped by Brodmann (1914) in a classic mosaic that is illustrated in Figure 7–15. Brodmann identified 52 discrete areas of human cerebral cortex. What makes these regions of particular interest is that there is evidence that regions of the brain are to some degree specialized for various functions. A map of some functions is shown in Figure 7–16. By comparing Figures 7–15 and 7–16, one can begin to establish correlations between anatomy and behavior. The term for such correlations is **functional localization**. Some neuroscientists believe that many behaviors can be highly localized, that is, a behavior is associated with activation of a discrete region of cortex. Others believe that behaviors, especially complicated ones like language, depend on the activation of large regions of the cortex. The study of localization has had a contentious history. In his 1805 book *Über die Verrichtungen des Gehirns* (On the Activities of the Brain), Franz Joseph Gall maintained that different parts of the brain serve different functions. However, he also believed that examination of the shape of a person's skull was a suitable method to study the brain. This led to the field of phrenology, which came to be rejected as baseless. Gall's reputation was demolished along with the method espoused by phrenology. He deserved better, but a recounting of his one big mistake is about all that is written about him in introductory books in psychology and neuroscience. In fact, modern neuroscience follows after Gall in some fundamental respects. Some repair to his reputation is due.

> ***"Gall has played a great role in deterministic thought about the functions of brain and mind—a long line stretching from the eighteenth century to this day, traveled by physicians and philosophers alike."***
>
> (Francis Schiller: *Paul Broca: Founder of French Anthropology, Explorer of the Brain*, 1992, p. 169. Oxford, England: Oxford University Press, 1992)

Different regions of the cortex are connected by fibers called **fasciculi** (singular form *fasciculus*). This communication network consists of two primary fiber types. **Association fibers** connect cortical areas on the same hemisphere and **commissural fibers** join a region of one hemisphere to a region of the other. Association fibers are of two types: short fibers that link adjacent gyri and long fibers that connect remote areas.

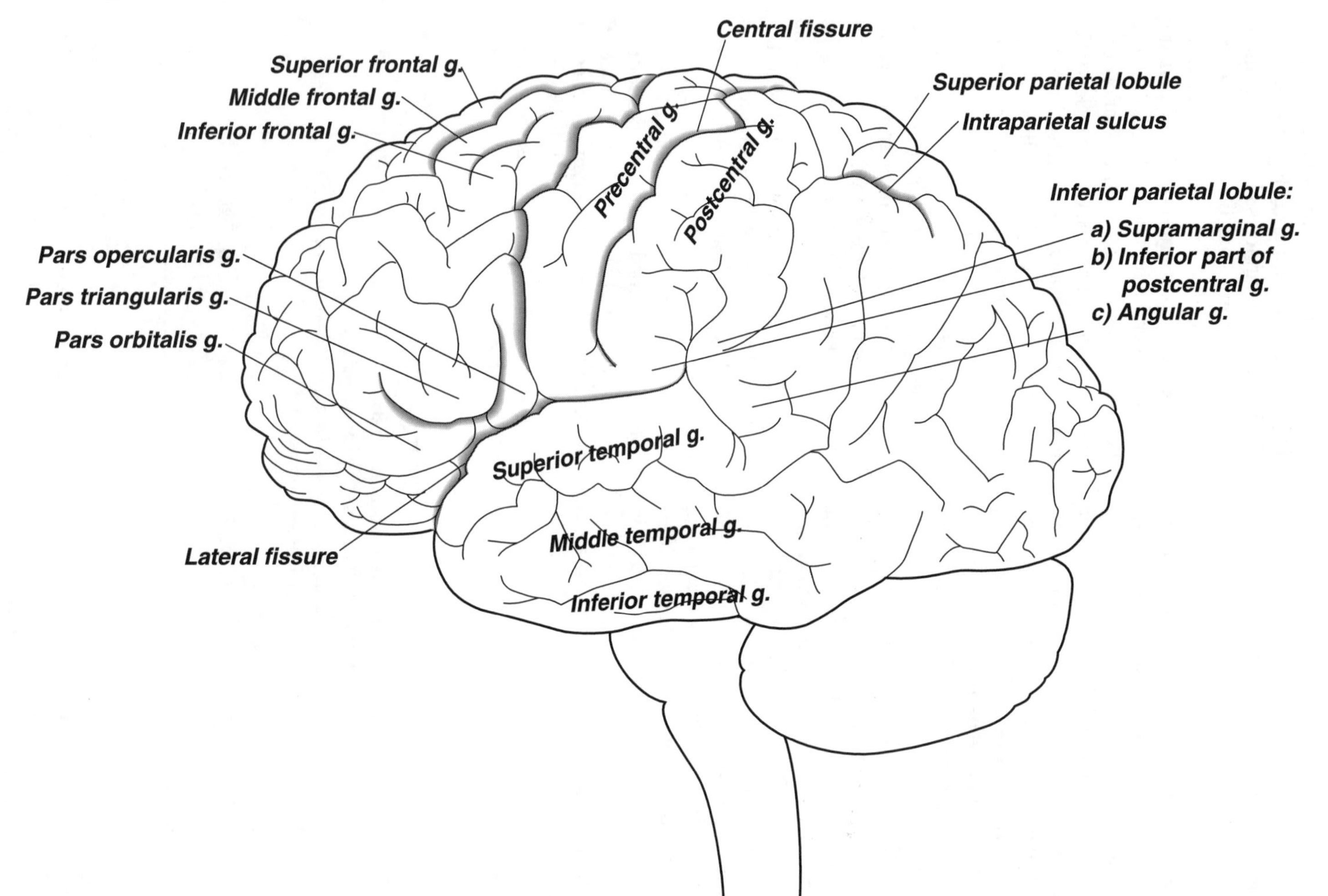

Figure 7–13. Major gyri (g.), fissures, and sulcus of the cerebral cortex. Lateral view of left cerebral hemisphere is shown.

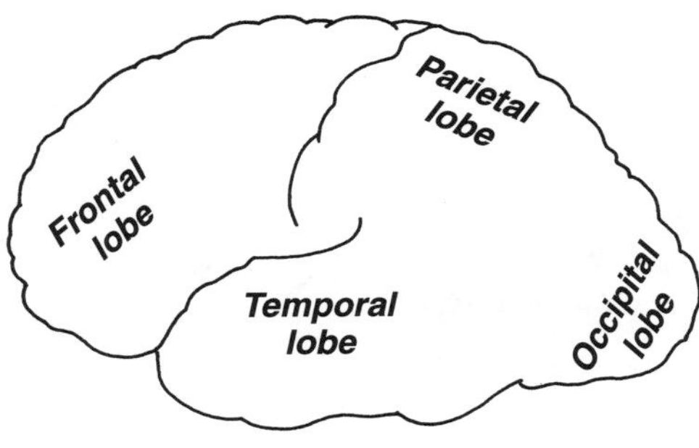

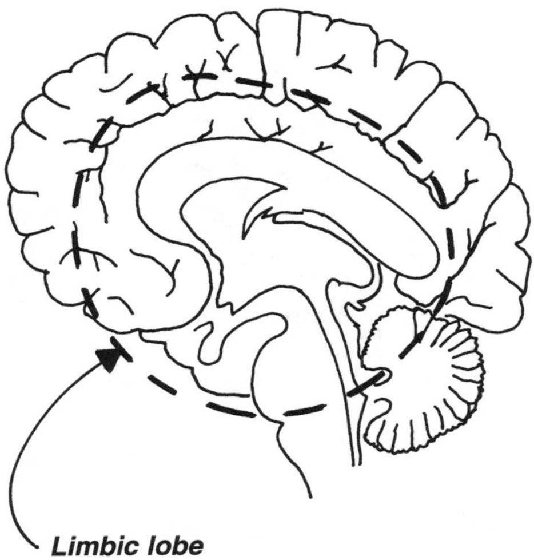

Figure 7–14. The lobes of the cerebrum visible on its outer surface. A fifth lobe, the limbic lobe, lies beneath the cerebral cortex.

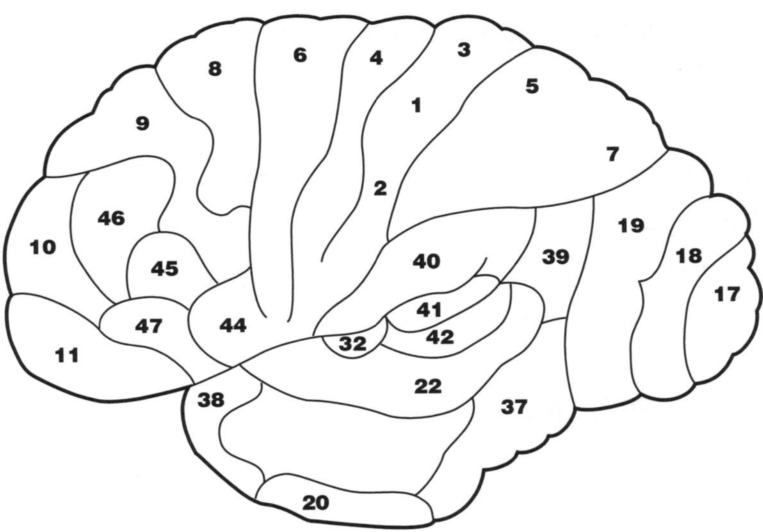

Figure 7–15. Selected Brodmann areas of the cerebral cortex.

Figure 7–17 illustrates the major long association fibers. The **superior longitudinal fasciculus** connects the cortex of the frontal, parietal, occipital, and temporal lobes. The **inferior longitudinal fasciculus** connects the temporal and occipital lobes. The **arcuate fasciculus** links parts of the frontal lobe with regions of the parietal and temporal lobes. Additional association fibers include the **cingulus**, which lies on the medial (inner) aspect of each hemisphere. This structure connects the frontal, parietal, and temporal lobes within each hemisphere. The **uncinate fasciculus** connects the temporal lobe with the frontal lobe.

The commissural fibers are found in four bundles: the large **corpus callosum**, the **an-**

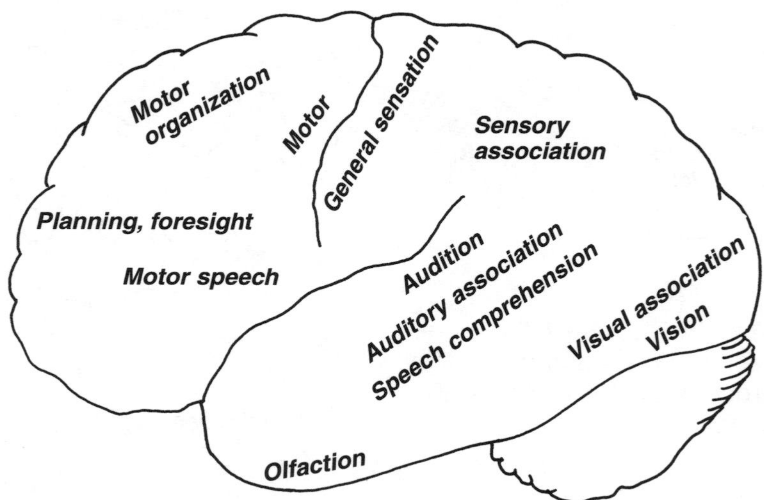

Figure 7–16. Map of cerebral cortex showing localization of selected functions.

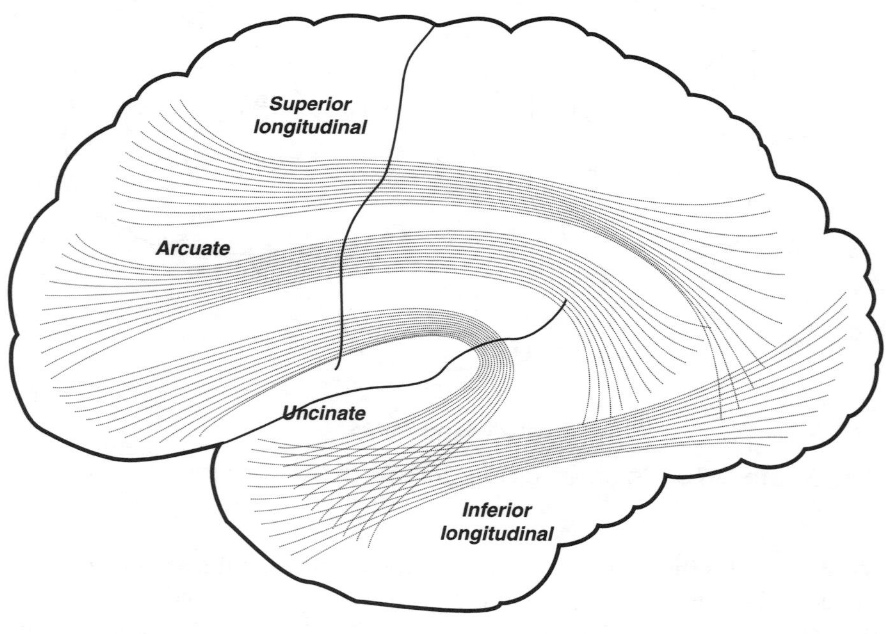

Fasiciculi

Figure 7–17. The major fasciculi of the cerebral cortex.

terior commissure, the **middle commissure**, and the **posterior commissure**. The corpus callosum, shown in Figure 7–18, is a major link between the hemispheres and connects homologous areas of the right and left cerebral hemispheres. If this fiber bundle is severed, as it sometimes is for surgical reasons, the two hemispheres are nearly without communication. The result is a so-called "split brain." Individuals who have undergone section of the corpus callosum have been valuable sources of information on the relative functions of the right and left hemispheres. The anatomic and functional asymmetry of the brain has been the subject of hundreds of published papers. It is difficult to distinguish reasonable conclusion from speculation in this complex literature, but for those who dare to attempt to make sense of it, some helpful readings are Geschwind and Galaburda (1987) and Kertesz (1989). It has been known for over a century that the two cerebral hemispheres are not equivalent in function, as explained in the following quotation (see also Schiller, 1992).

> ***"In 1865, 3 research papers were published, all purporting to show that the right and left hemispheres are not functionally equivalent. The best known of these papers was written by Paul Broca (1824-1880), the other 2 were written by Marc Dax (1770-1837) and his surviving son Gustave (1815-1893). Since no articles had been published on cerebral dominance prior to this time, 1865 can be rightfully thought of as a landmark year in neurology."***
>
> (S. Finger & D. Roe, "Gustave Dax and the Early History of Cerebral Dominance." *Archives of Neurology*, 1996, *53*, p. 806.)

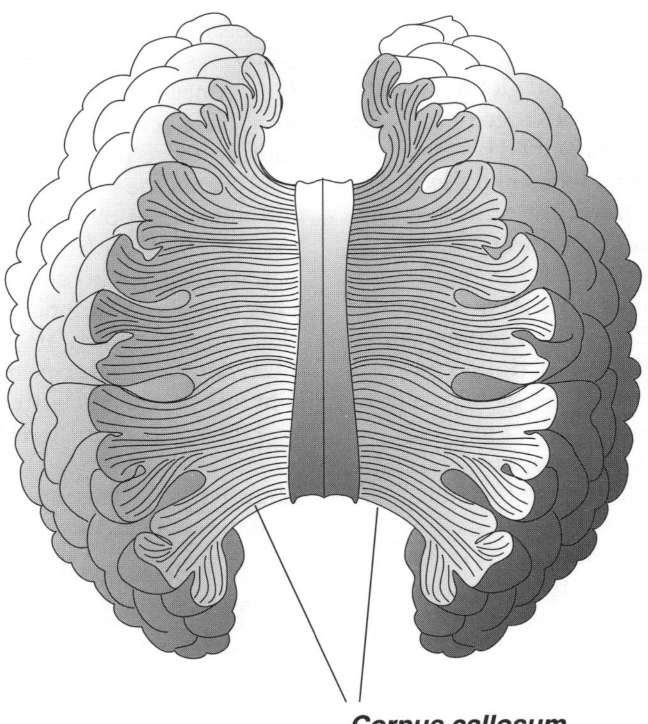

Figure 7–18. The corpus callosum.

Basal Nuclei

The **basal nuclei** are also known as the **basal ganglia** ("nerve knots"). Strictly speaking, the term *ganglia* should be reserved for aggregates of neuron cell bodies in the peripheral nervous system. However, the term basal ganglia is used with such frequency that there seems little point to arguing about the accuracy of the wording. The basal nuclei (or ganglia) are masses of neuron cell bodies that lie deeply within the brain. Figure 7–19 shows a coronal and sagittal section of the brain featuring the basal nuclei. There are several different nuclei included within the collective term basal nuclei, but the most important for the purposes of this book are the **caudate**, **putamen**, and **globus pallidus**. The caudate (from the Latin for tail) is a structure shaped like a shrimp with a large head and a curving tail. The putamen (Latin for stone) is a small rounded mass closely associated with the globus pallidus (Latin for pale globe). In a sagittal section of the brain, the putamen and globus pallidus are nestled within the C-shaped curve of the caudate. The putamen and globus pallidus are sometimes grouped together as the **lenticular nucleus**, so named because they form a structure that looks like a lens. The caudate and putamen are collectively referred to as the **striatum** (meaning striped), because of their appearance under microscopy. Connections of the basal nuclei to other brain structures are complex, but an important simplified description is: cerebral cortex → striatum → globus pallidus → thalamus → cerebral cortex. This circuit is the core of an important motor system to be described in a later section.

The basal nuclei are important in controlling motor functions of the body. One principal purpose may be to stabilize the large and complicated neural system that regulates movement. The basal nuclei also may be important in directing action and in interpreting sensory information to guide motor behavior. Recent theorizing emphasizes models of neural information processing in the basal nuclei (Alexander, Delong, & Strick, 1986; Graybiel, Aosaki, Flaherty, & Kimura, 1994). Damage to the basal nuclei results in a number of commonly recognized motor impairments. One of these is Parkinson's disease, which is characterized by slow movement, tremor, and rigidity.

Thalamus and Hypothalamus

The diencephalon consists essentially of the two structures discussed in this section. The **thalamus** (meeting place or chamber) is shaped like a small bird's egg (or actually two eggs, as the thalamus is paired). Its location is pictured in Figure 7–20. The thalamus is richly connected with the cerebral cortex and receives inputs from virtually every sensory system of the body (excluding only the sense of smell) and also monitors motoric information that is directed to the cerebral cortex. The thalamus has been likened to a major relay station between subcortical and cortical structures for sensory and motor information. However, the word *relay* may be inadequate to capture the critical role of this small but vital part of the brain. Among other things, the thalamus appears to be part of the brain systems that control language (Botez & Barbeau, 1971; Crosson, 1992). The thalamus contains a number of important nuclei, most of which are shown in Figure 7–21. Some of these nuclei are very important for speech. A selective listing of nuclei and their major functions follows:

- Anterior nucleus: involved in the brain's emotional circuits.
- Mediodorsal nucleus: also involved in emotion.
- Ventral anterior and ventral lateral nuclei: receive input from the basal nuclei and the cerebellum (discussed in the following section).

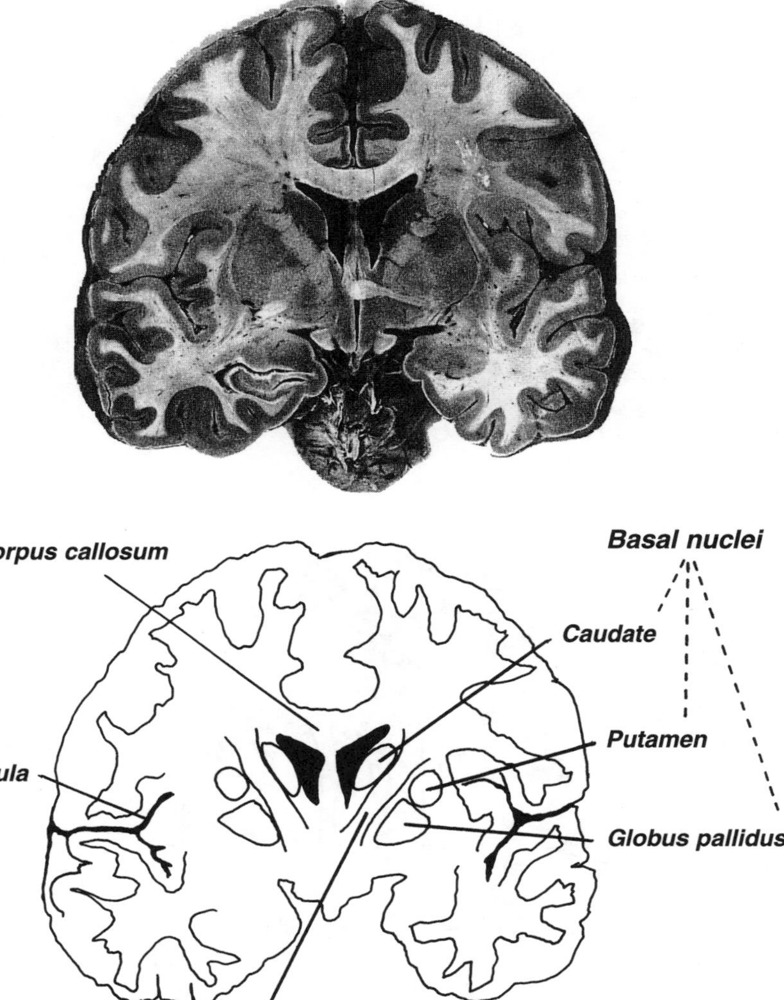

Figure 7–19. a. Coronal section of the brain, with accompanying drawing to identify the basal nuclei. *(continued)*

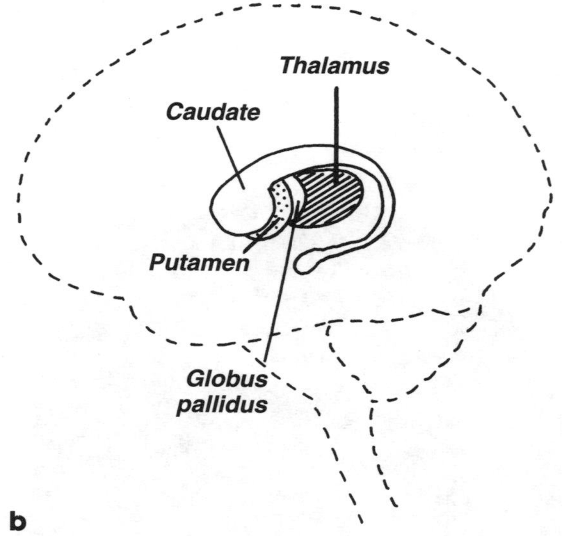

Figure 7–19. *(continued)* **b.** A drawing of a sagittal section of the brain to show the location of the basal nuclei.

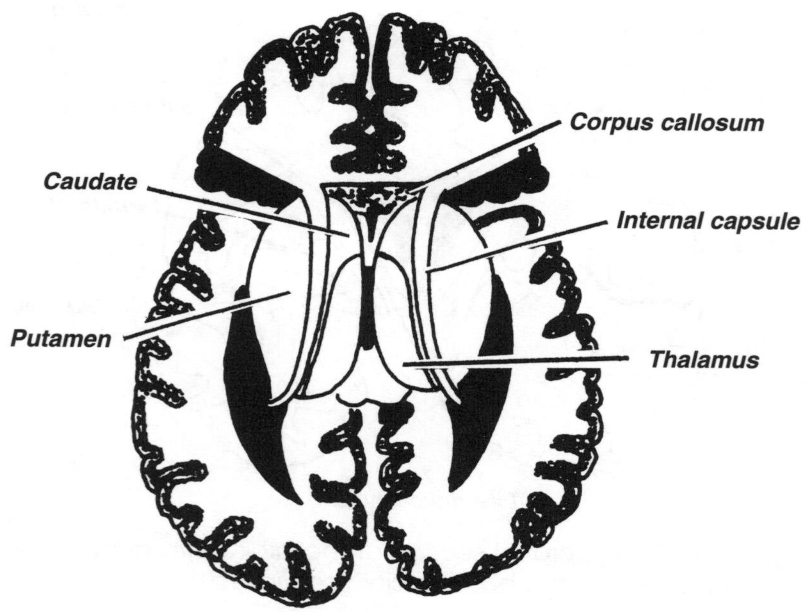

Figure 7–20. Transverse section of the brain to reveal the thalamus in relation to major structures of the basal nuclei. Compare with Figure 7–19.

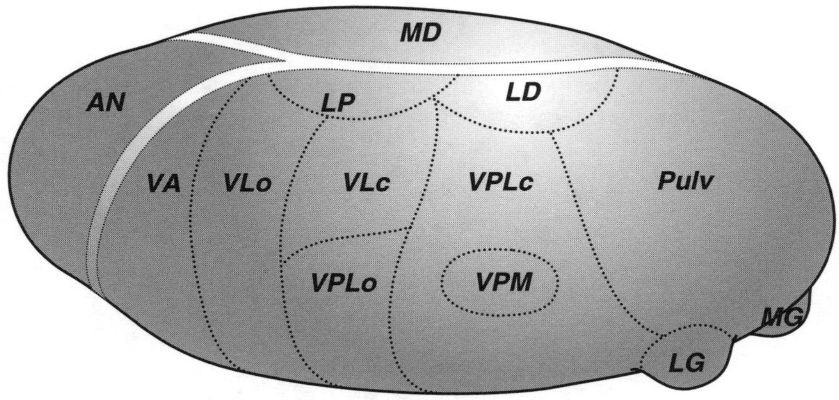

Figure 7–21. Major nuclei of the thalamus: Anterior nuclear group (AN), medial dorsal (MD), lateral dorsal (LD), ventral anterior nucleus (VA), ventral lateral nucleus (VL), ventral posterior lateral nucleus (VPL), ventral posterior medial nucleus (VPM), medial geniculate (MG), pulvinar (Pulv), and lateral geniculate (LG),

- Ventral posterior lateral nucleus and ventral posterior medial nucleus: relay information on general body sensation.
- Medial geniculate: processes auditory information.
- Lateral geniculate: processes visual information.

In contrast to the specific sensory and motor integration function of the thalamus, the **hypothalamus** is involved in endocrine, autonomic, and behavioral functions such as release of hormones, control of food and water intake, sexual behavior, diurnal (day/night) rhythms, and mediation of emotional responses. The hypothalamus is commonly divided into three regions including the supraoptic, tuberal, and mammillary regions. Although not directly involved in speech and language functions, the mammillary bodies are thought to play a role in the formation of memories. The hypothalamus may also act to mediate bodily functions via emotional factors.

Cerebellum

The **cerebellum** (Latin for little brain) is located at the base of the occipital lobe adjacent to the brainstem. It contains a considerable number of neurons, as much as half of the total neurons in the CNS. The cerebellum has a cortex constituted of narrow, leaflike folia that resemble the pages of a book (Figure 7–22). The cortex is the primary information-receiving part of the cerebellum. The information arrives by way of the middle and inferior **cerebellar peduncles** (*peduncles* means "little feet") that connect to pathways from the spinal cord, vestibular system, and motor control areas. The primary information-sending regions are three sets of paired deep cerebellar nuclei. Information from the deep cerebellar nuclei travels via the superior cerebellar peduncle to reach the spinal cord, thalamus, and cerebral cortex.

The role of the cerebellum in speech motor control is to coordinate the various muscle

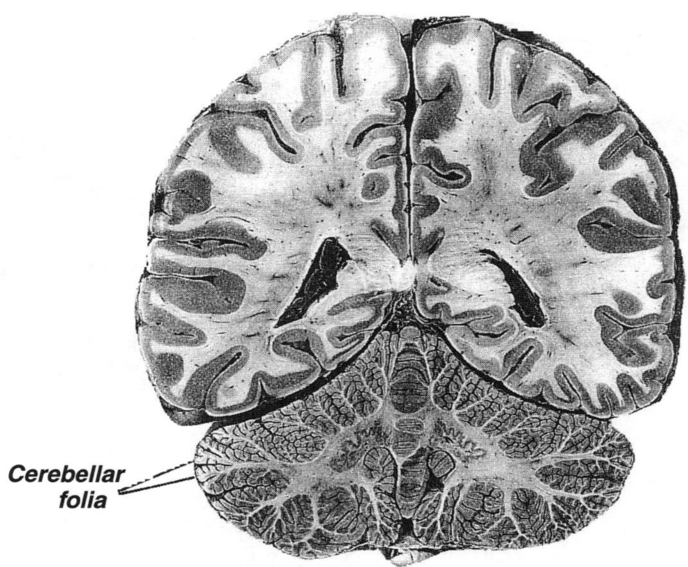

Figure 7–22. Coronal section through cerebrum and cerebellum. This section reveals the folia of the cerebellum.

groups to produce a smooth flow of movement. Lesions of the cerebellum can result in decomposition of movement into component parts as well as errors in rate and range of movement. Therefore, people with damage to the cerebellum may demonstrate a speech disorder that can cause them to sound inebriated. Because of the cerebellum's complex interconnections with the cortex and spinal cord, it has been hypothesized that the lateral cerebellum, which receives input from the premotor and association cortical areas, acts to preprogram a movement, whereas the intermediate cerebellum (a part called the vermis) acts to update an evolving movement via its input from the sensorimotor cortical and spinal inputs. Recent discussions of selected topics on cerebellar function are: (1) effects of cerebellar pathology (Diener & Dichgans, 1992); (2) cerebellar regulation of movement (Thach, Goodkin, & Keating, 1992); and (3) cerebellar function in computational, cognitive, and language skills (Chafetz, Friedman, Kevorkian, & Lovy, 1996; Daum & Ackermann, 1995; Leiner, Leiner & Dow, 1991; Silveri, Leggio, & Molinari, 1994). A new picture of cerebellar function may soon emerge, especially through neuroimaging studies (discussed in a later section).

Limbic System

The **limbic system** is one of the most recently described major structures of the human brain. The term *limbic* means border. The limbic lobe, as mentioned earlier, is a ring of cortex on the medial aspect of the cerebral hemispheres. Structures included as part of the limbic system are the limbic lobe, the hippocampus (seahorse), amygdala (almond), the septal (partition, or dividing wall) area, the mammillary (breastlike) bodies (sometimes including the entire hypothalamus), and the anterior nuclei of the thalamus. Several major structures of the limbic system are shown in Figure 7–23. The precise role of this structure in speech and language functions is unknown. However, the limbic system is thought to be important in emo-

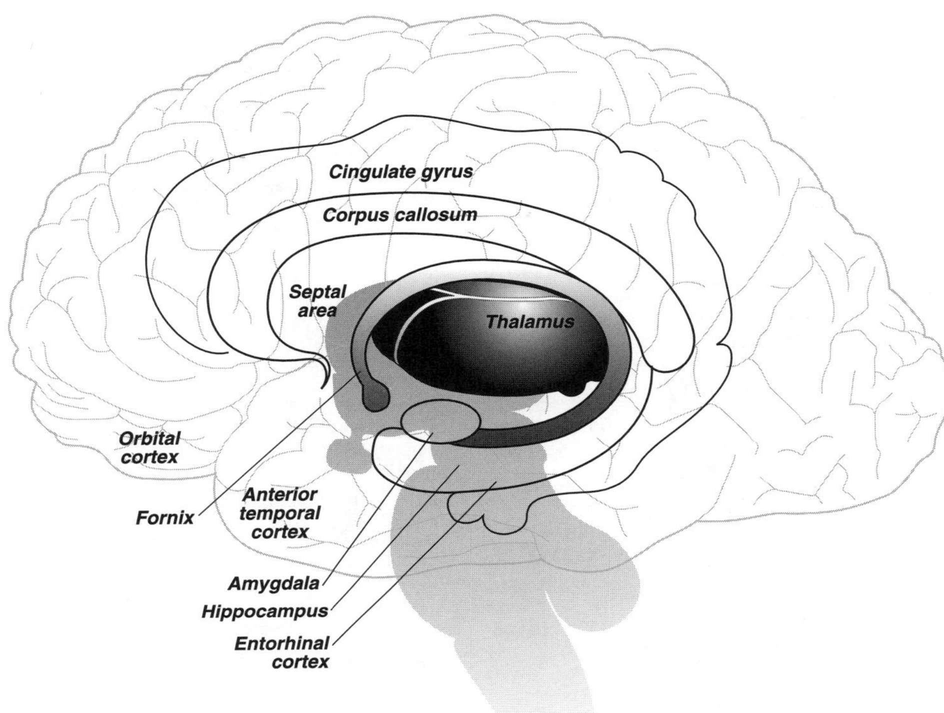

Figure 7–23. The limbic lobe of the cerebrum and structures of the limbic system.

tional and visceral responses and, therefore, may provide a motivational or intentional aspect to communication. Some types of damage to the limbic system result in **mutism** (lack of speech).

Brainstem

The structures of the **brainstem** (Figure 7–24) include the midbrain (mesencephalon), pons (metencephalon), and medulla (myelencephalon). Some authors also include the thalamus. The brainstem has been likened to the stem of a mushroom, with the cerebrum covering it much as the cap of a mushroom covers its stem. These structures serve essential life functions, including regulation of body temperature, respiration, swallowing, and digestion. Possibly, some of the brainstem centers that regulate behaviors such as swallowing and respiration are recruited in the control of speech. As is discussed later, the pons and medulla also are important because they contain the nuclei for the cranial nerves. Additional features of the brainstem are illustrated later in the chapter.

Spinal Cord

The spinal cord, along with the cranial nerves, constitute the peripheral nervous system. The spinal cord emerges from the skull through a large hole called the foramen magnum discussed in Chapter 5. This opening in the skull is the anatomic boundary between the medulla and the spinal cord. The cord is contained within the vertebral column. Its length in the adult male is about 42 cm and its diameter is about equal to that of the little finger. In cross section, the cord has a gray H-shaped core surrounded by white quadrants (Figure 7–25).

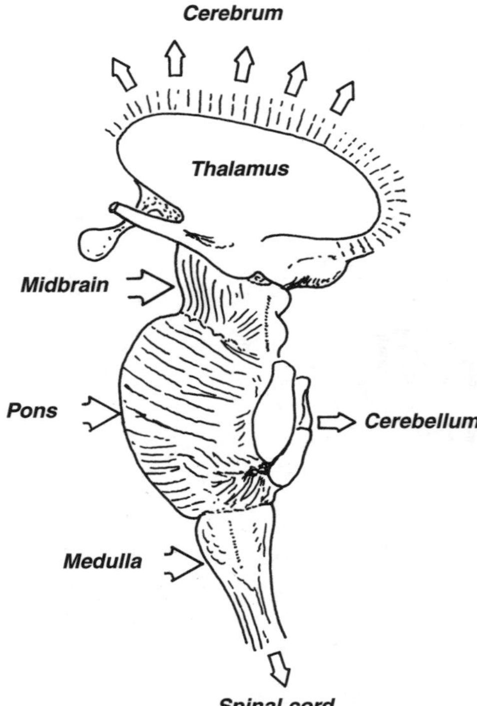

Figure 7–24. Lateral view of the brainstem.

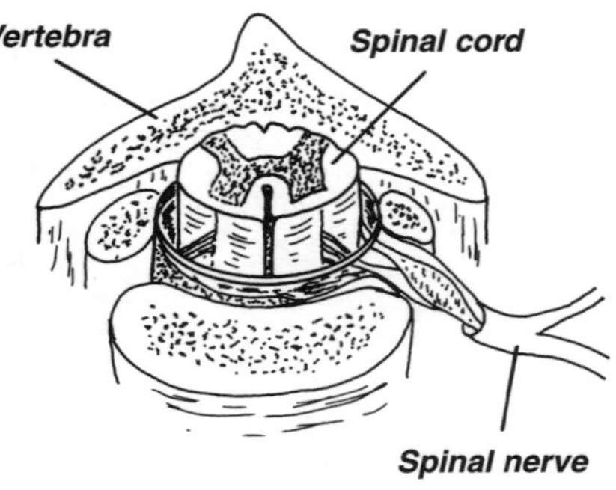

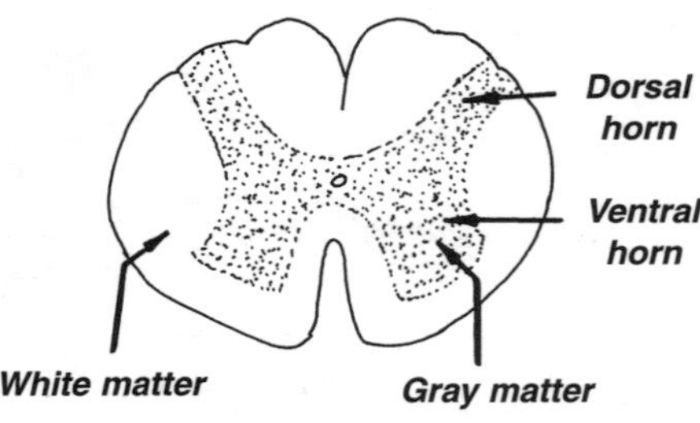

Figure 7–25. Top: Cross-section of spinal column to show vertebra, spinal cord, and spinal nerve. **Bottom:** Distribution of white and gray matter in a transverse section of the spinal cord.

The arms of the H are called horns, with two horns posterior and two anterior. The **posterior horns** are also called **dorsal horns**, and the **anterior horns** are also known as **ventral horns**. The cell bodies of spinal neurons are found in the gray matter and myelinated axons make up the white regions.

> ***"A comparison of the theoretical views of Karl Lashley with those of his contemporary, Wilder Penfield, reveals one of the most intriguing paradoxes in the annals of the neurosciences. On the one hand, Lashley, whose principal laboratory subject was the rat, looked upon the cerebral cortex as the dominant level of the nervous system, even though the rat is endowed with an underdeveloped cerebrum relative to that of primates. On the other hand, Penfield, who worked with humans whose cerebrums are maximally developed, viewed subcortical processes as taking precedence over neocortical processes for higher mental activities."***
>
> (R. Thompson, "Centrencephalic Theory, the General Learning System, and Subcortical Dementia." In *Brain Mechanisms: Papers in Memory of Robert Thompson. Annals of the New York Academy of Sciences*, 1993, *702*, p. 197.)

This quotation from Robert Thompson is a fitting close to this section on the CNS. The opposing views of Lashley and Penfield survive to the present in debates over the roles of cortical and subcortical structures in a wide range of behaviors, including speech and language, memory, and learning. This chapter tries to avoid making too sharp a functional divide between cortical and subcortical systems. Particularly for the understanding of speech, it is more important to understand the cooperation between cortical and subcortical systems than to segregate them by assigning to each presumed control over different speech functions.

Summary

The CNS, or neuraxis, consists of a number of structures, but primarily the cerebrum, thalamus and hypothalamus, basal nuclei, limbic system, brainstem, cerebellum, and spinal cord. These divisions of the CNS are associated with a variety of human functions including thought, language, emotion, consciousness, sensation, motor control, and regulation of basic body processes such as respiration and temperature. The primary neuronal constituent of the CNS is the interneuron, a multipolar neuron that is multiply connected to other neurons. The neurons of the CNS do not extend directly to innervate the sensory organs, glands, or muscles of the body. Rather, the neurons of the CNS connect with neurons of the PNS, which, in turn, innervate the sensory organs and the effectors (muscles and glands).

Peripheral Nervous System

"Nature, indeed, has had a triple end in view in the distribution of nerves: she wished to give sensibility to organs of perception, movement to organs of locomotion, and to all the others the faculty of recognising the experience of injury."

(Galen, 130–200 BC)

The PNS is discussed with respect to the two primary groupings of peripheral nerves: cranial nerves and spinal nerves.

Cranial Nerves

The 12 cranial nerves and their functions are summarized in Table 7–2. These nerves emerge from the base of the brain and penetrate the skull through various holes to reach their sensory or motor target tissues (Figure 7–26). For present purposes, the cranial nerves may be thought to serve either sensory, motor, or combined sensory/motor functions. Motor, or efferent, portions of cranial nerves originate in numerous brainstem nuclei and then proceed to exit the brainstem to innervate musculature of the head, neck, and shoulders as well as abdominal and thoracic viscera. In contrast, the afferent portions of the various cranial nerves carry sensory information from receptors located in the periphery to additional brainstem nuclei. Sensory information is then relayed via the thalamus (except for cranial nerve I) to the sensorimotor cortex.

One of the mnemonics that students use to remember the cranial nerves is the sentence, "On old Olympus towering top a Finn and German vended at hops." The first letters of the words recall the names of the cranial nerves, from CN I to CN XII: I = olfactory, II = optic, III = oculomotor, IV = trochlear, V = trigeminal, VI = abducens, VII = facial, VIII = acoustic, IX = glossopharyngeal, X = vagus, XI = accessory, and XII = hypoglossal. As might be inferred from Figure 7–26, the Roman numerals reflect the order of emergence of the nerves from the base of the brain, proceeding posteriorly.

Seven of the 12 paired cranial nerves are especially pertinent to speech production: cranial nerves V, VII, VIII, IX, X, XI, and XII. The cranial nerves most relevant to

Table 7–2. Cranial nerves, listed by Roman numeral, type (S = sensory, M = motor) and innervated region, and function.

Nerve	Type / Innervated Region	Function
CN I	S / olfactory epithelium	Sense of smell
CN II	S / ganglion cells of retina	Sense of sight
CN III	M / eye muscles	Eye movement
CN IV	M / eye muscles	Eye movement
CN V	S / skin and head, dura mater	Facial sensation
	S / muscle spindles and mechanoreceptors in jaw muscles	Proprioception
	M / jaw muscles, tensor tympani	Chewing, ear drum
CN VI	M / eye muscles	Eye movement
CN VII	S / outer ear	Sensation
	S / taste buds in anterior tongue	Taste
	S / portion of nasopharynx	Taste
	M / salivary glands, lacrimal gland	Secretion
	muscles of facial expression and stapedius	Facial expression, stapedial reflex
CN VIII	S / Organ of Corti and vestibular apparatus	Hearing and balance
CN IX	S / outer ear	Sensation
	S / taste of posterior tongue	Taste
CN X	S / carotid body and sinus mucosa	Sensation
	M / parotid gland	Secretion
	M / pharynx (stylopharyngeus)	Pharyngeal action in speech and swallowing
	S / outer ear	Sensation
CN XI	M / shoulder and neck muscles	Head and shoulder movements
CN XII	M / tongue muscles	Tongue movements

speech are shown in Figure 7–27, which shows for each nerve the approximate location of emergence from the brainstem and the sensory and motor functions. Additional details for these nerves are presented in an appendix; the information given here is intended as a basic introduction.

The **trigeminal nerve (CN V)** is motor to the muscles of mastication and sensory to the face and anterior parts of the head (including the teeth). This nerve has three branches, the ophthalmic, maxillary, and mandibular.

The **facial nerve (CN VII)** has an efferent role for the muscles of facial expression and an afferent role in mediating taste from the anterior two thirds of the tongue.

The **statoacoustic nerve (CN VIII)** was long thought to be purely sensory, but it is now recognized that it has efferent functions as well. CN VIII consists of both vestibular and cochlear portions for balance and hearing, respectively. The neural pathway for audition is considered in more detail later in this chapter.

The **glossopharyngeal nerve (CN IX)** is motor to muscles of the pharynx and sensory (for taste) to the posterior one third of the tongue. This cranial nerve also helps to regulate salivation.

The **vagus (CN X)** is a complex nerve with an extensive distribution. Its efferent portion innervates intrinsic laryngeal and pharyngeal muscles. The vagus also has efferent and afferent functions for the thoracic and abdominal viscera. Taste information from the epiglottis is mediated by the vagus.

The last two cranial nerves are exclusively motor. The **spinal accessory nerve (CN XI)** innervates the trapezius and sternocleidomastoid muscles of the neck and shoulder. This nerve also innervates muscles of the velum.

The **hypoglossal nerve (CN XII)** innervates all intrinsic muscles of tongue as well as select extrinsic muscles.

Why is the brain in the head, as opposed to the thorax, abdomen, or lower trunk? One reason may have to do with the cranial nerves, these important channels of neural information. Cherniak (1995) suggested that an important factor in accounting for the location of neural structures is the principle of "save wire." That is, it is wise to keep neural structures close to their place of work to minimize the lengths of nerves between the neural components and the tissues they innervate. The cranial nerves, with their huge numbers of sensory fibers for vision, olfaction, taste, audition, and equilibration, require massive connections to the brain. Therefore, it makes good design sense to put the brain close to the cranial nerves, so that the head becomes a kind of pod for the special senses. But the rest of the body is not neglected, for the organs located below the neck are reason-

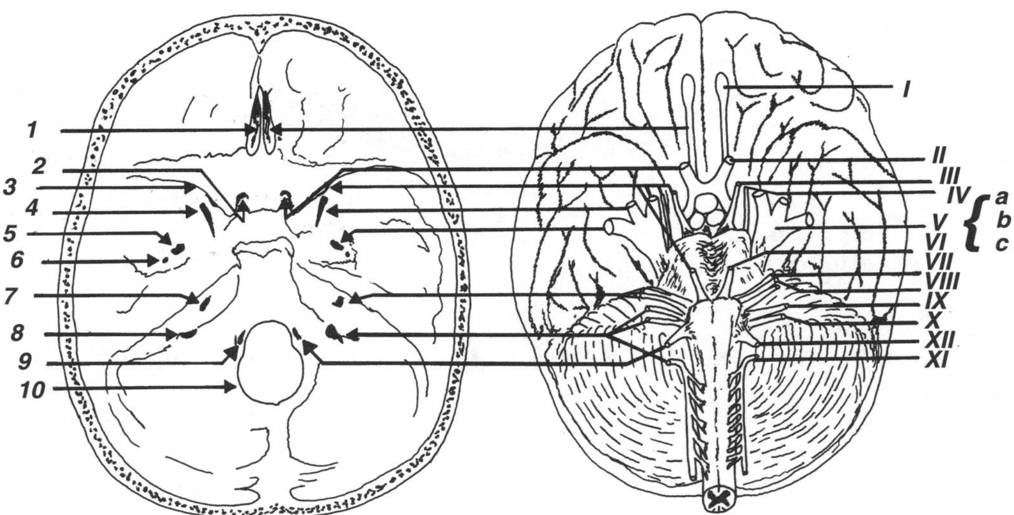

Figure 7–26. a. The right side of the drawing shows a superior view of base of skull, showing the holes in the skull through which cranial nerves exit to reach the body structures they innervate. The left side shows a basal view of the brain with cranial nerves labeled. *(continued)*

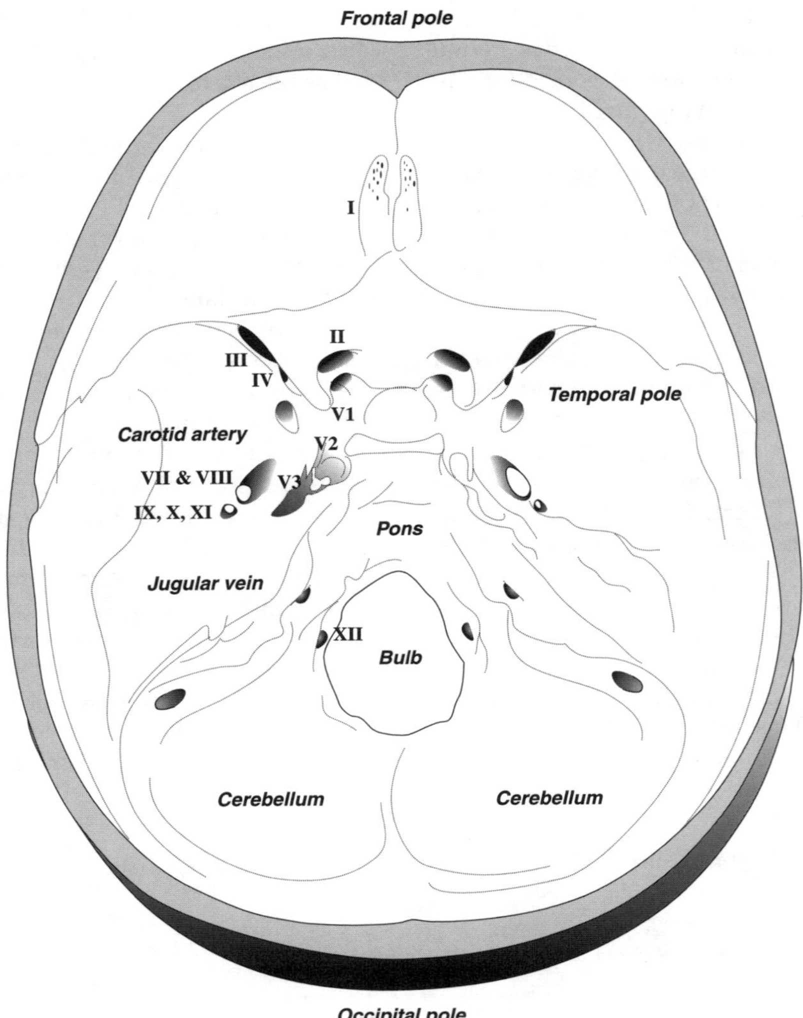

Figure 7–26. *(continued)* **b.** Superior view of base of skull showing exit points of cranial nerves.

ably close to another part of the CNS, the spinal cord.

Spinal Nerves

The 31 pairs of spinal nerves emerge from the spinal cord to innervate sensory and motor functions of the body. Each pair of spinal nerves contains a sensory and motor root (Figure 7–28). According to **Bell's law** (named after Charles Bell who wrote the *New Anatomy of the Brain*), the dorsal roots are sensory and the ventral roots are motor. Sensations from the body are passed to the dorsal (or posterior) horn of the spinal cord, from which the sensory information ascends along fiber tract systems to relay stations in the thalamic nuclei, which in turn pass the information to the cortex. The systematic emergence of these sensory nerves is linked with a segmented representation of body sensation. These segments are called **dermatomes** and are very useful in neurology in infer-

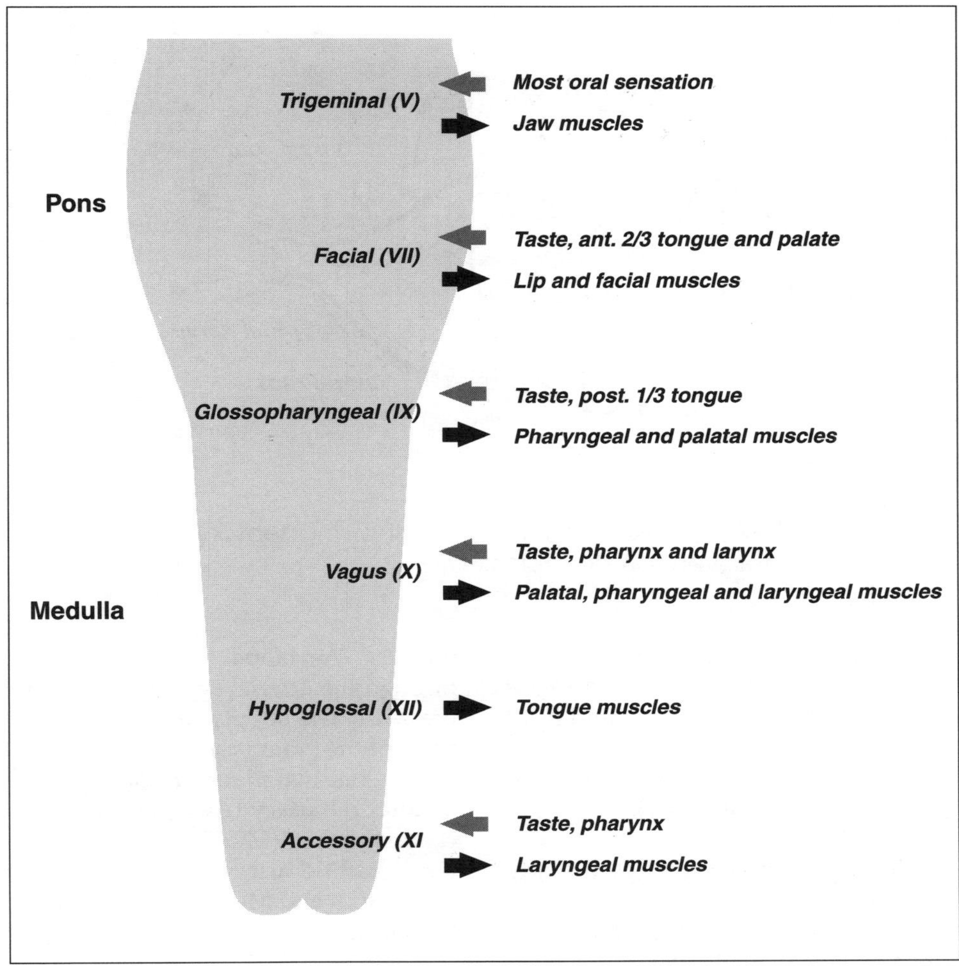

Figure 7–27. Schematic diagram of emergence of cranial nerves most relevant to speech. Motor and sensory functions are summarized.

ring site of damage to the spinal cord. The motor roots of the spinal nerves emerge from the ventral horn of the spinal cord to reach the muscles of the trunk and the limbs. The spinal cord has a slender waist that corresponds to the location of the spinal nerves that supply the axial musculature. The cord's diameter is largest in both the cervical and lumbar regions, where one finds the nerve fibers supplying the appendages. At its thickest, the spinal cord is about the diameter of an ordinary pencil or your little finger.

Nourishment and Protection of the Brain

Blood is a complex fluid with liquid and solid components. Its liquid component is a yellowish fluid called **plasma**. The solid components are various particulates, primarily **red corpuscles** (erythrocytes), **white corpuscles** (leukocytes), and **platelets** (thrombocytes). For the purposes of the present discussion, the red corpuscles are of greatest interest because these are

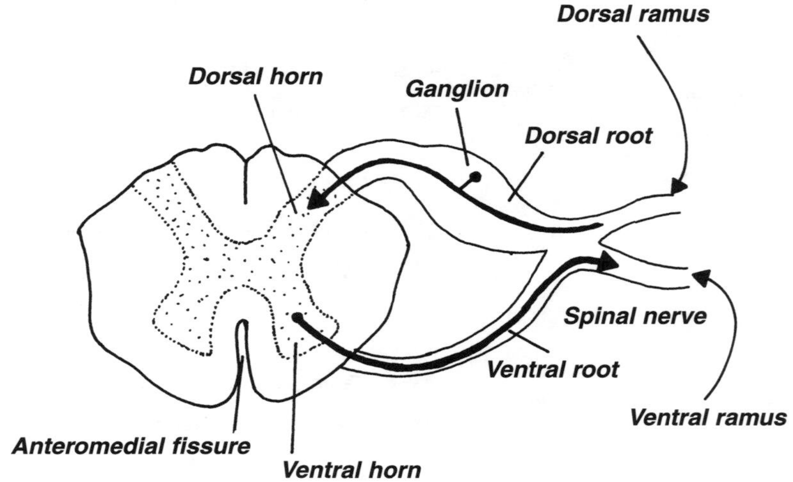

Figure 7–28. Section of spinal cord showing sensory (dorsal) and motor (ventral) structures.

the cells that carry oxygen from the lungs to the cells of the body. The red corpuscles are formed in the bone marrow and have an average life of about 120 days, after which they are removed by the spleen (an organ in the abdominal cavity).

The brain may not seem like a particularly active organ, but it requires about 20% of the blood pumped from the heart, even though the brain is only about 2% of body weight. We might say that the brain gets 10 times as much blood as might be expected on a weight-proportionate basis. Unlike many other types of cells in the body, the brain does not store **glycogen** (an energy source for metabolism) for future energy needs. Therefore, if the blood supply to a region of the brain is interrupted, the neurons quickly feel the loss of nutrients. If the interruption lasts for a few minutes, irreversible neuron death may occur. Neurons begin to die within about 5 minutes of a compete cardiac arrest. This cell death is called **necrosis**. It is a final death, because CNS neurons do not regenerate and they are not replaced.

The arteries that supply the neural tissues are thin-walled and possess relatively little muscle. The blood arrives at the brain through the arterial system shown in Figure 7–29. The supply of blood to various parts of the brain is shown in Figure 7–30. Notice that two major arteries, the **anterior cerebral artery** (ACA) and the **middle cerebral artery** (MCA) derive from the **internal carotid artery**. The course of blood to the ACA and MCA can be diagrammed as follows.

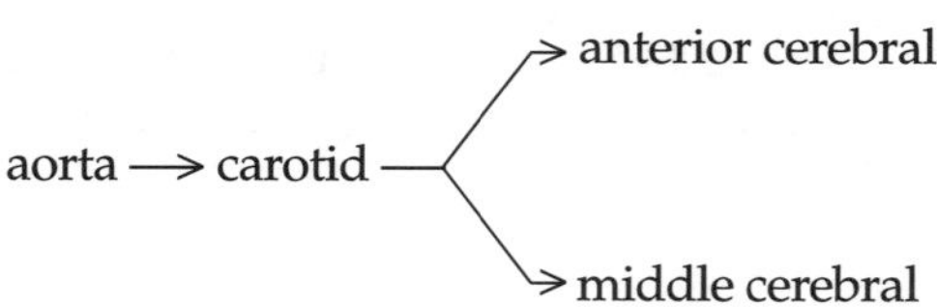

The **posterior cerebral artery** together with the **cerebellar arteries** are supplied by the **basilar artery**, which is formed by the confluence of the two **vertebral arteries**. Each vertebral artery arises from the **subclavian artery** on one side of the body. This pattern may be diagrammed as follows.

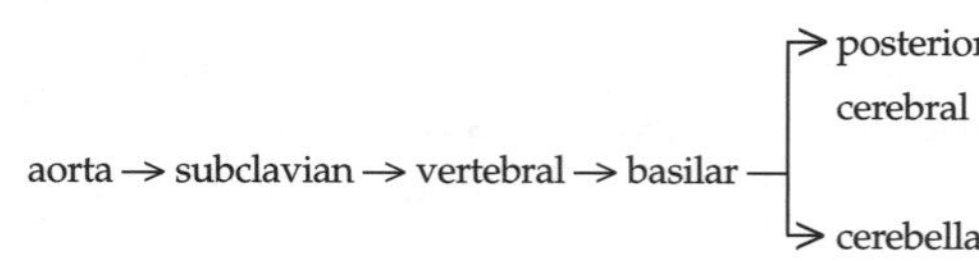

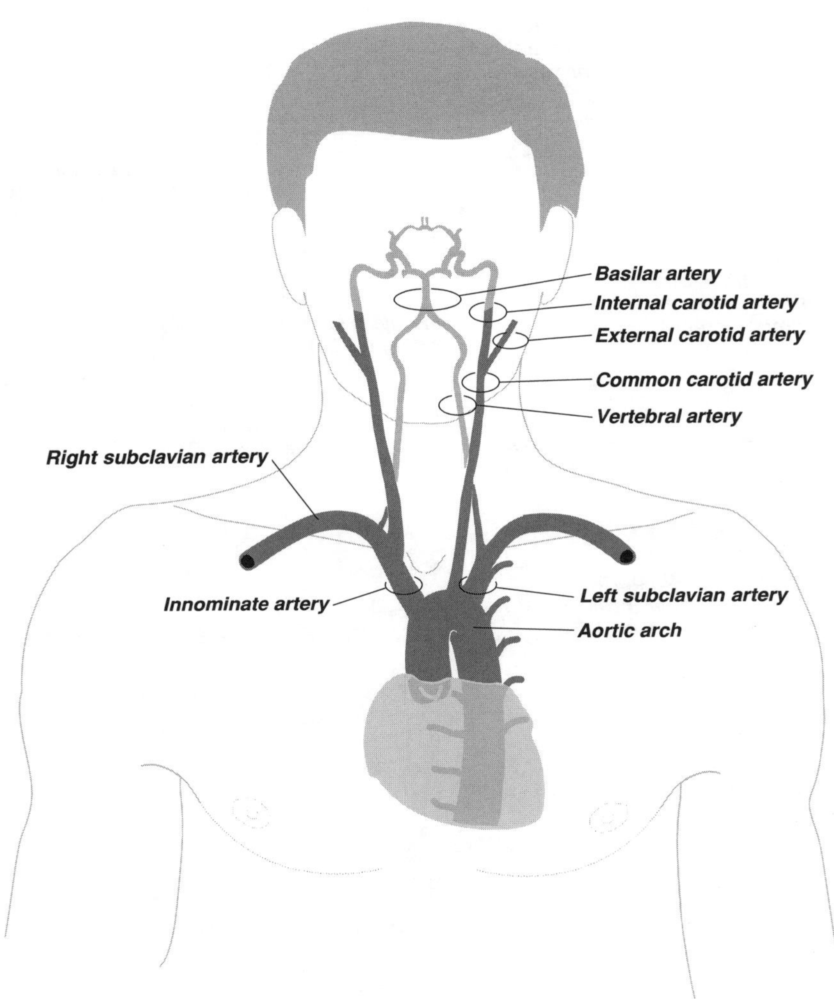

Figure 7–29. Major arterial blood supply to the brain.

The **middle cerebral artery** holds special significance for speech and language, because this artery supplies the regions of the brain that are most strongly implicated in linguistic functions (Buckingham, 1984; Caplan, 1987, 1994; Tikofsky, 1984). In addition, this artery is quite susceptible to strokes. A following section considers these speech and language centers in more detail.

Blood is returned to the heart and lungs through the venous system. The veins of the CNS do not have valves, because there is no back-flow problem created by gravity. Because the head normally is elevated with respect to the heart, blood return does not require a series of valves to prevent back-flow. The veins do not follow the course of the arteries, but rather follow a pattern of their own, as shown in Figure 7–31. Neurosurgeons seek to take advantage of the separate course of the venous system by using it as an alternate route of blood supply when part of the arterial system is damaged. Ultimately, the various sinuses drain into the jugular vein, which then returns blood to the heart.

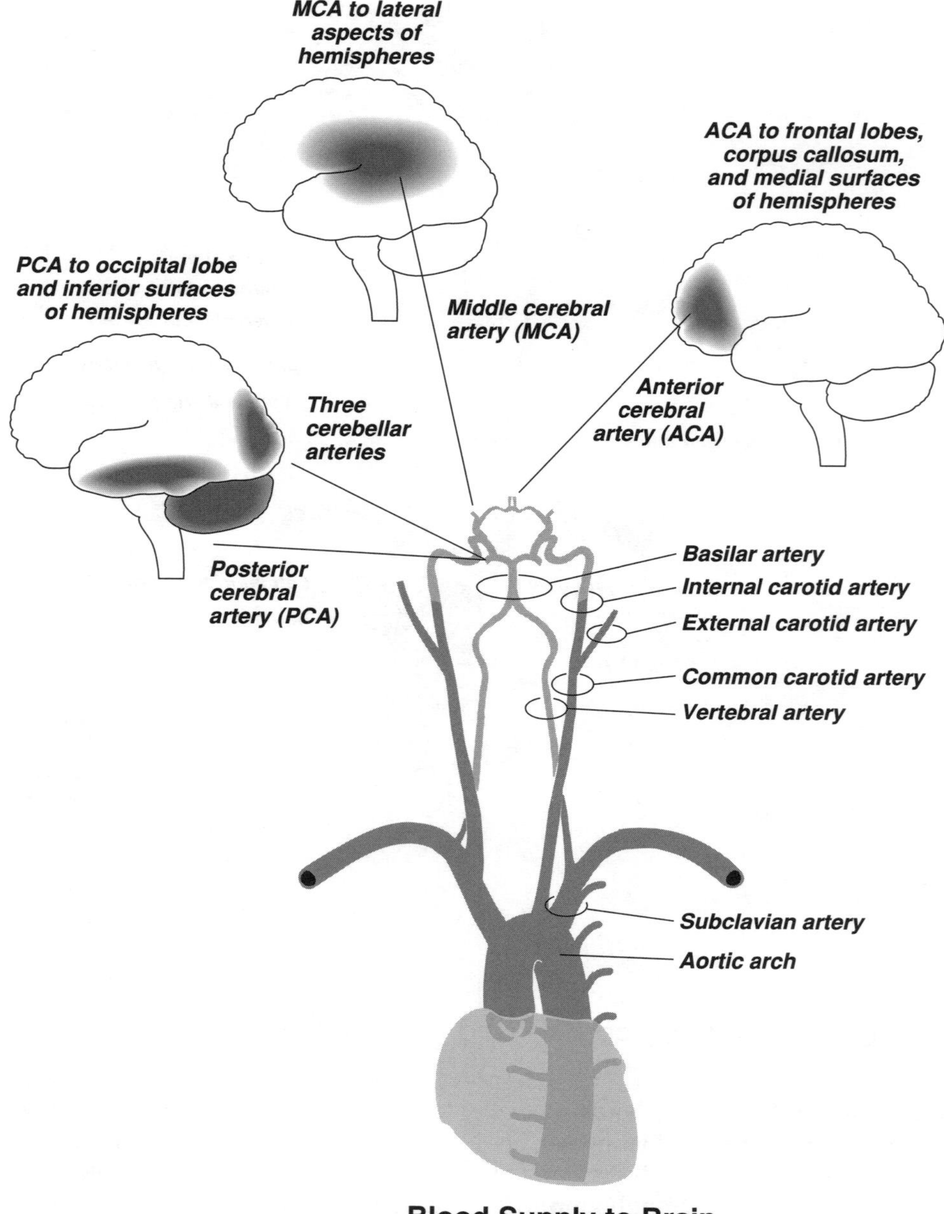

Figure 7–30. Blood supply to major regions of the cerebrum and cerebellum.

Protection of the precious 3 or 4 pounds of jellylike tissue called the brain comes from: the hard bone of the cranium that encloses the brain, the **meninges** (singular *meninx*) or wrappings of the brain, and the **ventricular system**, a series of internal cavities that contain the **cerebrospinal fluid**. Bone, meninges, and fluid constitute an ingenious packaging for the organ of intellect. The arrangement of these protective tissues can be seen in Figure 7–32. The bone of the skull is really a type of bone sand-

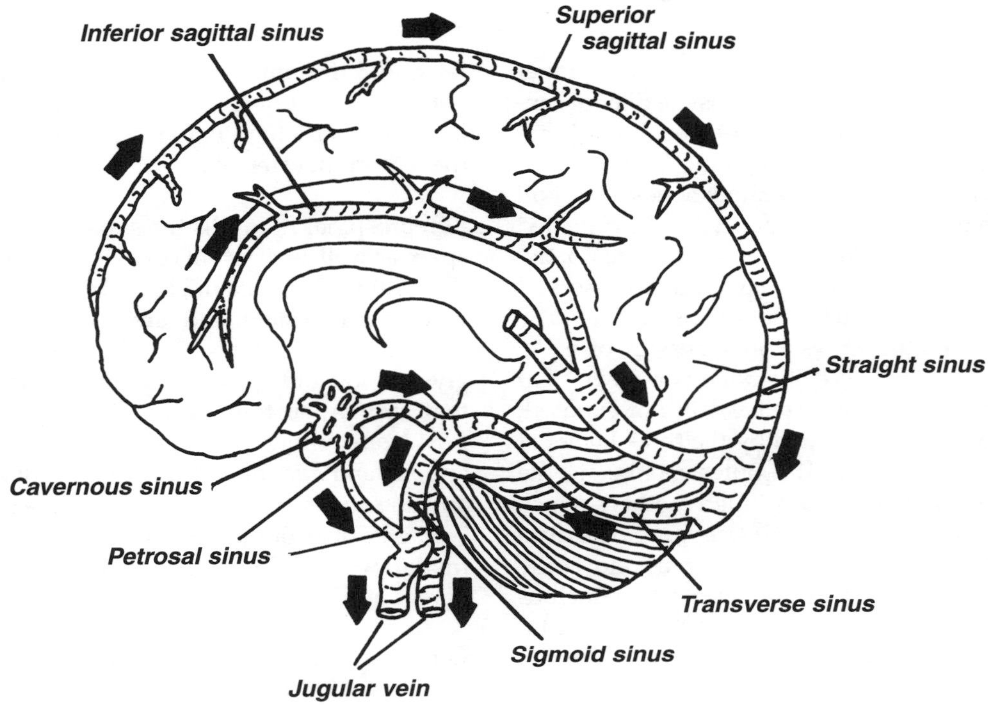

Figure 7–31. Venous system of the brain. Arrows indicate direction of blood return.

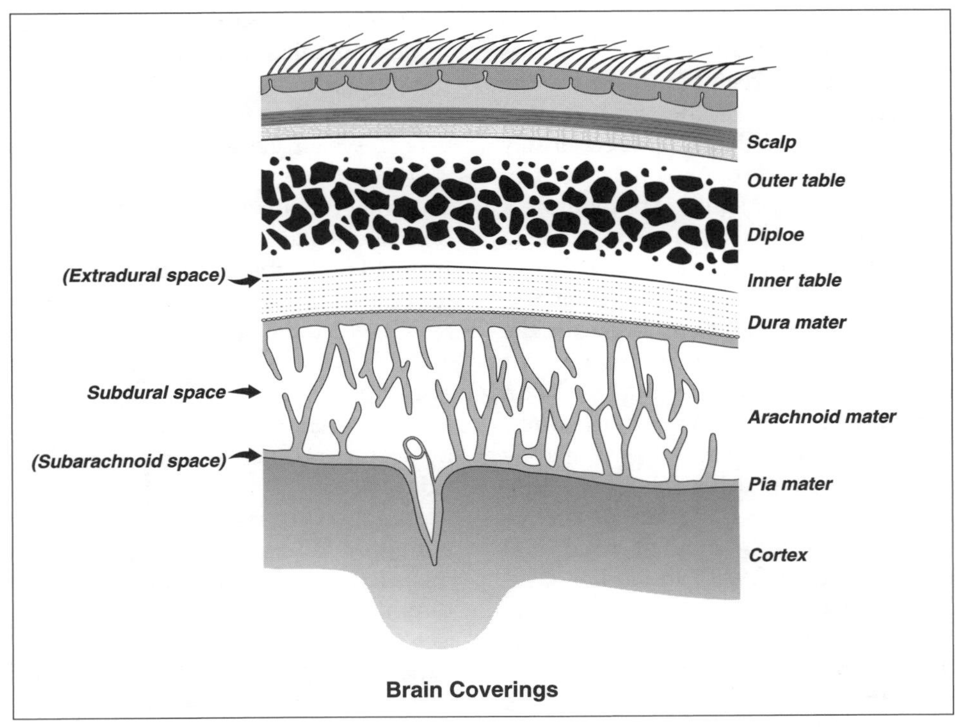

Figure 7–32. Skull and meningeal coverings of the CNS.

wich—a hard outer table and a hard inner table that enclose a collapsible filler of cancellous bone (the **diploe**). The diploe is not present in the infant skull, but develops with growth of the cranial bones. The skull may be likened to a super-hard corrugated cardboard. Physical blows that are not deflected by the outer table can be absorbed to some extent by the collapsible filler. The inner table serves a final measure of skeletal protection. If the bone is removed entirely, the brain itself is still not exposed, for it is surrounded by the three layers of the meninges. The outer meninx is the **dura mater** (literally tough mother), which is rather like a leather wrapping. The dura mater is invested with nerves and is the site of most intracranial sensation (including headaches). The brain itself is not locally sensitive; that is, the brain does not "feel" pain when a neurosurgeon removes brain tissue (although sensations may be felt elsewhere in the body). The middle meninx is the **arachnoid mater** (spider mother), which contains numerous tiny filaments that reach across a fluid-filled space to moor the brain much as a boat is moored in a pier. The inner meninx is the **pia mater** (delicate mother), which is a thin, delicate tissue that is applied closely to the cerebral cortex. As can be seen in Figure 7–32, several spaces are identified. The **extradural space** is situated between the skull and the dura mater. The **subdural space** is beneath the dura mater. Finally, the **subarachnoid space** is between the arachnoid mater and the pia mater. The dura mater plunges deeply into the brain to separate some of the major structures. The cerebral hemispheres are separated by the **falx cerebri**, which resembles a thin vertical wedge. It has important protective purposes, especially against rotational forces (Oldendorf, 1978). In similar fashion, the **falx cerebelli** separates the cerebellar hemispheres. The **tentorium cerebelli** is a horizontal dural plane that divides the cranial cavity into superior (cerebral) and inferior (cerebellar) regions. (See Exercise 7–5.) The terms **supratentorial** and **infratentorial** are used in neuroanatomy and neurology to describe the location of structures or damage relative to the tentorium cerebelli.

Cerebrospinal fluid fills the subarachnoid space as well as a system of cavities within the brain. These cavities constitute the **ventricular system** and are pictured in Figures 7–33, 7–34, and 7–35. Figure 7–33 gives an overall view of the fluid system that entirely surrounds the CNS. Figure 7–34 is an oblique view of the ventricular system and identifies the major cavities and the ducts that connect them. Figure 7–35 is a superior view of the ventricles, as though we were looking down on a transparent head.

Cerebrospinal fluid is produced in choroid plexus cells within the ventricles, especially the lateral ventricles. It flows from the lateral ventricles through the interventricular foramen into the third ventricle, from the third ventricle through the cerebral aqueduct into the fourth ventricle, and out through median and lateral apertures into the subarachnoid space where it envelopes the brain and eventually empties into the venous system at the superior sagittal sinus.

The total amount of cerebrospinal fluid is only about 125 ml. This fluid has both nutritional and protective functions. The latter relates to a kind of shock-absorber effect in which the brain is cushioned within a fluid mattress. The cerebrospinal fluid also affords a measure of protection against an expansion of some part of the intracranial contents. Such expansion carries considerable risk. Because the adult cranium is composed of tightly knit bone, it does not allow for expansion. If some intracranial element such as a hemorrhage or a tumor begins to enlarge, brain tissue is subject to damage. The **Monro-Kellie Doctrine** states that no part of the cranial contents can increase in volume except at the expense of some other part. Because the amount of cerebrospinal fluid can be regu-

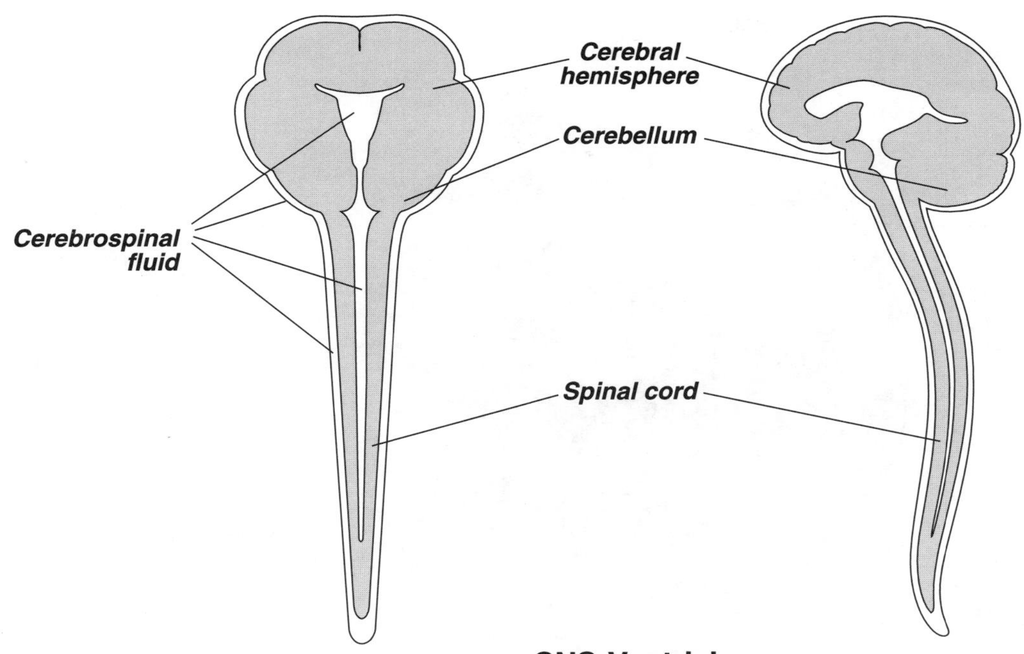

Figure 7-33. Overall view of the distribution of cerebrospinal fluid (in white) in the CNS.

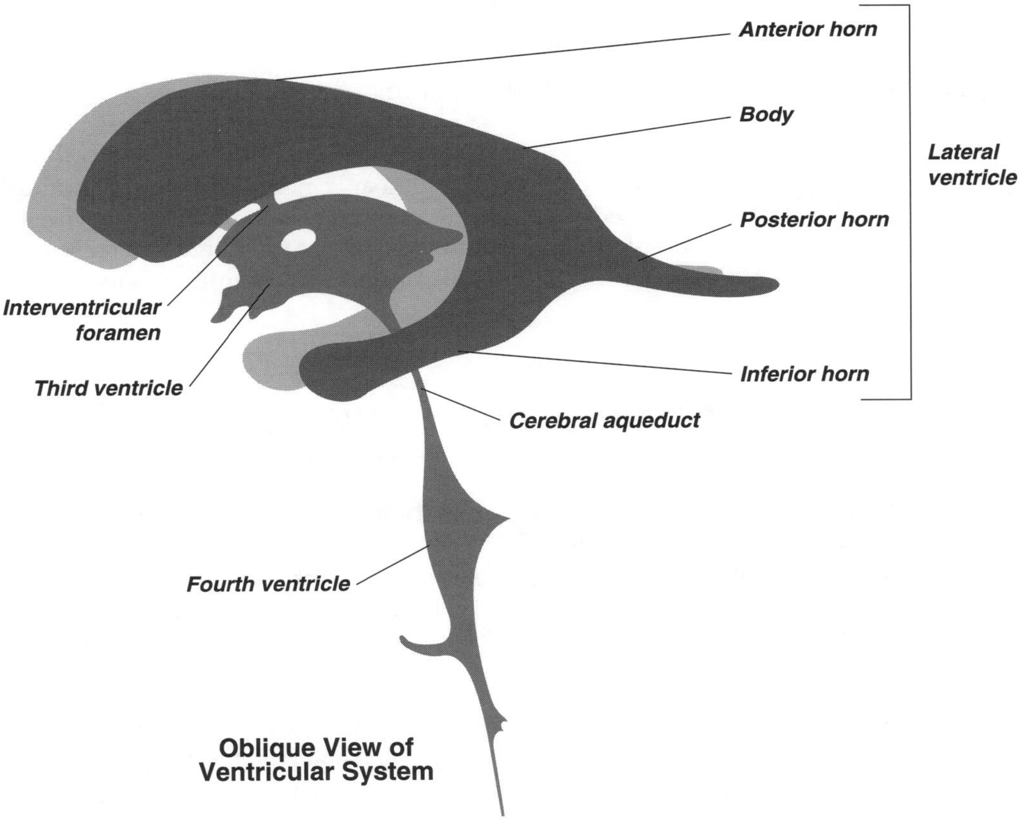

Anterior horn
Body
Lateral ventricle
Posterior horn
Interventricular foramen
Third ventricle
Inferior horn
Cerebral aqueduct
Fourth ventricle
Oblique View of Ventricular System

Figure 7-34. Oblique view of ventricular system of the brain. Left is anterior.

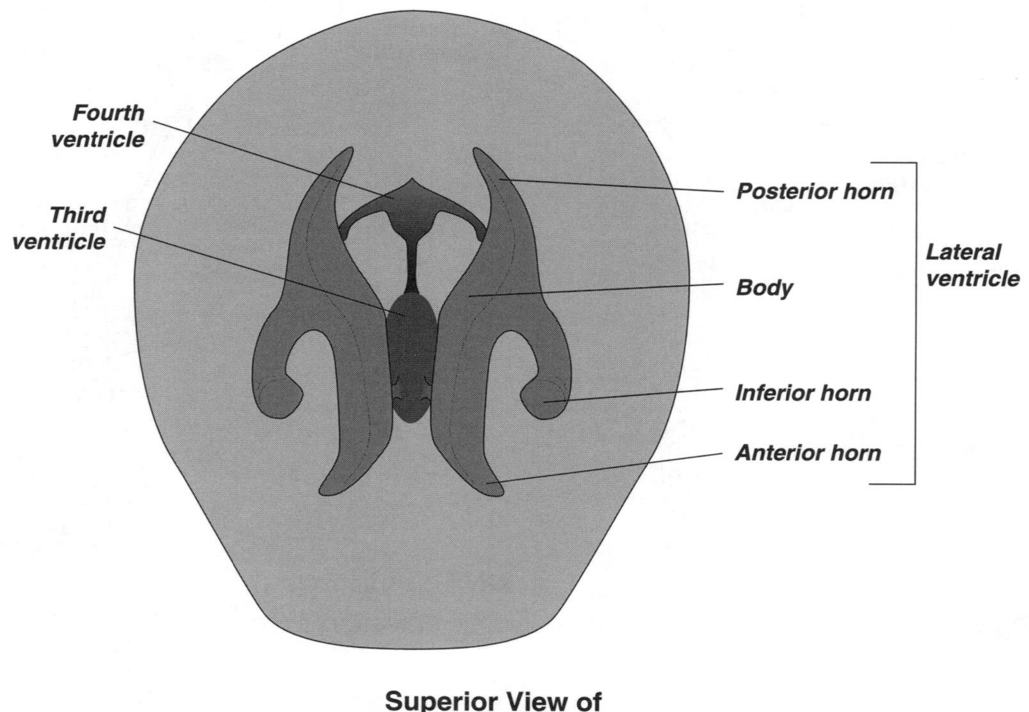

Figure 7–35. Superior view of ventricular system in the brain.

lated, a certain degree of expansion of an intracranial element can be tolerated. Cerebrospinal fluid can be sampled in a **spinal tap**, in which a needle is inserted in the lumbar region, just below the caudal extent of the spinal cord. The spinal nerves in this region are gathered in a loose bundle called the **cauda equina** (horse's tail).

NEUROIMAGING METHODS

Now that basic neuroanatomy and neurophysiology have been introduced, methods of **neuroimaging** or **brain imaging** can be discussed. Neuroimaging refers to methods that generate views of brain tissues. Generally speaking, they are not pictures in the sense of photographs, but rather images constructed from various types of physical data. These methods have resulted in dramatic advances in the understanding of the nervous system.

History

A brief review of the history of neuroimaging is helpful in understanding the revolutionary significance of this field in modern medicine and neurophysiology (Oldendorf, 1978; Taylor, 1990). First, it is necessary to understand that the X-ray shadow radiography invented by Roentgen in 1896 was successful for imaging bones in the limbs but not for imaging the brain. In

Roentgen's first use of X rays, he was able to image the bones in a hand. Generally, this type of X ray differentiates bone, water, and gas. X rays do not penetrate bone as readily as they do flesh or fluids, so the bones in the arms or legs leave prominent X-ray shadows. However, because the brain is encased in bone, it cannot be detected within the X-ray shadow of the cranium. Conventional X rays of the brain are simply noninformative, because they show only the continuous calcium of the skull.

One of the early origins of neuroimaging was the development of **pneumoencephalography** (*pneumo-* means air; *encephalography* means brain recording). Dandy in 1918 replaced the cerebrospinal fluid with air. The air in the ventricles reduced the scattering of X rays and therefore helped to create an image of the surrounding tissues. This method provided useful information and the patients usually survived. However, it caused excruciating pain. **Cerebral angiography** was introduced in 1927 by Egon Moniz. Moniz also pioneered the technique of **lobotomy**, in which the frontal lobes of the brain are severed as a treatment for psychiatric disorders. In 1949 he received the Nobel prize for his work on lobotomy, which is currently much disfavored in medicine (and discredited by Ken Kesey's book *One Flew Over the Cuckoo's Nest*). The citation for the Nobel prize did not even mention Moniz' contributions to angiography, which is used to this day. To accomplish angiography, Moniz injected a dye (strontium bromide) into the carotid arteries of living patients and then obtained X-ray pictures. This technique allowed the major arteries to be visualized. A refined version of this method is still very much in use.

Radioactive substances were first used in about 1950, when it was recognized that the **blood-brain barrier**, which normally prevents various chemical substances from passing from blood to brain, fails in diseased neural tissues. Therefore, fluorescent or radioactive dyes injected into the blood can diffuse into the region of damage. In the early experiments with this method, a Geiger counter ("counts" radioactivity) was simply held in various positions around the patient's head to determine where the dyes accumulated. The clinical application of this technique was reported by Moore in 1947 and 1948. His pioneering work was a forerunner of a major approach described below.

Modern Methods

We now turn to the most commonly used modern methods of neuroimaging. Neuroimaging is used for two basic purposes: to image structure (anatomy) or function (physiology). Common methods used to study structure are **computerized axial tomography (CAT)** and **magnetic resonance imaging (MRI)**. CAT is an X-ray technique in which a computer is used to process data obtained from a rotating X-ray apparatus. It was discovered in 1973 by Hounsfield. CAT uses an external source of X rays and differs from more conventional X-ray methods in its use of computer processing. MRI relies on an intense magnetic field, which causes electrons to assume a particular orientation of spin around their axes. A brief pulse of radiofrequency energy then knocks the electrons slightly off the axis of spin. When the pulse of energy is turned off, the electrons emit a weak burst of energy as they return to their original spin. This weak burst, a kind of echo, is used to construct the images in MRI. The first application in imaging was described by Lauterbur in 1973. Because MRI does not depend on ionizing radiation, it is regarded as a safe technique for repeated use or for application with children. Figure 7–36 shows a MRI section of an infant's head. This sagittal slice shows the neuraxis (central nervous system). Lefkowitz and Netsell (1993) published a

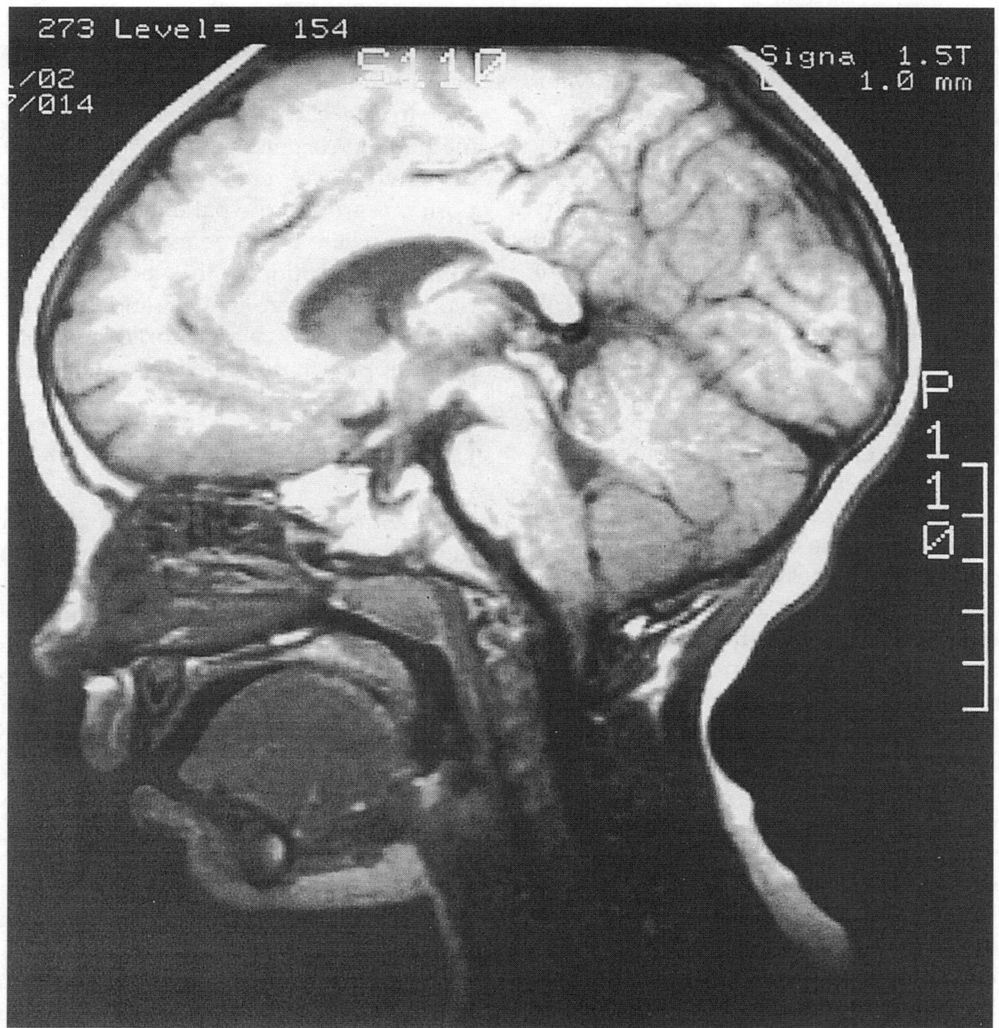

Figure 7–36. Magnetic resonance image of a child's head. Several brain structures are visible in this sagittal section.

useful MRI atlas pertinent to the neuroanatomy of speech.

Physiology or function can be studied with a variety of other techniques. Among the most frequently used are **positron emission tomography (PET)**, **electroencephalography (EEG)**, and **functional magnetic resonance imaging (fMRI)**. PET images are produced by a procedure in which the source of X rays is placed inside the body. This is accomplished by the use of radioisotopes (radioactive elements) that can be injected into the bloodstream or inhaled as a gas. The basic theory is that the isotopes will concentrate in regions of high metabolism or regions of breakdown of the blood-brain barrier. Therefore, external detectors can determine brain regions that are highly activated or damaged. The seminal work leading to this method was reported by Kuhl and Edwards (1964), who generated images of radioisotope distribution in a single slice of the brain. The technique of fMRI can sense blood flow because of the iron content in the blood's hemoglobin. This method therefore can be used to track blood flow in the brain. It is one of the most promising of the newly developed methods of brain imaging.

The technique of EEG is similar to the bioelectrical recordings discussed earlier in this chapter. The first person to record brain electrical activity from the intact human skull was Hans Berger in 1929. His paper, *Über das Elektrenkephalogram des Menschen*, was initially neglected but came to more deserved recognition 5 years after its publication when it was endorsed by Lord Adrian, a prominent British neurologist. Berger went on to describe four major rhythms of electrical activity: **alpha** (8–13 Hz, dominating when the brain is at rest); **beta** (13 Hz or higher, prominent during conscious attention), **theta** (4–8 Hz, occurring especially in a drowsy state); and **delta** (less than 4 Hz, characteristic of deep sleep).

Some modern EEG techniques use computer processing to gather the data and display the results in color-coded images (sometimes called **quantitative electroencephalography**, or **qEEG**). Different colors are used to represent different levels of activity. A recent method of studying EEG is based on chaos theory (discussed in Chapter 2) and uses a measure called the *correlational dimension*, which reflects the complexity of EEG dynamics and, perhaps as well, the complexity of the underlying neurophysiological processes from which the EEG is generated. Using this approach Anokhin, Birbaumer, Lutzenberger, Nikolaov, and Voge (1996) demonstrated that complexity in brain dynamics increases with age, despite a decline in some metabolic and memory functions. As we age, we might find some comfort in this finding.

The last method of functional imaging is fMRI. This technique is similar to the MRI method described previously, but it is specially designed to be sensitive to blood flow, specifically to the iron contained in the blood. This method is being rapidly improved and already is producing extremely important data on brain function.

Because these techniques will play a pivotal role in the future understanding of the nervous system, it is well to have at least a basic idea of how they work. For a more extended discussion of these methods in relation to the study of speech, language, and hearing, see Lauter (1995). Sarter, Berntson, and Cacioppo (1996) consider the potentials and pitfalls of neuroimaging as a tool for the study of cognitive science, and Poeppel (1996) criticizes PET studies that have sought to identify brain regions associated with phonological processing.

AFFERENT AND EFFERENT NEURAL PATHWAYS

This section considers the afferent and efferent neural pathways most relevant to hearing and speech. In so doing, it adds detail to previous sections and examines the sensory and motor functions of selected neural structures. Many of these structures will be discussed in relation to Figure 7–37, which illustrates lateral and posterior aspects of the brainstem and diencephalon. A number of structures are labeled in these drawings, some of which have been mentioned previously. Figure 7–37a gives a general orientation to the brainstem, showing divisions into diencephalon, midbrain, pons, and medulla. This figure also shows the location of ventricular structures in the brainstem. Figure 7–37b identifies several nuclei, including the thalamus, caudate, med-

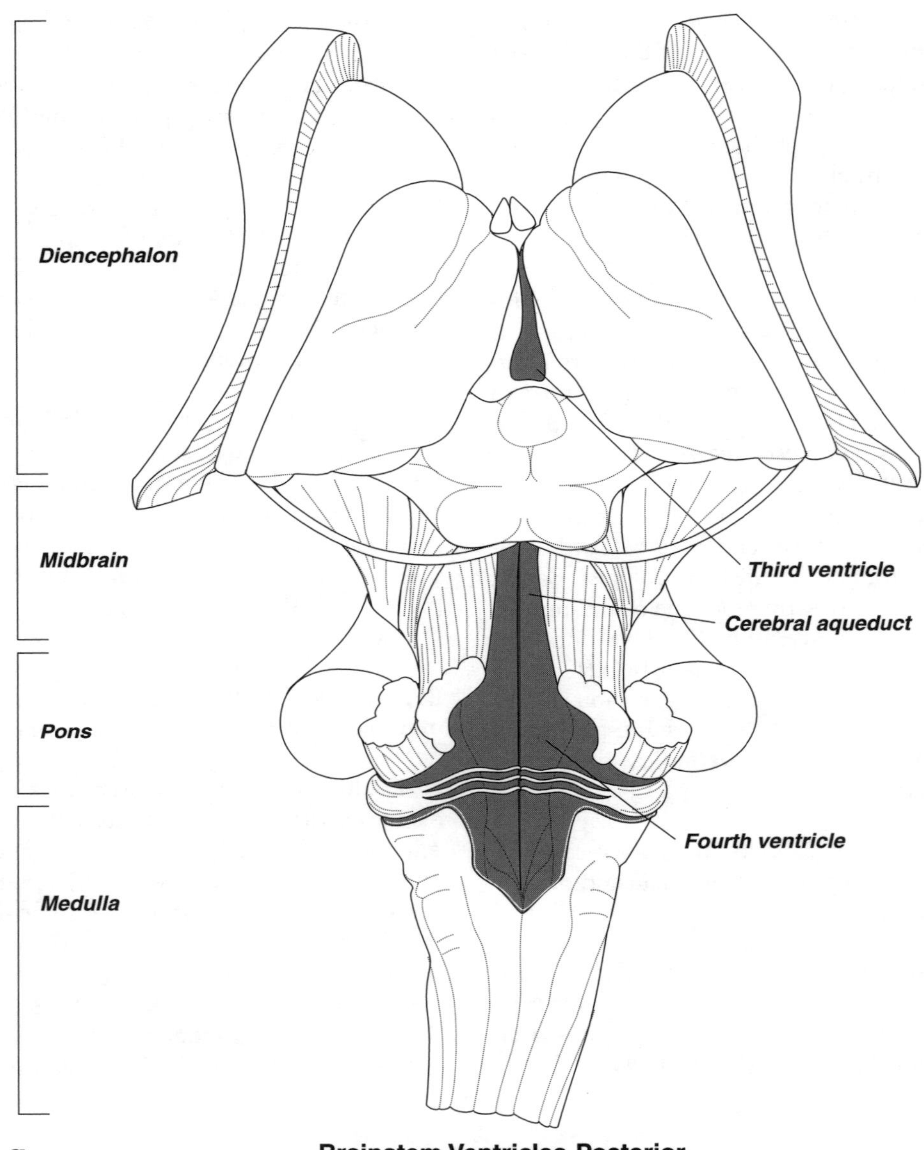

Figure 7–37. The brainstem and diencephalon: **a.** Posterior view showing location of ventricular spaces. *(continued)*

ial geniculate of the thalamus, and the superior and inferior colliculi. In addition, it shows the three paired peduncles by which the cerebellum attaches to the brainstem. The **corona radiata** is a fanlike system of fibers that connects the thalamus with the cortex. It is also called the **thalamocortical radiation**. Figure 7–37c, the lateral aspect of the brainstem, illustrates the emergence of several cranial nerves.

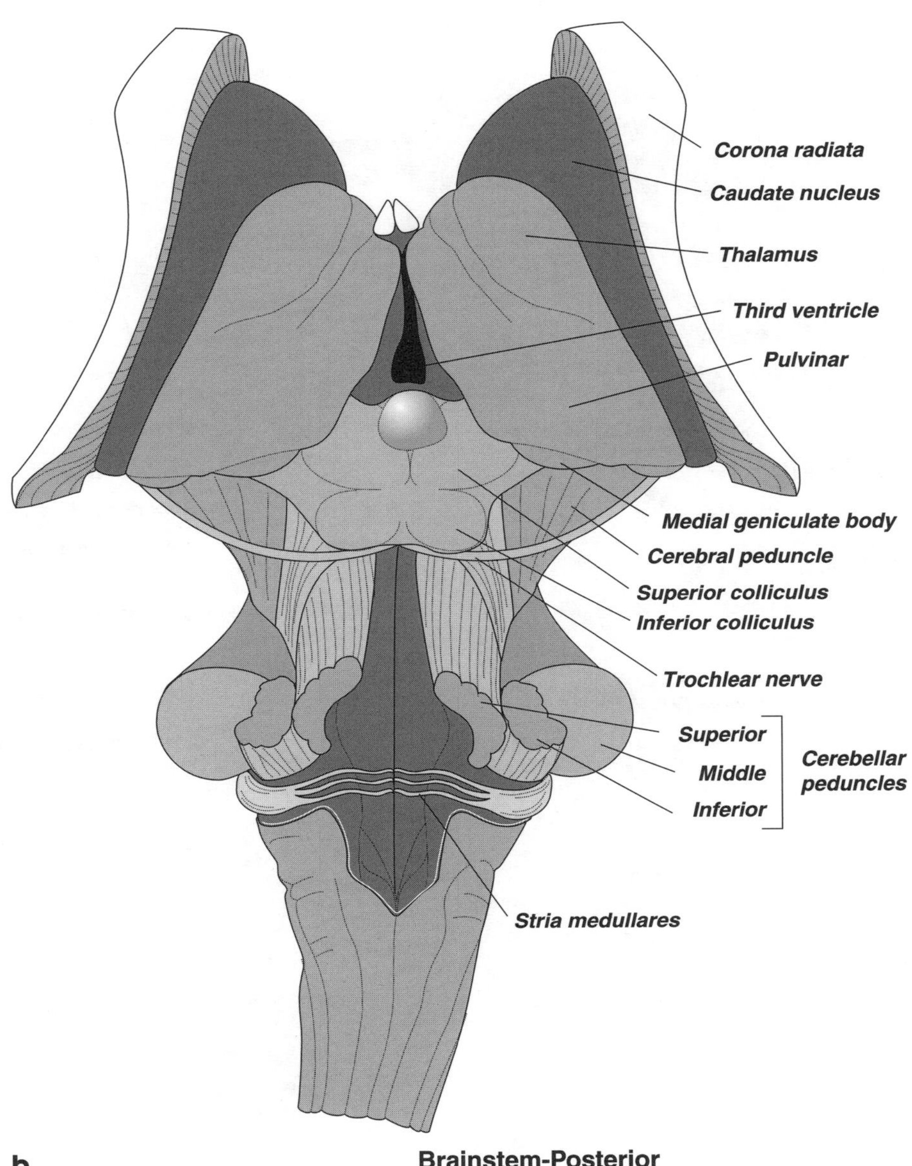

b. Posterior view with major structures labeled. *(continued)*

Cortical Representation of Somatosensation and Motor Function

As noted earlier, the cortex can be divided into functional fields. Among the fields that have been most intensively studied are strips of cortex that lie on either side of the central fissure. The strip that lies anterior to the fissure is called the **motor strip, motor cortex**, or **primary motor cortex**. It corresponds to Brodmann Area 4 in Figure 7–15. This is the cortical region in which body movements are represented. Stimu-

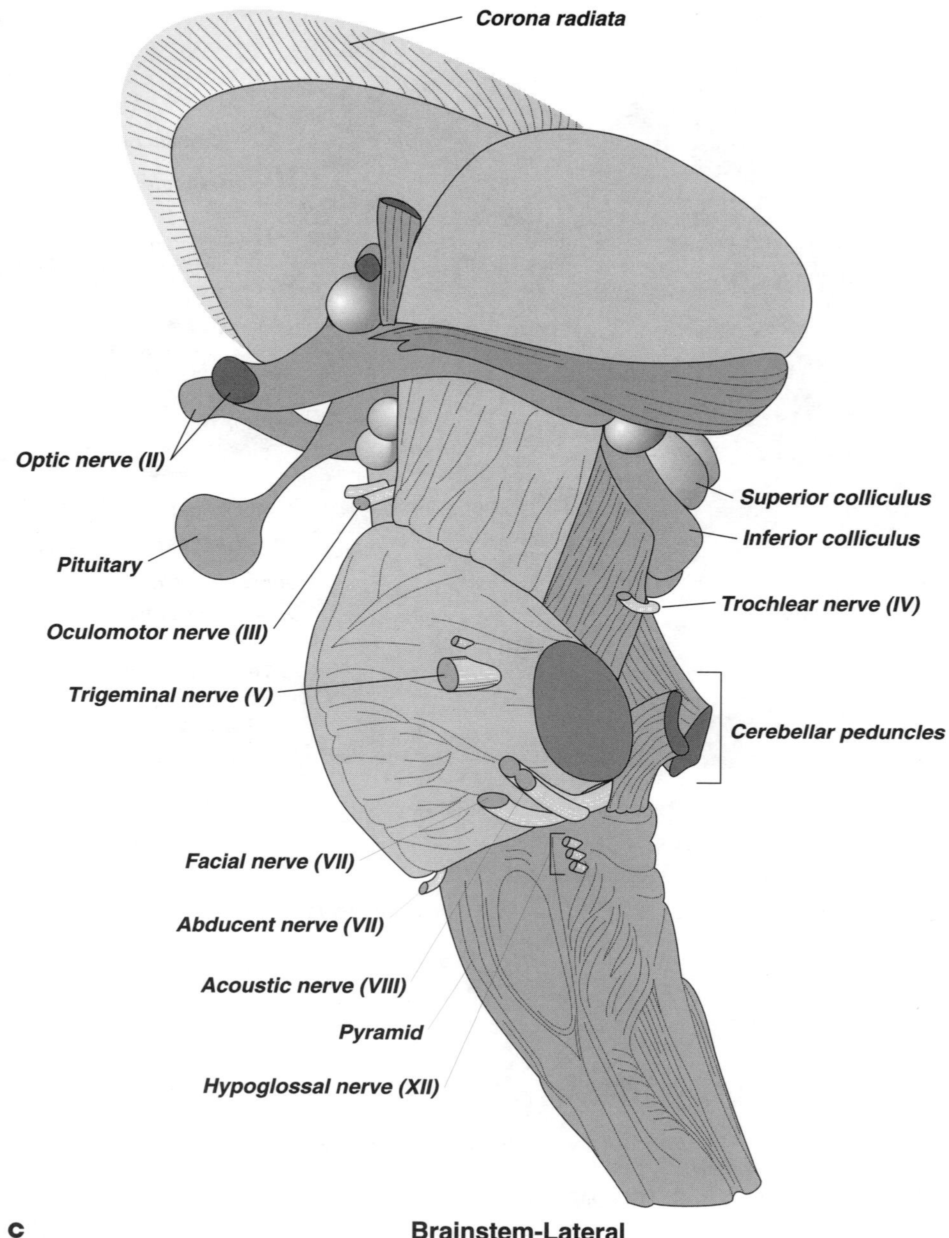

Figure 7–37. *(continued)* **c.** Lateral view with major structures labeled.

lation of this cortex can result in movement of a part of the body. The body is represented along this cortical region as shown in Figure 7–38. The strip that lies posterior to the central fissure is called the **sensory strip, primary sensory cortex**, or **somatosensory cortex** (*somato-* means body, so *somatosensory* means "body sensation"). This cortical region corresponds to Brodmann Areas 1, 2, 3, and 5 in Figure 7–15. Like the motor strip, the sensory strip contains a representation of the body.

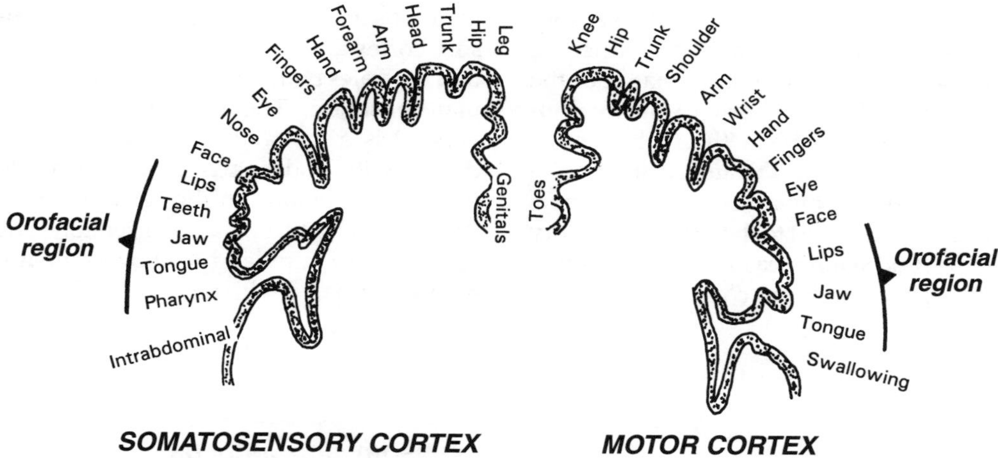

Figure 7–38. Somatosensory and motor cortex in a coronal section of cerebrum. Localization of selected body parts is shown.

Notice from Figure 7–38 that the orofacial structures (face, lips, tongue, pharynx) command a relatively large region of cortical tissue. More is said about this in a following section. For the present, it should be noted that the amount of cortical tissue allocated to a structure is an index of the potential for sophisticated motor control or for rich sensory information. The orofacial tissues have privileged access to large amounts of both motor and sensory cortex.

The General Somatic Sensory Pathway

The various senses have their own neural pathways and can differ from one another in, for instance, the number of synapses that constitute the pathway from periphery to cortex. As a matter of reference, it is helpful to consider the most general plan of the sensory neural pathway, the pathway that serves the general senses of touch and pressure. This is the sense of somatosensation mentioned earlier. The pathway is a three-neuron system as shown in Figure 7–39. The **first-order sensory neuron** has its cell body in either a cranial nerve nucleus or a dorsal root ganglion of

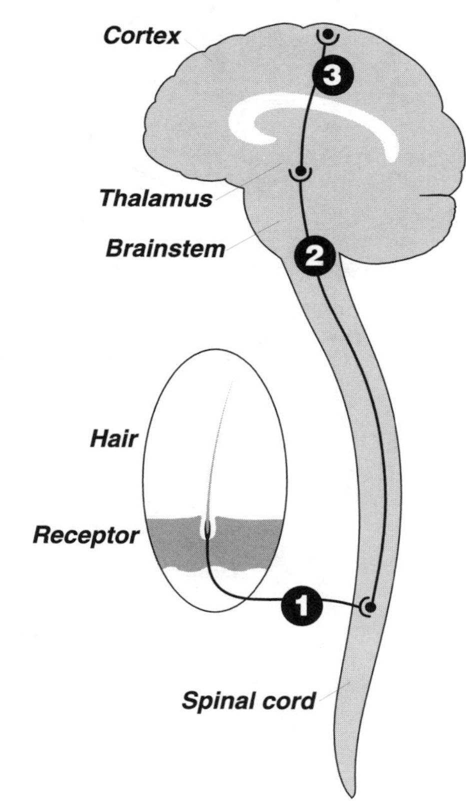

Figure 7–39. Diagram of the general somatosensory nervous pathway. The three neurons of the pathway are illustrated.

the spinal cord. The **second-order sensory neuron** has a cell body located in either the brainstem or the dorsal gray matter of the spinal cord. The **third-order sensory neuron** has a cell body in the thalamus. Its axon projects via the thalamocortical radiation (a major pathway between thalamus and cerebral cortex) to the primary sensory cortex, Brodmann areas 1, 2, and 3). Figure 7–40 shows the basic components of somatosensation, including the somatosensory cortex and the three-neuron pathway that mediates both deep and superficial somatosensation. The **homunculus** (little person) is a cartoonlike character that is drawn with body parts proportionate to their representation in the sensory cortex (Penfield & Boldrey, 1937). Therefore, the orofacial structures and the fingers are immense compared with the trunk or limbs.

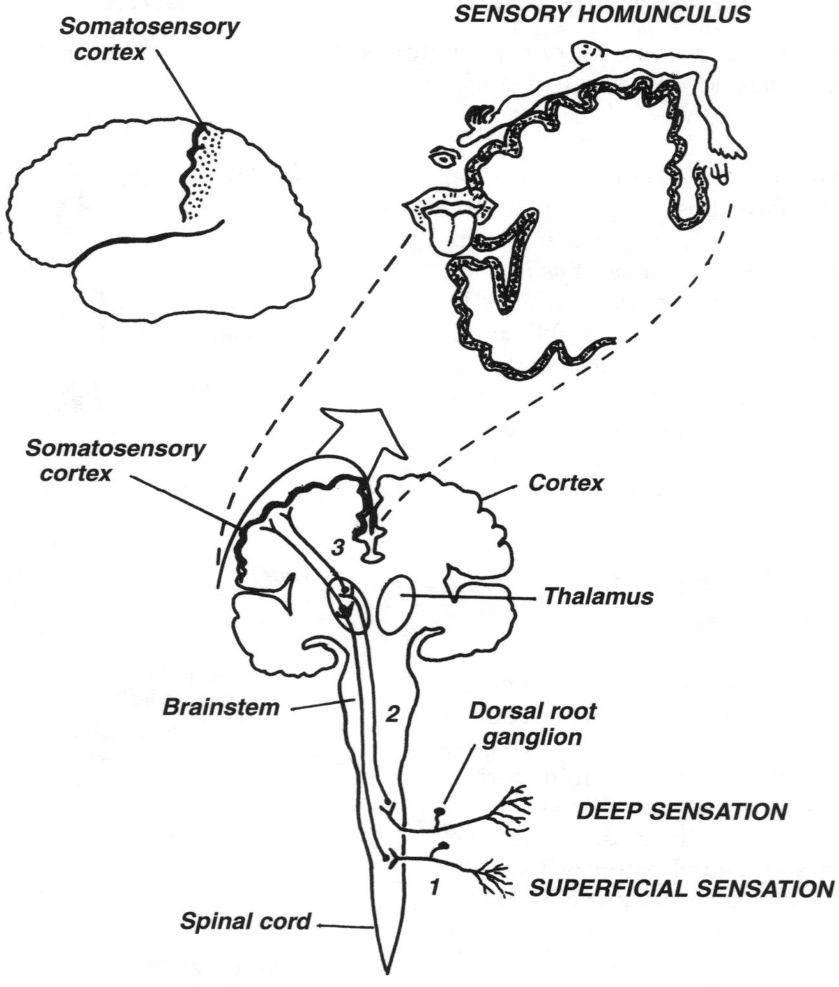

Figure 7–40. Neural pathway of the somatosensory system, including the three sensory neurons and the somatosensory cortex (with the "sensory homunculus").

The Neural Pathway of Audition

Most sensory systems have relatively little in the way of subcortical processing. Vision, olfaction, taste, and somatosensation rely largely on the cerebral cortex for the processing and interpretation of the signals they transmit. But audition is different. The neural pathway of audition is well endowed with subcortical nuclei, actually more than 50 (Masterton, 1992). Furthermore, it appears that these nuclei accomplish a great deal of sensory processing, including basic analysis of sound components, detection of many kinds of patterns, and localization of sounds in space. The auditory cortex receives a highly processed neural signal. Moreover, the neural pathways of audition are highly interlaced with the pathways that serve vocalization. As Huffman and Hanson (1990) put it, "The interface between auditory and vocalization centers is distributed to all levels of the brain" (p. 314).

But to learn 50 subcortical nuclei is a formidable task, especially for an introductory text. Therefore, we follow a tradition of convenience and simplicity and assume that there are only about five major nuclei in the subcortical neural pathway of audition. In the past, these nuclei were compared to way stations that did little more than to guarantee that the signals they received were sent on to the next station. The modern understanding assigns much more important roles to these nuclei. In many respects, they are the "hearing" parts of the nervous system. Masterton (1992) observed that these groups of neurons have important "distributive functions" and each group differs from every other group in its efferent targets and the brain chemicals (neurotransmitters and neuromodulators) that are used in its projection terminals.

Figure 7–41 identifies the major structures being considered in this selective account. Figure 7–42 is a schematic representation of the auditory nervous system and complements Figure 7–40. As discussed in Chapter 6, the sensory end organ of hearing is in the cochlea. Neural information from the cochlea passes to the CNS by way of CN VIII, the statoacoustic nerve. The first CNS structure is the **cochlear nucleus** which receives ipsilateral input from the cochlea. The cochlear nucleus is not a single homogenous structure, but rather a combination of related structures. For this reason, it is sometimes called the **cochlear nuclear complex** and consists primarily of the **dorsal cochlear nucleus**, **anterior ventral cochlear nucleus**, and **posterior cochlear nucleus**. An important point is that information from the cochlea is represented in three different divisions of the cochlear nucleus, thus providing redundancy of neural analysis at this level.

Most of the neural fibers from the cochlear nucleus pass to the contralateral **superior olivary complex**, which is a cluster of small nuclei. This the lowest level in the auditory nervous system where information from the two ears comes together. Not surprisingly, then, the superior olivary complex is involved in binaural interaction for purposes such as sound localization.

The **lateral lemniscus** is a large tract consisting of the axons of the second-order neurons. In fact, it is not a single tract, but six parallel pathways that project primarily to the **inferior colliculus**. The inferior colliculus is an important point of convergence of auditory information, gathering information from the different pathways of the lateral lemniscus. Although the function of the inferior colliculus is not clearly known, it has been suggested that it can process biologically significant sounds. Casseday and Covey (1996) wrote that, "Neurons in the inferior colliculus are filters for sounds that require immediate action, such as certain sounds made by prey, predators, or conspecifics" (p. 311). The authors believe that this structure is

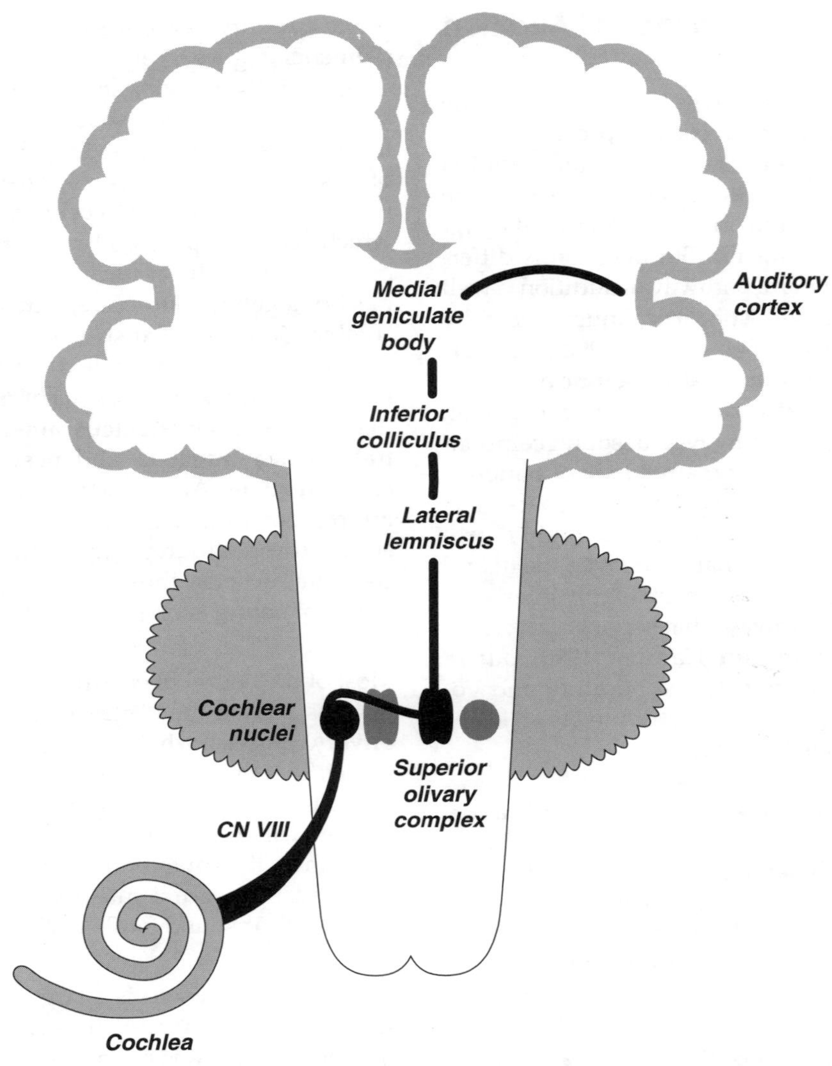

Figure 7–41. Simplified representation of the auditory nervous system.

capable of tuning processes related to biologically significant sounds and that it represents a change in timing properties from rapid input to slowed output. The slowed output may relate to specific behaviors, such as those associated with escape, attack, or approach. The inferior colliculus projects to the **medial geniculate**, which is a point of divergence, sending information broadly to cortex, primary auditory cortex, and auditory association cortex.

Interestingly, the medial geniculate has been implicated in certain language disorders, such as reading disability. Musiek and Lamb (1992) is a good source of additional information on the neuroanatomy and neurophysiology of the auditory nervous system.

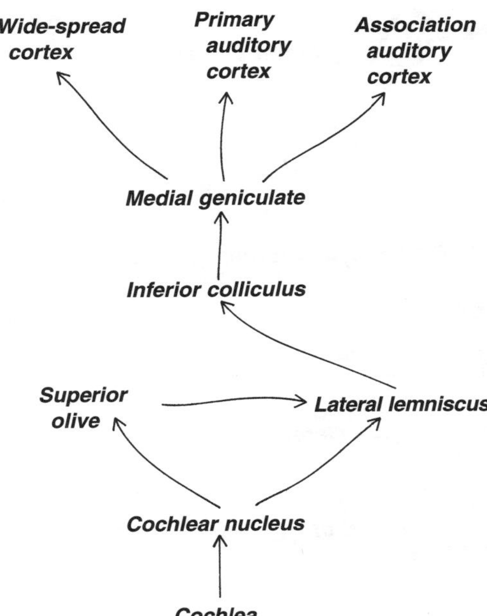

Figure 7–42. Schematic diagram of major pathways in the auditory nervous system.

The Neural Pathways of Motor Control

It is customary pedagogy in neuroscience to state that the neural pathway of motor control is actually two pathways or systems that cooperate with one another. One reason to recognize the two systems is that this classification is used in diagnosing neurological disorders of movement. In fact, it can be quite difficult to distinguish them because both systems are continuously active. As a first step, in distinguishing these systems, their anatomic features are described.

Pyramidal Motor System

The **pyramidal motor system** (or **pyramidal motor pathway**) (Figure 7–43) is often called the major system of voluntary motor control. That is, it is this system that is involved when we will a movement. However, this statement can be misleading, because the other motor system to be described also is involved in regulating voluntary movements. As we will see, the most important thing is to understand how the two systems work together. The cortical origin of the pyramidal motor system is primarily, but not exclusively, in the motor cortex (Brodmann area 4). The remaining neurons (about 40%) originate in the premotor cortex or even the sensory cortex (Davidoff, 1990). As mentioned earlier, the neurons in the motor cortex ("motor strip") and the adjacent sensory cortex ("sensory strip") are systematically organized to reflect the body regions they innervate (Figure 7–38). Moreover, the proportion of cortex assigned to various parts of the body is not commensurate with the size of the parts, but rather with the apparent need for precise motor and sensory information. Therefore, the fingers, tongue, lips, and larynx have a disproportionate allocation of cerebral cortex considering their relatively small size. The axons of the cortical neuron then pass down to the level of the medulla where about 90% of them decussate (cross over) in a structure called the medullary pyramids. It is this structure that gives the pyramidal system its name. The axons then synapse with a second neuron, which runs to the muscles. Although the pyramidal system originally was thought to be exclusively motor, the recent view is that the pyramidal tract contains many fibers that originate in the cortex and affect sensory transmission at the subcortical and spinal levels. Another change in the understanding of the pyramidal tract is that it is now recognized that movement does not begin in the motor cortex, but rather the motor cortex is a funnel for information derived from various cortical and subcortical sites.

In a highly simplified sense, the pyramidal motor system can be conceived of as a two-neuron system, as illustrated in Figure 7–43. The **upper motor neuron** is con-

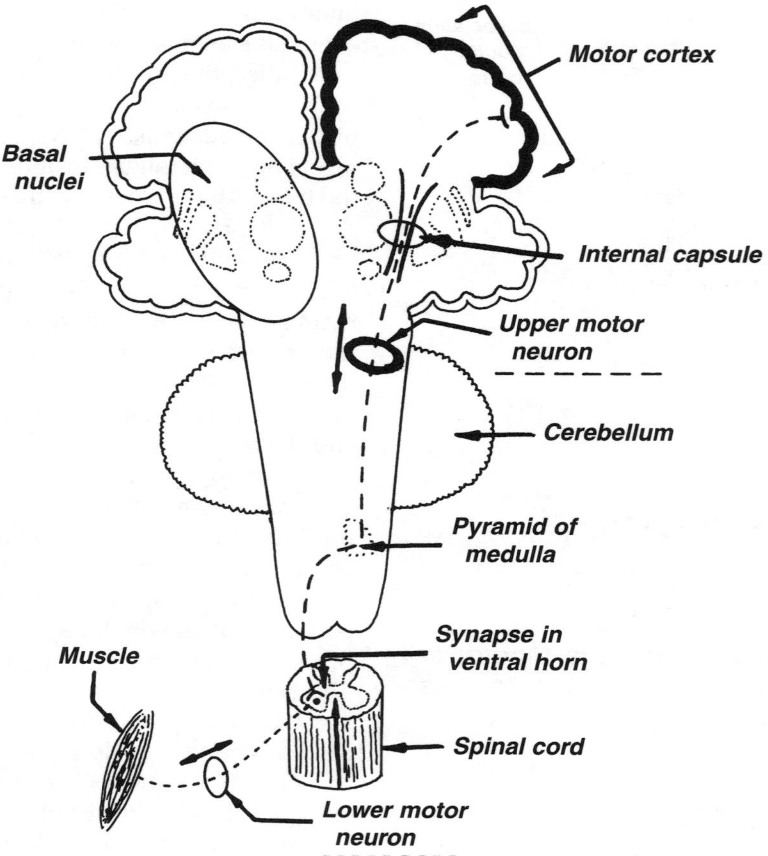

Figure 7–43. Pyramidal motor system represented as an upper motor neuron and lower motor neuron. The upper motor neuron originates in the motor cortex and passes through the internal capsule. It decussates at the pyramids of the medulla and then synapses with a lower motor neuron.

tained entirely within the central nervous system, taking its origin in the cerebral cortex and then typically crossing over at the level of the medullary pyramids (named for their pyramidal shape). This fact has an important consequence: One side of the brain largely controls the opposite side of the body (Figure 7–44). This principle of **contralateral innervation** is very useful in neurological diagnosis of problems such as paralysis. The **lower motor neuron** is innervated by the upper motor neuron (typically, in fact, by many upper motor neurons) and directly innervates the muscles. The lower motor neuron is called the **common pathway** because all motor instructions must pass through it. The concepts of upper motor neuron and lower motor neuron are motivated more by clinical usefulness than by anatomic accuracy. An important type of neurological disorder is called upper motor neuron lesion (or upper motor neuron syndrome). This lesion can result in spastic paralysis, exaggerated reflexes, and increased muscle tone (**hypertonia**, or elevated resting activity in the muscle). Another important type of neurological disorder is called lower

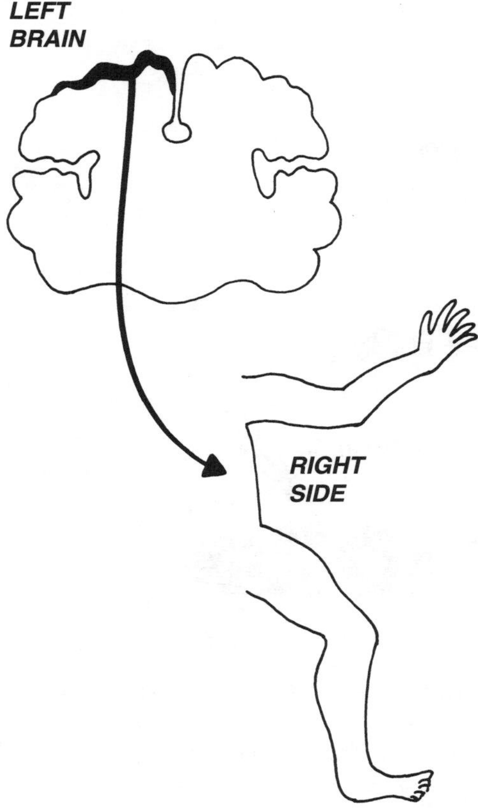

Figure 7–44. Principle of contralateral innervation of motor control.

motor neuron lesion (or lower motor neuron syndrome). This type of lesion typically results in flaccid paralysis, absent or reduced reflexes, decreased muscle tone, and atrophy of the affected muscles.

A lower motor neuron is illustrated in Figure 7–45. The neuron has its cell body in the ventral horn of the spinal cord. Its axon passes through the ventral root. The motor neuron innervates a number of muscle fibers collectively called the **motor unit**. Motor units can be described in terms of their **innervation ratios**, or the number of muscle fibers innervated by a single lower motor neuron. In large powerful muscles, such as those of the thigh, a single motor neuron may innervate hundreds of fibers. But in small, delicate muscles capable of precise action, the innervation ratio is very low, with only a few muscle fibers innervated by a motor neuron. Eye muscles and some speech muscles have low innervation ratios. In Figure 7–45, axon terminals are shown ending on several fibers in a striated (skeletal) muscle. The enlargement shows the neuromuscular junction, which is where the motor neuron makes functional contact with muscle tissue. Myasthenia gravis is a neurological disorder that interferes with neurotransmitters in the neuromuscular junction.

Extrapyramidal Motor System

Described in its full anatomic complexity, the **extrapyramidal motor system** (or **extrapyramidal motor pathway**) is formidable indeed. The description presented here is a simplified version and is shown schematically in the progressive illustration of Figure 7–46. The principal structures of this system are the basal nuclei described earlier. The structures include the caudate, putamen, and globus pallidus. We begin the discussion with the connections among these three nuclei. Recall that the caudate and putamen together are called the striatum in recognition of their striated appearance. The input to this system is first sent to the caudate, which in turn projects to the putamen. The putamen projects to the globus pallidus, which is the motor outflow of the extrapyramidal system. As shown in the sequential illustrations, the input to the basal nuclei is from both the thalamus and the cerebral cortex. The pathways between the basal nuclei and the cortex and between the basal nuclei and the thalamus complete the basic circuit of the extrapyramidal system. Actually, several other structures also are involved, and some of these are shown in the final figure of the progressive illustration. The extrapyramidal motor system influences the motor instructions sent to the periphery. As noted in the discussion of the basal nuclei, one role of the basal nuclei may be to stabilize the large and compli-

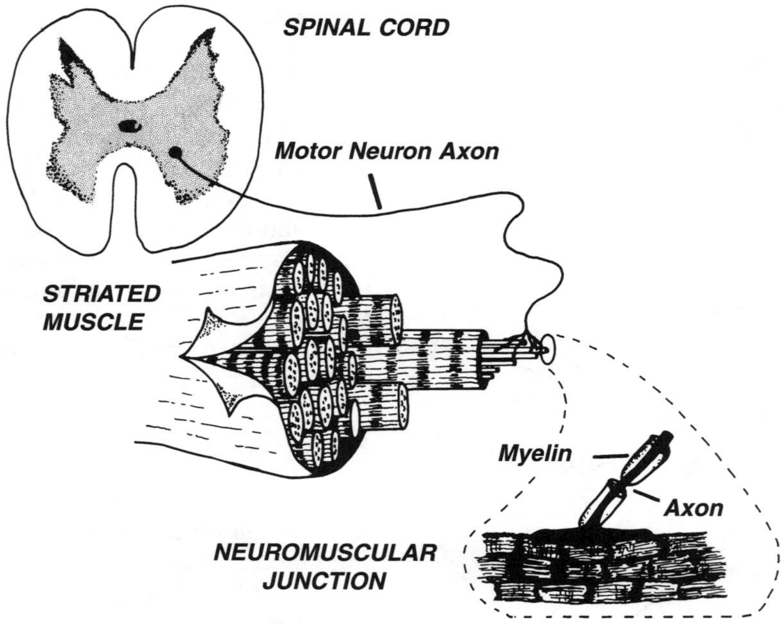

Figure 7–45. Drawing of the lower motor neuron. Its cell body is in the ventral column of the spinal cord and its axon extends to innervate muscle fibers. The neuromuscular junction is illustrated in the enlargement.

cated neural system that regulates movement. In addition, the basal nuclei may help to direct action and to interpret sensory information. Part **c** of Figure 7–46 shows both the pyramidal and extrapyramidal systems that function as a unit to regulate motor behavior.

Sensorimotor Regulation

It is somewhat artificial to speak of sensory and motor functions as separate processes because they are closely integrated in behavior. In general, motor function is predicated on sensory information. It is particularly interesting to consider the role of sensory information in speech because speech production generates several possible forms of afference. Also some of the principle structures involved in speech are extraordinarily sensitive.

Speech is movement and it therefore generates afference in the form of **kinesthesia** (the movement sense). Kinesthetic information is relayed by several specialized receptors including **joint receptors** (such as those found in the temporomandibular joint) and various receptors found in muscle, including **free nerve endings**, **Golgi tendon organs**, and **muscle spindles**. Joint receptors supply information on joint position, such as rotation around the joint. Free nerve endings located in or around muscle can provide information on muscle state. Golgi tendon organs are located in musculo-tendinous junctions and are sensitive to muscle tension. Muscle spindles are receptors in striated (skeletal) muscle that are sensitive to the degree of stretch in the muscle. The spindles are innervated by efferent neurons, enabling them to be biased or preset for a particular movement. The muscle spindle is encapsulated, as

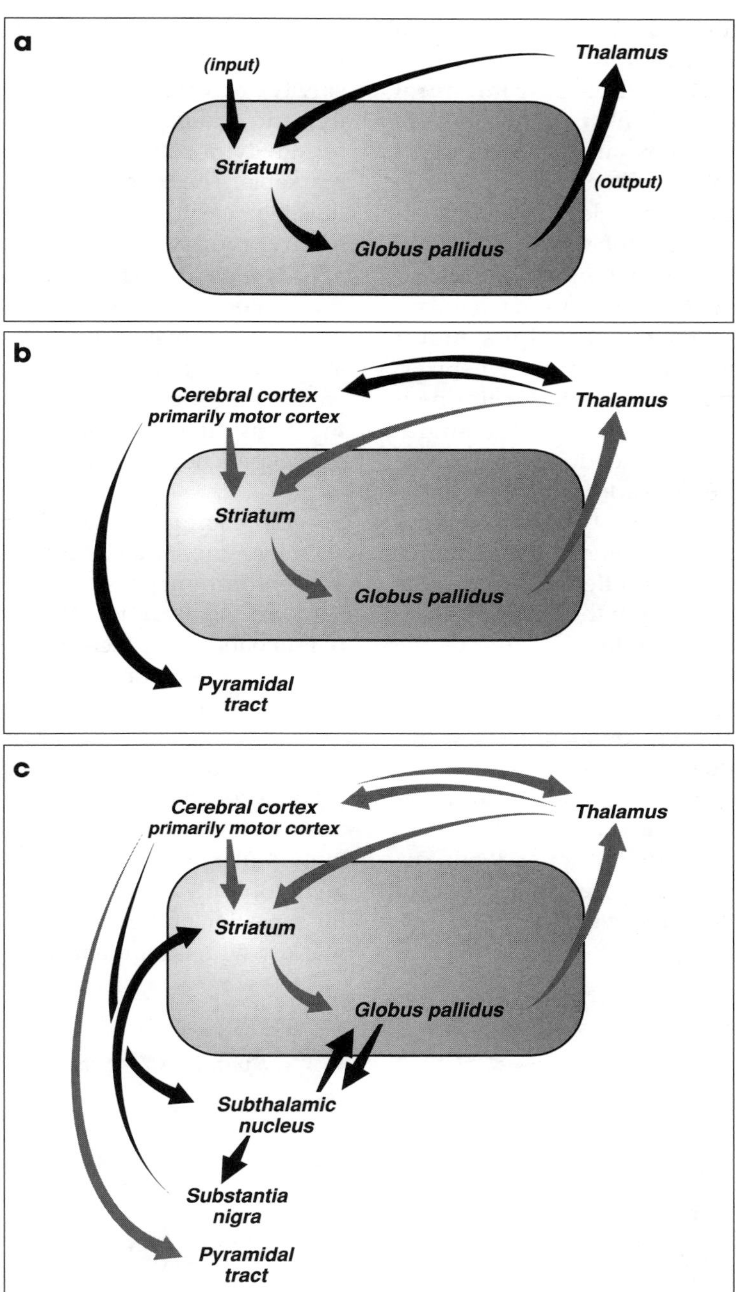

Motor Control

Figure 7–46. Progressive diagram of the extrapyramidal and pyramidal motor systems. The basic circuit of the extrapyramidal system is shown in **a**, the cerebral cortex and pyramidal pathway are added in **b**, and additional structures of the extrapyramidal pathway are shown in **c**.

shown in Figure 7–47. It consists of several relatively short fibers that run parallel to other muscle fibers. The term **intrafusal fibers** identifies the fibers of the muscle spindle. The term **extrafusal fibers** refers to the main muscle fibers that lie outside and parallel to the muscle spindle. The efferent innervation to the muscle spindle is by means of **gamma motor neurons**, or **gamma efferents**. This gamma neurons system complements the **alpha motor neurons**, which are the primary neurons of muscle action. The gamma motor neurons regulate the contraction of the intrafusal fibers and, in so doing, allow the muscle spindle to be adjusted to the status of the extrafusal fibers. This kind of regulation enhances the sensitivity of motor control. The gamma efferent system has been of great interest in the study of skeletal movement generally. The role of the gamma efferent system in speech is a matter of continuing investigation. Muscle spindles have been found in several important muscles involved in speech, including muscles of the jaw (Smith & Macarian, 1967), lips (Kadanoff, 1956), tongue (Bowman, 1971; Cooper, 1960), larynx (Lucas-Keene, 1976), respiratory system (Kennedy, 1970) and velopharynx (Liss, 1990).

Speech production also generates afference in the form of **taction** (touch or pressure sensitivity), **baroreception** (air pressure sensivity), and audition. The tactile or cutaneous sensitivity of some speech structures is remarkable. The tongue tip and lips are exquisitely sensitive to touch stimuli. This sensitivity certainly is useful in eating but it also affords a great deal of afference in speech production. Baroreceptors in the tracheobronchial tree may help speakers to regulate air pressures in speech. Audition is a preeminent sensory channel, as evidenced by the great difficulty that children who are deaf experience in learning to speak.

Speech, then, generates plurimodal afference: kinesthesia, taction, baroreception, and audition are major sensory channels that support the learning of speech and the maintenance of speech skills. What would happen if these normal channels were disrupted? An experiment that attempted to answer this question examined speech production in subjects who wore **bite blocks** (appliances that held the jaw in clenched position), had anesthesia of the temporomandibular joint (to reduce joint afference), were topically anesthetized (to reduce tactile sensation of the oral mucosa), and were masked with high-intensity noise (Kelso &

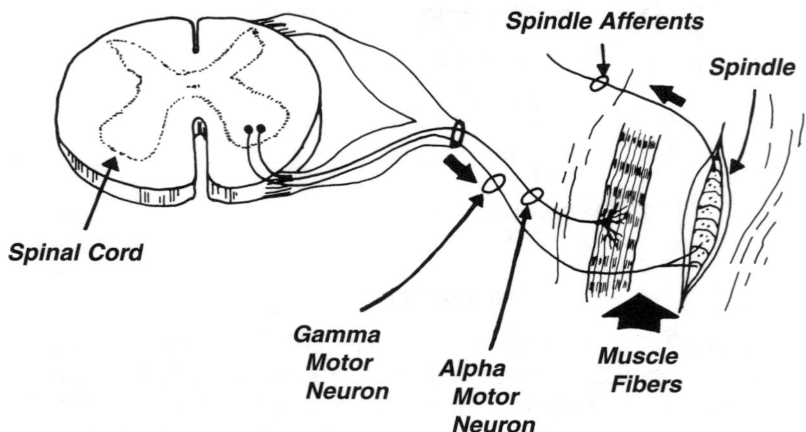

Figure 7–47. Drawing of the muscle spindle and the gamma-efferent system.

Tuller, 1983). The consequences on speech production were negligible. But this outcome does not mean that speech production is indifferent to afference. Because speech is a highly practiced motor activity (some might say overpracticed), speakers probably do not need continuous feedback information from all sensory channels. Therefore, short-term disruptions can be tolerated with little difficulty. Long-term disruptions may be more damaging. In addition, it appears that sensory information is important to speech development in children and that some kinds of sensory disruption may interfere with speech production (Kent, Martin, & Sufit, 1990).

CENTERS AND CIRCUITS FOR THE NEURAL CONTROL OF SPEECH

This section considers contemporary evidence for brain structures that have been hypothesized to control spoken language. A particular objective is to weigh the evidence for parts of the brain that might be regarded as control centers. As a first step, it is helpful to identify brain regions thought to be of primary importance in speech and language. Most of these regions are shown in Figures 7–48 and 7–49. Some of these are examined in more detail later in the chapter.

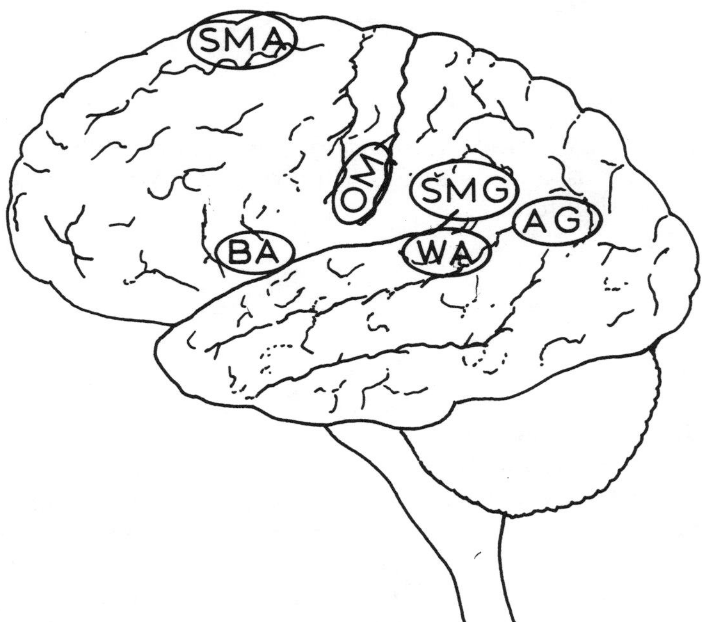

Figure 7–48. Lateral aspect of the left cerebral hemisphere, with major speech-language areas labeled. BA = Broca's area, WA = Wernicke's area, AG = angular gyrus, SMG = supramarginal gyrus, SMA = supplementary motor area, and OM = orofacial motor cortex.

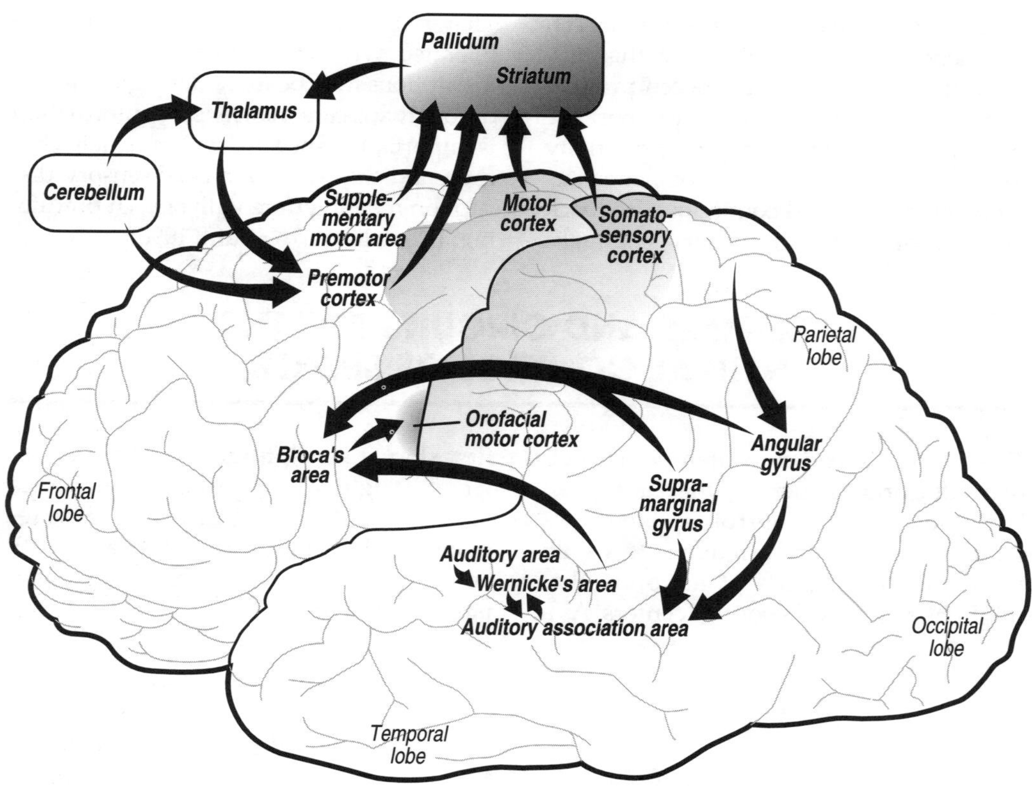

Flow Chart

Figure 7–49. The basic speech and language circuits of the cerebral cortex, basal nuclei, thalamus, and cerebellum. The arrows indicate primary flows of information among structures.

The **primary auditory cortex** (Brodmann area 41) is also known as **Heschl's gyrus**, or **transverse gyrus**. It is located in the lateral fissure, two-thirds posterior on the upper surface of the temporal lobe. The number of gyri varies from one to three across individual brains. This is the region of cortex responsible for the primary processing of auditory signals. It receives information from the thalamus via the thalamocortical radiations.

The **planum temporale** is the cortical region that extends posteriorly from Heschl's gyrus to the endpoint of the lateral fissure. It is typically larger on the left hemisphere, at least in right-handed persons. It is thought to be involved in auditory language processing.

The **supramarginal gyrus** (Brodmann area 40) is the fold of cortex that curves around the end of the lateral fissure. It responds to acoustic stimulation and is presumably involved in language processing. Damage to this gyrus and its pathways frequently disturbs the formulation of written language. Lesions to this area are associated with **agraphia** (disorder of writing). However, recent evidence from PET studies also points to a possible role of this structure, particularly its inferior portion, in phonological storage (Demonet, Fiez, Paulesu, Petersen, & Zatorre, 1996).

The **angular gyrus** (Brodmann area 39) is immediately posterior to the supramarginal gyrus. Damage to this area is frequently associated with reading difficulties (dyslexia).

Wernicke's area is a region on the superior part of the temporal lobe (usually described as Brodmann areas 22, 41, and 42). It presumably is involved in the auditory comprehension of language. It is named after Carl Wernicke, a 19th century neurologist.

Broca's area (also known as the **opercular part of the inferior frontal gyrus**; Brodmann area 44) has been traditionally identified as the cortical center for motor speech. It is named after Paul Broca, a 19th century neurologist and anthropologist.

The aforementioned regions often have been considered as centers of speech and language in the brain. These regions and their connecting pathways (such as the arcuate fasciculus) have been the critical components in most neural models of language comprehension and production. These regions connect with other sensory and motor parts of the brain, including the primary auditory cortex, the **supplementary motor area** (Brodmann area 6) and the primary motor area (Brodmann area 4).

With this background, we now turn to some recent evidence on the participation of selected cortical regions in speech and language.

Broca's Area

One of the earliest cerebral regions to be associated with speech is Broca's area (Figures 7–48 and 7–49). In fact, this area was one of the first to have been associated with any behavioral function, which was, therefore, a milestone in the history of neurology. Most historical accounts attribute the discovery of this region as a speech center to the French surgeon and anthropologist Paul Broca. Broca's discovery was reportedly the first demonstration of a behavioral function that could be localized to a discrete region of the brain. As noted earlier in this chapter, he also is usually credited with the first report that the two hemispheres are not functionally equivalent. Broca's work was of immense historical significance. (Perhaps credit really should go, at least in part, to Broca's medical and scientific predecessors, including Alexander Hood, who in 1824, "did a better job of analyzing expressive language functions and correlating them to frontal lobe anatomy" [Whitaker, 1995, p. 165]).

Broca discovered this brain region in his examinations of a patient with a severe form of expressive aphasia, that is, the patient had extremely limited spoken language. So severe was the disorder than Broca's patient could say only a single word—"tan." Ever since, this cortical area has been regarded by many specialists as an important region for the production of fluent, articulate speech. "Broca's aphasia" is classically described as nonfluent, effortful speech comprising short, agrammatic phrases. Broca's inference of a discrete cortical area underlying spoken language is all the more remarkable given that Tan had extensive brain damage that invaded the frontal, parietal, and temporal lobes. However, evidence has not been entirely consistent with the classic view. Alexander, Naeser, and Palumbo (1990) introduced a revised classification system for Broca's aphasia in which three distinct categorizations are associated with site and extent of lesion, as well as speech symptomatology.

The clinical studies of Broca's area are complemented by recent studies of brain activity in normal speakers. Functional neuroimaging techniques have been used to study Broca's area in relation to various speech tasks performed by typically speaking subjects. Some investigators did not observe significant increases in regional cerebral blood flow (rCBF) in Broca's area during automatic naming tasks (Ingvar & Schwartz, 1974; Larsen, Skinhoj, & Lassen, 1978). But other researchers reported increased rCBF in Broca's area in subjects reading both silently and aloud (Lassen, Ingvar, & Skinhoj, 1978; Leblanc, Meyer, Bub, Zatorre, & Evans, 1992; Menard, Kosslyn, Thompson, Alpert, & Rauch, 1996; Wise et al., 1991). These contradictory results may be explained partly by differences in techniques. Further studies are needed to show exactly what role Broca's area plays in controlling speech. Possibly, Broca's area is involved in general processes of motor planning and selection, especially hierarchical organization. Its role in phonological processing or speech production remains uncertain.

Wernicke's Area

This cortical region (Figures 7–48 and 7–49) is like Broca's area in having a long history in studies of the neural representation of language. The classic view is that Wernicke's area is a center for language comprehension, possibly the storage center of sounds or the phonological representations of words (Caplan, 1987). Damage to this region is thought to result in deficits in language comprehension as well as expressive deficits characterized by fluent, incomprehensible speech (called jargon). This disorder has been termed Wernicke's aphasia. The bulk of evidence in which structural imaging techniques have been used to examine lesions relative to behavioral and cognitive tests suggests that a language center is located in the general cortical area of Wernicke's area. However, this area is thought to differ in both size and relative location across individuals (Caplan, 1987; Howard et al., 1992).

Neuroimaging studies have been an important recent source of information on Wernicke's area. In one study of this region, the brain imaging technique of PET was used to investigate blood flow while subjects performed two different tasks (Petersen, Fox, Posner, Mintun, & Raichle, 1988). One task was merely listening to spoken words while looking at a cross-hair. The other task was looking at the cross-hair without listening to words. Increased blood flow was observed in Wernicke's area for the task that involved listening to words. However, in another study (Howard et al., 1992) no single cortical area showed significant increases in blood flow while subjects either read words or repeated them. The authors concluded that representations of word meanings are not discretely localized, but rather depend on the activation of semantic features and connections between these features that are distributed over a large region of cortex. These results are not easy to reconcile. And, to complicate interpretations even further, Spitzer et al. (1995) concluded that different cortical regions become active during the recognition of words from different semantic categories, such as fruit, furniture, animals, and tools.

These results are presented to show that, when the results of several different studies are considered, it is not necessarily an easy matter to reach compelling conclusions about the ways in which language is regulated by the brain. However tantalizing the results of any single study may be, it is a good idea to maintain a skeptical attitude and seek agreement across several studies. Brain imaging studies bring exciting new data to the neuroscience of communication, but much remains to be done to consolidate the various reports into a coherent view of how language, complex in itself, is processed by the immensely complicated networks of the brain.

Supplementary Motor Area

Another cortical region that may be relevant to speech control is the supplementary motor area (SMA) or the premotor area designated as Brodmann Area 6 (Figures 7–48 and 7–49). Activity in this area has been recorded while subjects performed a variety of motor tasks (Deiber et al., 1991). SMA activity was observed especially for tasks that required the internal generation of movement, rather than tasks in which movement was based on external cues. Speech generally is believed to be based on internally generated movements, and it is therefore expected that speech would be associated with activation of the SMA. In related studies of cerebral blood flow, increased flow was observed in the SMA during the performance of repetitive, sequential motor tasks (Orgogozo, Larsen, Roland, Malamed, & Lassen, 1979; Roland, Larsen, Lassen, & Skinhoj, 1980). These results may mean that the SMA is involved in the regulation of complex, sequential movements. In studies on the monkey, Tanji and Shima (1994) reported that the SMA is involved in the planning of learned movements.

Jonas (1981) reported on the brain scans of two patients who had expressive speech deficits marked by short phrases of reduced intensity, dysfluencies, and periods of muteness. The brain scans showed regions of abnormally high activity in the left SMA. Caplan (1987) reviewed studies on the SMA and concluded that it plays a role in the control of activation and initiation of speech. Studies of normal speakers also point to a possible role of the SMA in language. Increased regional cerebral blood flow has been observed in the SMA during verbal and nonverbal naming tasks (Posner, Petersen, Fox, & Raichle, 1988; Wise et al., 1991). In their classic study of electrical stimulation of the exposed cerebral cortex in humans, Penfield and Welch (1951) noted that the SMA was the most effective site of stimulation to elicit vocalization.

Supramarginal Gyrus

Although damage to this structure has been thought to result especially in written language, a recent assessment of its activity in PET studies points to a possible role in phonological storage (Demonet et al., 1996). This role is particularly linked to the inferior part of this gyrus. Possibly, the supramarginal gyrus is involved in both written and spoken language, and it may serve a common phonological role for these two forms of expression.

Large-scale Cortical Networks

If speech and language were compactly represented in the brain, then it should be possible to stimulate the exposed brain electrically and evoke spoken language. But when the brain is electrically stimulated, as during neurosurgery, the primary effect is either to evoke very simple vocalizations (Penfield & Roberts, 1959) or to disrupt ongoing vocalization (Ojemann, 1983). But electrical stimulation at any single site does not evoke phrases, words, or even the simple consonant-vowel syllables heard in an infant's babbling. In contrast, electrical stimulation of the limbic system and other structures in monkeys can elicit almost the entire sound repertoire (Larson, 1988).

Why is it not possible to elicit speech from stimulation of the brain in humans? One reason is that speech may be represented in the brain in distributed neural networks, such that no single area is sufficient to produce even a single syllable. Some support for this idea comes from brain imaging studies of human speech perception and production. From observations of cerebral activity using PET, Friston, Frith, Liddle, and Frackowiak (1991) proposed a network model of intrinsic versus extrinsic word generation. Their model consists of three neuronal systems including: (1) a pool that stores word representations in a distributed mode, (2) an afferent system that conveys sensory input to this pool, and (3) a modulating system that regulates the sensitivity or responsivity of neurons in the pool. The distributed word store was hypothesized to be in the left superior temporal region (Wernicke's area) and the modulation site in the left dorsolateral prefrontal cortex (DLPFC). The DLPFC was thought to modulate the responsivity of a neural system in the superior temporal gyrus. In addition, the DLPFC may have a part in regulating the attentional and intentional states that underlie the intrinsic generation of words. Damasio (1989) has described one model for multiregional activation of the brain.

Gender Differences

There is also evidence that males and females differ in the cortical representation of language (Harasty, Double, Halliday, Kril, & McRichie, 1997; Shaywitz et al., 1995). Generally, females have a more bilateral representation of language, and it appears that language processing in women activates both hemispheres to a greater degree than in men (Shaywitz et al., 1995). Furthermore, observations by Harasty et al. (1997) indicate that women have proportionately larger language-related cortical regions of the left (language-dominant) hemisphere. For example, the planum temporale was 30% larger in women than men and Broca's area was 20% larger. These differences in language-related neural regions are interesting in view of the several studies that point to generally superior language abilities in women (reviewed in Chapter 1). This issue is further considered in Chapter 13, especially in respect to theories on the evolution of the nervous system.

Localization or Not?

It is not a simple matter to synthesize the various studies of cortical localization for speech and language. Some studies point to relatively discrete regions of primary activity associated with functions such as speaking words. This tradition, which began in Broca's time, continues to be influential. Caplan (1994) advocates a general position of localization. He notes that "despite [some] variation, there are strong tendencies for most components of the language processing system to be located in the left hemisphere and for particular language processing components to be localized in particular areas of the left perisylvian cortex" (Caplan, 1994, p. 1043). In contrast, Damasio (1989) proposes multiregional activation for language processing. Even relatively simple language tasks can involve extensive regions of cortex. For that matter, it appears that even in birds, vocalization may be controlled by multiple pathways in the nervous system (Williams, 1989). It would not be surprising to find even more complexity in the neural pathways that regulate human speech.

One reason for the disagreement is that language is not a unitary activity that is easily dissociated from other higher cortical processing. By its nature, language relates to personal experience, and it can be highly evocative and provocative. Because language has cognitive roots, it has the potential to induce activity in regions of the brain that may not be strictly necessary for language in the narrowest sense. Furthermore, the spoken message is multidimensional in its informational character. Language carries phonetic, prosodic, paralinguistic, personal, and transmittal information, as mentioned in Chapter 1. These various types of information can be processed in different regions of the brain. Depending on the nature of any given utterance, various sites of cortex may be activated to process its acoustic, linguistic, affective, and cognitive aspects.

Another theoretical issue to be considered is if language is **modular** (Fodor, 1983). Although definitions of modularity vary, Fodor (1983) described a modular cognitive system as "domain specific, innately specified, hardwired, autonomous, and not assembled" (Fodor, 1983, p. 37). Briefly, a module is a functional system that operates on its own informational domain and makes the products of its computation available to other systems. The essence of modularity is its informational encapsulation, that is, the segregation of informational privileges from other types of information. Modules are quasi-independent systems that insure the rapid, mandatory, and efficient processing of information in a restricted domain. Fodor, among many others, argues that language is modular. Some believe that this cognitive property implies a restricted neural representation. However, this is a strong assumption. Even if language is modular, its neural representation could be complex and diffuse. Furthermore, some of the evidence put forward to support the modularity of language (such as preservation of linguistic ability in some persons with severe mental retardation) has been disputed (Levy, 1996). This issue is too complex to be considered in any depth here, but it is an example of the difficulty of conceptualizing the neural correlates of human faculties.

Another difficulty in determining which cortical regions are associated with specific language functions is that studies do not always result in compatible or convergent conclusions. For example, Poeppel (1996) concluded that published PET studies of phonological processing do not show the expected agreement. Cortical activity associated with phonological processing was reported in several different regions, including frontal, parietal, and temporal lobes. In responding to Poeppel's criticisms, Demonet et al. (1996) argued that Poeppel overstated the divergence of results and that several studies point to activation of one well-defined cortical region, the inferior part of the left supramarginal gyrus.

LIFE COURSE CONSIDERATIONS

As noted earlier in this chapter, the full complement of neurons is present by about 5 months gestational age. But much remains to be done to bring the nervous system to maturity. During the remainder of the gestational period, a major event is the migration of early forms of neurons (**neuroblasts**) to their ultimate destination. For example, neuroblasts originally found in the periventricular region (i.e., the region surrounding the ventricles) migrate outward to form the cerebral cortex. Of course, simply having neurons in the right locations is not sufficient for a functional nervous system. The neurons must form connections, and **synaptogenesis**, meaning formation of synapses, is the means by which the neurons come together in networks. Synaptic connections are formed especially during early childhood. It has long been recognized that children's brains are highly plastic compared to adults' brains, and that children can tolerate brain injuries that would be devastating to adults. One particular example of the extraordinary plasticity of the developing brain is that children often overcome serious unilateral brain lesions, even hemispherectomy (removal of one hemisphere) (Aram, 1988; Sugishita, Otomo, Koike, Segawa, & Nomura, 1992).

Another important maturational event is the formation of myelin in both the PNS and CNS. The earliest myelin development is in the sensory and motor roots of the spinal cord. Among the latest structures to be myelinated are the long association tracts of the cerebrum. Table 7–3 summarizes the chronology of myelination for some structures in the CNS. Note that the development of myelination continues until young adulthood. Additional details of neural development are noted in Chapter 14.

The extended process of neural maturation gives the brain considerable flexibility and allows environmental factors to influence the development of the nervous system. One of the fundamental questions pertaining to language is whether there is a sensitive period (sometimes called the *critical period*) of neural development during which language is optimally acquired. The sensitive period hypothesis was noted in Chapter 1. The essential argument is that the brain possesses the flexibility for language representation only during the years of early childhood. Presumably, if a child passes through this period without learning language, then it is not likely that the child will ever develop normal linguistic abilities. Until very recently, the oldest reported age at which a child first began to speak was 6 years. It was generally believed that language development beyond the age of 6 years was unlikely. But a report by Vargha-Khadem et al. (1996) described a boy who began to speak at the age of 9.5 years, following surgery to remove his damaged left hemisphere. After the surgery, the boy made remarkable progress in language development and was capable of the fluent production of long, well-formed sentences.

Table 7–3. Approximate age of onset and completion of myelination for several structures of the nervous system.

Structure	Onset	Completion
Motor roots of spinal cord	5th month GA	2nd month
Sensory roots of spinal cord	6th month GA	6th month
Optic nerve and tract	9th month GA	3rd–4th year
Somesthetic radiations	9th month GA	1st year
Pyramidal tracts	10th month GA	2nd year
Optic radiations	Birth	5th month
Acoustic radiations	Birth	3rd–4th year
Reticular formation	1st month	15+ years
Cingulum	2nd month	11th month
Striatum	3rd month	1st–2nd year
Great cerebral commissures	4th month	10th year
Intracortical association fibers	4th month	20+ years

Source: Drawn from data in, "The Myelogenetic Cycles of Regional Maturation of the Brain," by P. Yakovlev and A. Lecours (pp. 3–70) in A. Minkowski (Ed.), *Regional Development of the Brain in Early Life.* Oxford, England: Blackwell Scientific.

Although neurons are lost continuously and irrevocably after we are born, the rate of loss is very small compared to the tremendous number of neurons that we have to begin with. But eventually the loss of neurons has its effects. In advanced age, the rate of loss can increase, and the brain actually shrinks. Some diseases also accelerate the rate of neuronal loss. One of the most devastating diseases in this respect is **Alzheimer's disease**, which is the major cause of dementia in the elderly.

CONCLUSION

Although certain structures and regions of the nervous system have been historically emphasized in the neural control of speech and language, it appears that the most accurate conception is one of large-scale distributed networks. Perhaps some neural structures play particularly critical roles in some aspects of regulation, but they do not seem to work in isolation. Therefore, it can be misleading to describe selective parts of the nervous system as the sufficient components for speech and language. Although certain structures such as Wernicke's area and Broca's area are prominently mentioned in almost every account of how the brain controls spoken language, it is well to keep in mind that these areas are highly interconnected with other areas. Language may draw on substantial neural resources, and it is therefore fitting that its representation in the brain is potentially widely distributed.

On The Reference Shelf

Readings for those who seek a wider or deeper coverage.

Barlow, S. M., & Farley, G. R. (1989). Neurophysiology of speech. In D. P. Kuehn, M. L. Lemme, & J. M. Baumgartner (Eds.), *Neural bases of speech, hearing, and language* (pp. 146–200). Boston: College-Hill Press.
A concise, though somewhat dated, discussion of the topic.

Edelman, G. M. (1992). *Bright air, brilliant fire: On the matter of mind*. New York: Basic Books.
The Nobel laureate describes how the grouping of nerve cells accounts for human behavior.

Finger, S. (1994). *Origins of neuroscience: A history of exploration into brain function*. New York: Oxford University Press.
A rich historical account of investigations into the brain.

Hellige, J. B. (1993). *Hemispheric asymmetry*. Cambridge, MA: Harvard University Press.
Extensive coverage of this much-studied aspect of the nervous system.

Kean, M.-L. (1988). Brain structures and linguistic capacity. In F. J. Newmeyer (Ed.), *Linguistics: The Cambridge Survey. II. Linguistic theory: Extensions and implications* (pp. 74–95). Cambridge, UK: Cambridge University Press.
A thoughtful essay on issues in basic neurolinguistics.

Lauter, J. L. (1995). Visions of speech and language: Noninvasive imaging techniques and their applications to the study of human communication. In H. Winitz (Ed.), *Human communication and its disorders* (pp. 277–390). Timonium, MD: York Press.
Systematic review of neuroimaging methods related to speech, language, and hearing.

Liebman, M. (1991). *Neuroanatomy made easy and understandable*. Gaithersburg, MD: Aspen Publishers.
This book, illustrated with simplified informal drawings, can help a novice understand basic neuroanatomy. Perhaps neuroanatomy is never really easy, but this book certainly helps.

Love, R. J., & Webb, W. G. (1992). *Neurology for the speech-language pathologist* (2nd ed.). Boston: Butterworth-Heinemann.
This overview of basic neurology for speech-language pathologists is a good introduction to neurogenic disorders of communication including dysarthria, aphasia, and apraxia.

Oldendorf, W. H. (1978). The quest for an image of the brain: A brief historical and technical review of brain imaging. *Neurology, 28*, 517–523.
The title explains the article.

Nieuwenhuys, R. (1994). The neocortex: An overview of its evolutionary development, structural organization and synaptology. *Anatomy and Embryology, 190*, 307–337.
Concise but informative overview of this part of the nervous system that is highly developed in humans.

Schiller, F. (1992). *Paul Broca: Founder of French anthropology, explorer of the brain*. Oxford, England: Oxford University Press.
The only biography of the great 19th century anthropologist and surgeon, this book describes the social and scientific milieu of Broca's work and his manifold contributions to science and medicine.

Webster, D. B. (1995). *Neuroscience of communication*. San Diego: Singular Publishing Group, Inc.
A good introduction to the neuroanatomy and neurophysiology related to spoken language. It is particularly recommended for its summary of the auditory nervous system.

Chapter References

Alexander, G. E., Delong, M. R., & Strick, P. L. (1986). Parallel organization of functionally segregated circuits linking basal ganglia and cortex. *Annual Review of Neuroscience, 9*, 357–381.

Alexander, M., Naeser, M., & Palumbo, C. (1990). Broca's area aphasias: Aphasia after lesions including the frontal operculum. *Neurology, 40*, 353–362.

Anokhin, A. P., Birbaumer, N., Lutzenberger, W., Nikolaov, A., & Vogel, F. (1996). Age increases brain complexity. *Electroencephalography and Clinical Neurophysiology, 99*, 63–68.

Aram, D. (1988). Language sequelae of unilateral brain lesions in children. In F. Plum (Ed.), *Language, communication, and the brain* (pp. 171–197). New York: Raven Press.

Botez, M. I., & Barbeau, A. (1971). Role of subcortical structures, and particularly of the thalamus, in the mechanisms of speech and language. *International Journal of Neurology, 8*, 300–320.

Bowman, J. P. (1971). *The muscle spindle and neural control of the tongue: Implications for speech*. Springfield, IL: Charles C. Thomas.

Brodmann, K. (1914). Physiologie des Gehirns, in die Allgemeine Chirurgie der Gehirnkrankheiten. *Neue Deutsche Chirurgia (Vol. 11*, p. 1). Stuttgart: Ferdinand Enke Verlag.

Buckingham, H. W. (1984). Localization of language in the brain. In R. C. Naremore (Ed.), *Language science* (pp. 243–280). San Diego: College-Hill Press.

Caplan, D. (1987). *Neurolinguistics and linguistic aphasiology*. Cambridge, UK: Cambridge University Press.

Caplan, D. (1994). Language and the brain. In M. A. Gernsbacher (Ed.), *Handbook of psy-*

cholinguistics (pp. 1023–1053). San Diego: Academic Press.

Casseday, J. H., & Covey, E. (1996). A neuroethological theory of the operation of the inferior colliculus. *Brain, Behavior and Evolution, 47*, 311–336.

Chafetz, M. D., Friedman, A. L., Kevorkian, C. G., & Lovy, J. K. (1996). The cerebellum and cognitive function: Implications for rehabilitation. *Archives of Physical Medicine and Rehabilitation, 77*, 1303–1308.

Cherniak, C. (1995). Neural component placement. *Trends in Neuroscience, 18*, 522–527.

Cooper, S. (1960). Muscle spindles and other receptors. In G. H. Bourne (Ed.), *Structure and function of muscle*. New York: Academic Press.

Crosson, B. A. (1992). *Subcortical functions in language and memory*. New York: Guilford Press.

Damasio, A. R. (1989). Time-locked multiregional retroactivation: A system-level proposal for the neural substrates of recall and recognition. *Cognition, 33*, 25–62.

Dandy, W. H. (1918). Ventriculography following injection of air into the cerebral ventricles. *American Surgeon, 68*, 5–11.

Daum, I., & Ackermann, H. (1995). Cerebellar contributions to cognition. *Behavioural Brain Research, 67*, 201–210.

Davidoff, R. A. (1990). The pyramidal tract. *Neurology, 40*, 332–339.

Demonet, J. F., Fiez, J. A., Paulesu, F., Petersen, S. E., & Zatorre, R. J. (1996). PET studies and phonological processing: A critical rely to Poeppel. *Brain and Language, 55*, 352–379.

Demonet, J. F., Price, C., Wise, R., & Frackowiak, R. S. (1994). Differential activation of right and left posterior sylvian regions by semantic and phonological tasks: A positron-emission tomography study in normal human subjects. *Neuroscience Letters, 182*, 25–28.

Dieber, M. P., Passingham, R. E., Colebatch, J. G., Friston, K. J., Nixon, P. D., & Frackowiak, R. S. J. (1991). Cortical areas and the selection of movement. A study with positron emission tomography. *Experimental Brain Research, 84*, 393–402.

Diener, H.-C., & Dichgans, J. (1992). Pathophysiology of cerebellar ataxia. *Movement Disorders, 7*, 95–108.

Finger, S., & Roe, D. (1996). Gustave Dax and the early history of cerebral dominance. *Archives of Neurology, 53*, 806–813.

Fodor, J. A. (1983). *The modularity of mind*. Cambridge, MA: MIT Press.

Friston, K. J., Frith, C. D., Liddle, P. F., & Frackowiak, R. S. (1991). Investigating a network model of word generation with positron emission tomography. *Proceedings of the Royal Society of London: Biological Sciences, 244*, 101–106.

Geschwind, N., & Galaburda, A. M. (1987). *Cerebral lateralization*. Cambridge, MA: MIT Press.

Graybiel, A. M., Aosaki, T., Flaherty, A. W., & Kimura, M. (1994). The basal ganglia and adaptive motor control. *Science, 265*, 1826–1831.

Harasty, J., Double, K. L., Halliday, G. M., Kril, J. J., & McRitchie, D. A. (1997). Language-associated cortical regions are proportionately larger in the female brain. *Archives of Neurology, 54*, 171–176.

Hounsfield, G. N. (1973). Computerized transverse axial scanning (tomography): Part 1. Description of system. *British Journal of Radiology, 46*, 1016–1022.

Howard, D., Patterson, K., Wise, R., Brown, W. D., Friston, K., Weiller, C., & Frackowiak, R. (1992). The cortical localization of the lexicons. *Brain, 115*, 1769–1782.

Huffman, R. F., & Hanson, O. W., Jr. (1990). The descending auditory pathway and acousticomotor systems: Connections with the inferior colliculus. *Brain Research Reviews, 15*, 295–323.

Ingvar, D. H., & Schwartz, M. S. (1974). Blood flow patterns induced in the dominant hemisphere by speech and reading. *Brain, 97*, 273–288.

Jonas, S. (1981). The supplementary motor region and speech emission. *Journal of Communication Disorders, 14*, 349–373.

Kadanoff, D. (1956). Die sensiblen Nervenendigungen in der mimischen Musculatur des Menschen. *Zeitschrift für mikroskopische anatomische Forschung, 62*, 1–15.

Karbe, H., Wurker, M., Herholz, K., Ghaemi, M., Pietrzyk, U., Kessler, J., & Heiss, W. D. (1995). Planum temporale and Brodmann's area 22: Magnetic resonance imaging and high-resolution positron emission tomography demonstrate functional left–right asymmetry. *Archives of Neurology, 52*, 869–874.

Kelso, S., & Tuller, B. (1983). "Compensatory articulation" under conditions of reduced afferent information: A dynamic formulation. *Journal of Speech and Hearing Research, 26*, 217–224.

Kennedy, W. R. (1970). Innervation of normal human muscle spindles. *Neurology, 20,* 463–476.

Kent, R. D., Martin, R. E., & Sufit, R. L. (1990). Oral sensation: A review and clinical prospective. In H. Winitz (Ed.), *Human communication and its disorders. A review—1990* (pp. 135–191). Norwood, NJ: Ablex.

Kertesz, A. (1989). Hemispheric dominance: Its development and relation to speech disorders. *Folia Phoniatrica, 41,* 61–88.

Kuhl, D. E., & Edwards, R. Q. (1964). Cylindrical and section radioisotope scanning of the liver and brain. *Radiology, 83,* 926–932.

Larsen, B., Skinhoj, E., & Lassen, N. A. (1978). Variations in regional cortical blood flow in the right and left hemispheres during automatic speech, *Brain, 101,* 193–209.

Larson, C. R. (1988). Brain mechanisms involved in the control of vocalization. *Journal of Voice, 2,* 301–311.

Lassen, N. A., Ingvar, D. H., & Skinhoj, E. (1978). Brain function and blood flow. *Scientific American, 239,* 62–71.

Lauter, J. L. (1995). Visions of speech and language: Noninvasive imaging techniques and their applications to the study of human communication. In H. Winitz (Ed.), *Human communication and its disorders* (pp. 277–390). Timonium, MD: York Press.

Lauterbur, P. (1973). Image formation by induced local interaction. Examples employing nuclear magnetic resonance. *Nature, 342,* 190–194.

Leblanc, R., Meyer, E., Bub, D., Zatorre, R. J., & Evans, A. C. (1992). Language localization with activation positron emission tomography scanning. *Neurosurgery, 31,* 369–373.

Lefkowitz, D., & Netsell, R. (1993). Neuroanatomy of speech: An MRI atlas. *Journal of Medical Speech-Language Pathology, 1,* 3–26.

Leiner, H. C., Leiner, A. L., & Dow, R. S. (1991). The human cerebro-cerebellar system: Its computing, cognitive and language skills. *Behavioral and Brain Research, 44,* 113–128.

Levy, Y. (1996). Modularity of language reconsidered. *Brain and Language, 55,* 240–263.

Lidsky, T. I., Manetto, C., & Schneider, J. S. (1985). A consideration of sensory factors involved in motor functions of the basal ganglia. *Brain Research Reviews, 9,* 133–146.

Liss, J. M. (1990). Muscle spindles in the human levator veli palatini and palatoglossus muscles. *Journal of Speech and Hearing Research, 33,* 736–746.

Lucas-Keene, M. F. (1976). Muscle spindles in human laryngeal muscles. *Journal of Anatomy, 95,* 25–29.

Masterton, R. B. (1992). Role of the central auditory system in hearing: The new direction. *Trends in Neuroscience, 15,* 280–285.

Menard, M. T., Kosslyn, S. M., Thompson, W. L., Alpert, N. M., & Rauch, S. L. (1996). Encoding words and pictures: A positron emission study. *Neuropsychologia, 34,* 185–192.

Moore, G. E. (1947). Fluoroscein as an agent in the differentiation of normal and malignant tissues. *Science, 106,* 130–131.

Moore, G. E. (1948). The use of radioactive diiodofluorescein in the diagnosis and localization of brain tumors. *Science, 107,* 569–571.

Moniz, E. (1927). L'encephalographie arterielle. Son importance dans la localisation des tumeurs cerebrales. *Revue Neurologie, 34,* 72–84.

Musiek, F. E., & Lamb, L. (1992). Neuroanatomy and neurophysiology of central auditory processing. In J. Katz, N. Stecker, & D. Henderson (Eds.), *Central auditory processing: A transdisciplinary view* (pp. 11–38). St. Louis: Mosby-Year Book.

Ojemann, G. A. (1983). Brain organization for language from the perspective of electrical stimulation mapping. *Behavioral and Brain Sciences, 6,* 189–230.

Oldendorf, (1978). The quest for an image of the brain: A brief historical and technical review of brain imaging. *Neurology, 28,* 517–533.

Ono, M., Kubik, S., & Abernathy, C. D. (1990). *Atlas of the Cerebral Sulci.* New York: Thieme.

Orgogozo, J. M., Larsen, B., Roland, P. E., Melamed, E., & Lassen, N. A. (1979). Further studies on the supplementary motor area in man with rCBF method. *Acta Neurology Scandinavia, 60*(Suppl. 72), 8–9.

Penfield, W., & Boldrey E. (1937). Somatic motor and sensory representation in the cerebral cortex of man as studied by electrical stimulaion. *Brain, 60,* 389–397.

Penfield, W., & Roberts, L. (1959). *Speech and brain mechanisms.* Princeton, NJ: Princeton University Press.

Penfield, W., & Welch, K. (1951). The supplementary motor area of the cerebral cortex. *Archives of Neurology and Psychiatry, 66,* 289–317.

Petersen, S. E., Fox, P. T., Posner, M. I., Mintun, M., & Raichle, M. E. (1988). Positron emission tomographic studies of the cortical anatomy of single-word proccessing. *Nature, 331*, 585–589.

Poeppel, D. (1996). A critical review of PET studies of phonological processing. *Brain and Language, 55*, 317–351.

Posner, M. I., Petersen, S. E., Fox, P. T., & Raichle, M. E. (1988). Localization of cognitive operations in the human brain. *Science, 240*, 1627–1631.

Roland. P. E., Larsen, B., Lassen, N. A., & Skinhoj, E. (1980). Supplementary motor area and other cortical areas in organization of voluntary movements in man. *Journal of Neurophysiology, 43*, 118–136.

Sarter, M., Berntson, G. G., & Cacioppo, J. T. (1996). Brain imaging and cognitive neuroscience. *American Psychologist, 51*, 13–21.

Shaywitz, B. A., Shaywitz, S. E., Pugh, K. R., Constable, R. T., Skudlarski, P., Fulbright, R. K., Bronen, R. A., Fletcher, J. M., Shankweiler, D. P., & Katz, L. (1995). Sex differences in the functional organization of the brain for language. *Nature, 373*, 607–609.

Schiller, F. (1992). *Paul Broca: Founder of French anthropology, explorer of the brain*. Oxford, England: Oxford University Press.

Silveri, M. C., Leggio, M. G., & Molinari, M. (1994). The cerebellum contributes to linguistic production: A case of agrammatic speech following a right cerebellar lesion. *Neurology, 44*, 2047–2050.

Smith, R. D., & Macarian, H. Q. (1967). The neuromuscular spindles of the lateral pterygoid muscle. *Anatomischer Anzeiger, 120*, 47–53.

Spitzer, M., Kwong, K. K., Kennedy, W., Rosen, B. R., & Belliveau, J. W. (1995). Category-specific brain activation in fMRI during picture naming. *Neuroreport, 6*, 2109–2112.

Sugashita, M., Otomo, K., Koike, A., Segawa, M., & Nomura, Y. (1992). Long-term effects of early unilateral brain lesions upon intelligence and language skills. *Brain Dysfunction, 5*, 301–309.

Tanji, J., & Shima, K. (1994). Role for supplementary motor area cells in planning several movements ahead. *Nature, 371*, 413–415.

Taylor, R. (1990, May). Evolutions: Brain imaging. *The Journal of NIH Research, 2*, 103–104.

Thach, W. T., Goodkin, H. P., & Keating, J. G. (1992). The cerebellum and the adaptive coordination of movement. *Annual Review of Neuroscience, 15*, 403–442.

Tikofsky, R. S. (1984). Contemporary aphasia diagnostics. In N. J. Lass (Ed.), *Speech and language: Advances in basic research and practice* (Vol. 11, pp. 1–111). New York: Academic Press.

Vargha-Khadem, F., Carr, L. J., Isaacs, E., Brett, E., Adams, C., & Mishkin, M. (1997). Onset of speech after left hemispherectomy in a 9-year-old boy. *Brain, 120*, 562–567.

Whitaker, H. A. (1995). Roots: 5 notes on the history of neurolinguistics. In K. Elenius & P. Branderud (Eds.), *Proceedings of the XIIIth International Congress of Phonetic Sciences* (Vol. 2, pp. 164–171). Stockholm: Royal Institute of Technology and Stockholm University.

Williams. H. (1989). Multiple representations and auditory-motor interactions in the avian song system. In M. Davis, B. L. Jacobs, & R. I. Schoenfeld (Eds.), *Modulation of defined vertebrate neural circuits. Annals of the New York Academy of Sciences, 563*, 148–164.

Wise, R., Chollet, F., Hadar, U., Friston, K., Hoffner, E., & Frackowiak, R. (1991). Distribution of cortical neural networks involved in word comprehension and word retrieval. *Brain, 114*, 1803–1817.

Exercises

7-1. Match the brain divisions at the left with the structures at the right.

telencephalon	thalamus and hypothalamus
diencephalon	midbrain
mesencephalon	cerebral hemispheres
metencephalon	medulla oblongata
myelencephalon	pons

7-2. The figure below shows the lateral surface of the left cerebral hemisphere. Identify the following regions: lateral fissure, central fissure, precentral gyrus, postcentral gyrus, frontal lobe, parietal lobe, occipital lobe, and temporal lobe. Then, mark the locations of the following: Broca's area, Wernicke's area, angular gyrus, supramarginal gyrus, supplementary motor area, and orofacial motor area.

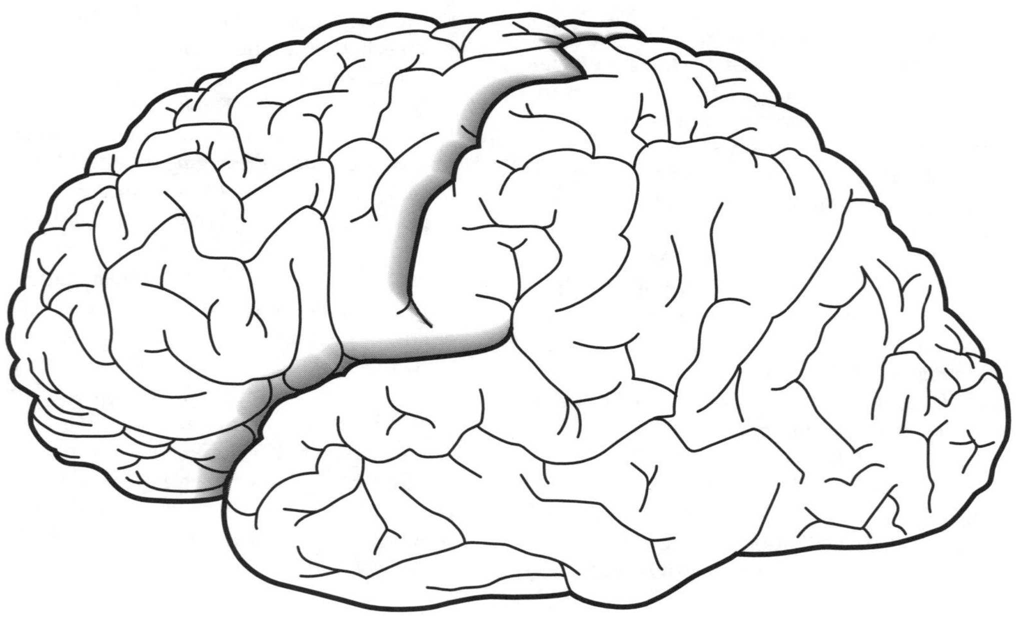

7-3. The figure on the next page shows two coronal sections of the brain. The one labeled **a** is anterior to the one labeled **b**. Match the letters in part **a** to the following regions and structures.

cortex of temporal lobe
pon
insula
Sylvian (lateral) fissure
corpus callosum
thalamus
cerebral aqueduct
cerebellum
lateral ventricle
cerebral peduncle
median longitudinal fissure

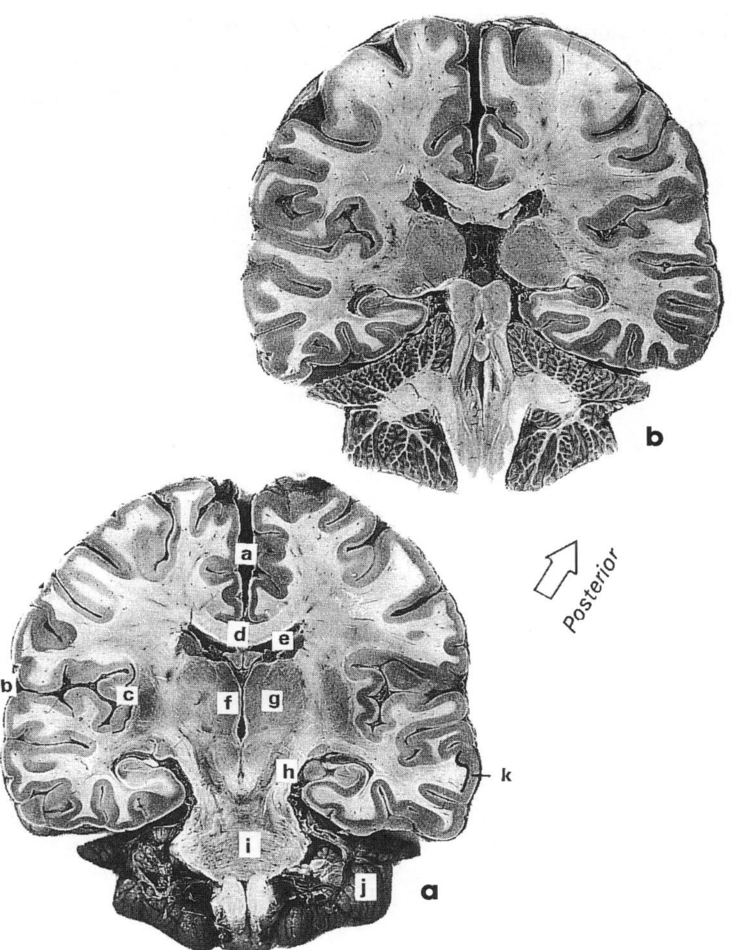

7-4. Using part **b** in this figure, locate the following: medial longitudinal fissure, corpus callosum, Sylvian (lateral) fissure, thalamus, cerebellum.

7-5. This is a simple exercise often used in teaching neuroanatomy. Cut along the lines in the figure on the right to form two shields consisting of the falx cerebri, falx cerebelli, and tentorium cerebelli. Using slots **a** and **b**, fit these shields together at an angle of about 90° to form the three-dimensional structure of the falx cerebri and the tentorium cerebelli. When the two shields are oriented perpendicularly, they form a model of the dural sheaths that divide the cranial cavity into its major portions.

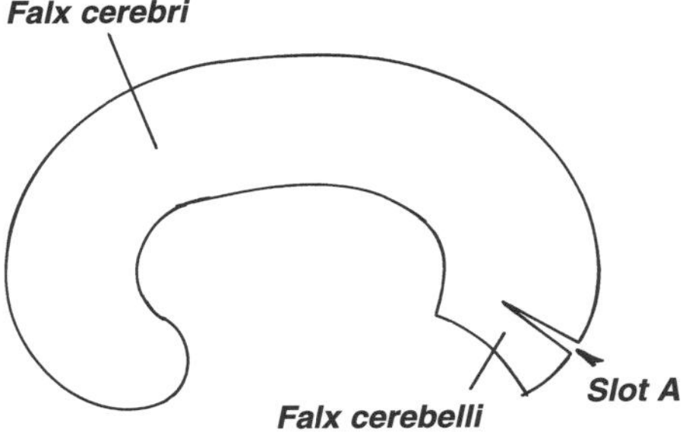

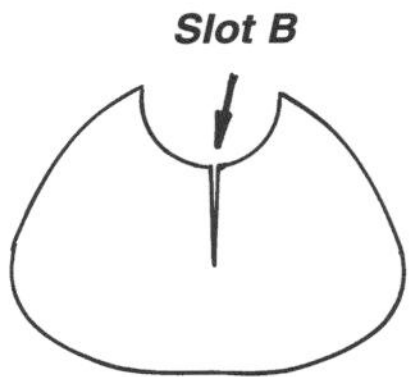

7-6. Discuss the functional significance of the following (i.e., what is the major role of each?): pyramidal motor control system, extrapyramidal motor control system, basal nuclei, limbic system, primary sensory cortex, primary motor cortex, supplementary motor region, angular gyrus, and brainstem.

APPENDIX

Cranial Nerve Supplement

PART A. Detailed Listing of Cranial Nerves Important in Speech and Hearing

CN V—Trigeminal nerve

Sensory: Somatosensation from the face, cornea, nose sinuses, teeth, mouth, meninges, eardrum, and temporomandibular joint

Motor: Muscles of mastication (masseter, temporalis, internal pterygoid, external pterygoid), extrinsic larynx (anterior belly of digastric, mylohyoid), middle ear (tensor tympani), and velopharynx (tensor veli palatine)

CN VII—Facial nerve

Sensory: Taste from the anterior two-thirds of tongue

Motor: Muscles of facial expression (orbicularis oculi, orbicularis oris, buccinator, platysma), middle ear (stapedius), extrinsic larynx (posterior belly of digastric, stylohyoid)

Other: Salivary and tear glands

CN VIII—Acoustic-vestibular nerve

Sensory: Special senses of audition and balance

CN IX—Glossopharyngeal nerve

Sensory: Taste from posterior one third of tongue
Somatosensation from back of tongue and pharynx

Motor: Stylopharyngeus muscle and possibly pharyngeal constrictors (along with CN X)

Other: Innervation of salivary glands

CN X—Vagus nerve

Sensory: Somatosensation from larynx, pharynx, thoracic and abdominal viscera

Motor: Muscles of larynx (all intrinsic laryngeal muscles, muscles of pharynx (except stylopharyngeus) and velopharynx (pharyngeal constrictors, palatoglossus, palatopharyngeus, salpingopharyngeus, uvular, and levator veli palatine)

Other: Innervation of autonomic structures of thorax and abdomen (heart, stomach, intestines, glands)

CN XI—Spinal accessory nerve

Motor: Sternocleidomastoid and trapezius muscles

CN XII—Hypoglossal nerve

Motor: Muscles of tongue (all intrinsic lingual muscles plus styloglossus, hyoglossus, genioglossus) and strap muscles of neck (sternohyoid, sternothyroid, geniohyoid, thyrohyoid, and anterior belly of omohyoid)

Part B. Summary of Innervation of Major Structures and Systems in Speech Production

Structure or System	*Cranial Nerve*
Mandibular muscles	V
Lip muscles	VII
Other facial muscles	VII
Palatal muscles	V and X
Pharyngeal muscles	IX and X
Laryngeal muscles	X
Lingual muscles	XII

Part C. Classifications of Cranial Nerves

Branchial nerves are the nerves derived from the branchial arches of the embryo (see Chapter 14). These are: V, VII, IX, X, XI.

Bulbar nerves are the nerves that emerge from the bulb (medulla). These are: IX, X, XI, XII.

The **branchial/bulbar nerves** are the nerves derived from the branchial arches and that emerge from the medulla: IX, X, XI.

The **vagal group** includes IX, X, and XI, which are closely related in their embryology, brain stem emergence, and some innervation patterns (see previous).

The **sensory nerves** are those with exclusively or predominantly sensory function. These are: I, II, VIII (except for efferent pathways, noted in Chapter 6).

The **motor nerves** are those with exclusively motor function. These are: III, IV, VI, XI, XII.

The **mixed sensory/motor nerves** have both sensory and motor functions. These are: V, VII, IX, X.

CHAPTER 8

Physiological Phonetics

> ***"All the theories of phonemics and phonetics assume articulate language as the medium to be considered. Even the basic phonemic distinction of 'la langue et la parole' [language and speech] was made within the domain of articulate language. 'Ce qu'on s'imagine prononcer,' [imagined pronunciation] 'ce qu'on prononce en realité [actual pronunciation] both assume the process of pronouncing, either in physiological or mental terms . . . Since mentalism has been abandoned in the main in phonology, articulate language in action is the concrete medium for observation and for experimentation which can be repeated."***
>
> (R. H. Stetson, *Motor Phonetics,* reprinted in J. A. S. Kelso and K. G. Munhall (Eds.), *R. H. Stetson's Motor Phonetics: A Retrospective Edition.* Boston: Little, Brown, 1988, p. 35.)

The field of physiological phonetics, also known as speech physiology, may well be defined by Stetson's words, "articulate language in action is the concrete medium for observation and for experimentation which can be repeated." Raymond H. Stetson was the quintessential speech physiologist. He received his bachelor's degree in chemistry in 1893 from Oberlin College, his master's in zoology in 1896 from the same college, and his doctorate in psychology in 1906 from Harvard University (making him only the 12th Harvard doctorate in psychology). Between 1903 and 1949, Stetson published some 30 papers in scientific journals, two books, four monographs, and eight reviews. He was a consummate laboratory scientist who devised instruments to study the dynamic and mostly hidden attributes of speech production. His influence on the field of speech science was profound. The span of his knowledge was considerable. It was said of him at Oberlin that he could "teach any course on campus, given 10 minutes notice" (Sperry, 1988, p. 12).

But perhaps the founder of experimental phonetics was Wolfgang von Kempelen, whose writings included a book *Mechanismus der menschlichen Sprache* (Mechanisms of Human Speech) (1791) which helped to define a physiology of speaking. Eberhard and Kurt Zwirner's *Principles of Phonometrics* (1970) is a scholarly account of the early history of experimental phonetics. Readers who want to trace the history of the field would do well to begin with this book, which appeared in its original German edition *Grundfragen der Phonometrie* in 1936.

The discussion in this chapter includes a brief overview of some of the most commonly used techniques in physiological phonetics. First, however, we will consider the motivation for the use of these techniques. That is, what is it we want to know? In the broadest sense, we want to know how it is that a thought can be expressed as speech. In a highly influential and brilliant paper, Karl Lashley (1951) took speech as a particular example of the problem of the serial control of behavior. He proposed three physiological mechanisms for control:

- A *determining tendency*, or idea, governs the whole operation and relates it to a person's goals and desires. That is, we speak to express a thought. It is quite an accomplishment that we can convey these thoughts to one another through the medium of sound. As is discussed in Chapter 13, this is perhaps the ultimate triumph of humankind.
- *A priming of expressive units* is the selection and arousal of the units that will be used in the actual speech production. Lashley recognized that the units to be expressed are selected in advance of their execution. In addition, they are activated to prepare them for their imminent role in producing speech. This idea continues to be a part of contemporary models of speech and language behavior.
- A *schema of order*, or syntax of the act, puts the selected and aroused elements into the proper serial order. This seriation is fundamental to a behavior that is presumably controlled by discrete units and is realized as a temporal pattern of movements.

In brief, to speak out a thought, first, we need to hold the thought as a governing superstructure for behavior; second, we select and activate the units that will be used in expressing the thought as a spoken message; and, third, we put the activated units into the intended sequence. Of course, this is not the whole story, as it is also important to account for the sensory and motor processes that actually generate a sequence of movements. But Lashley's insight helps us to formulate the basic questions about how language can be realized as speech. The next section discusses additional aspects of this process, focusing on basic questions about speech as movement.

ISSUES IN SPEECH PHYSIOLOGY

One lesson learned from previous chapters is that speech production involves the regulation of a complex system. When we produce speech, we somehow orchestrate the components of this system to convert an intended linguistic message to a sequence of muscular contractions that results in a desired pattern of aerodynamic and acoustic events. A complete understanding of this process might include a physiological description of each component, for example, the chest wall, vocal folds, mandible, tongue, and velopharynx. Assuming that we had such a complete description (which we do not), one might then ask the broader question: How are these diverse structures controlled for the purpose of speech? Attempts to answer this question may very well lead to the conclusion that the whole is greater than the sum of the parts. The study of speech physiology rests partly on a detailed study of the components of speech production, but it also demands an examination of the ways in which the complete system works together.

Speech physiology addresses the concrete physical processes by which speech is formed. It therefore complements the methods of linguistics, which focus on abstract units and concepts. If speech is movement (as Stetson declared), then one way of investigating speech is to study its movements. The study of movements has been essential to progress in fields such as kinesiology and physical therapy. Can the study of movements lead to progress in speech and related fields such as linguistics? Let us briefly consider three questions that are examples of what might be learned.

The first question is: What is the unit of speech? The identification of the unit would be a significant advance for language science generally. As Eberhard and Kurt Zwirner (1970) commented, "The verification of the concept of the unit of speech sounds would provide the foundation for a systematic science of language statistics, and indeed could serve as a basis for any kind of quantitative linguistics" (p. 7). Unless scientists have a unit of some kind to record and analyze, it is difficult to study any natural phenomenon. For centuries, those who have studied speech have presumed some kind of unit, but the definition of unit varies among those who have written about it. Perhaps speech physiology can answer this most basic question: What is the unit of speech? The answer could lie in careful observations of movement patterns in the respiratory, laryngeal, and supralaryngeal subsystems. Because movements are not haphazard, their organization may be transparent to the units of control.

The second question is: How are the various components of speech production coordinated to produce fluent speech? This is a difficult question, and considerable effort has been focused on the coordination of movements within the individual subsystems. Even the most mundane speech behavior, such as a cheery "Good morning!" entails the activation of numerous muscles to produce a variety of movements. A major effort in speech physiology has been to investigate how muscles or movements are coordinated in the typical speaker, how a child learns this coordination, and how coordination can be disturbed in individuals with speech or voice disorders. A secure knowledge of coordination is needed to evaluate important questions such as: (1) To what degree can a child's progress in coordination of movement explain the usual order of sound acquisition? (2) Does stuttering reflect a basic disorder of coordination? (3) Do learned patterns of coordination for a particular language interfere with the learning of later languages?

The third question is: Given that speech is produced by means of aerodynamic forces, how can aerodynamic variables such as volume, pressure, and flow be used to study speech production? As discussed in Chapters 4 and 5, the respiratory, laryngeal, and supralaryngeal systems can be described in part by their actions on aerodynamic variables. That is, the movements of speaking result in basic aerodynamic events such as expiration of a volume of air, generation of air pressure beneath the vocal folds, or regulation of airflow through a groove in the tongue to produce a fricative sound. If aerodynamic variables could be recorded during the production of speech then valuable information would be available to describe the processes by which speech sounds are formed. This information would be useful to basic speech science, but it also could be used clinically in the assessment of individuals with speech or voice disorders.

To answer these and other questions, a number of ingenious methods have been developed for the study of speech physiology. These methods permit the examination of even the most hidden movements of speech. It is convenient to describe some of the most commonly used methods before taking a further look at their application to basic and applied questions in the study of speech.

METHODS OF SPEECH PHYSIOLOGY

The physiology of speech covers the biophysical mechanisms that are involved in the production of speech. There are several such mechanisms and a variety of ways of monitoring the physiological activity associated with speech. The following discussion is keyed to Table 8–1, which is a general outline of the levels of observation of speech physiology. The table shows that questions about speech production can be framed at several different levels, beginning at the highest levels of neural organization and proceeding to the final levels of sound generation.

Neural Impulses

It is convenient to begin the discussion of physiology in the nervous system with a look at the generation of neural impulses that are transmitted to the muscles. These neural instructions to the musculature are called **motor commands** and are covered in the following section. It is usually supposed that when we want to speak, we either retrieve stored motor commands or formulate appropriate motor commands for the task at hand. Theorists are divided as to whether retrieval of previously assembled commands or formulation of task-specific commands is the more accurate view. But, in either case, the neural system issues commands to the appropriate muscles. It was explained in Chapter 7 that the neural instructions for speech articulation are transmitted primarily along the corticobulbar pathway of the pyramidal motor system. By means of this pathway, neural instructions from cortical-subcortical neural circuits are issued to the motor nuclei of the cranial nerves. The available motor resources are called the **motor neuron pool**, or the reserve of motor neurons controlling individual muscles. Recall from Chapter 7 that a given motor neuron is associated with a motor unit that may include large numbers of individual motor fibers, typically from tens to hundreds. The task of the motor control system is to select the appropriate motor units and activate them in an effective sequence to perform the desired act. Because more than 100 different muscles can be called on to produce speech, the motor control task is not triv-

Table 8–1. Levels of observation in the study of speech, accompanied by a listing of common techniques for each level.

Level of Observation	Techniques
Neural	Brain imaging methods: electroencephalography, evoked potentials, positron emission tomography, functional magnetic resonance imaging
Motor command	Electromyography
Structural movement	Strain gauges, panendoscopy, photoelectric and optical methods, X-ray techniques such as videofluoroscopy, magnetometry, ultrasonography, palatography (electopalatography)
Aerodynamic events	Airflow, air pressure, air volume, and calculated entities

ial. Even though the full complement of these muscles is not used every time we speak, the muscles that are selected must be precisely regulated to ensure the proper sequence of muscular contractions.

In practice it is very difficult to record the actual neural signals prepared in the brain and sent to the muscles of speech. As discussed in Chapter 7, modern methods of brain imaging permit investigators to learn which brain structures are active during speech production and speech perception. For example, methods such as PET, EEG, and fMRI can be used to study brain activity associated with speech events. In addition, recordings of electrical activity at various sites in the nervous system can be used to determine the elapsed time between activity in the orofacial region of the motor cortex and the contraction of a muscle in part of the speech production system.

Motor Commands

Motor commands result in sequences of muscle contractions in the respiratory, laryngeal, and upper airway systems of speech production. Contraction of muscles is the aggregate effect of the contraction of the individual motor fibers innervated by the activated motor units. Muscle contractions, in turn, result in forces that create structural movements, such as displacement of the diaphragm in the respiratory system, adduction of the vocal folds in the larynx, and lowering of the jaw in the upper airway. Many of these movements can generate air pressures and flows in various parts of the speech system. Other movements introduce changes in vocal tract shape and thereby effect different resonator possibilities, as is discussed in Chapter 9.

Muscle contractions can be studied with the technique of **electromyography**, or EMG. EMG is one method of recording electrical activity generated by the body. Other methods are electrocardiography (EKG) and electroencephalography (EEG). EKG is a recording of electical activity in heart muscle. EEG, as mentioned in Chapter 7, is a recording of electrical activity in the brain. Because contracting muscles produce electrical activity, electrodes can be used to monitor these electrical signals as an index of muscular activation. Three primary types of electrodes, **microelectrodes**, **needle electrodes**, and **surface electrodes**, are shown in Figure 8–1. Microelectrodes, as their name implies, are the smallest and are capable of recording the activity from individual motor units. Needle electrodes are sharp needles, insu-

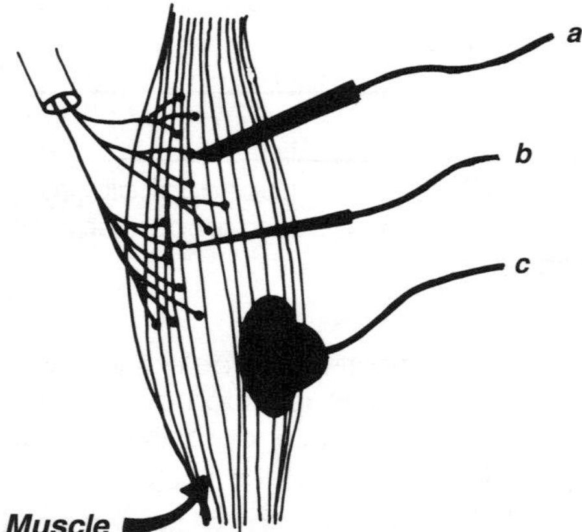

Figure 8–1. Three types of electrodes used to record electrical activity from muscle: a = needle electrode, b = microelectrode, and c = surface electrode. A motor unit is shown at the left of the drawing.

lated except at their tips. They typically record activity from a number of motor units in the vicinity of the electrode. Both microelectrodes and needle electrodes penetrate the skin to reach the muscle fibers. Surface electrodes resemble discs that are applied on the skin over the muscles of interest. They pick up the activity of numerous muscle fibers and are therefore a gauge of overall muscle activity in the proximity of the electrode.

A type of electrode frequently used in speech research is the **hooked-wire electrode**, which is similar to needle electrodes in its selectivity. The hooked-wire electrode is made by stripping the insulation from a thin flexible wire. The wire is inserted through a hypodermic needle, and the wire is bent back over the tip of the wire to form a hook. When the needle is inserted into a muscle and then withdrawn, the hooked wire remains embedded in the muscle and can be used to record electrical activity generated in its vicinity. When the recording is completed, a gentle tug on the hooked wire usually removes it easily. This type of electrode permits good selectivity, but it cannot be repositioned once it is inserted.

A large-scale electromyographic study of speech requires that numerous electrodes be placed to sample the various muscles involved. Once an electrode is inserted or attached, its placement is verified by looking for muscle activity in a task that is thought to require the use of the muscle in question. For example, if the cricothyroid muscle is being recorded, the examiner might ask the subject to make a large change in fundamental frequency of phonation.

EMG is particularly useful in determining the activity in a small group of selected muscles, especially if the muscles of interest are bundled (i.e., not intermixed with other muscles). Because it can involve substantial subject preparation in electrode placement and can encumber the subject with electrode wires, EMG is not easily used for casual recordings by inexperienced individuals. Typically, the signals require considerable postprocessing, such as averaging across several recordings to eliminate noise components. This method has been an important source of information on muscle activation in speech. It has been used in all of the major systems of speech production, respiratory, laryngeal, and upper airway.

Structural Movements

Structural movements in speech are of several types, some of which are easily visible (lip or jaw movements, for example) and others that are difficult or impossible to visualize without special instruments (vocal fold adjustments, for example). The reader may well appreciate the difficulties involved from the anatomical descriptions of the speech structures in Chapters 4 and 5. Because the movements of interest differ greatly in their accessibility and biomechanical properties, there is no single method that is universally applicable to study the structural movements of speech. Table 8–1 lists a number of different techniques that are discussed in this section. Before these techniques are described, brief mention will be made of some questions for which answers are sought.

Kinesiology is the study of movement. Speech kinesiology, then, is the study of speech movements. Because a large number of movements in speech may be simultaneous, or nearly so, one general objective of the study of speech movements is to determine the timing patterns between movements. At the level of an individual articulator, such as the lip, tongue, or mandible, the speech scientist may seek to determine how movement variables, such as magnitude and speed, are regulated. In Chapter 9 it is shown that the total time for the formant transitions associated with a stop-to-vowel sequence is about 50 ms. This constancy of transition duration is maintained across articulatory movements that vary considerably in total distance to be covered. How does the movement control system accomplish this durational constancy when varying distances are involved? Another research issue pertains to the accuracy of positioning of a given articulator. For example, what is the accuracy with which the tongue tip makes contact with the alveolar ridge to produce the fricative /s/?

Now we turn to specific techniques that can be used to address these and other questions.

Strain gauges are thin strips of piezoelectric material bonded to a support plate. They produce differential electric signals when the plate is deformed by external forces. Strain gauge assemblies have been used especially for the study of lip and jaw movements and also for movements of the respiratory system. Because these techniques do not present hazards to the subject, they are effective as a general laboratory method for the study of speech movements. However, they are not suitable for the study of complex movements, such as those of the tongue. An example of a cantilever system for recording lip and jaw movements is shown in Figure 8–2, which shows a strain gauge system used to record movements of the upper lip, lower lip, and mandible. This technique was adapted to speech research in the 1970s (Abbs & Gilbert, 1973) and, with continuing refinements, has been used as a major tool for the study of labial and mandibular movements and forces (Barlow & Abbs, 1983).

Oral panendoscopy permits visualization of internal structures by means of an optical viewing system, such as fiberoptics. The system has a self-contained light source to illuminate the field of view. This method can provide information on ordinarily invisible movements, such as the pattern of closure of the velopharynx. As was discussed in Chapter 5, velopharyngeal closure can be achieved in several ways (Croft, Shprintzen, & Rakoff, 1981; Shprintzen, 1992; Skolnick, McCall, & Barnes, 1973). Panendoscopy was helpful in identifying the various patterns of velopharyngeal closure, such as coronal, sagittal, circular, and circular with Passavant's ridge. Because panendoscopy does not present hazards such as radiation, it is a valuable clinical tool in speech-language pathology and otolaryngology. It can be used to examine the interior of the oral and pharyngeal cavities. The panendoscope permits observation of structures at rest and of certain kinds of movement. However, calibration of the device to enable the collection of quantitative data with an absolute reference can be difficult. In general, this method is more suitable to the derivation of relative values of motion.

Photoelectric, or **optical, tracking** systems also have been used to study speech movements. In one such system, a light-emitting

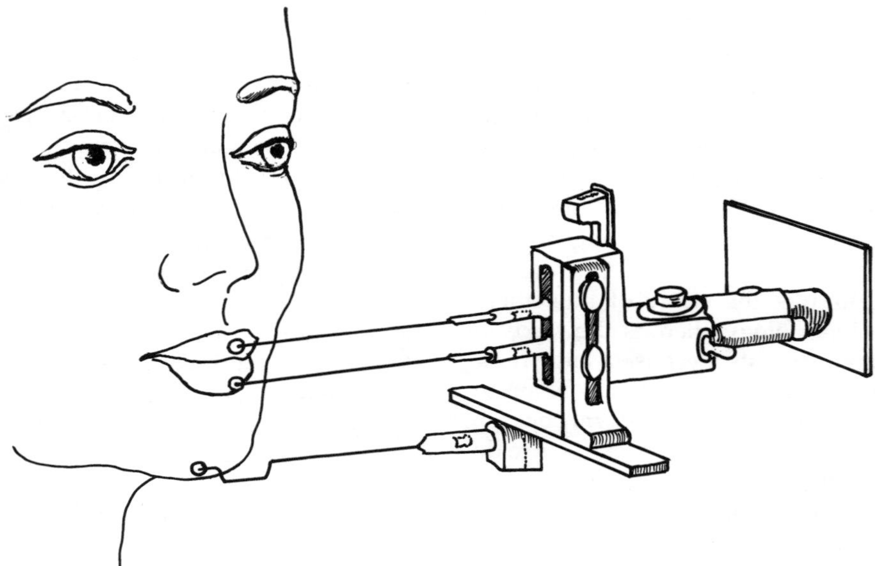

Figure 8–2. Strain gauge system used to record movements of the upper lip, lower lip, and mandible. (Based on drawings in "A Strain Gauge Transduction System for Lip and Jaw Motion in Two Dimensions," by J. Abbs and H. Gilbert, 1973, *Journal of Speech and Hearing Research, 16,* pp. 248–256; and "Force Transducers for the Evaluation of Labial, Lingual, and Mandibular Motor Impairments," by S. Barlow and J. Abbs, 1983, *Journal of Speech and Hearing Research, 26,* pp. 616–621.)

diode (LED) is attached to the structure to be studied (e.g., the lip). A specialized receiver is then used to record the motion of the LED. Although this approach cannot be used for all structures involved in speech, it can be used with great effectiveness to record lip and jaw movements.

X-ray methods such as **fluoroscopy** employ ionizing radiation to obtain images of internal structures. X-ray techniques have a long history in speech research, but their use is severely limited because of the biohazard of radiation exposure. **Still X rays** produce an image of a single posture or configuration. A lateral perspective often is used to obtain an image of the vocal tract. Figure 8–3 is a drawing of vocal tract structures derived from an X ray. A permanent X-ray motion picture film or video can be obtained through the use of **cinefluorography** or **videofluorography**, respectively. Cinefluorography was used extensively in the 1960s and 1970s to investigate the movements of speech (Moll, 1960). High-speed cinefluorography (i.e., with speeds greater than the conventional 24 frames per second) was especially revealing of the rapid movements of speech (Kent & Moll, 1972; Moll, 1960). A highly specialized X-ray system that is used to study oral movements with a computer-controlled X-ray microbeam was developed at the University of Wisconsin-Madison. Because the X-ray beam is sharply focused and is controlled to follow radiodense markers placed on the articulators, it collects large amounts of data with relatively little radiation to the subject.

Magnetometry is a method that uses miniature receivers and coils to produce a mag-

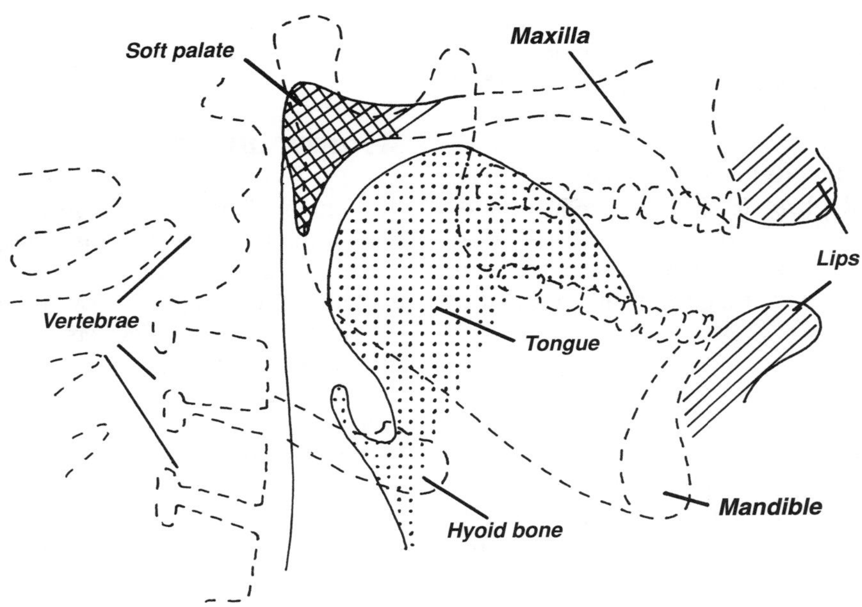

Figure 8–3. Tracing of articulatory structures from a lateral X ray of the vocal tract. Although the clarity of structures can vary markedly, it is generally possible to visualize both bony structures (e.g., maxilla, mandible, teeth, and vertebrae) and soft tissues (e.g., lips, tongue, soft palate, and posterior wall of the pharynx).

netic field. Movements of the coil within the field produce variations in the signal picked up by the receivers. Magnetometry systems for the study of speech articulation were developed only within the last decade (Perkell et al., 1992; Schonle et al., 1987). This technique has excellent potential for future development and may become a fairly standard laboratory apparatus for recording speech movements. It presents no apparent risks to subjects and therefore can be used repetitively with subjects who vary widely in age. It is limited to the tracking of midline motions of discrete points represented by the coils.

Ultrasonography (or **ultrasound**) uses sound signals above the frequency range of human hearing. Ultrasonography in clinical applications typically uses a frequency above 1 MHz (1 MHz = 1,000,000 Hz). Sound waves are emitted from a specialized transducer that is placed in close contact with the body in the region to be visualized. As the sound waves pass through the body, they encounter different tissues and air spaces. At the boundaries between different tissues, part of the sound beam is reflected. These reflected waves, or echoes, are the means by which ultrasound can be used to examine the internal organs of the body. This procedure is used to image fetuses in medical examinations of pregnant women. The resolution is adequate to permit a determination of the baby's sex after a few weeks gestational age. As mentioned in Chapter 6, ultrasound can even be used to judge a fetus' response to sound.

Ultrasound was first used in the study of speech about three decades ago (Kelsey, Minifie, & Hixon, 1969; Minifie, Hixon, Kelsey, & Woodhouse, 1970). Since then it has been used to investigate several aspects of speech, including motions of the vocal folds, tongue, and lateral pharyngeal walls. Examples of recent applications are the study of cross-sectional tongue shapes during the production of fricatives (Stone, Faber, Raphael, & Shawker, 1992), the determination of tongue motions during speech and swallowing (Stone, 1990; Sonies, 1991), and imaging of the vocal tract (Stone, 1991).

Some methods do not record movement per se but rather articulatory contacts. **Palatography** is one such method. The original method of palatography used a coating of cornstarch that was applied to a speaker's palate. When the speaker produced a sound involving lingual contact against the palate, the tongue removed the cornstarch from the area of contact. The investigator then viewed or photographed the subject's palate to see where the articulatory contact was made. Although this method provided some important information, it was limited in its precision and could be used only for individual isolated sounds. It was essentially a static method used to determine regions of articulator contact. A more modern approach, developed about three decades ago (Fletcher, McCutcheon, & Wolf, 1975; Hardcastle, 1972; Palmer, 1973) is **dynamic palatography**, or **electropalatography** (EPG). This method uses a pseudopalate (false palate) that is embedded with tiny electrodes. When the speaker touches the tongue to the pseudopalate, the electrodes record the regions of contact. In modern applications of EPG, a computer is used to process the data (Hardcastle, Gibbon, & Nicolaidis, 1991). EPG analyses for selected English consonants studied by Stone and Lundberg (1996) are shown in Figure 8–4. This illustration demonstrates how EPG can reveal variations in tongue contact with the palate, including a central groove for the fricatives, complete oral closure for the nasals [n] and [ŋ], lateral opening for [l], and considerable midline opening for the glides and the rhotic.

Aerodynamics

As mentioned in Chapter 2, aerodynamics is part of the larger field of fluid mechanics. Aerodynamics is the study of the motion of air. During speaking, we move air through the speech production system, and the air movements are therefore a useful means of representing the process of speech production. Aerodynamic recordings have a long history in speech research and they are used today for both research and clinical purposes (Shadle, 1997; Warren, 1996). Figure 8–5 shows some of the possible aerodynamic quantities that might be studied in speech. This illustration pertains to measures of air pressure and airflow. The air pressures include: alveolar air pressure (the pressure within the alveoli of the lungs), subglottal air pressure (the pressure recorded beneath the vocal folds), intraoral air pressure (the pressure within the oral cavity), and intranasal (or nasal) air pressure (the pressure within the nasal tract). The airflow quantities include: transglottal airflow (the airflow through the glottis), oral airflow (the airflow through the oral cavity), and nasal airflow (the airflow through the nares).

Table 8–2 lists the primary functional significance for the aerodynamic variables shown in Figure 8–5. The essential idea is that these variables can reveal much about basic processes of speech and voice production.

The quantities of air pressure and airflow can be used to derive other quantities of interest, especially volume and resistance. A volume is a quantity of air and is often calculated by integrating (summing) airflow values. For example, the volume of air expired during a speech event is obtained by integrating the instantaneous airflow during the event. Aerodynamic resistance refers to the opposition to airflow

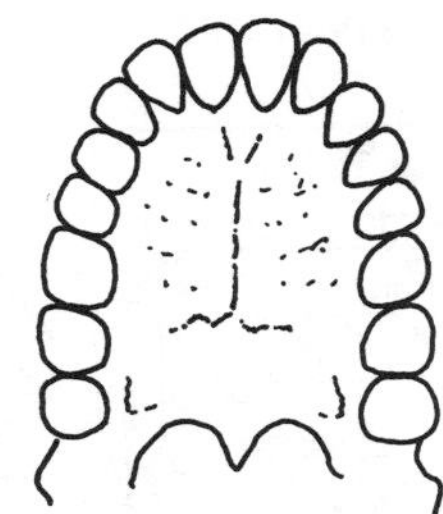

Inferior view of hard palate

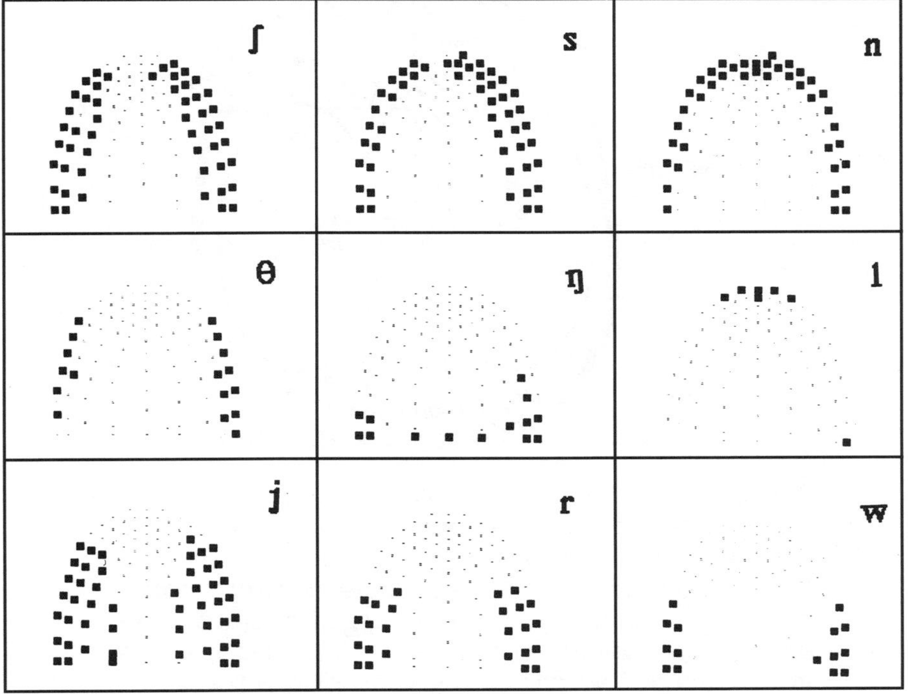

EPG patterns for selected English consonants

Figure 8–4. Palatal contact regions for selected consonants, based on data obtained by electropalatography. (The contact regions shown in the bottom of the illustration are reprinted from "Three-Dimensional Tongue Surface Shapes of English Consonants," by M. Stone and A. Lundberg, 1996, *Journal of the Acoustical Society of America, 99*, p. 3734. Reprinted with permission from the American Institute of Physics.)

at some region of the speech production system. Among the most commonly used measures of aeodynamic resistance in speech are laryngeal resistance and velopharyngeal (nasal) resistance. These resistance measures have been used clinically to assess the efficiency of vocal fold vibration or the adequacy of velopharyngeal function.

A device commonly used to measure airflow or volume during speech is the **pneu-**

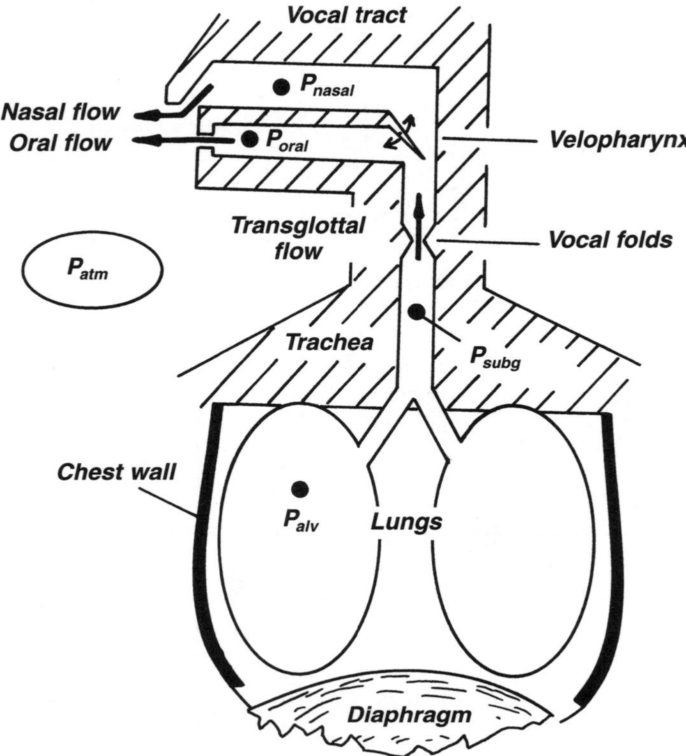

Figure 8–5. Schematic illustration of various pressures and flows that can be used to study speech production. The pressures are symbolized with a filled circle and the flows with an arrow. The air pressures are: alveolar (lung) air pressure, P_{alv}; subglottal air pressure, P_{subg}; intraoral air pressure, P_{oral}, and intranasal air pressure, P_{nasal}. The flows are transglottal air flow, oral airflow, and nasal air flow.

motachograph, pictured in Figure 8–6. Air pressures typically are recorded with a pressure transducer connected to a tube that inserts into a suitable part of the speech production system. Figure 8–7 shows three pressures that can be recorded simultaneously to study speech production: esophageal pressure, or $P_{esophageal}$, (measured by a balloon that is swallowed and held in the esophagus), intraoral pressure, or P_{oral}, (measured by an open-ended tube inserted into the oral cavity), and subglottal pressure, or $P_{subglottal}$, (measured by an open-ended tube inserted through a tracheal puncture). Intraoral air pressure is discussed further later in this chapter.

The aerodynamic quantities can be used to study specific functions of parts of the speech system, as follows.

Phonatory airflow (mean airflow during vowel production) is one index of the efficiency of phonation. An inefficient larynx often allows excessive loss of air during vocal fold vibration. An efficient larynx maintains vibration with a moderate flow of air. The airflow used in normal phonation by adult males and females is about 110 ml/s and 100 ml/s, respectively. During whisper, the airflow increases severalfold over the value obtained for phonation. A person with severe breathy or hoarse

Table 8–2. Major aerodynamic variables and their functional significance in the study of speech production.

Aerodynamic Variable	Significance
Air Pressure	
Alveolar air pressure	Respiratory driving pressure measured in the lungs
Subglottal air pressure	Respiratory driving pressure measured below the glottis (approximates the alveolar air pressure)
Intraoral air pressure	Pressure recorded within the oral cavity (approximates the subglottal air pressure when the vocal folds are abducted, but is typically less than subglottal air pressure when folds are adducted)
Intranasal air pressure	Pressure recorded within the nasal cavity
Airflow	
Transglottal airflow	Airflow through the glottis
Oral airflow	Airflow through the oral cavity
Nasal airflow	Airflow through the nasal cavity

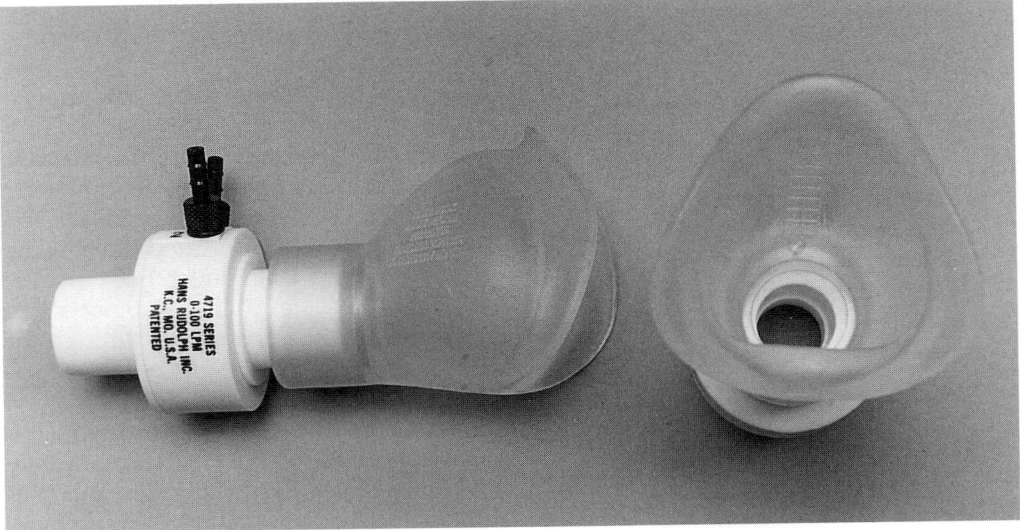

Figure 8–6. Photograph of a pneumotachograph, a device used to obtain measurements of airflow. (Reproduced with permission from Hans Rudolph, Inc., 7200 Wyandotte, Kansas City, MO.)

voice quality often has very high flow values and therefore a less efficient voice production system. Phonatory airflow is fairly easily measured by means of a mask that fits over the subject's mouth and terminates in a pneumotachograph (as shown in Figure 8–6).

Phonation air volume (the total volume of air used in a specified speech task) can be

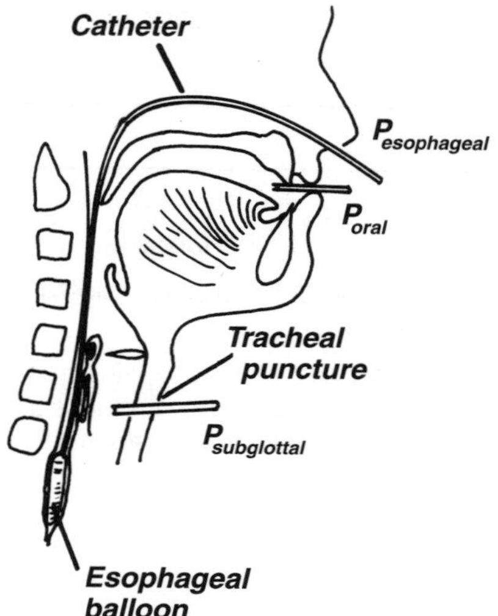

Figure 8–7. Illustration of techniques used to make simultaneous recordings of intraoral air pressure, tracheal (subglottal) air pressure, and esophageal air pressure.

used to assess respiratory capacity and function. A speaker with an impaired respiratory system may have a reduced capacity to move air into and out of the lungs. For example, an individual with a partially paralyzed respiratory system may have a diminished ability to push air out of the lungs. Phonation air volume is integrated (accumulated) airflow. The integration can be accomplished by special hardware instruments or by a computer.

Intraoral air pressure (the level of air pressure that is impounded behind an articulatory obstruction in the oral cavity) can be measured to determine the effectiveness of velopharyngeal function for oral consonants and to determine if the lungs have delivered sufficient air pressure for speech articulation. If the velopharynx fails to close tightly, the speaker typically cannot produce high levels of intraoral air pressure, because air escapes through the velopharynx. Intraoral air pressure is often measured for the **pressure consonants** (consonant sounds that are associated with high values of intraoral air pressure, such as the consonants in the word *showstopper*). The usual method of recording intraoral air pressure is to insert a small tube into the mouth behind the point of articulatory obstruction, as shown in Figure 8–7. The tube is then connected to a pressure transducer that converts the air pressure signal to a voltage signal that can be recorded or displayed.

Nasal airflow (the flow recorded at the nares) is an index of nasalization or nasal emission. In normal speech, nasal airflow is observed only in connection with nasal breathing or with the production of nasal consonants. But individuals who have abnormalities in velopharyngeal function may exhibit nasal flow even for oral consonants. Recording of nasal airflow is a valuable technique to evaluate the function of the velopharyngeal system of speech production. Nasal airflow can be recorded by means of a nose mask connected to a pneumotachograph.

Subglottal air pressure (the pressure developed below the vocal folds) is a measure of the respiratory driving pressure. This pressure can be used to determine if a speaker has a weakened respiratory system. It is not easily measured directly and noninvasively. One direct but invasive method for determining subglottal air pressure is to insert a needle through the tracheal wall at a point just below the larynx (Figure 8–7). A more indirect method is to record the maximum intraoral air pressure developed during voiceless consonants, under the assumption that this pressure approximates the air pressure below the vocal folds. Esophageal air pressure (Figure 8–7) also has been used to estimate subglottal air pressure, but a correction for lung volume is required to obtain accurate information.

Many laboratories that record aerodynamic quantities use a combination of pressures, flows, and volumes. A simple example of airflow and air pressure recording is shown in Figure 8–8. This schematic drawing

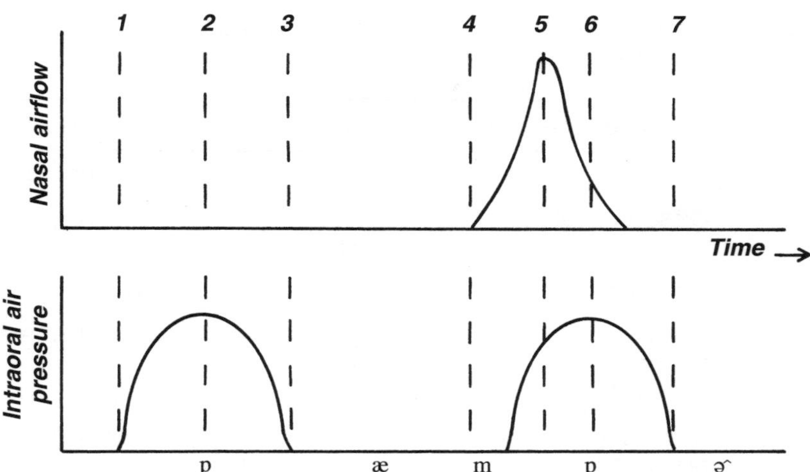

Figure 8–8. Schematic drawing of nasal airflow and intraoral air pressure during production of the word *pamper*. The numerals 1–7 represent the following aerodynamic events: 1 = formation of bilabial closure, evidenced by increase in intraoral air pressure; 2 = maximum of intraoral air pressure; 3 = release of bilabial closure, evidenced by drop of intraoral air pressure to baseline level for vowel; 4 = opening of velopharynx, as indicated by onset of nasal airflow; 5 = maximum of nasal airflow; 6 = maximum of intraoral air pressure; and 7 = release of bilabial closure, evidenced by drop of intraoral air pressure to baseline level.

shows nasal airflow and intraoral air pressure during production of the word *pamper*. Notice in particular: Intraoral air pressure builds up during the bilabial closures for the [p] sounds, and nasal airflow reaches its peak during the [m] sound. The [mp] requires a highly coordinated action of the lips and velopharynx, and this coordination is reflected in the aerodynamic recording.

Table 8–3 summarizes selected aerodynamic properties for major classes of speech sounds. The properties include oral airflow, nasal airflow, intranasal air pressure, and intraoral air pressure.

In summary, a variety of physiological signals can be used to study speech, including regional activity in the central nervous system, neural impulses from the peripheral nerves, electrical signals from contracting muscles, forces developed by contracting muscles, displacements of body structures, and air pressures and flows. Techniques have been developed to record each of these types of signals. The remainder of the chapter discusses selected problems in speech physiology and summarizes quantitative data that have been obtained from physiologic studies.

PHYSIOLOGICAL REQUIREMENTS OF SPEECH PRODUCTION

One general line of inquiry is to determine the physiological requirements of speech. This issue is noted briefly in previous chapters. For example, it is mentioned in Chapter

Table 8–3. Summary of physiologic properties of major sound classes. OR = oral; NA = nasal; IO = intraoral; IN = intranasal.

Sound Class	Degree of Constriction	Airflow	Air Pressure
Vowels	Open vocal tract	Low OR flow	Minimal IO pressure
Stops	Closed vocal tract	No OR flow during closure	High IO pressure during closure
Nasals	Open nasal tract	Low NA flow	Minimal IN pressure
Fricatives	Constricted to narrow opening	High OR flow	High IO pressure
Affricates	Closed, then narrowed	No OR flow, then high OR flow	High IO pressure
Glides	Nearly as open as for vowels	Low OR flow	Minimal IO pressure

4 that speech is not particularly taxing as far as normal respiratory function is concerned. In most individuals, the maximum respiratory capability for air volume, flow, or pressure far exceeds the typical requirements of speech. Is this true for other aspects of speech production? A partial answer to this question is given in Table 8–4, which shows the speech requirements and biophysical maxima for several variables relevant to speech. In general, the requirements for speech fall comfortably within the maximum physiological range (Kent, Kent, & Rosenbek, 1989). The respiratory system can move considerably more air and generate much higher air pressures than are needed for speech, the vocal folds can adjust to a much wider range of vocal frequencies than typically occurs for speech, the respiratory-phonatory system can produce greater sound pressure levels than are usually needed for communication, and the articulatory system can produce greater compression forces than are routine for speech production. However, this statement should be qualified somewhat for young children and the elderly. For these individuals, the physiological reserve may not be great compared to the demands of speech.

Ordinary speech does approach the physiological limit for one aspect: the production of serial elements. Whether measured in segments, syllables, or movements per second, speech of the routine variety is produced at a rate that nearly matches the fastest possible rate. Furthermore, the maximum rates were typically obtained for a simple repetition task, such as saying the syllable [tə] as fast as possible in a repetitive train. It is remarkable that conversational speech, with all its phonetic variation, can be produced at a rate that is about as fast as that for rapid repetition of the same syllable. One interpretation is that we often talk at close to a maximal rate, perhaps in the interest of speedy communication.

Rapid syllable repetition is also called **diadochokinesis**. This task often is used in speech pathology to assess a speaker's ability to make rapid alternating movements of the articulators. Adults typically can produce about 6 to 7 [tə] syllables in one second. Children tend to be slower than adults until the age of puberty. Data on the maximum rate of [tə] repetition are shown in Figure 8–9. The circles and diamonds represent data for children reported in

Table 8–4. Biophysical requirements for speech compared to maximum physiologic capability for healthy young adult men.

	Speech Requirement	Biophysical Capability
Air volume	25–40% vital capacity (1–2 liters of air)	100% vital capacity (4–5 liters of air)
Vocal frequency	75–200 Hz (1 octave)	50–1000 Hz (3–4 octaves)
Sound pressure	85 dB SPL re 20 μPa	100–120 dB SPL re 20 μPa
Air pressure	1.3–2.2 kPa	10–20 kPa
Mechanical force	Less than 2 N	20 N
Sound repetition rate	4–7 syllables/s 8–14 sounds/s	4–7 syllables/s 8–14 sounds/s
Phonation time	1–10 s	20–35 s

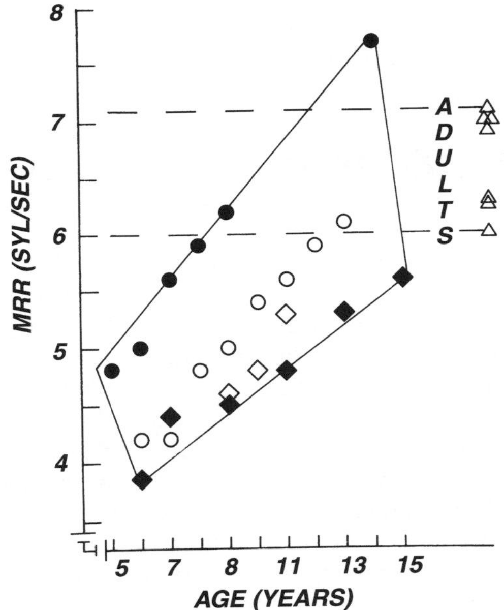

Figure 8–9. Mean diadochokinetic (syllables per second) for the syllable (tə) produced by children of various ages, by men, and by women. (Reprinted from "Maximum Performance Tests of Speech Production," by R. D. Kent, J. F. Kent, and J. C. Rosenbek, 1987, *Journal of Speech and Hearing Disorders, 52,* p. 380. Reprinted with permission from the American Speech-Language-Hearing Association.)

◇ = data from "Diadochokinetic movements of nine, ten, and eleven-year-old children," by B. Blomquist (1950) *Journal of Speech and Hearing Disorders, 15,* pp. 159–164.

● = data from "Clinical measurements of the speed of tongue and lip movements in British children with normal speech," by B. Canning and M. Rose (1974) *British Journal of Disorders of Communication, 9,* 45–50.

◆ = data from "Time-by-count measurement of diadochokinetic syllable rate," by S. Fletcher (1972) *Journal of Speech and Hearing Research, 15,* 763–770.

○ = data from "Norms and maximum repetitive rates for certain sounds established with the sylrater," by J. V. Irwin and D. Becklund (1953) *Journal of Speech and Hearing Research, 18,* 149–160.

△ = means reported in several studies of adults; see Kent et al. (1987) for sources.

three different studies cited in the figure caption. The triangles represent mean data for adults from several different studies. Apparently, the rate of syllable repetition increases from the age of 5 years to at least the age of 9 years. But it is also evident that the mean rates differ considerably across the different studies. This variance in results limits the usefulness of this task. However, the data indicate that almost any speaker from the age of 5 years through adulthood should be able to produce at least 4 syllables/s. This rate can be taken as a minimum requirement for speech production at normal rates.

Producing speech at faster rates in terms of phonetic events per second does not necessarily mean that the actual rates of articulatory movement are increased. Speakers may accomplish the diadochokinetic task "by adopting relatively stable articulatory configurations or postures that appear to be functionally advantageous for rapid formation and release of constrictions" (Westbury & Dembowski, 1993, p. 23). In particular, many speakers produce faster rates of syllable repetition by minimizing the articulatory distance to be covered in the alternating movements. To speak faster, they move the articulators a shorter distance. For example, for [tə], the speaker may hold the tongue close to the alveolar ridge so the consonant-to-vowel movement is minimized. Westbury and Dembowski (1993) speculated that some abnormal performances by individuals with speech disorders may actually be a failure to assume optimal postural solutions for the rapid rate task. Perhaps young children also do not assume these optimal solutions, which could partially explain why children have slower diadochokinetic rates than adults.

COMMONLY USED PHYSIOLOGICAL INDEXES OF SPEECH

The preceding section discussed various maximal biophysical efforts compared to biophysical measures of speech. Because speech typically does not require anywhere near the maximal physiologic capability for airflow, air pressure, or mechanical force, measures of maximal effort are not necessarily highly informative about speech production. For many practical purposes, it is desirable to have measures that relate more directly to typical speech production. The following measures are examples of such practically directed indexes.

Intraoral Air Pressure

A practical index for intraoral air pressure is the "5 for 5 rule" (Netsell, 1985; Netsell & Hixon, 1978). This rule states that a subject should be able to maintain 5 cm H_2O for 5 s. This pressure index is suitable to support the production of a moderately loud sentence of at least 20 words or so. If equipment is not available to measure intraoral air pressure, then the simple method described in Exercise 2–2 can be used. The subject simply blows into a straw or tube that is immersed to a depth of 5 cm in a glass of water. The "5 for 5 rule" requires that the subject be able to blow a steady stream of bubbles through the straw for a period of 5 s. This rule permits a straightforward assessment of respiratory power for speech. The same apparatus can have clinical value as a means of training for individuals who lack respiratory control for speech.

Airflow

As noted previously, the oral airflow for vowel production is about 110 ml/s for men and 100 ml/s for women. These are the expected values for a task of sustained phonation and normal voice quality. Whispered or breathy voice has higher flow. Therefore, oral airflow can be used to study disorders of voice (considered further in Chapter 12). The consonants with the highest airflow are the voiceless fricatives in the words *see* ([s]) and *she* ([ʃ]). A speaker should be able to produce a sustained fricative [s] or [ʃ] with an airflow between 300–500 ml/s.

Rate of Speech Sound Production

Normal adult speakers should be capable of producing at least four syllables per second for repetitions of [tə] (*tUH*) or [pə] (*pUH*). The evaluation of velopharyngeal valving can be done with words that require a rapid sequence of velopharyngeal closure and opening. For example, rapid repetitions of a word like *pamper* or *bumper* can be used to assess velopharyngeal function. Normal speakers should be able to produce at least one word per second with these test words. Tests of syllable repetition are useful clinically to assess movement disorders.

MULTIARTICULATE RECORDINGS OF SPEECH PRODUCTION

A multiarticulate system is one that has multiple articulations. Speech production is accomplished with several articulators, many of which can be simultaneously active. This manifold potential for movement is one of the challenging aspects to the study of speech physiology. Ideally, the investigator would be able to record movements of the tongue, jaw, lips, velum, and related structures so that their composite effects can be determined. Few methods afford such a rich opportunity for data collection. X-ray methods have been particularly useful in speech research, but must be used with great caution because of the danger posed by radiation. Sample data from X-ray recordings are used here to demonstrate the multiarticulate nature of speech.

As a first look at the multiarticulate properties of speech, we consider the phoneme /r/. Phoneticians have written extensively about this sound, especially because it appears to be quite variable in the way it is produced. Although various types of articulation have been described, two major types are the retroflex and the bunched, as mentioned in Chapter 3. The retroflex variant of /r/ is made with a backward pointing of the tongue, and the bunched variant is made with a blunt shaping of the tongue blade. Figure 8–10 shows the bunched form of /r/ as it occurs in the syllables [ra] and [ri]. Notice that, even for this one type of /r/ articulation, the tongue assumes somewhat different positions. Apparently, the location of the bunched articulation is influenced by the vowel following /r/, such that /r/ before /a/ is relatively back and /r/ before /i/ is relatively forward. Figure 8–10 also shows that this form of

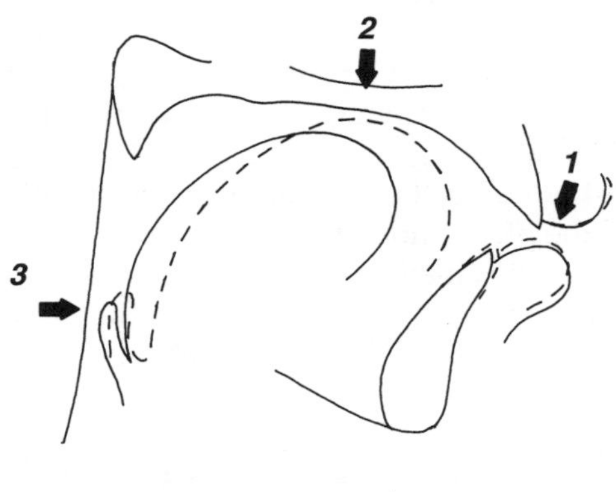

Figure 8–10. X-ray tracings of the bunched form of phoneme /r/. Articulatory positions are shown for the /r/ in two different syllables: (ra) and (ri). The numerals 1, 2, and 3 point to three regions of constriction commonly formed in /r/ production.

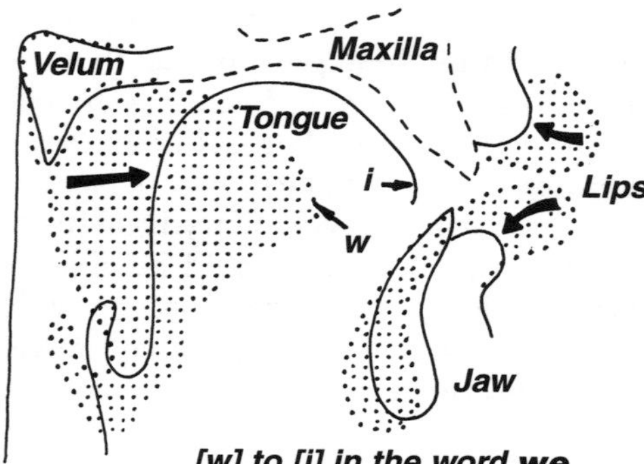

Figure 8–11. The articulatory configurations for the onglide of (w) and the steady-state of vowel (i) in the word *we*. The configurations were obtained from cinefluorography of an adult female.

/r/ is produced with three regions of vocal tract constriction: (1) labial, (2) midpalatal, and (3) pharyngeal. The X-ray method is quite suitable for studying variations in vocal tract shaping, even though the information typically pertains to a single plane, the midsagittal section.

To make matters more complex, we next consider the production of a single syllable. The syllable [wi], as in the word *we*, is a good example, because it is produced with coordinated movements of the tongue and lips. A diagrammatic example of this articulation was given in Chapter 3. Figure 8–11 depicts the articulatory adjustments in the production of this syllable, as determined by cinefluorography (X-ray motion pictures). In the transition from the glide [w] to the vowel [i], the body of the tongue moves forward, the lips go from a protruded to a retracted configuration, and the jaw closes slightly. The position of the velum changes very little because both phonetic elements are nonnasal. An interesting feature of this syllable is that the movements of the tongue and lips are tightly coordinated. They begin to move at the same time and they complete their movement at the same time.

Of course, articulatory patterns become considerably more complex in the case of words, phrases, and sentences. Figure 8–12 shows movements of several articulators during production of the sentence, *Soon the snow began to melt*. The movement data were obtained from cinefluorography with a filming rate of 150 frames/s, so that articulatory positions were sampled at intervals of 6.7 ms. The multiple-parameter graph in Figure 8–12 illustrates only part of the complexity of speech production because it does not show data for the respiratory or laryngeal systems. However, the graph suffices to show that speech involves simultaneous movements of several vocal tract structures.

Careful study of Figure 8–12 reveals several examples of coarticulation. The first word *soon* involves a sequence of oral consonant + vowel + nasal consonant. Because the nasal consonant requires velopharyngeal opening, the velum must descend for this sound. As Figure 8–12 shows, the actual descending motion of the velum begins shortly after the /s/ sound is produced. Therefore, the vowel is nasalized.

MULTISYSTEM PHYSIOLOGICAL RECORDINGS

If we wish to obtain data for the entire process of speech production, it is necessary to make recordings of activity in the respiratory, laryngeal, and supralaryngeal systems. No single technology is suited for this purpose. Therefore, such studies may use several technologies, such as electromyography, aerodynamics, movement transduction, and acoustics. Subject preparation can be time consuming, and the data can present a formidable challenge to analyze.

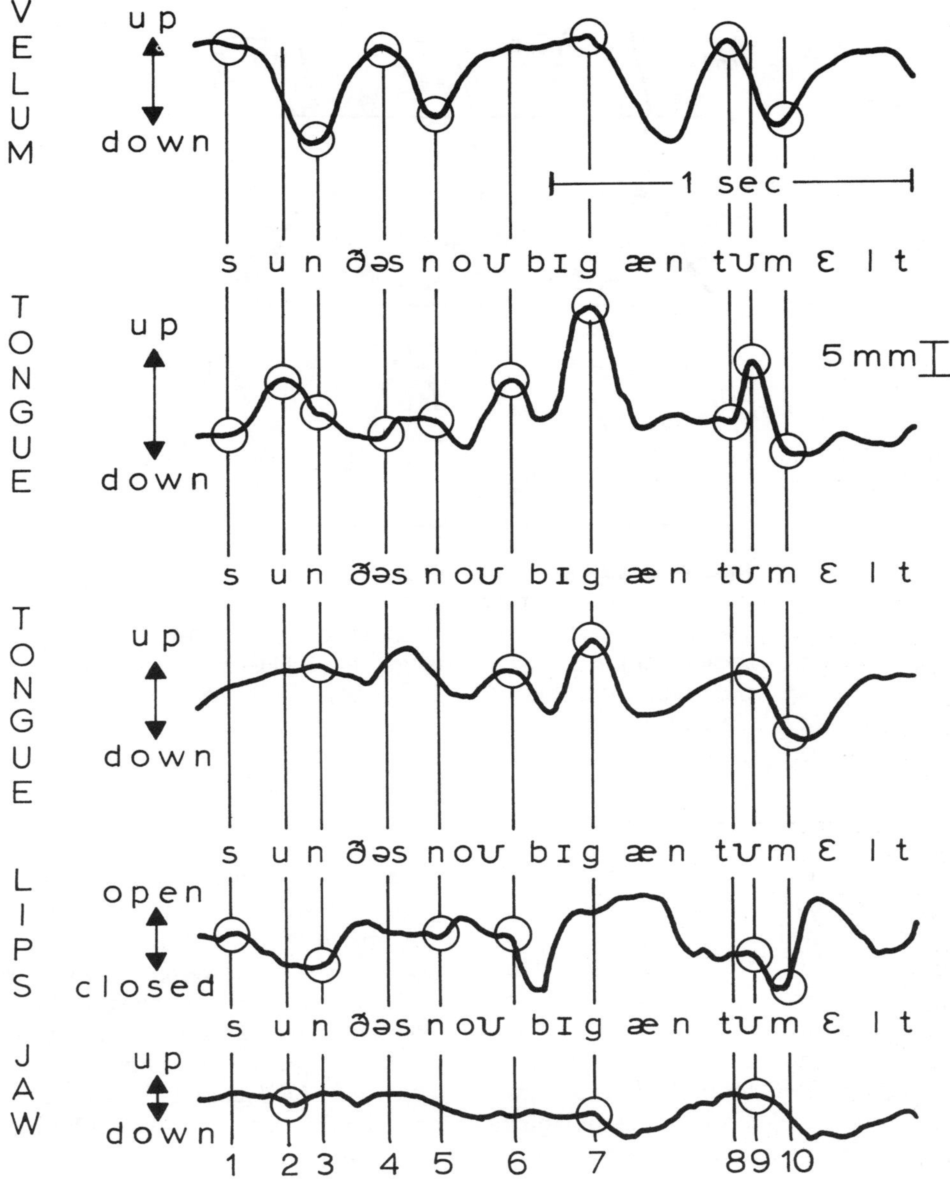

Figure 8–12. Multiparameter articulatory record obtained from measurements of a cinefluorographic film of the sentence, *Soon the snow began to melt*. Data are shown for vertical movements of the velum, vertical movements of the tongue body, vertical movements of the tongue blade, opening and closing motions of the lips, and opening and closing movements of the mandible. The small circles and vertical lines indicate important points in coordination of the articulatory events. Some of the numbered events are used in Exercise 8–4.

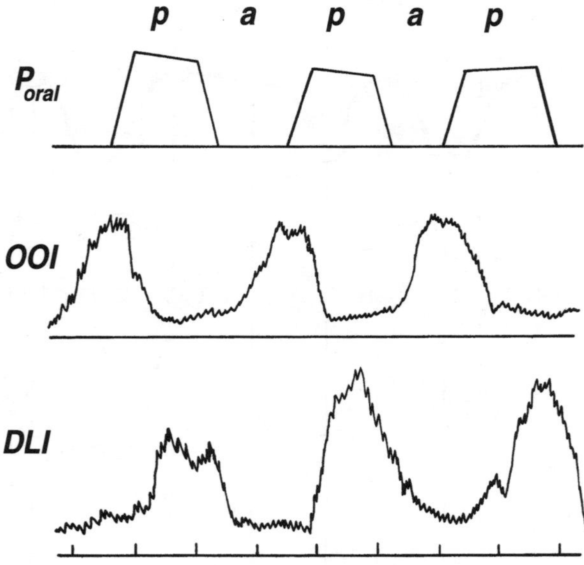

Figure 8–13. Example of combined aerodynamic and electromyographic recordings of speech production events. Idealized data are shown for intraoral air pressure (P_{oral}), EEG from orbicularis oris inferior (OOI), and EEG from depressor labii inferior (DLI). Contraction of OOI closes the lips, and contraction of DLI opens the lips. See text for additional description.

However, when a small number of techniques are used in a directed way, the information obtained can be highly valuable. Figure 8–13 shows three data channels that might be used to study the events associated with production of the syllable [pa]. The channels are, from top to bottom, intraoral air pressure, EMG for orbicularis oris inferior (OOI), and EMG for depressor labii inferior (DLI). The trace for intraoral air pressure defines the intervals of bilabial closure, given that the air pressure increases when the lips close and decreases when the lips open. The trace for OOI shows the muscle activity associated with closure of the lips, and the trace for DLI shows activity associated with opening of the lips. Note that the activity for OOI and DLI is essentially reciprocal: When OOI is active, DLI is inactive (and vice versa).

CONCLUSION AND SUMMARY

Speech physiology complements perceptual and acoustic analyses of speech (both of which are considered in later chapters) by providing information on (1) individual structures involved in speaking, (2) the interaction of different structures or systems, and (3) fundamental processes such as muscle contraction, air pressure regulation, or different ways of closing the velopharyngeal port. Because no single technique can answer all relevant questions for all structures used in speech, a number of different techniques have been developed. As a result, the understanding of speech physiology reflects a synthesis of several different kinds of data. These methods also have clinical application for individuals with speech or voice disorders.

Through the efforts of many speech scientists, the physiology of speaking is now understood in several general respects. However, much more needs to be learned about this process to give a full account. This chapter pertains to some methods that are most commonly employed for the study of speech physiology. The methods themselves are being continually improved; and, as the improvements are made, valuable sets of data are being collected to illuminate this field of study. The scope of the possible laboratory observations is considerable, including bioelectrical signals, structural movements, and aerodynamic events. Each of these methods can give the speech scientist a glimpse into the functions of speech production. Each technique has its advantages and disadvantages, and these should be carefully considered in designing a study or interpreting data. These laboratory techniques can be coupled with another powerful analysis considered in the next chapter, the acoustic analysis of speech.

On The Reference Shelf

Recommended to readers who seek additional discussion of the basic issues introduced in this chapter.

Baken, R. J. (1987). *Clinical measurement of speech and voice*. San Diego: Singular Publishing Group.
A thorough discussion of basic instrumental procedures in the study of speech and voice; a valuable reference book.

Stone, M. (1997). Laboratory techniques for investigating speech articulation. In W. Hardcastle & J. Laver (Eds.), *The handbook of phonetic sciences* (pp. 11–32). Oxford, England: Blackwell.
A contemporary summary of basic tools for the study of speech movements.

Warren, D. W. (1996). Regulation of speech aerodynamics. In N. J. Lass (Ed.), *Principles of experimental phonetics* (pp. 46–92). St. Louis: Mosby.
A thorough discussion of aerodynamics in speech production.

Zwirner, E., & Zwirner, K. (1970). *Principles of phonometrics*. [Trans. H. Bluhme.] University, AL: University of Alabama Press.
A scholarly account of the history of experimental phonetics.

Chapter References

Abbs, J., & Gilbert, B. (1973). A strain gauge transduction system for lip and jaw motion in two dimensions. *Journal of Speech and Hearing Research, 16*, 248–256.

Barlow, S., & Abbs, J. (1983). Force transducers for the evaluation of labial, lingual, and mandibular motor impairments. *Journal of Speech and Hearing Research, 26*, 616–621.

Croft, C. B., Shprintzen, R. J., & Rakoff, S. J. (1981). Patterns of velopharyngeal valving in normal and cleft palate subjects: A multi-view videofluoroscopic and nasendoscopic study. *Laryngoscope, 91*, 265–271.

Fletcher, S., McCutcheon, M., & Wolf, M. (1975). Dynamic palatometry. *Journal of Speech and Hearing Research, 18*, 812–819.

Hardcastle, W. (1972). The use of electropalatography in phonetic research. *Phonetica, 25*, 197–215.

Hardcastle, W., Gibbon, F., & Nicolaidis, K. (1991). EPG data reduction methods and their implications for studies of lingual coarticulation. *Journal of Phonetics, 19,* 251–266.

Kelsey, C. A., Minifie, F. D., & Hixon, T. J. (1969). Applications of ultrasound in speech research. *Journal of Speech and Hearing Research, 12,* 564–575.

Kent, R. D., Kent, J. F., & Rosenbek, J. C. (1987). Maximum performance measures of speech production. *Journal of Speech and Hearing Disorders, 52,* 367–387.

Kent, R. D., & Moll, K. L. (1972). Cinefluorographic analysis of selected lingual consonants. *Journal of Speech and Hearing Research, 15,* 453–473.

Lashley, K. S. (1951). The problem of serial order in behavior. In L. A. Jeffress (Ed.), *Cerebral mechanisms in behavior* (pp. 112–136). New York: Wiley.

Minifie, F., Hixon, T., Kelsey, C., & Woodhouse, R. (1970). Lateral pharyngeal wall movement during speech production. *Journal of Speech and Hearing Research, 13,* 584–594.

Moll, K. L. (1960). Cinefluorographic techniques in speech research. *Journal of Speech and Hearing Research, 3,* 227–241.

Netsell, R. (1985). Treating the dysarthrias. In J. Darby (Ed.), *Speech and language evaluation in neurology: Adult disorders* (pp. 363–392). Orlando, FL: Grune & Stratton.

Netsell, R., & Hixon, R. (1978). A noninvasive method for clinically estimating subglottal air pressure. *Journal of Speech and Hearing Disorders, 43,* 326–330.

Palmer, J. (1973). Dynamic palatography. *Phonetica, 28,* 76–85.

Perkell, J., Cohen, M., Svirksy, M., Matthies, M., Garabieta, I., & Jakson, M. (1992). Electromagnetic midsagittal articulometer (EMMA) systems for transducing speech articulatory movements. *Journal of the Acoustical Society of America, 92,* 3078–3096.

Schonle, P., Grabe, K., Wenig, P., Hohne, J., Schrader, J., & Conrad, B. (1987). Electromagnetic articulography: Use of alternating magnetic fields for tracking movements of multiple points inside and outside of the vocal tract. *Brain and Language, 31,* 26–35.

Shadle, C. H. (1997). The aerodynamics of speech. In W. Hardcastle & J. Laver (Eds.), *The handbook of phonetic sciences* (pp. 33–64). Oxford, England: Blackwell.

Shprintzen, R. J. (1992). Assessment of velopharyngeal function: Nasopharyngoscopy and multiview videofluoroscopy. In L. Brodsky, L. Holt, & D. H. Ritter-Schmidt, *Craniofacial anomalies: An interdisciplinary approach* (pp. 196–207). St. Louis: Mosby-Year Book.

Skolnick, M. L., McCall, G. N., & Barnes, M. (1973). The sphincteric mechanism of velopharyngeal closure. *Cleft Palate Journal, 10,* 286–305.

Sonies, B. (1991). Ultrasound imaging and swallowing. In M. Donner & B. Jones (Eds.), *Normal and abnormal swallowing: Imaging in diagnosis and therapy* (pp. 237–260). New York: Springer.

Sperry, R. (1988). Recollections of R. H. Stetson. In J. A. S. Kelso & K. G. Munhall (Eds.), *R. H. Stetson's motor phonetics: A retrospective edition* (pp. 12–14). Boston: College-Hill Press.

Stone, M. (1990). A three–dimensional model of tongue movement based on ultrasound and x-ray microbeam data. *Journal of the Acoustical Society of America, 87,* 2207–2217.

Stone, M. (1991). Imaging the tongue and vocal tract. *British Journal of Disorders of Communication, 26,* 11–23.

Stone, M., Faber, A., Raphael, L., & Shawker, T. (1992). Cross-sectional tongue shape and linguopalatal contact patterns in [s], [ʃ], and [l]. *Journal of Phonetics, 20,* 253–270.

Stone, M., & Lundberg, A. (1996). Three-dimensional tongue surface shapes of English consonants. *Journal of the Acoustical Society of America, 99,* 3728–3737.

Warren, D. W. (1996). Regulation of speech aerodynamics. In N. J. Lass (Ed.), *Principles of experimental phonetics* (pp. 46–92). St. Louis: Mosby.

Westbury, J., & Dembowski, J. (1993). Articulatory kinematics of normal diadochokinetic performance. *Annual Bulletin, Research Institute of Logopedics and Phoniatrics, University of Tokyo, 27,* 13–36.

Zwirner, E., & Zwirner, K. (1970). *Principles of phonometrics.* [Trans. H. Bluhme.] University: University of Alabama Press.

Exercises

8-1. Describe the relative patterns of labial movement, voicing, and velopharyngeal valving for the following words: *bomb, mom, mob, mop, pom,* and *pop*. For example, for the word *bomb,* the lips make closure for the initial consonants, the entire word is voiced, and the velopharyngeal valve opens for the final [m]. It may be helpful to describe the events with a chart such as the one below.

	b	a	m
Labial Movement	close ———	open ———	close
Voicing	voicing ———	———	———
Velopharyngeal Valving	valve closed ———	———	open

8-2. Explain the EPG patterns shown for English consonants in Figure 8–4. For example, the contact patterns for [s] might be explained as follows: The tongue is closed against the palate except for a narrow midline groove. This groove is the point of generation of turbulence noise.

8-3. Draw a graph that represents the expected patterns of intraoral air pressure and nasal air flow for the following words: *popping, mopping,* and *pumping*. Use Figure 8–8 as a guide.

8-4. Using the data in Figure 8–12, interpret the movements shown to give an articulatory description for the following phonetic events: event 1, [s] in *soon;* event 2, [u] in *soon;* event 5, [n] in *snow,* event 7, [g] in *began;* event 8, [t] in *to;* and event 10, [m] in *melt*. For example, for [s] in *soon,* the data show that (a) velum is raised, (b) the tongue body and blade are in relatively low positions, (c) the lips are mid-open, and (d) the jaw is mid-open.

8-5. With reference to Figure 8–5, describe the aerodynamic events (air pressures and flows) for the word *snowballing*. *Hint:* Begin with the alveolar air pressure and then describe the aerodynamic requirements for each sound in the word.

8-6. Speech sounds are only a part of human sound-producing capability. We also make a variety of nonspeech sounds, such as chirps, honks, roars, and hisses. Some people become highly proficient in making these sounds. Accomplished sound-makers can produce a variety of sound effects, including machinery and animals. A good source for nonspeech soundmaking is *Mouth Sounds* by Frederick R. Newman (New York: Workman Publishing, 1980). As an exercise in describing the physiology of nonspeech sound production, try to describe how a few nonspeech sounds are produced. Practice making a few sounds until you have a fairly good production. Then provide a description of articulatory, laryngeal, and respiratory actions for each. You might compare your analyses with others who have produced the same sounds.

CHAPTER 9

Acoustic Phonetics

> *"We open our mouths, force air from our lungs into our larynx, our voice box, and through an opening between our vocal cords, which vibrate. And then we speak . . . It seems so simple, but it's made it possible for empires to rise and fall; for children to reach small workable armistices with their parents, for corporations to control a nation as it were a great big wind-up bathtub toy; for lovers to run the emotional rapids of courtship, for societies to express their loftiest dreams or lowest prejudices."*
>
> (Diane Ackerman, *A Natural History of the Senses.* New York: Random House, 1990, p. 182.)

Speech and sound are so intimately connected in human communication that it can be difficult to imagine speech without sound. Frequently, only acoustic information is available about speech, as when we hear someone talking on the telephone or when we hear a recording of another person's speech. We are highly adept at retrieving a linguistic message from the acoustic signal. Obviously, then, the information needed for linguistic interpretation is latent in the sound stream of speech. Decades of research into speech acoustics have revealed how a listener is able to retrieve a linguistic message from the acoustic signal that a talker generates. Understanding has progressed to the point that computers are being programmed to "produce" and "understand" speech with a degree of accuracy that was only imagined 20 years ago. The field of acoustic phonetics has supplied the basic information that has enabled the development of speech technologies such as speech synthesis and computer speech recognition. Work in acoustic phonetics also has prepared the way for the investigation of disorders and dialects. This chapter summarizes some of the major discoveries in the field of acoustic phonetics. The chapter is divided into three major sections: acoustic theory of speech production, methods of acoustic analysis, and acoustic correlates of information sources in speech.

ACOUSTIC THEORY OF SPEECH PRODUCTION

This discussion begins with a very simple version of a vocal tract and then progress through gradual modifications of this simple version until the result is very close to the human vocal tract. The general direction is from relatively simple ideas to more complex ideas. A major tool of science is **modeling**, or the construction of some replica of the actual physical object under study. Physical objects, whether galaxies, brains, plants, or vocal tracts are often too complex to be studied in their full natural detail. The scientist gains initial understanding by working with a simplified model of the physical system. If the model is carefully chosen, it can provide important insights into the real system. Much of what follows is based largely on work by Fant (1960), a principal contributor to the modern acoustic theory of speech production.

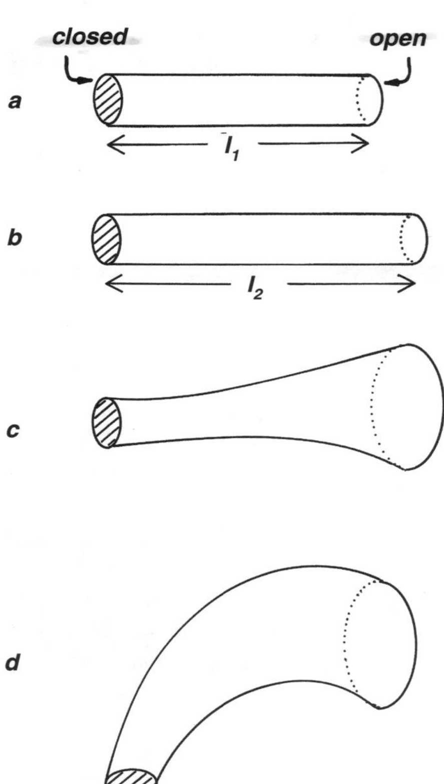

Figure 9–1. Simple acoustic pipe models: **a.** A uniform straight tube of length l_1 closed at one end and open at the other. **b.** A uniform straight tube of length l_2 closed at one end and open at the other. **c.** A straight tube of varying cross-sectional diameter. **d.** A bent tube of varying cross-sectional diameter.

Figure 9–1 is an overview of the modeling process summarized in this chapter. The initial model is a tube or pipe with a uniform diameter along its length, as shown in part **a** of the illustration. This tube is closed at one end and open at the other. The closed end represents the glottis, which, for initial purposes, can be regarded as tightly closed. That is, the vibrating vocal folds act like a closed end of the tube. The open end represents the lips separated for the production of vowel sounds. The first modification of this simple model is to vary the length of the tube, to make it shorter or longer. Lengthening is shown in part **b** of Figure 9–1 by an increase in tube length, l. The pipe in part **b** has a length l_2 that is greater than the length l_1 of the pipe in part **a**. The next modification is to shape the pipe so that its diameter varies along its length (part **c**). Now, instead of having a uniform cross-sectional diameter, the tube flares at its open (lip) end. The final modification is to bend the tube (part **d**) until it resembles the distinctive right-angled configuration described in Chapter 5. Imagine that the bent pipe in part **d** is fitted into the supralaryngeal system (surrounded by muscles, bones, ligaments, and other tissues) and you have the basic idea of acoustic modeling.

A major premise of this discussion is that important physical laws and relations unify the various vocal tract models in Figure 9–1. In particular, this chapter discusses resonances that can be determined from the dimensions of the different tube models. As will be clear in the final section of the chapter, these resonances are a primary molder of the sound stream that we hear as the acoustic signal of speech.

The Simple Pipe Model: Modeling One Vowel

The first vocal tract model is extremely simple and it has a simple pattern of resonance. The tube illustrated in Figure 9–1a is closed at one end, open at the other, and is 17.5 cm long. Like any tube of this nature, this tube will exhibit resonance under the right physical conditions. These conditions depend on the relation between the frequency of a sound source and the length of the tube. The relation is known as the **odd-quarter wavelength** relation. As explained in Chapter 2, the wavelength of a sound is the "distance traveled by a sound wave during one period of vibration." The wavelength, therefore, depends on two physical quantities, the frequency of vibration and the speed of sound. The equation for wavelength is given below,

$$\lambda = s / f \qquad \text{Equation 9–1}$$

where λ is the wavelength in meters,
s is the speed of sound in meters/sec, and
f is the frequency in hertz.

Equation 9–1 tells us that the wavelength of a sinusoid can actually be measured in physical space. For example, the wavelength of a 1 kHz tone is about 0.34 meters. If this tone were played into a hallway and we could visualize its wave motion, then the same point on the wave would be encountered every .34 meters. In this sense, the wavelength is a spatial phenomenon.

The odd-quarter wavelength relation describes the relation between a sound source and a resonating tube. To show how resonance is created, we use the situation shown in Figure 9–2. A sound source, a pure tone or sinusoid, is located just outside the open end of the tube. The tube has a length l and the tone has a wavelength of $4l$ (i.e., the wavelength of the tone is exactly four times the length of the tube). The sinusoid can be conceptualized as a wave of condensation and a wave of rarefaction separated by one-half wavelength. Therefore, the opening of the tube will receive a train of condensations and rarefactions. In the diagram labeled **a**, the condensation **C** is just entering the tube with a particle motion from left to right. This condensation is followed by a rarefaction **R** with particle motion from right to left. As shown in part **b**, when condensation **C** reaches the closed end of the tube, it is reflected as a condensation with reversed particle motion (from right to left). Because the length of the tube is one-quarter wavelength, this reflected condensation will return to the open end

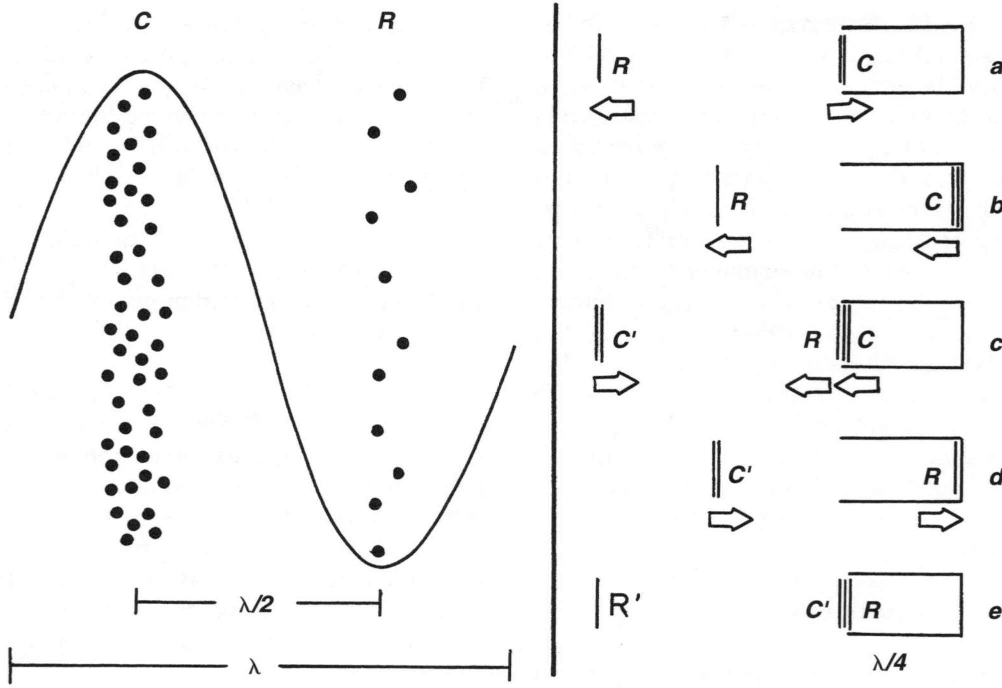

Figure 9–2. Diagram to show resonance in a simple pipe. C and R designate condensation and rarefaction, respectively. The pipes labeled **a–e** represent different patterns of condensation and rarefaction waves in the pipe. See text.

at the same instant that rarefaction **R** enters the pipe (part **c**). Another condensation, **C'**, can be seen following the rarefaction **R**. Note that the reflected condensation **C** and the entering rarefaction **R** have the *same* direction of particle motion, from right to left. The condensation reflected from the closed end now is reflected at the open end as a rarefaction, combining with the rarefaction **R** just entering the tube. The result is a rarefaction of increased amplitude (the condition of resonance). This strengthened wave is reflected at the closed end as a rarefaction (particle motion of left to right), as shown in part **d**, and then at the open end as a condensation (particle motion of left to right). What are the directions of particle motion in part **e**? The rarefaction **R'** will have a motion of right to left, the condensation **C'** will have a motion of right to left and the reflected rarefaction **R** will have a motion of right to left. Therefore, a condensation of increased amplitude will be observed at the opening of the tube.

This example demonstrates how resonance is created when the dimensions of a tube are adjusted to the wavelength of a tone. Other resonances occur at odd-number multiples of the quarter-wavelength relationship. Therefore, the tubes shown in Figure 9–1 actually have an infinite number of resonances spaced at regular intervals. Because the energy of human speech is contained at relatively low frequencies, the higher areas can be neglected. In fact, the emphasis in this chapter is only on the first three resonances. In the study of speech, these vocal tract resonances are called **formants** and their frequencies are called **formant frequencies**. The formants are identified by formant number. The first formant, abbreviated F1, is the lowest-frequency formant. The second formant, F2, is the next highest formant, and the third formant, F3, is the formant immediately above F2.

For a given tube of length l, the formant frequencies can be computed with the following formula, which is based on the odd-quarter wavelength relation:

$F_n = (2n - 1)\ c\ /\ 4l$, Equation 9–2
where F_n is the formant number (e.g., F1, F2, F3),
(2n – 1) is a term that generates the set of odd integers,
c is the speed of sound, which will be approximated in this text as 350 m/s,
and l is the tube length as discussed above.

This equation pertains to a pipe of uniform cross-sectional area that is open at one end and closed at the other. It can be used to estimate the formant frequencies of a vowel produced so that the cross-sectional area of the vocal tract is nearly uniform along its length. This vowel can be described as having a mid-central tongue position. If we assume a vocal tract length of 17.5 cm (typical for an adult male), then the frequencies of the first three formants would be as follows using Equation 9–2:

F1 = 500 Hz,
F2 = 1500 Hz, and
F3 = 2500 Hz.

Summary

A tube closed at one end and open at the other will resonate with maximum amplitude a tone whose wavelength is one-fourth the length of the pipe. Tones with odd-integer multiples of this wavelength also will be resonated. Therefore, this simple tube has a number of resonances equally spaced in frequency. Furthermore, this tube is analogous to one vowel in human speech, the mid-central vowel, as described in Chapter 3.

Adjusting the Length of the Tube Model: Modeling Vowels of Men, Women, and Children

The first modifications of the simple tube model are changes in the length of the tube. Figure 9–1b illustrates lengthening of the original tube. We know from the odd-quarter wavelength relation that the length of the tube determines the frequencies of its resonances. The lengthened tube has lower resonance frequencies than the original pipe, and the shortened tube has higher resonance frequencies than the original tube.

Pretend for a moment that a tube can grow, much as a child does. A short tube would then represent a baby, a moderately long tube would be an older child, and the longest tube would be an adult. In fact, this is essentially what happens with the human vocal tract. An infant has a short vocal tract, about 8–10 cm long. For the purposes of calculation, let us take the example of a newborn with a vocal tract length of 8 cm. An adult female has a vocal tract length of about 15 cm and, as noted earlier, the adult male has a vocal tract length of about 17.5 cm. The resonance frequencies calculated for these three tubes of different length are listed in Table 9–1 as theoretical values. From an acoustic point of view, these three tubes of uniform cross-section

Table 9-1. Calculated formant frequencies (F1, F2, F3) for a central vowel produced by a neonate (vocal tract length of 8 cm), a woman (vocal tract length of 15 cm), and a man (vocal tract length of 17.5 cm).

	F1	F2	F3
Neonate	1094	3282	5470
Woman	583	1749	2915
Man	500	1500	2500

correspond to one vowel, the so-called neutral, or central, vowel, in which the tongue and other articulators are positioned so that the vocal tract has a uniform cross-sectional area from glottis to lips (Figure 9–1a). As the values in Table 9–1 demonstrate, this "same" vowel produced by a newborn, an adult female, and an adult male has different formant frequencies.

Summary

Adjusting the length of the straight tube alters its resonance frequencies. A longer tube has lower resonance frequencies and a shorter tube has higher resonance frequencies. As related to human speech, this means that speakers with the shortest vocal tracts (young children) will have the highest formant frequencies, speakers with somewhat longer vocal tracts (women) will have somewhat lower formant frequencies than the children, and speakers with the longest vocal tracts (men) will have the lowest formant frequencies.

If acoustic theory went no further than this in accounting for speech sounds, there would not be much interest in it. But acoustic theory goes much further. To continue the story, we need to make further modifications of the tube model.

Adjusting the Cross-sectional Area of the Tube: Making More Vowels

For vowel production, the vocal tract is an air-filled tube. The resonances of this tube are determined by its length, as we already have seen and by variations in its cross-sectional area over its length (some sections of the tube are narrow and others are wide). To model vowels other than the one shown in Figure 9–1a, we need to depart from the simple tube of uniform cross-sectional area. Four vowels are taken as examples to continue the discussion. These are /i/ (as in "he"), /u/ (as in "who"), /ɑ/ (as in "ha"), and /æ/ (as in "had"). (The virgules, or slashes, / /, are used in this chapter to denote a general phoneme class of speech sounds.) These four vowels are among the most frequently occurring in the world's languages, and they define the corners of the classic vowel quadrilateral as discussed in Chapter 3.

To modify the pipe model for these four vowels, the major change required is to vary the tube's cross-sectional area so that it resembles the vocal tract configurations of the vowels. The principles are illustrated in Figure 9–3. For vowel /i/, the back cavity is enlarged relative to the front cavity. For vowel /u/, there is a constricted interval about midway along the tube and also at its mouth. For vowel /ɑ/, the front cavity is enlarged relative to the back cavity. For vowel /æ/, the front cavity is relatively enlarged compared to the back cavity, but the back cavity is larger than for /i/. It is possible to compute the resonances of these modified tubes using formulas from acoustics, but these formulas are beyond the scope of this discussion.

If we plot the formant frequencies for F2 (second-formant frequency) versus F1 (first-formant frequency), we have the result shown in Figure 9–4 for vowels produced by men and by women. Recall from the earlier section that women's vowels will have higher formant frequencies because their vocal tracts are shorter than men's. Figure 9–4 is the F1–F2 plot (or F1–F2 chart), one of the most frequently used graphs in acoustic studies of speech. When the corner vowels are plotted in the F1–F2 plane, the result is the **acoustic vowel quadrilateral**, a four-sided figure that defines the acoustic space of vowel production. This acoustic vowel quadrilateral corresponds to the articulatory vowel quadrilateral discussed in Chapter 3. This geometric similarity can be explored further by asking if the articulatory dimen-

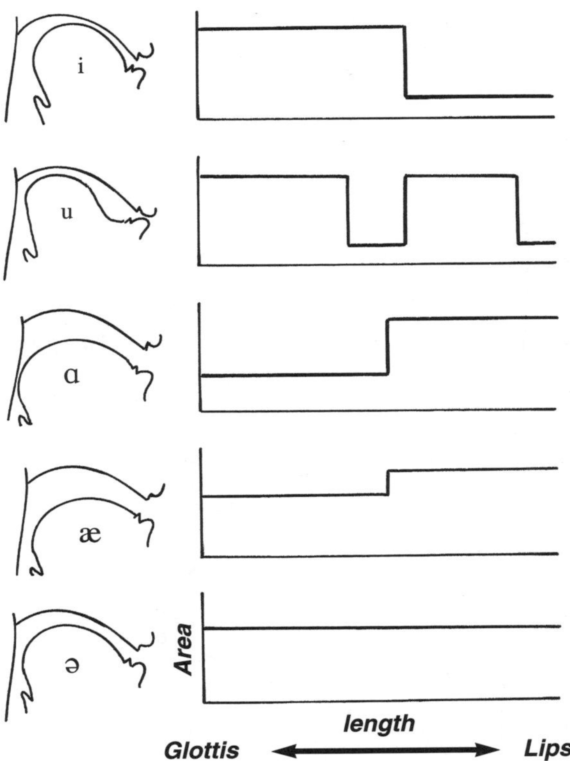

Figure 9–3. Vowels represented by stylized vocal tract configuration and area functions.

sions of the vowel quadrilateral can be interpreted acoustically. The articulatory dimensions are tongue height (from low to high) and tongue antero-posterior position (from front to back). The acoustic dimensions are the frequencies of F1 and F2. Note the following:

1. The high vowels /i/ and /u/ have a low F1 frequency, but the low vowels /æ/ and /ɑ/ have a high F1 frequency. Therefore, the relative value of F1 is associated with tongue height.
2. The back vowels /u/ and /ɑ/ have a low F2 frequency, but the front vowels /i/ and /æ/ have a high F2 frequency. Therefore, the relative value of F2 is associated with the antero-posterior position of the tongue.

With these two rules in mind, we can complete the F1–F2 chart with the other vowels of American English, as shown in Figure 9–5. This illustration has two parts: The left panel (**a**) shows the F1–F2 chart with ellipses that enclose the data for a large number of speakers including men, women, and children (Peterson & Barney, 1952). Note that a logarithmic frequency axis is used for F2. The formant-frequency values vary with age and sex, as described above. Despite these variations, there is an orderly arrangement of the formant-frequency data. Note that the new vowels, that is, the ones other than the corner vowels, are effectively inserted into the quadrilateral defined by the corner vowels. In this sense, the corner vowels define the overall acoustic space.

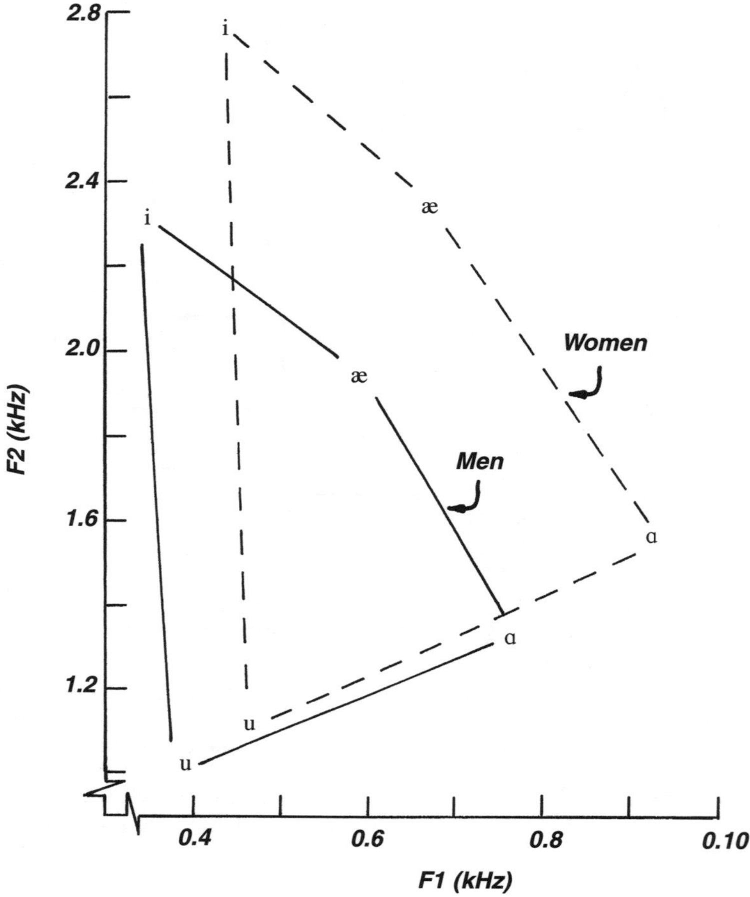

Figure 9–4. F1–F2 plot for the corner vowels produced by men and women. The frequency of the first formant (F1) is plotted on the horizontal axis, and the frequency of the second formant (F2) is plotted on the vertical axis.

The right panel **(b)** shows key words for the 10 vowels arranged to approximate their location in the F1–F2 chart. If you do not know the phonetic symbols used in panel a, then panel b should help. Reading the keywords clockwise beginning with *heed* and ending with *heard* will put your tongue through the following exercise. Reading *heed* to *had* lowers your tongue while keeping it in the front of the mouth. In going from *had* to *hod*, your tongue will move from a front to a back articulation. Now, in reading the sequence *hod, hawed, hood*, and *who'd*, your tongue will remain in the back position but will elevate progressively across the sequence. Finally, the words *heard* and *hud* require that the tongue be positioned in the mid-central region. This little walk with the tongue has circled the quadrilateral and ended in dead center of the vowel plane.

Mean formant frequencies for vowels produced by men and women are compiled in Tables 9–2 and 9–3, respectively. These tables summarize the data obtained in two

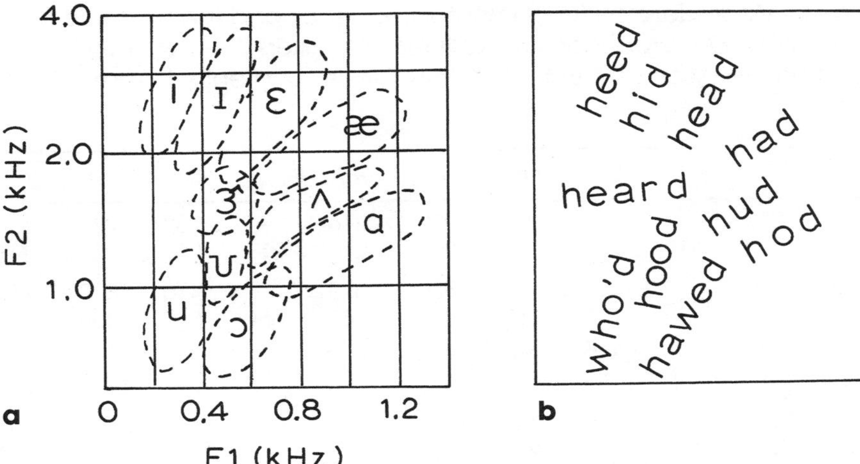

Figure 9–5. F1–F2 plot for 10 vowels. *Left panel:* The ellipses enclose the formant-frequency values for a large group of men, women, and children. *Right panel:* Key words for the vowels shown in the left panel.

Table 9–2. Mean data on fundamental frequency and the first three formant frequencies for vowels produced by adult male talkers. The first entry in each cell is a value from Peterson and Barney (1952). The second entry is from Hillenbrand et al. (1995).

	/i/	/ɪ/	/e/	/ɛ/	/æ/	/ɑ/	/ɔ/	/o/	/U/	/u/	/ʌ/	/ɝ/
F_0	136	135	—	130	12	124	129	—	137	141	130	133
	138	135	129	127	123	123	121	129	133	143	133	130
F1	270	390	—	530	660	730	570	—	440	300	640	490
	342	427	476	580	588	768	652	497	469	378	623	474
F2	2290	1990	—	1840	1720	1090	840	—	1020	870	1190	1350
	2322	2034	2089	1799	1952	1333	997	910	1122	997	1200	1379
F3	3010	2550	—	2480	2410	2440	2410	—	2240	2240	2390	1690
	3000	2684	2691	2605	2601	2522	2538	2459	2434	2343	2550	1710

large studies of vowel formant frequencies, a classic paper by Peterson and Barney (1952) and a recent replication by Hillenbrand, Getty, Clark, and Wheeler (1995). Data also are reported on mean fundamental frequency. From an inspection of the fundamental frequency data, one can see evidence of a general pattern: Vocal fundamental frequency varies with vowel height, such that high vowels have a higher frequency than low vowels. For example, in the Hillenbrand et al. data, the fundamental frequency for vowel /u/ is 20 Hz higher than it is for vowel /ɑ/.

The fact that vowel formant frequencies vary with vocal tract length (and therefore with characteristics such as age and sex) presents a basic problem in acoustic phonetics: How do we achieve the same pho-

Table 9–3. Mean data on fundamental frequency and the first three formant frequencies for vowels produced by adult female talkers. The first entry in each cell is a value from Peterson and Barney (1952). The second entry is from Hillenbrand et al. (1995).

	/i/	/ɪ/	/e/	/ɛ/	/æ/	/ɑ/	/ɔ/	/o/	/U/	/u/	/ʌ/	/ɝ/
F_0	275	232	—	223	210	212	216	—	232	231	221	218
	270	224	219	214	215	215	210	217	230	235	218	217
F1	310	430	—	610	860	850	590	—	470	370	760	500
	437	483	536	731	669	936	781	555	519	459	753	523
F2	2790	2480	—	2330	2050	1220	920	—	1160	950	1400	1640
	2761	2365	2530	2058	2349	1551	1136	1035	1225	1105	1426	1588
F3	3310	3070	—	2990	2850	2810	2710	—	2680	2670	2780	1960
	3372	3053	3047	2979	2972	2815	2824	2828	2827	2735	2933	1929

netic classification for vowels that do not have the same acoustic properties? This is the problem of **speaker (vocal tract) normalization**. A number of solutions have been proposed, most of which apply some kind of nonlinear transformation to the formant-frequency values. One example of a nonlinear transformation is the **Bark scale**, which is based on the nonlinear properties of human audition. Using this scale, Syrdal and Gopal (1986) determined the **Bark differences** that can be used to classify different vowels. These values are given in Table 9–4. For example, the table shows that for vowel /i/ there is a small difference between F1 and f_0, a large difference between F2 and F1, and a small difference between F3 and F2.

The Voice Source: Giving Sound to the Resonators

All the resonating tubes discussed so far would be silent were it not for some source of energy activating the resonators. Tube resonances do not create energy in themselves. They are latent properties of a tube and their effects are evidenced only when a sound source is present. For much of speech, the sound source is the periodic (or, more correctly, quasi-periodic, because vocal fold vibration is not exactly periodic) energy generated by the vibrating vocal folds discussed in Chapter 4. Recall from that chapter that the vocal fold opening and closing produces a glottal waveform that is roughly the shape of a series of triangular pulses. The spectrum of this voice source, the laryngeal flow spectrum, is shown in Figure 9–6a, and its waveform is shown in Figure 9–6b. The spectrum is an example of a **harmonic spectrum** in which the acoustic energy is located at harmonic intervals. In the spectrum shown in Figure 9–6a, the first harmonic is the fundamental frequency and all the higher harmonics are integer multiples of that fundamental. So, for example, if the fundamental frequency is 125 Hz (typical for an adult male), then the next three harmonics would have frequencies of 250, 375, and 500 Hz, respectively. If the fundamental frequency is 250 Hz (typical for an adult female), then the next three harmonics would have frequencies of 500, 750, and 1000 Hz, respectively. But not only does the harmonic spectrum vary across individuals, it also varies within individual speakers. Although we tend to produce speech at a typical fundamental frequency (which is heard as habitual voice pitch), we can adjust the fundamen-

Table 9–4. Vowel classification based on critical distance features in five Bark-difference dimensions (Syrdal & Gopal, 1986).

Vowel	F1–f_0 < 1 Bark	F2–F1 < 3 Bark	F3–F2 < 3 Bark	F4–F3 < 3 Bark	F4–F2 < 1 Bark
/ i /	+	–	+	+	+
/ ɪ /	+	–	+	–	+
/ ɛ /	–	–	+	–	+
/ æ /	–	–	+	–	+
/ ɛ /		–	+	–	–
/ ʌ /	–	–	–	–	+
/ a /	–	+	–	–	+
/ ɔ /		+	–	–	+
/ U /	+	–	–	–	+
/ u /	+	–	–	–	+

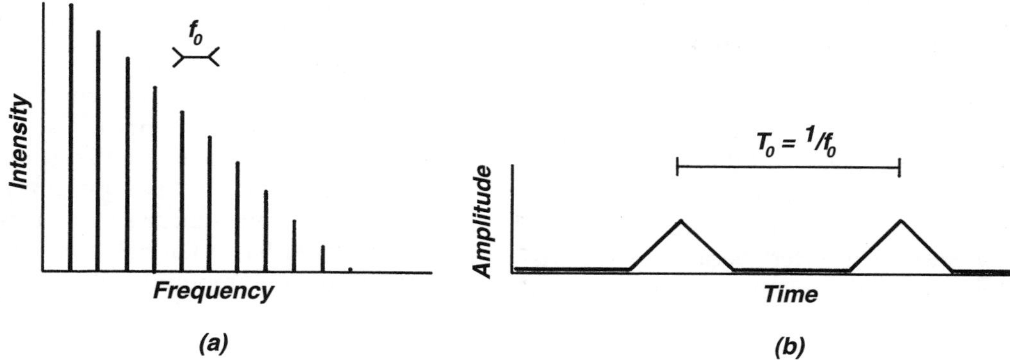

Figure 9–6. The laryngeal source represented as a harmonic spectrum (**b**) and a triangle-pulse waveform (**a**). The harmonics in **a** are spaced at intervals equal to the fundamental frequency f_0. The glottal pulses in **b** are spaced at intervals equal to the fundamental period T_0.

tal frequency over a considerable range. For instance, a man who has an average fundamental frequency of 125 Hz may increase his fundamental frequency to 250 Hz, in which case his harmonics would have the same values as those listed earlier for a woman.

The harmonic spectrum of the voice source is the energy that activates the formants. Because human voices are rich in harmonic energy, several formants can be strongly activated. However, most of the energy in the voice source is at relatively lower frequencies. The reason is that the amplitudes of the harmonics decrease at roughly 12 dB/octave, as illustrated in Figure 9–6a. That is, for every doubling of frequency, the harmonic amplitude is reduced by 12 dB. Most of the energy in voiced speech is contained in the lowest three formants, F1, F2, and F3, which are somtimes called the **main vowel formants**. The frequency range of these formants fits fairly well within the standard bandwidth used in the telephone industry (500–3500 Hz). Our ability to understand one another over the telephone is everyday confirmation of the principle that the acoustic signal of speech does not need to be transmitted in its full frequency range of physical energy. A bandwidth of about 3000 Hz is sufficient to represent the primary acoustic information that reflects phonetically significant adjustments of the vocal tract.

The Source-Filter Theory of Speech Production

So far we have examined two major aspects of the acoustics of speech production: the resonator and the source energy. For vowels, the resonator can be modeled as a pipe such as shown in Figure 9–1. The resonator is a **filter**, because energy is passed in a frequency-selective manner. When source energy happens to occur in the frequency region of a resonance, then the resonance will enhance the source energy. But if source energy occurs outside (or between) resonance regions, then that energy will not be increased by resonance. The vocal tract is an acoustic filter, the characteristics of which depend on the length and shaping of the vocal tract. When speakers produce different vowels, they are changing the filter characteristics of the vocal tract.

As mentioned earlier, the source energy for voiced speech is the harmonic spectrum of voicing, that is, the fundamental frequency and its harmonics. For vowel production, this source spectrum is the acoustic energy that activates the formants.

The **source-filter theory of vowel production** (Fant, 1960; Stevens & House, 1961) is illustrated in Figure 9–7. Essentially, the theory states that energy from the *source* (the vibrating vocal folds) is modified by the resonance characteristics of the *filter* (the vocal tract). Figure 9–7 shows the source spectrum, or laryngeal flow spectrum, drawn near the vocal folds and the formants (also called a **transfer function**) drawn near the vocal tract. One additional term needs to be added to complete the theory. Notice that in Figure 9–7, a term called the **radiation characteristic** exerts a final shaping on the acoustic signal. This characteristic takes into account the way in which the vocal tract opens into the atmosphere (called a **baffle** effect). The radiation characteristic can be modeled very simply as a +6 dB increase for every octave. Because the source energy has a –12 dB/octave characteristic, we can combine the source characteristic and radiation characteristic as a resultant –6 dB/octave fall-off in energy. The output or final product is the radiated pressure spectrum. This output spectrum has a harmonic energy distribution, but the amplitudes of the harmonics have been shaped by the formants and the radiation characteristic. It is in this sense that the source energy is filtered by the vocal tract.

Extending the Theory to Consonants

To show how the acoustic theory can be extended to consonants, we consider two general classes of consonant production: fricatives and nasals. Let us begin with a voiceless fricative, such as /s/ in *see*. The energy source for a voiceless fricative is

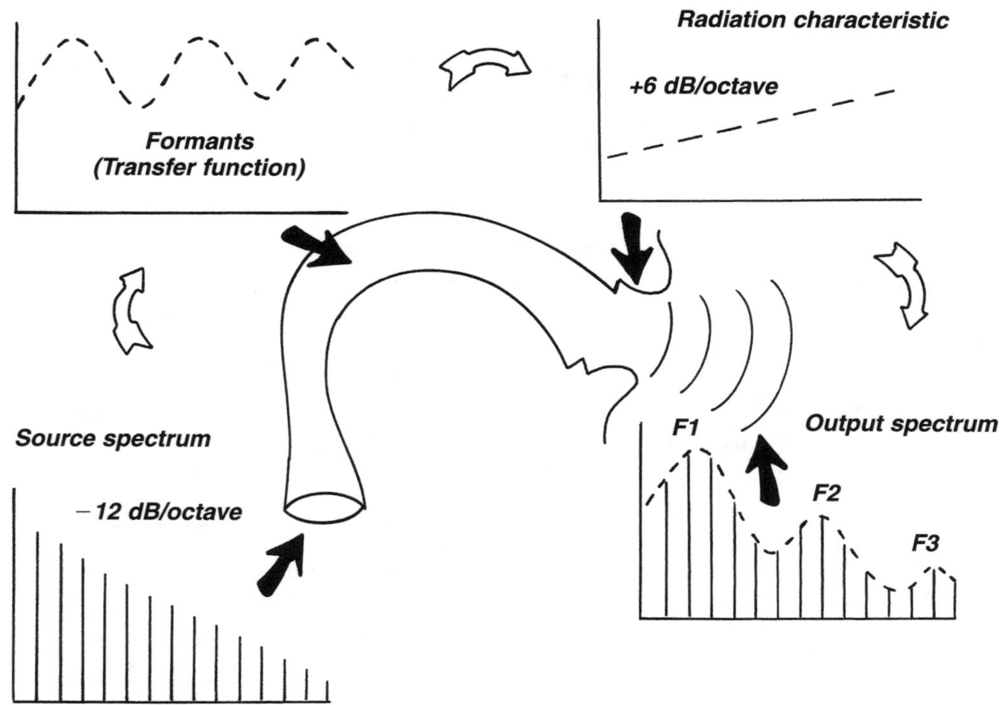

Figure 9–7. Diagrammatic summary of the source-filter theory of speech production.

not vocal fold vibration, but turbulence noise generated at some location along the vocal tract. The model for production of a fricative, using /s/ as in *see* as an example, is shown in Figure 9–8. The turbulence noise is generated at the constricted region of the model. The cavity that lies in front of the noise source is the primary determinant of the resonant shaping of the noise. In particular, the length of the front cavity determines the lowest frequency resonance. If the length is very short, as it is with the labio-dental and lingua-dental fricatives, then the lowest frequency resonance of the front cavity is so high in frequency that it contributes relatively little spectral shaping. As a result, the noise spectrum of the radiated fricative is flat. But if the length of the front cavity is increased so that it approximates the front cavity for production of the fricative /s/, then the lowest frequency resonance is low enough to give substantial shaping to the noise energy. Under certain conditions, the back cavity also can contribute to the resonance shaping of the noise. When this happens, a condition of **coupling** between front and back cavities is said to occur.

A major difference between the vocal tract filtering for vowels and for fricatives is that filtering for fricatives is determined not only by formants, but also by **antiformants**. Antiformants are essentially the opposite of formants in that they result in a *loss* of sound energy rather than an enhancement of sound energy transmision. The difference between a formant and antiformant is shown schematically in Figure 9–9. In this drawing, a formant and an antiformant with the same center frequency f_c are shown in part **a** and **c**, respectively.

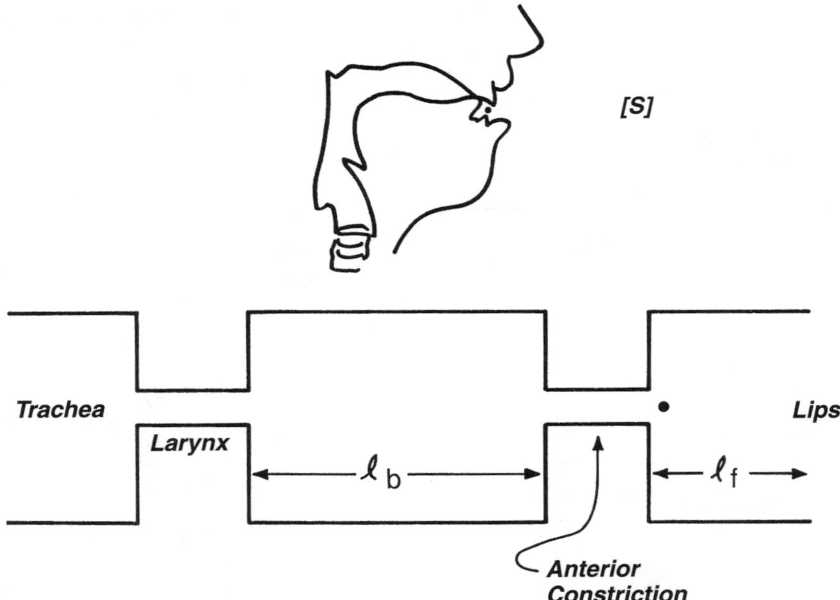

Figure 9–8. Model for the generation and filtering of frication noise. The small dot located to the right of the anterior constriction is the point of noise generation. The noise is shaped by resonances of the front cavity, and sometimes also by resonances of the back cavity.

The effect of each is shown for a harmonic spectrum similar to that for voiced speech. The formant enhances the harmonic components, so that when the formant interacts with the harmonic spectrum (part **a**), the result is a modified harmonic spectrum with a peak at or near f_c (part **b** of Figure 9–9). The antiformant weakens the amplitudes of the harmonic components. Therefore, when the antiformant interacts with the harmonic spectrum (part **c**), the result is a modified harmonic spectrum with a dip at or near f_c (part **d** of Figure 9–9). Frequency regions influenced by antiformants are those in which the sound is not transmitted through the vocal tract.

Antiformants arise in two general conditions: (a) when the vocal tract is radically constricted, as in the case of stops or fricatives, or (b) when the vocal tract is bifurcated, or split, into two passages (such as the oral and nasal passages formed during nasal sounds). Sounds formed under either of these two conditions have a filtering function that is determined by both formants and antiformants. In the case of fricatives, the formants are determined by the length of the entire vocal tract from glottis to lips. Therefore, the formants in fricative production are approximately the same as vowel formants for a vowel with a similar vocal tract configuration. The antiformants in fricative production are determined by the size of the back cavity and the size of the constriction itself. Because these two cavities are smaller than the vocal tract as a whole, the antiformants are more widely spaced than the formants. One consequence is that formants and antiformants tend to occur closely to each other at low frequencies, but further apart at higher frequencies. Therefore, at low frequencies, their effects cancel (rather like adding a postive and negative number of the same magnitude), but not at higher frequencies where they are more widely separated.

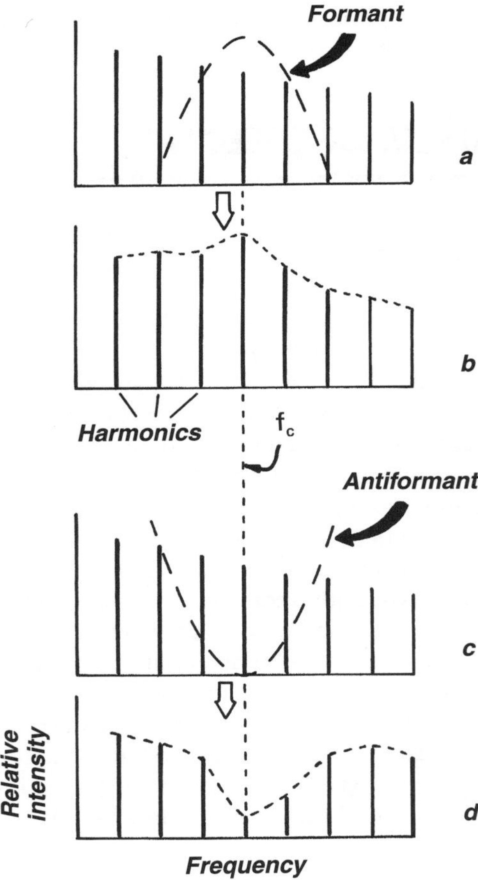

Figure 9–9. Schematic illustration of the effects of a formant and an antiformant on a harmonic spectrum: **a.** Formant and harmonic spectrum shown separately. **b.** Output spectrum resulting from interaction of formant and harmonic spectrum. **c.** Antiformant and harmonic spectrum shown separately. **d.** Output spectrum resulting from interaction of antiformant and harmonic spectrum.

Nasals, like fricatives, have a vocal tract filtering in which formants and antiformants interact. Nasalized vowels, or vowels produced with nasalization, have a filter function composed of oral formants, nasal formants, and antiformants introduced by the vocal tract bifurcation. In addition, because the nasal cavities are lined with soft and convoluted mucous membranes, they tend to absorb sound energy. Therefore, nasalized vowels are less intense than nonnasal vowels.

For nasal consonants, constriction of the oral cavity produces antiformants that reduce the radiation of energy through the nasal passages for frequencies near the antiformant frequency. The antiformants associated with nasal consonant production are determined primarily by the length of the cavity. The coupling of the nasal passages to the vocal tract also increases the overall length of the tract, which lowers formant frequencies generally. A distinctive feature of nasal consonants is a low-frequency formant in the vicinity of 250–300 Hz for adult male speakers. This resonance is referred to as the **nasal murmur** or **nasal formant**. The acoustic evidence of this murmur is considered later.

As is probably evident, the acoustic theory for fricatives and nasals is quite complex. Only a few general features have been discussed in this chapter. Perhaps the most important point is that the acoustic theory of speech production has been developed to account for all classes of speech sounds.

METHODS OF ACOUSTIC ANALYSIS

In about the middle of the 20th century, the acoustic analysis of speech was greatly enhanced by a fundamental form of acoustic analysis called the **spectrograph**, which produces visible patterns of acoustic energy called **spectrograms** (Koenig, Dunn, & Lacy, 1946; Potter, Kopp, & Green, 1947). Before turning to a closer look at the acoustic properties of various speech sounds, we examine the spectrogram and see why it is a useful tool for the study of speech acoustics.

THE ACOUSTIC ANALYSIS OF SPEECH

Spectrographic Analysis

A major problem encountered in the acoustic analysis of speech is that the acoustic signal changes rapidly and nearly continuously, even for simple utterances. Therefore, a long-term average spectrum is not informative about the dynamics of speech. The waveform captures the dynamics but is not easily interpreted because its characteristics are not especially transparent to the important phonetic properties of speech sounds. For example, it is very difficult to determine vowel identity by looking at waveforms. What is needed is a short-term running spectrum, that is, a dynamic analysis that reveals spectral features in a nearly continuous fashion. That is what the spectrogram achieves. It is a running short-term spectrum, or, in other words, a continuously changing spectral pattern.

To understand what the patterns in a spectrogram mean, we must begin by describing the dimensions of the spectrogram. These dimensions are in fact the essential dimensions of acoustics—time, frequency, and intensity (Figure 9–10). Time is represented along the horizontal axis, so that the phonetic elements can be read from left to right. Frequency is scaled along the vertical axis, with frequency increasing in the upward direction. Intensity is represented by the gray scale or as variations in darkness. A dark region is a region of energy. The frequency components of the dark region can be determined by reference to the frequency (vertical) axis. The temporal location and duration of the dark region can

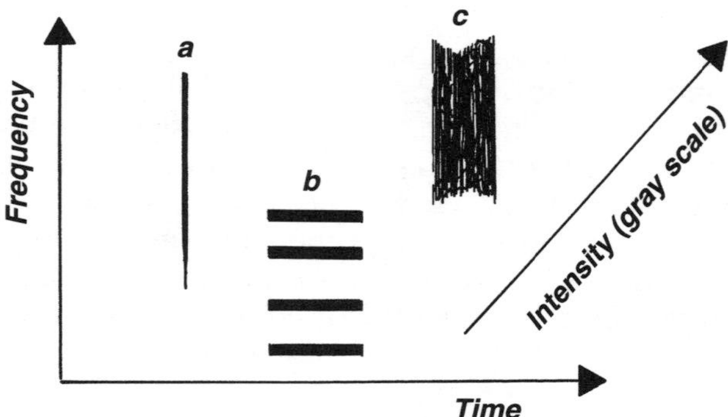

Figure 9–10. Diagram showing the dimensions of a spectrogram: time on the horizonal axis, frequency on the vertical axis, and intensity on the gray (darkness) scale. Stylized spectrographic patterns are shown for (**a**) a burst of noise, (**b**) a vowel with four formants, and (**c**) a noise with high-frequency energy.

be determined by reference to the time (horizontal) axis.

A sample spectrogram and a highly stylized replica are shown in Figure 9–11. The spectrogram follows the production of the word *science* by an adult male. This word is transcribed phonetically as [s aɪ ə n s], that is, a sequence of a fricative, diphthong, short vowel, nasal, and a final fricative. Major properties useful in describing these phonetic segments are shown in the stylized pattern at the bottom of the illustration. The initial and final fricative are associated with intervals of noise. This noise energy has a fine temporal structure and its frequency location is primarily above about 3 or 4 kHz. The diphthong is associated with bands of energy that run roughly horizontally across the spectrogram, but tilting slightly upward or downward to reflect the changing formant frequencies over time. Each band is identified with a formant, F1, F2, F3, F4, and so on. A **voice bar** is seen at the very bottom (low-frequency portion) of the spectrogram. This

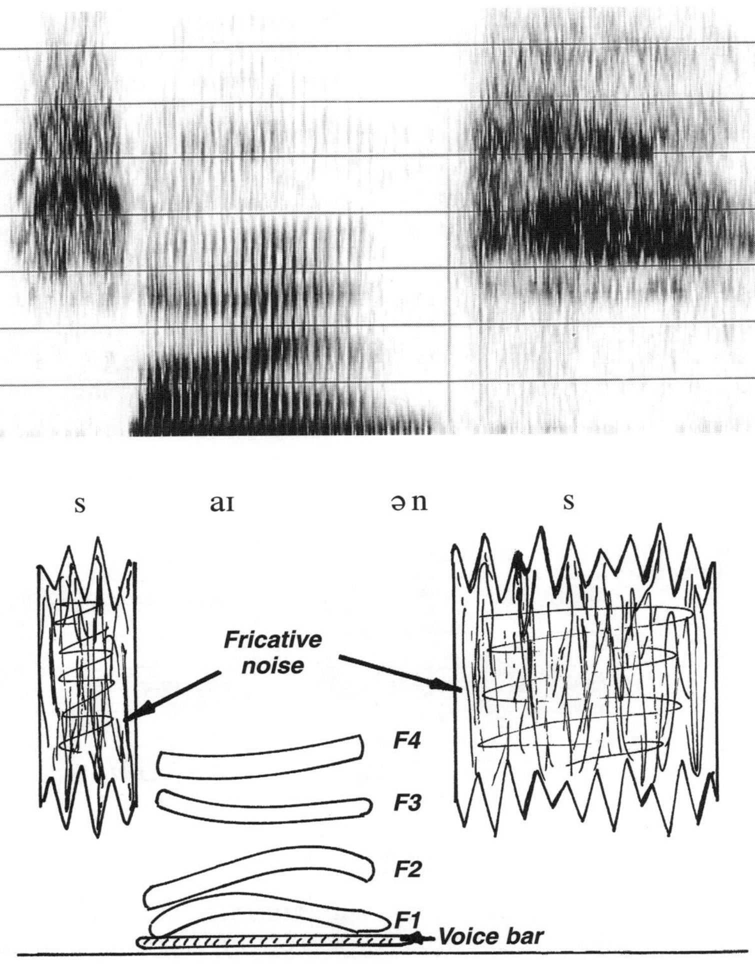

Figure 9–11. Actual spectrogram (*top*) and stylized spectrogram (*bottom*) for the word *science*.

bar reflects the energy of the fundamental frequency of voicing.

The spectrogram in Figure 9–11 is a type of spectrogram called the **wide-band spectrogram**, meaning that the analyzing filter is relatively wide (usually about 300–400 Hz). Such a wide analyzing filter is well suited to display formant energy, because formants have a rather wide spread of acoustic energy. What would happen if we used a **narrow-band spectrogram**, that is, a spectrogram produced with a narrow analyzing filter? The result is shown in Figure 9–12. Notice that the narrow filter accomplishes a much finer resolution in frequency—fine enough, in fact, to display the harmonics of the source spectrum of voicing. The wide and narrow-band spectrograms are complementary analyses. The choice between them depends on the purpose of our analyses. Generally, if we are interested in estimating formant frequencies or in looking at short-time dynamic events such as noise bursts, then we use the wide-band spectrogram. But if our interest is in finer frequency resolution, then the narrow-band spectrogram is preferred.

Digital Signal Processing of Speech

The spectrograph introduced in about the middle of the 20th century was a major advance in the study of speech acoustics. It was followed about two decades later by the expanding use of digital computers to analyze the acoustic patterns of speech. This era of digital signal processing made possible the flexible and efficient analysis of even large amounts of speech. We now take a quick look at the essence of digital signal processing, because it is the core of almost all modern analysis systems. It is also the means by which personal computers (and larger ones as well) are able to store, retrieve, and modify human speech.

The basic objective in digital signal processing is to convert the analog acoustic signal (the waveform that appears in panel **a** of Figure 9–13) to a digital form, that is, a series of numbers. Digital computers operate on discrete numbers, not on a continuously varying pattern such as a waveform. How then, do we get a speech waveform into a digital computer? The process is

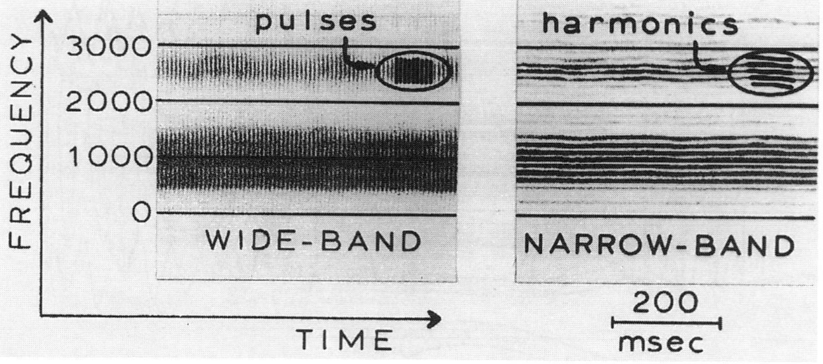

Figure 9–12. A sample of vowel (ɑ) analyzed with a wide-band and narrow-band spectrogram. Voice energy is analyzed as glottal pulses in the wide-band spectrogram and as spectral harmonics in the narrow-band spectrogram.

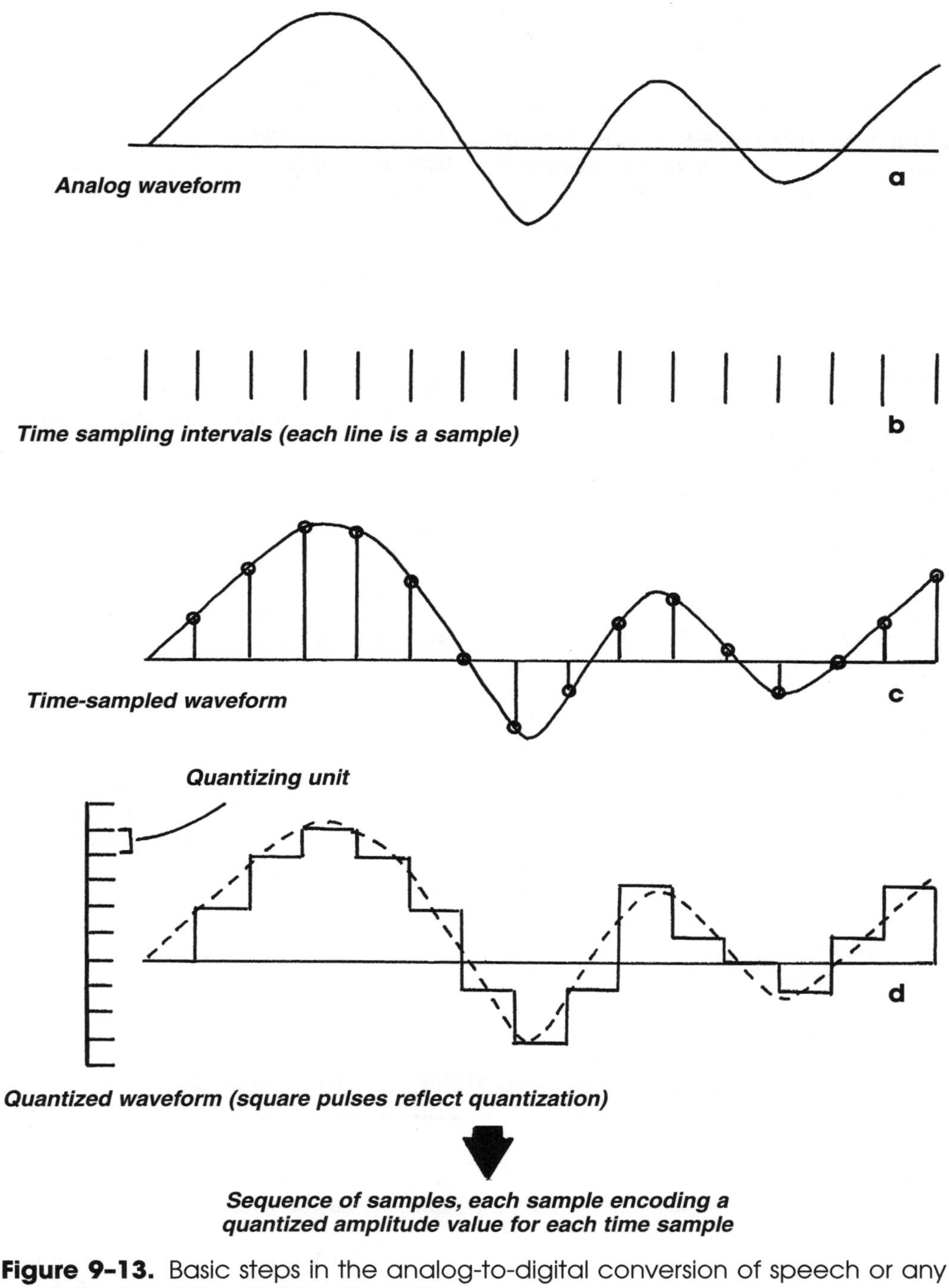

Figure 9–13. Basic steps in the analog-to-digital conversion of speech or any acoustic signal. See text for discussion.

called **analog-to-digital** (A–D) conversion. A–D conversion results in discrete samples of time and amplitude. To obtain discrete samples in time, the computer samples the waveform at a selected rate called the **sampling rate**. This process is illustrated in Figure 9–13. Typically, a constant sampling rate is selected for a given A–D task. Therefore, the sampling rate can be represented as a series of pulses such as shown in panel **b** of Figure 9–13. The interesting thing about this process is that the waveform can be sampled only at certain points *without loss of information*. That is, if the proper sampling rate is used, the waveform can be reconstructed accurately and unambiguously even though the digital information pertains to selected time points and not the entire waveform. The sampling rate chosen for this purpose must be at least twice the desired bandwidth of analysis (this sampling rate is called the **Nyquist frequency**). For example, if we wish to sample a recording of speech with a bandwidth of 5000 Hz (i.e., a range of 0 to 5000 Hz), then the sampling rate should be 10,000 Hz. The basic idea is that two sampling points are required for the highest frequency (shortest period) of interest. It is not necessary to sample more frequently than this. In fact, it is not desirable because the additional information would simply require more computer memory but would not define the signal any more accurately. The time-sampled data are shown in panel **c** of Figure 9–13.

Next, to make the amplitude variations discrete, a process of **quantization** is used. As shown in panel **d** of Figure 9–13, quantization simply chops the amplitude dimension into discrete steps. Modern computers permit quantization levels that ensure excellent quality of the digitized waveform. Quantization is a nonlinear process that converts a continuous waveform into discrete amplitude values.

Finally, as shown in panel **e** of Figure 9–13, the processes of sampling and quantization yield a sequence of samples, each of which preserves information on the quantization value for a particular sampling point. These samples can be stored in a digital computer and retrieved as needed for analysis of the signal or for playback. If playback is desired, then the process of **digital-to-analog conversion** is used to reconstruct an analog waveform from the digital data.

Digital signal processing is a highly sophisticated field, largely outside the scope of this introductory book. But because digital methods are used extensively in various applications, it is important to know at least the basic principles. More detailed information for the general reader is available in Kent and Read (1992).

ACOUSTIC CORRELATES OF INFORMATION SOURCES IN SPEECH

Chapter 1 began with a description of information sources in speech. These information sources have been reiterated at several points in this book, and we are about to do so again. Ideally, acoustic analysis would enable us to study phonetic quality, affective quality, personal quality, and transmittal quality. The remainder of this chapter gives examples of how this objective can be realized.

With the background given in the first two sections of this chapter, we are ready to list the major acoustic correlates for the following classes of speech sounds: vowels, stops, nasals, fricatives, affricates, glides, and liquids. This summary will be selective and brief; for more details, see Fant (1960); Fujimura and Erickson (1997); Kent, Dembowski, and Lass (1996); Kent and Read (1992); or Pickett (1980).

Phonetic Quality: Vowels

In line with the phonetic summary given in Chapter 2, the acoustic correlates are discussed for the vowel classifications: front, back, and central. Recall that these classifications are based on the relative position of the tongue in the oral cavity. Reference to Tables 9–2, 9–3, and 9–4 may be helpful.

Front Vowels

Selected front vowels are shown as idealized spectrograms (first two formants only) in Figure 9–14. As a group, the front vowels have a large separation between F1 and F2 (they also have a relatively small separation between F2 and F3). The front vowels vary in their F1 frequency such that the frequency of F1 reflects the relative tongue height for the vowel. As can be seen in Figure 9–14, the F1 frequency increases in the order /i ɪ ɛ æ/. Another acoustic correlate of tongue height is the difference between F1 and f_0, with high vowels having a small F1–f_0 difference and low vowels having a large F1–f_0 difference.

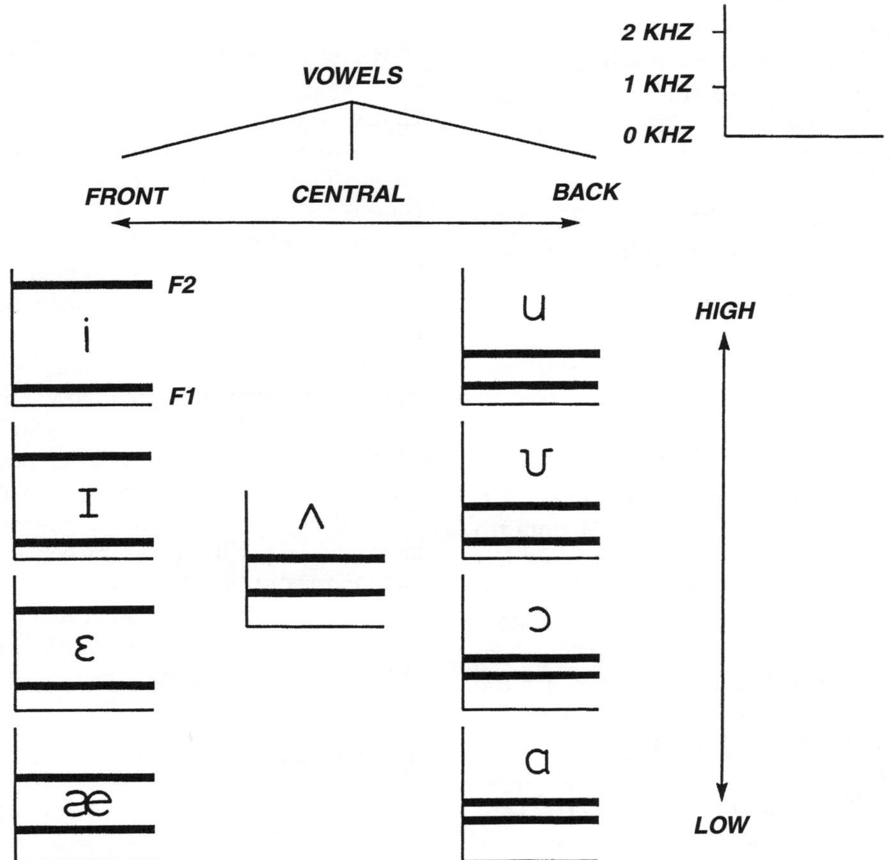

Figure 9–14. Stylized two-formant spectrograms for front, central, and back vowels.

As noted earlier, on the average, high vowels have a higher f_0 than low vowels, and this is one reason for the small F1-f_0 difference for the high vowels.

To summarize, the front vowels have a large F1–F2 separation, a small F2–F3 separation, and a variable F1–f_0 difference reflecting tongue height.

Back Vowels

Selected back vowels are shown as idealized spectrograms in Figure 9–14. Back vowels as a group have a small separation between F2 and F1 (and a large separation between F3 and F2). As in the case of the front vowels, the back vowels vary in the frequency of F1, which is related to vowel height. The height of the vowel also is correlated with the F1–f_0 difference, with high vowels having a small difference and low vowels having a large difference.

To summarize, the back vowels have a small F1–F2 separation, a large F2–F3 separation, and a variable F1–f_0 difference reflecting tongue height.

Central Vowels

Figure 9–14 shows an idealized spectrogram of a central vowel. The primary formant correlate of centrality is a uniform formant pattern in which the formant frequencies tend to be equally spaced, with the important exception of a low F3 for the r-colored vowels /ɝ/ and /ɚ/ (giving them a relatively small F2–F3 difference). For the ideal central vowel, the formants are equally spaced in frequency. Deviations from true centrality introduce departures from uniform formant spacing. The central vowels of English are produced with a moderate jaw opening and therefore a mid-range value of F1.

Other Acoustic Correlates of Vowels

In addition to the major groups of front, back, and central vowels, the vowels also differ in length and in lip rounding. The acoustic correlate of length is duration. The inherently long vowels are /i e æ ɑ u o ɔ/. These are sometimes called tense vowels. The inherently short vowels are /ɪ ʊ ə ʌ ɛ/. These are sometimes called lax vowels. In English, back vowels tend to be rounded, but front vowels are not. The acoustic correlate of rounding is a lowering of all formant frequencies. The reason, as explained earlier, is that rounding of the lips lengthens the vocal tract. As the vocal tract is lengthened, its formant frequencies become lower.

Phonetic Quality: Consonants

Consonants differ greatly among themselves in their acoustic characteristics. Some are vowel-like. For instance, the sounds /j/ (y) and /w/ (w) are sometimes called **semivowels** in recognition of their similarity to vowels. Other consonants are characterized by frication noise. The /s/ in the word *say* is a good example of a consonant that possesses frication noise as a primary acoustic cue. Other consonants, like the /t/ in *two* can have several acoustic cues, including a brief interval of silence, a brief burst of noise, and a set of formant transitions. Given these variations among consonants, the discussion will proceed by considering them in major phonetic classes, specifically stops, nasals, fricatives, affricates, glides, and liquids. The major acoustic features for each class are discussed.

Stop Consonants

Examples of spectrograms of stop consonants in syllable-initial position are shown in Figure 9–15. The acoustic cues include a silent, or low-energy, interval; burst; transi-

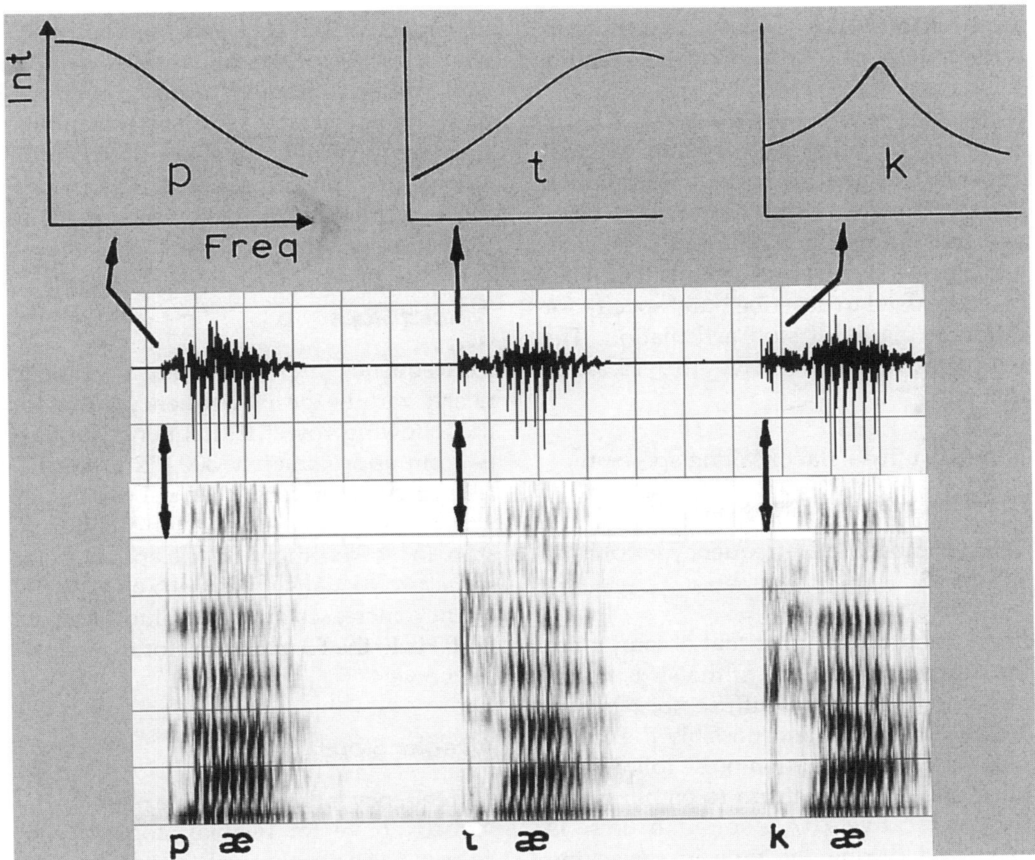

Figure 9–15. Spectrograms of the voiceless stop consonants in consonant-vowel syllables. The stylized spectra at the top of the figure illustrate the shape of the burst spectrum.

tion; and various cues associated with the voicing feature. Because stops are associated with a number of potential acoustic cues, the analysis of these sounds involves a variety of measures (Kent & Read, 1992; Klatt, 1975). Furthermore, the pertinent cues vary with context, especially syllable or word position. For brevity, the syllable-initial position is assumed in the following discussion.

The silent (or low-energy) interval is a period of markedly reduced acoustic energy associated with the articulatory event of oral constriction, that is, the closure of the lips for the stop /b/. This is also called a **stop gap** because it resembles a gap in the acoustic analysis. The stop may be essentially silent for voiceless stops. But for voiced stops, voicing energy may be present during part or all of the stop gap. The voicing energy is evident in a spectrogram as the low-frequency **voice bar** illustrated in Figure 9–11.

The burst is created when the articulatory constriction for the stop is released. The impounded air pressure escapes in a brief interval of noise, about 10–30 ms in duration. Bursts are nearly always evident for syllable-initial stops and also occur with high reliability for medial stops. But the burst may not occur for stops in syllable-final position.

Although the burst is a very brief event, it appears to signal important information about the place of stop articulation. Stevens and Blumstein (1978) and Blumstein and Stevens (1979) proposed that templates could be used to describe burst spectra for different places of stop articulation. The templates, illustrated in Figure 9–15, are as follows:

Bilabial: diffuse, flat or falling spectrum;

Alveolar: diffuse, rising spectrum;

Velar: compact (mid-frequency emphasis) spectrum.

In addition to the burst that accompanies the articulatory release of the stop, voiceless stops also have a diffuse noise generated at the larynx and possibly the lower pharynx. This aspiration noise follows the burst and has a spectrum resembling that for the fricative /h/. Aspiration noise is generated during the time in which the vocal folds move from an abducted (open) state for the voiceless stop to an adducted (closed) state for a following voiced sound. Aspiration does not occur for voiceless stops that follow the fricative /s/, as in the consonant sequences in the words *spot, stop*, and *skip*.

The **formant transitions** are bends in the formant pattern that occur in the interval corresponding to the articulatory movement from stop closure to the open vocal tract for a following sound such as a vowel (Figure 9–16). Formant transitions usually are easier to detect for voiced stops than for voiceless stops, because of the continuity of voicing energy between voiced stops and following voiced sounds. Each formant can assume a rising, falling, or relatively flat pattern during a stop-to-vowel transition. The direction and magnitude of frequency shift depends on the place of articulation for the stop and the vocal tract configuration for the following vowel. Because of the combined influence of consonant and vowel on the formant transitions, the rules governing the shape of stop transitions are a bit complicated. The following is a brief summary for each place of stop consonant articulation.

Bilabial Stops (/ p b /)

F1 frequency increases from a value of nearly zero to the F1-frequency value for the following vowel. F2 frequency increases from approximately 800 Hz to the F2-frequency value for the vowel (that is, F2 almost always has a rising transition from stop to vowel; the only exception is for some productions of vowel /u/). F3 frequency increases from a value of about 2200 Hz to the F3 frequency for the following vowel.

Alveolar Stops (/ t d /)

F1 frequency follows the same patterns described above for bilabial stops. F2 frequency has a starting value of about 1800 Hz and moves toward the F2-frequency value for the following vowel. Therefore, the direction of F2 movement varies with vowels. Typically, F2 frequency has a rising transition for the high-front vowels, a flat transition for mid-front vowels, and a falling transition for all other vowels.

Velar Stops (/ k g /)

F1 frequency follows the pattern described above for bilabials and alveolar stops (the stereotypic F1 pattern is important because it suggests that the F1 transition is a cue for *manner of production*. F2 frequency has at least two starting values: a low-frequency of about 1300 Hz and a higher frequency of about 2300 Hz. Typically, the F2 and F3 frequencies begin very close together but separate during the transition, so that the combined F2–F3 pattern has a wedge shape.

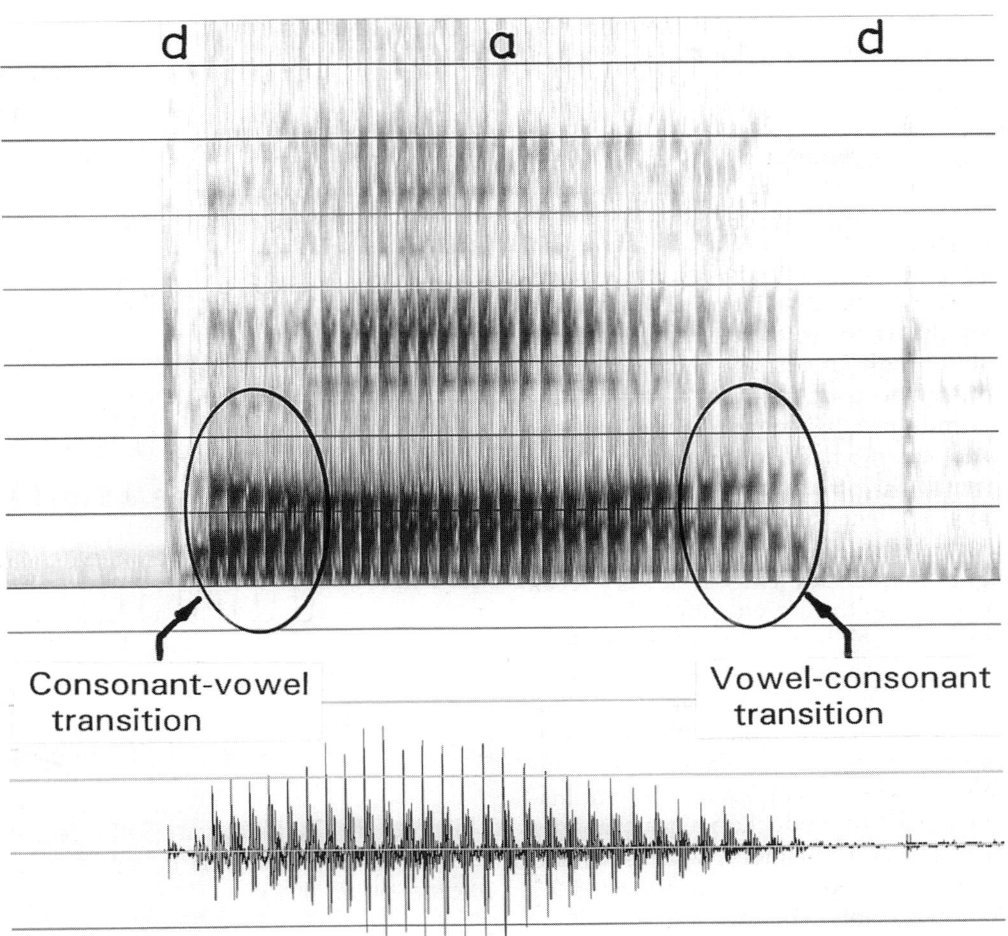

Figure 9–16. Spectrogram of the syllable (d ɑ d) labeled with consonant-vowel and vowel-consonant formant transitions.

In it simplest sense, **voicing** is a binary (two-valued) phonetic property. The stops are said to be either voiced (/b d g/) or voiceless (/p t k/). However, this simple phonetic characterization is realized acoustically in a complex fashion. Among the acoustic cues that signal voicing for stops are voice onset time (VOT), closure duration of the stop, duration of the following vowel, and even the fundamental frequency pattern at the moment of stop release. Rather than detail all the possible cues, the following discussion emphasizes VOT and vowel duration.

VOT is especially important for stops in utterance-initial position. **VOT** is defined as the interval between release of the stop (marked acoustically by the release burst) and the onset of voicing (marked acoustically by the appearance of glottal pulses, or vertical striations in a spectrogram). Voiced stops in English can assume different VOT values: (a) **prevoicing**, in which the voice onset slightly precedes the release burst; (b) **simultaneous voicing**, in which the voice onset is simultaneous with the release burst; or (c) **short lag**, in which voice onset slightly follows the release burst. Voiceless stops in initial position usually have a **long lag**, or relatively long interval between the burst release and the onset of voice. These VOT possibilities are shown schematically in Figure 9–17. VOT is considered further in Chapter 10, which deals with speech perception.

Nasal Consonants

Sample spectrograms of nasal consonants in syllable-initial position are shown in Figure 9–18. Nasal consonants are produced with nasal radiation of acoustic energy, that is, the sound energy is transmitted through the nasal cavity. The two primary acoustic cues for nasals are the **murmur** and the formant transitions. The nasal murmur has a spectrum that is dominated by low-frequency energy, especially a low-frequency resonance less than about 0.5 kHz for adult male speakers. Energy at higher frequencies tends to be very weak compared to the aforementioned low-frequency energy band that reflects the lowest nasal resonance. The three nasal consonants have murmurs that are similar but not exactly alike. Indeed, the acoustic differences among them are not always sufficient for reliable identification. Discrimination of place of production relies primarily on the formant transitions, which essentially follow the same rules just described for stop consonants. The murmur is most effective as a cue for manner of production.

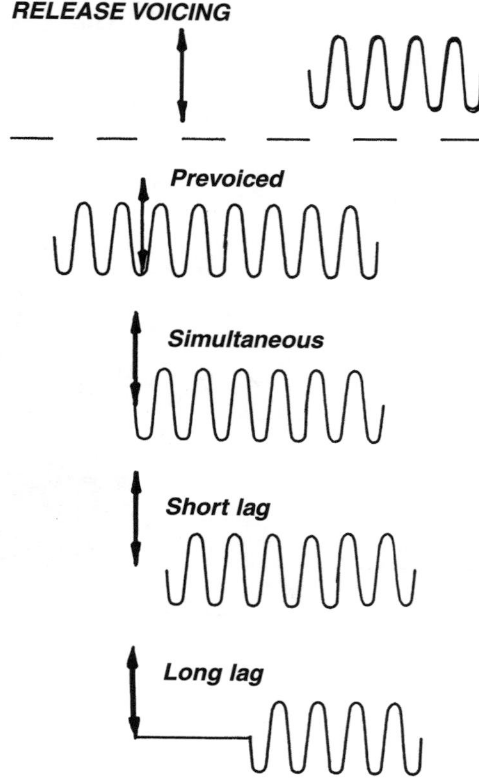

Figure 9–17. Diagrammatic representation of different possibilities of voice onset time (VOT).

The spectrum of a murmur is actually quite complex because nasal sounds have not only formants but also antiformants, as discussed earlier in this chapter. Recall that antiformants are opposite in effect to formants because they result in a loss of energy. In addition, acoustic transmission through the nasal cavity is associated with substantial damping, both because the length of sound travel is great (from larynx through the nasal cavities) and because the convoluted tissues that line the nasal cavities absorb sound energy. Figure 9–19 is a spectrogram of a sustained production of the nasal consonant [n]. The signal was amplified to reveal the complexity of the nasal murmur. The presence of several formants is indicated by the dark bands in the spectrogram, similar to the formants of vowels discussed earlier. In addition, the spectrogram shows the presence of a distinctive region of reduced energy—a horizontal white streak in the spectrogram. This frequency region of reduced energy is most likely the result of an antiformant. Actually determining the precise frequency of an antiformant is difficult, because formants and antiformants can interact in a complex manner.

Nasals are ordinarily voiced in English, with the exception of whispered speech.

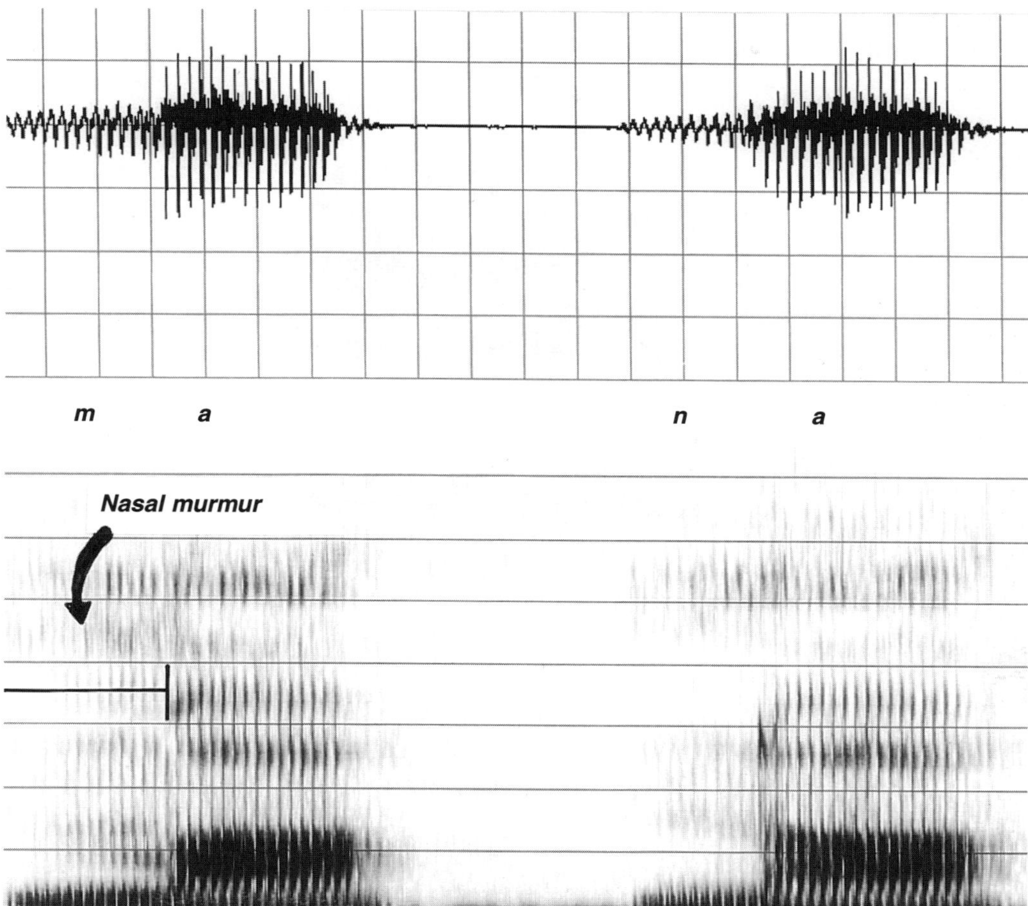

Figure 9–18. Spectrograms of the syllables (m ɑ) and (n ɑ) to illustrate acoustic features of nasal consonants. The interval of nasal murmur is marked for (m ɑ).

Fricative Consonants

A spectrogram of a complex fricative sound is shown in Figure 9–20. The fricative sound was produced by slowly changing the place of constriction by pulling the tongue backward across the following places of articulation: lingua-dental, lingua-alveolar, lingua-palatal, and lingua-velar. One of the most conspicuous features of the spectrogram is that the lower frequency limit of the noise energy generally decreases across the sound complex. That is, the frontal fricatives have a relatively high value of the lower margin of acoustic energy. Therefore a sound such as /s/ in *see* sounds higher in pitch than a sound such as /ʃ/ in *she*. The difference between these two fricatives is apparent in Figure 9–21. This figure contains two kinds of acoustic analysis for the fricatives /s/ and /ʃ/: a waveform at the top and a wide-band spectrogram at the bottom. The waveform has a random fine structure, and the spectrogram has a "salt and pepper" appearance. These are the typical acoustic patterns of noise energy.

The fricatives are distinguished from other consonants by the presence of a rather

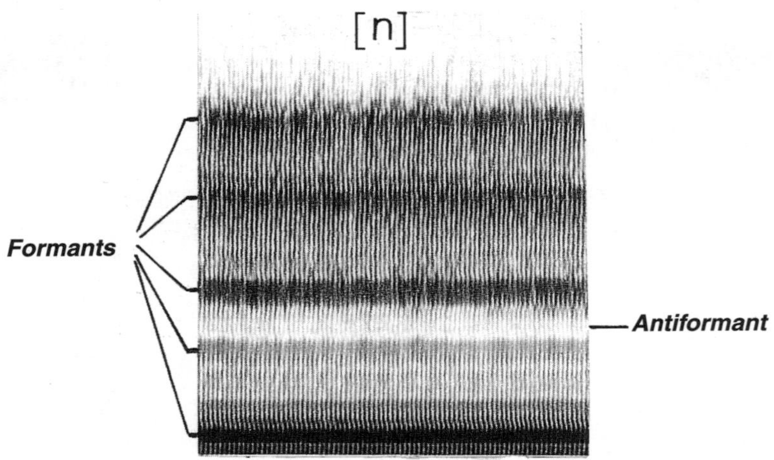

Figure 9–19. Spectrogram of a sustained nasal (n) to illustrate formants and antiformants.

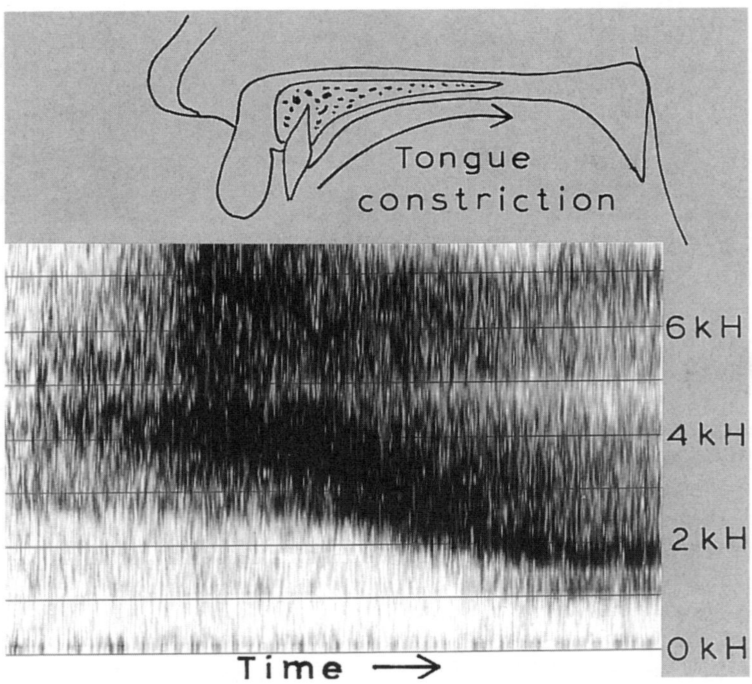

Figure 9–20. Spectrogram showing changing pattern of fricative noise energy as the tongue is moved posteriorly in the manner illustrated at the top of the figure.

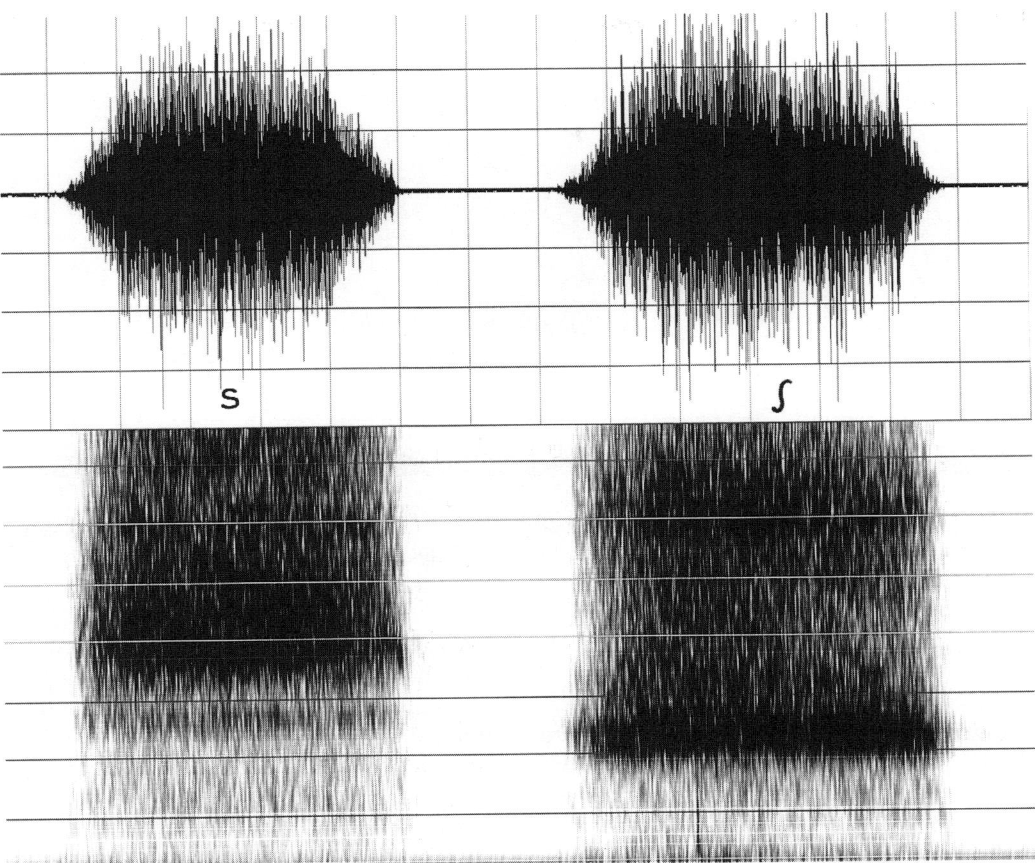

Figure 9–21. Waveform (*top*) and spectrogram (*bottom*) for the fricatives (s) as in *see* and (ʃ) as in *she*.

lengthy noise interval (frication). The spectrum of the noise is a major acoustic cue for fricative identification, but formant transitions also can be important. As discussed in Chapter 2, noise energy is generated when air is forced through a narrow constriction. Therefore, a primary feature of fricative production is a specific location at which turbulence occurs. The turbulence noise is filtered by the vocal tract, especially the cavity in front of the constriction. The role of the cavity behind the constriction depends on the geometry of the vocal tract. Characterization of the spectrum of fricative noise is not straightforward. The following summaries rely on a very general description of the major spectral features for each place of fricative production.

Labiodental fricatives (/ f v /) have low-energy, flat, and diffuse spectra. Because the front cavity is short, it has relatively little filtering effect on the noise energy (i.e., the lowest resonance frequency is so high that it is not perceptually significant).

Linguadental fricatives (/θ ð/) have low-energy, flat, and diffuse spectra. The short front cavity gives relatively little shaping to the spectrum.

The similarity of the labiodental and linguadental fricatives can be seen in Figure 9–22, which shows a spectrogram of the word *thief* spoken in isolation by a woman. Notice that the frication intervals that

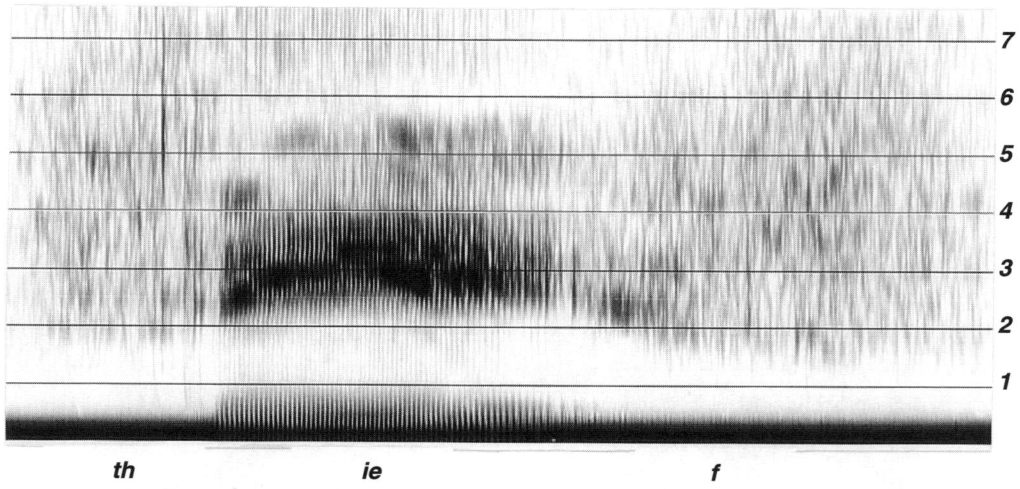

Figure 9–22. Spectrogram of the word *thief* spoken by a woman.

begin and end the word are very much alike.

Lingua-alveolar fricatives (/s z/) have high-energy noise spectra with most of the energy lying in the high frequencies (above 4 kHz for adult male speakers and above 5 kHz for adult female speakers). The front cavity is sufficiently long that it contributes to the distinctive spectral shaping.

Linguapalatal fricatives (/ʃ ʒ/) have intense noise spectra with most of the energy lying in the mid to high frequencies (above 2 kHz for men and above 3 kHz for women). The front cavity has a significant resonance effect.

The glottal fricative /h/ has a low-energy, flat, and diffuse spectrum, resembling that for the labio-dentals and lingua-dentals. Because the turbulence noise is generated in the larynx and pharynx, the sound is filtered by the vocal tract as a whole. Therefore, vowel-like formant patterns often are evident in the radiated noise.

Formant transitions can be observed for fricative consonants. The transitions are most important perceptually for the weak fricatives (labio-dentals, lingua-dentals, and the glottal). Voicing for fricatives presumably reflects whether or not the vocal folds are vibrating during the period of turbulence noise production. However, things are not quite that simple, because voicing can be signaled by other cues, including the duration of a following vowel.

Affricate Consonants

An example of the affricate /dʒ/ is shown in Figure 9–23 as a waveform and spectrogram for the word *judge*. Affricate consonants (/tʃ dʒ/) have a stop gap (silence, or low-energy interval) followed by intense frication. The stop gap marks the interval of articulatory closure. The following frication segment is generated in much the same way as the frication noise for fricatives. Transition and voicing cues are similar to those described for the preceding consonant classes.

Glide Consonants

Waveforms and spectrograms of glides (semivowels) are shown in Figure 9–24 for the words *you* and *we*. Glide consonants (/j w/) have a gradual transition (hence the

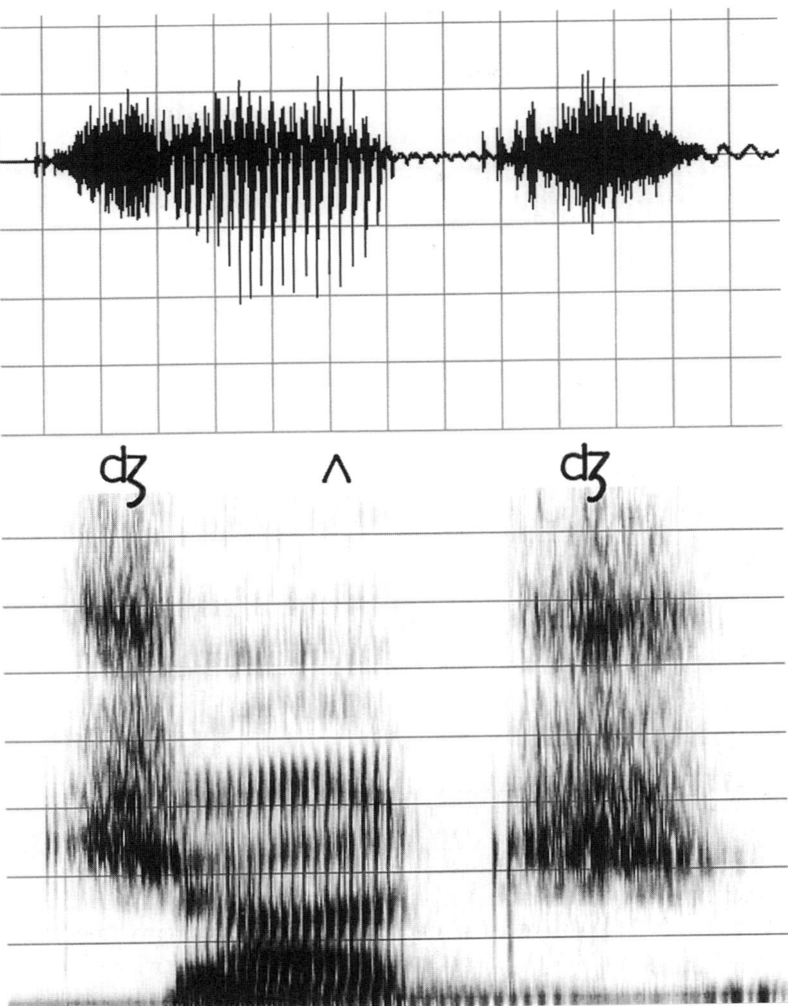

Figure 9–23. Waveform (*top*) and spectrogram (*bottom*) for the word *judge,* which contains the affricate (dʒ) in initial and final word position.

name *glide*) that appears on a spectrogram as a slowly changing formant pattern. The formant transitions typically have durations in the range of 75 to 150 ms, compared to a duration of about 50 or 75 ms for stop transitions.

Liquid Consonants

Spectrograms of the liquids (/l r/) are shown in Figure 9–25 for the words *rye* and *lie*. For liquids, the formant pattern (steady-state and transition) is the primary acoustic cue. The steady-state formant pattern is the combination of formants (and, for /l/, antiformants) that pertains to a prolongation of the /l/ or /r/ sound. The steady-state formant values for /l/ are as follows for an adult male: 360 Hz for F1, 1300 Hz for F2, and 2700 Hz for F3. Liquid /r/ has about the same steady-state frequencies for F1 and F2 but has a much lower F3 frequency of about 1600 Hz. A low frequency F3 is a distinctive acoustic property of rhotic (r-

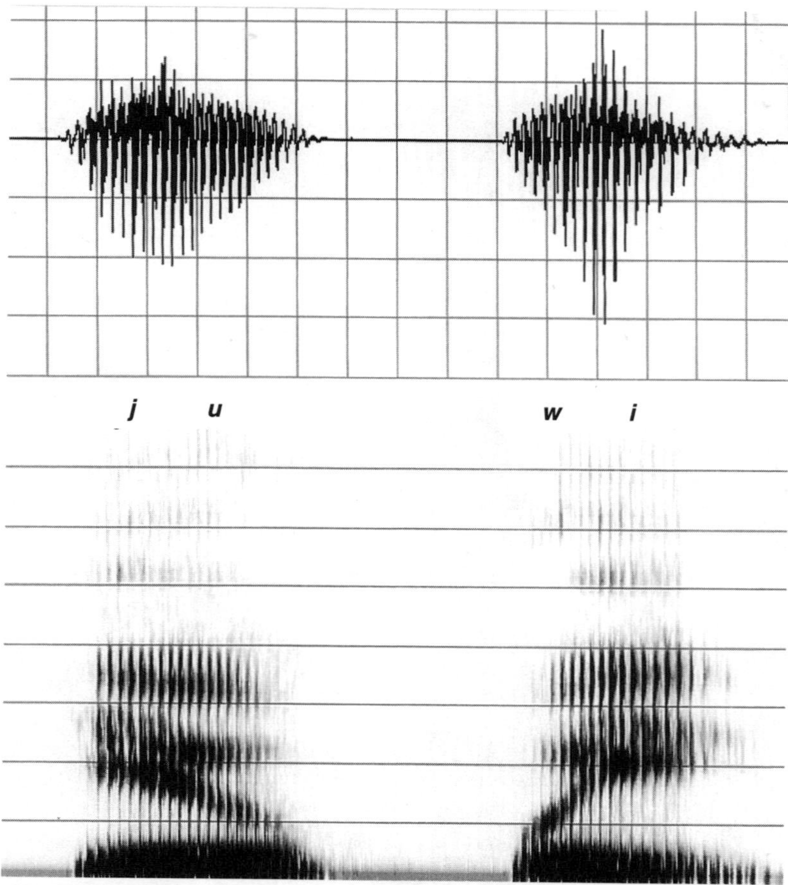

Figure 9–24. Waveform (*top*) and spectrogram (*bottom*) for the words *you* and *we* to illustrate acoustic features of the glides /j/ and /w/.

colored) sounds, for both consonants and vowels. Because /l/ is produced with a bifurcated vocal tract, with sound energy radiated on either side of the midline tongue closure, it has a complex filter function consisting of both formants and antiformants. The acoustic energy for /l/ is largely in the low frequencies.

Liquid consonants are not always produced with a steady state that is visible on a spectrogram or other acoustic analysis. Because the steady-state portion is not necessarily present, the formant transitions are the most reliable acoustic cue for auditory identification. However, the information on steady-state formant patterns summarized above is useful in defining the initial part of the formant patterns for the liquids. The formant frequencies begin with these values and then move in directions determined by the following sound.

Phonetic Quality: Suprasegmentals

The information discussed to this point in the chapter pertains to the phonetic properties of speech, that is, the segments that are used to make up syllables and words.

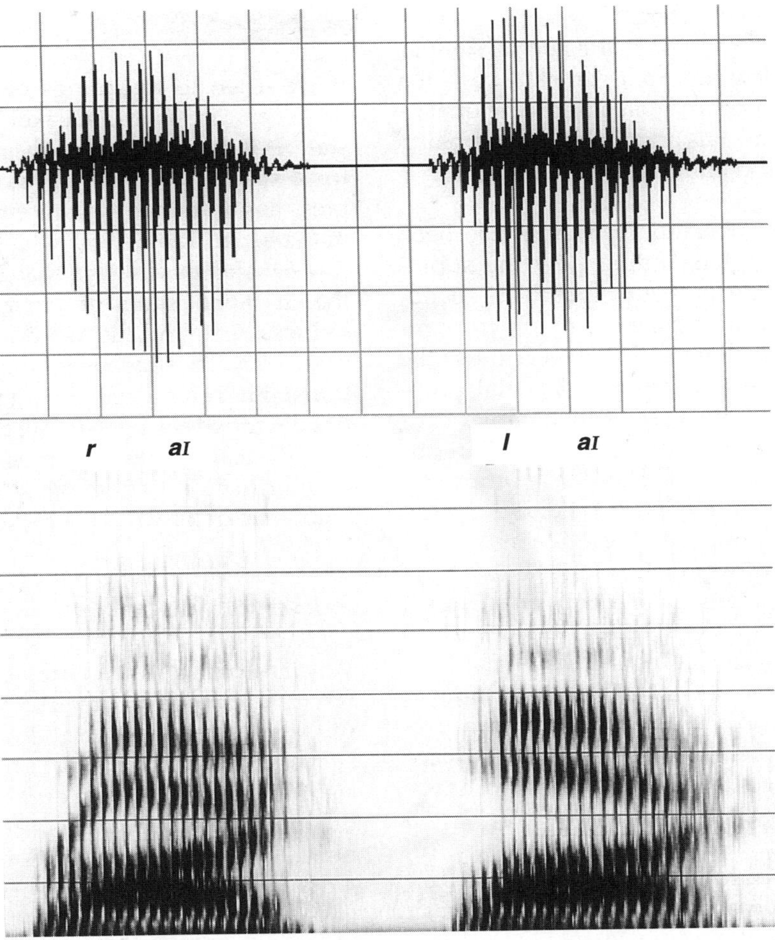

Figure 9–25. Waveform (*top*) and spectrogram (*bottom*) for the words *rye* and *lie* to illustrate acoustic features of the liquids /r/ and /l/.

But speech also consists of properties such as speaking rate, pitch, intonation, stress, and rhythm. These properties are called suprasegmentals, because their influence often extends beyond the boundaries of individual phonetic elements. The acoustic cues for the suprasegmentals are intermingled with the acoustic cues for segmental properties of speech.

It is difficult to conceive of speech without suprasegmental properties, because they are always present in some form. But to give some idea of how suprasegmentals contribute to speech, we begin with a speech pattern that is relatively neutral in its suprasegmental makeup. Imagine a speech sample produced with a monopitch, an average speaking rate, and without emphasis on any particular word. Early attempts at synthesized speech sometimes were characterized as having this kind of quality. Such a sample of speech may sound rather colorless, as though it lacks the dynamism of typical speech. Now imagine that the same phonetic sequence is produced with an altered suprasegmental pattern, that is, with pitch variations, with either a slow or rapid speaking rate, and with emphasis on one particular word. In contrast to the neutral sample, this sample with suprasegmental variation will have a richer, more interesting quality. Suprasegmentals add flavor to speech and they can also influence the meaning.

Although substantial progress has been made in understanding how the suprasegmental properties of speech are encoded in the acoustic signal, much work remains to be done in this area. Because the relations between suprasegmental properties and acoustic cues are complex, this issue is not discussed in any detail in this book. For the most part, these properties involve adjustments in fundamental frequency (average level or dynamics), the durations of segments, and the intensity of the components of speech. For example, when we speak at different pitch levels (such as when mothers talk to infants as opposed to adults), a long-term adjustment is made in vocal fundamental frequency. When a speaker wishes to place greater stress (emphasis) on a word, a typical strategy is to give the stressed word an (a) increased fundamental frequency, (b) increased duration, and (c) increased intensity. However, different speakers may not use the three adjustments to the same degree. Changes in speaking rate involve, at the minimum, a reduction in the average segment durations of a speech sample. But changes in speaking rate also tend to be accompanied by phonetic changes, especially a reduction in the range of acoustic values (reflecting a reduction in the range of articulatory movements at rapid speaking rates).

These changes in suprasegmental phonetic quality are superimposed on the acoustic cues that transmit information on the phonetic quality for the vowels and consonants in the utterance. Somehow the listener is able to distinguish these sources of information.

Affective Quality

If we listen to recordings of speech, we often can discern the speaker's emotional state. Is it possible to identify acoustic cues for a speaker's affect? Considerable progress has been made in this effort, as summarized in Table 9–5, which identifies some major parameters that differentiate the emotional states of anger, happiness, sadness, fear, and disgust (Murray & Arnott, 1993). These acoustic adjustments are transmitted along with the phonetic qualities described earlier in this chapter. Therefore, the listener must "peel off" the acoustic information pertaining to a speaker's emotional quality.

Personal Quality

We all recognize voices, sometimes identifying a telephone caller we have not talked with for several years. Obviously, the acoustic signal contains information sufficient to identify a speaker. This prompts the question if acoustic analyses might permit objective determination of an individual speaker's identity. This possibility gave rise to the use of **voiceprints** for individual identification. The term *voiceprint* was coined in 1944 by Gray and Kopp and reintroduced about two decades later by Kersta (1962). Kersta was an early advocate of the possibility of speaker recognition through comparisons of visual patterns. The "voiceprint" was considered by some authorities to be analogous to the fingerprint. Others preferred the term *voicegram* to avoid the suggestion that voice analyses were as individual as fingerprints. A fingerprint is in fact a direct physical impression of a finger that touches a surface. In contrast, a voice sample becomes a visual representation only through a series of transformations that convert acoustic energy to some kind of analysis printed on paper. In addition, the acoustic

Table 9–5. Selected speech and voice correlates of human vocal emotion.

	Anger	Happiness	Sadness	Fear	Disgust
Speech Rate	Slightly faster	Faster or slower	Slightly slower	Much faster	Very much slower
Pitch Average	Very much higher	Much higher	Slightly lower	Very much higher	Very much lower
Pitch Range	Much wider	Much wider	Slightly narrower	Much wider	Slightly wider
Intensity	Higher	Higher	Lower	Normal	Lower
Voice Quality	Breathy, chest tone	Breathy, blaring	Resonant	Irregular voicing	Grumbled chest tone
Pitch Changes	Abrupt, on stressed syllables	Smooth, upward inflections	Downward inflections	Normal	Wide, downward terminal inflections
Articulation	Tense	Normal	Slurring	Precise	Normal

Source: Based on data from Toward the Simulation of Emotion in Synthetic Speech by I. R. Murray and J. L. Arnott, 1993. *Journal of the Acoustical Society of America, 93,* 1097–1108.

signal of speech is influenced by many factors, including the phonetic constituents of a particular utterance, the prosodic properties of the utterance, accompanying emotional features, and even the state of the speaker's health (Kent & Chial, in press). Voice identification involves a large number of variables that must be carefully considered in its application to situations such as criminal investigations. This subject is discussed briefly in Chapter 12. For a recent review of this field, see Nolan (1997) and Kent and Chial (in press).

Transmittal Quality

Transmittal quality gives the listener perspectival information on the talker's location, including such things as the distance from the listener, the speaker's orientation in space, the presence of background sounds, and the influence of environmental acoustics that may introduce effects such as reverberation. These issues are not discussed here, but are extremely important factors in speech communication.

Phrases and Sentences

The complexity of speech becomes increasingly evident as we consider the acoustic patterns of phrases and sentences. A spectrogram of a simple sentence, *We were away a year ago*, is shown in Figure 9–26. Because the phonetic constituents of this utterance are predominantly vowels and glides, the spectrogram is characterized especially by changing formant patterns. Several features are of interest. First, notice that, in general, word boundaries are not particu-

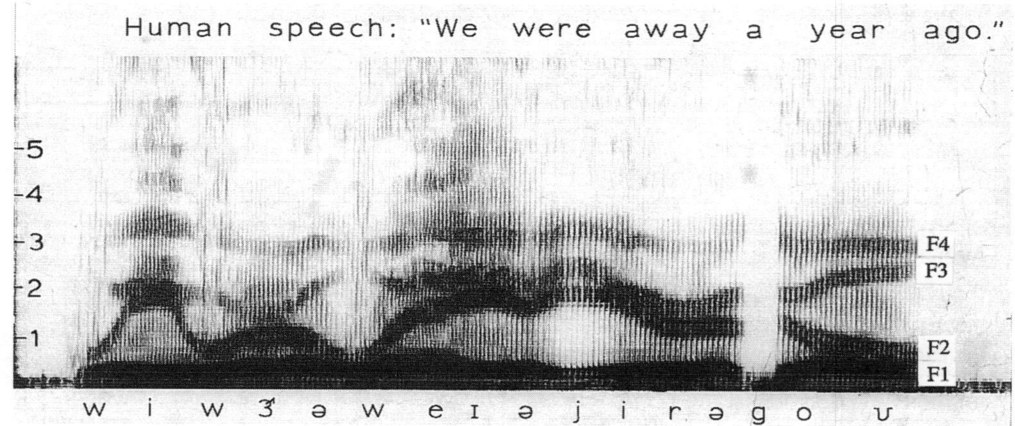

Figure 9–26. Spectrogram of the sentence *We were away a year ago* spoken by a man.

larly obvious. The formants tend to weave nearly continuously across the utterance, and they are not even interrupted by a word boundary. Only occasionally is there a fairly clear acoustic correlate of a boundary between words. Second, the boundaries between adjacent phonemes are also rather obscure. Because the formant changes are generally gradual, it is difficult to identify distinct time points at which one segment definitely ends and another begins. Probably the most striking acoustic event is the stop gap for /g/ in *ago*. Third, this spectrogram shows how F1, F2, and F3 frequencies vary from segment to segment.

The utterance represented in Figure 9–26 is a good example of continuously changing formants. Other acoustic constrasts are illustrated in the spectrogram of Figure 9–27, which pertains to the utterance, *The amplitude of speech varies widely.* The vertical lines represent the approximate locations of the word boundaries, as judged by the author. This spectrogram illustrates how the spectrogram changes for a variety of phonetic segments, including vowels, liquids, stops, fricatives, and nasals. The tracing at the top of the spectrogram is the waveform (amplitude versus time) and is useful for both (a) segmenting the utterance into words or phonetic elements, and (b) viewing the intensity differences across the utterance.

In our increasingly technological world, we sometimes hear speech produced by machines as well as by humans. Machine speech, or synthetic speech, resembles natural speech in its overall acoustic characteristics. What does computer-synthesized speech look like in a spectrogram? Figure 9–28 is a spectrogram of an early form of speech synthesis. (This sample should not be taken as representative of more sophisticated recent efforts, which are discussed in Chapter 12.) The utterance shown in Figure 9–28 is, suitably enough, *I am a computer.* The spectrogram of this sample of synthesized speech has a rough resemblance to a spectrogram of human speech. However, notice that the most variable acoustic patterns occupy a limited bandwidth, below about 3 kHz. Acoustic patterns above that frequency are both weak in energy and almost invariant in spectral properties. The first three formants, F1, F2, and F3, are readily visible. The synthesized speech is highly stylized and lacks

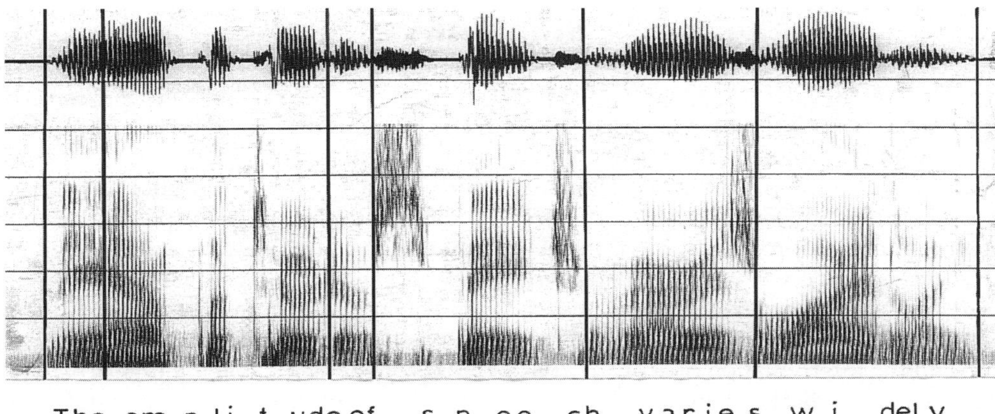

Figure 9–27. Spectrogram of the sentence *The amplitude of speech varies widely* spoken by a man.

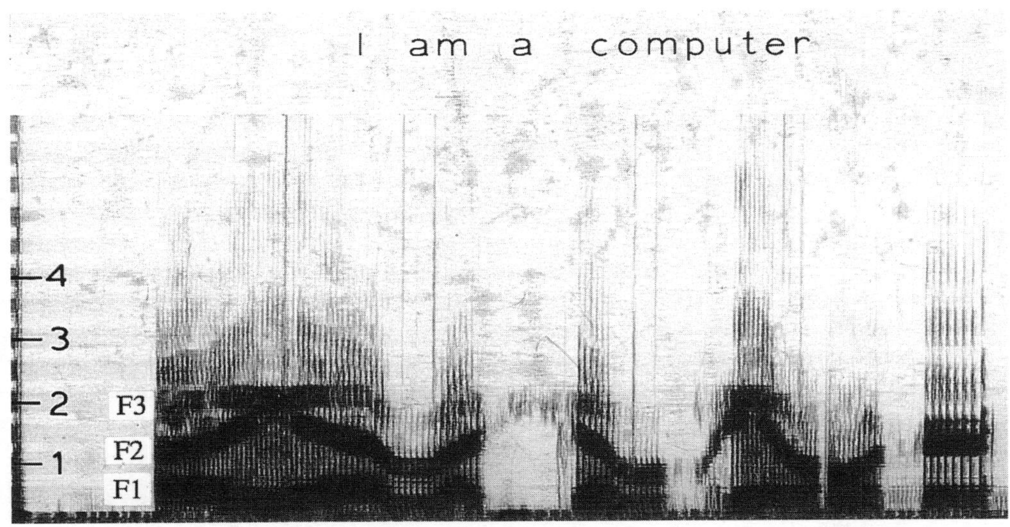

Figure 9–28. Spectrogram of the sentence *I am a computer* produced by a speech synthesizer.

the rich redundancy of human speech. The auditory impression of this sample was that it had a rather mechanical quality. It sounded like a machine. A much higher quality can be obtained with newer methods of speech synthesis, some of which are discussed in Chapter 12.

SUMMARY

Speech acoustics has been discussed from three general perspectives: acoustic theory of speech production, methods of acoustic analysis of speech, and acoustic correlates of information sources in speech. In fact, these three perspectives are closely related. Methods of acoustic analysis typically are based on an understanding of acoustic theory, and the interpretation of acoustic cues for speech sounds also depends on a theory of speech sound production. Acoustic analyses of speech make very clear the differences among infants, children, women, and men. These differences should be taken into account in theories of speech production and in application of acoustic methods to the study of speech. For most intents and purposes, the acoustic signal is the *sine qua non* of speech. Speech must be heard for it to be known that it exists. A primary value of acoustic analysis is that it focuses on the signal that intervenes between speaker and listener. Accordingly, this analysis can tell us much about both speech production and speech perception. The latter is the subject of the next chapter.

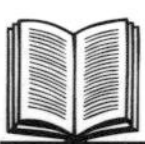

On The Reference Shelf

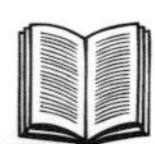

References for the reader who seeks extended discussions of the acoustic characteristics of speech.

Fant, G. (1960). *Acoustic theory of speech production.* The Hague: Mouton.
A classic treatise on the source-filter theory of speech production and its implications.

Fujimura, O., & Erickson, D. (1997). Acoustic phonetics. In W. Hardcastle & J. Laver (Eds.), *The handbook of phonetic sciences* (pp. 65–115). Oxford, England: Blackwell.
A general introductory discussion of the field, with many spectrograms.

Kent, R. D., & Read, W. C. (1992). *The acoustic analysis of speech.* San Diego: Singular Publishing Group.
A nonmathematical introduction to general issues in speech acoustics, including the acoustic theory of speech production, methods of acoustic analysis, and acoustic properties of speech sounds.

Chapter References

Blumstein, S. E., & Stevens, K. N. (1979). Acoustic invariance in speech production: Evidence from measurements of the spectral characteristics of stop consonants. *Journal of the Acoustical Society of America, 66,* 1001–1017.

Fant, G. (1960). *Acoustic theory of speech production*. The Hague: Mouton.

Fujimura, O., & Erickson, D. (1997). Acoustic phonetics. In W. Hardcastle & J. Laver (Eds.), *The handbook of phonetic sciences* (pp. 65–115). Oxford, England: Blackwell.

Gray, C. H., & Kopp, G. A. (1944). *Voiceprint identification.* (Bell Telephone Laboratories Technical Report 1, 1–14). Murray Hill, NJ: Bell Laboratories.

Hillenbrand, J., Getty, L. A., Clark, M. J., & Wheeler, K. (1995). Acoustic characteristics of American English vowels. *Journal of the Acoustical Society of America, 97,* 3099–3111.

Kent, R. D. (1993). Vocal tract acoustics. *Journal of Voice, 7*, 97–117.

Kent, R. D., & Chial, M. R. (in press). Voice spectrography ("Voiceprints"). In D. L. Faigman, D. Kaye, M. J. Saks, & J. Sanders (Eds.), *Modern scientific evidence.* St. Paul: West Publishing Co.

Kent, R. D., Dembowski, J., & Lass, N. J. (1996). Acoustic characteristics of the sounds of American English. In N. J. Lass (Ed.), *Principles of experimental phonetics* (pp. 185–225). St. Louis: C. V. Mosby.

Kent, R. D., Netsell, R., Osberger, M. J., & Hustedde, C. G. (1987). Phonetic development in twins who differ in auditory function. *Journal of Speech and Hearing Disorders, 52*, 64-75.

Kent, R. D., & Read, W. C. (1992). *The acoustic analysis of speech.* San Diego: Singular Publishing Group.

Kersta, L. G. (1962). Voiceprint identification. *Nature, 196*, 1253–1257.

Klatt, D. H. (1975). Voice onset time, frication and aspiration in word-initial consonant clusters. *Journal of the Acoustical Society of America, 18*, 686–706.

Koenig, W., Dunn, H. D., & Lacy, L. Y. (1946). The sound spectrograph. *Journal of the Acoustical Society of America, 17*, 19–49.

Murray, I. R., & Arnott, J. L. (1993). Toward the simulation of emotion in synthetic speech: A review of the literature on human vocal emotion. *Journal of the Acoustical Society of America, 93*, 1097–1108.

Nolan, F. (1997). Speaker recognition and forensic phonetics. In W. Hardcastle & J. Laver (Eds.), *The handbook of phonetic sciences* (pp. 744–767). Oxford, England: Blackwell.

Pickett, J. M. (1980). *The sounds of speech communication*. Baltimore: University Park Press.

Peterson, G. E., & Barney, H. E. (1952). Control methods used in a study of vowels. *Journal of the Acoustical Society of America, 24*, 175–184.

Potter, R., Kopp, G., & Green, H. (1947). *Visible speech.* New York: Van Nostrand Reinhold (reprinted in 1966 by Dover Press, New York).

Stevens, K. N., & Blumsten, S. E. (1978). Invariant cues for the place of articulation in stop consonants. *Journal of the Acoustical Society of America, 64*, 1358–1368.

Stevens, K. N., & House, A. S. (1961). An acoustical theory of vowel production and some of its implications. *Journal of Speech and Hearing Research, 4*, 303–320.

Syrdal, A. K., & Gopal, H. S. (1986). A perceptual model of vowel recognition based on the auditory represention of American English vowels. *Journal of the Acoustical Society of America, 79*, 1086–1100.

Exercises

9-1. By referring to Table 9–2 or 9–3, describe the differences in formant structure for the word pairs listed below. Notice that only the vowels are different in each word pair.

Example:

seat	suit

[The /i/ in seat has a higher F2 and higher F3 frequency; F1 is nearly the same]

hat	hot
fit	foot
heat	hat
her	hoe
hoot	hot

9-2. Describe the major acoustic events that are expected for the phonetic sequence in the word *cats. Hint:* Begin with the phonetic transcription [k æ t s] and then determine the acoustic cues for each phonetic element.

9-3. Although speech usually is readily understood as an auditory signal, it can be very difficult to make phonetic sense of the visual representation of speech in a spectrogram. This is an exercise in manual segmentation, that is, the division of a spectrogram into its phonetic components. The figure below is a spectrogram of the word *yesterday*. Draw vertical lines to segment the spectrogram into its presumed phonetic elements. Compare your segmentation with that of another person. How well did you agree?

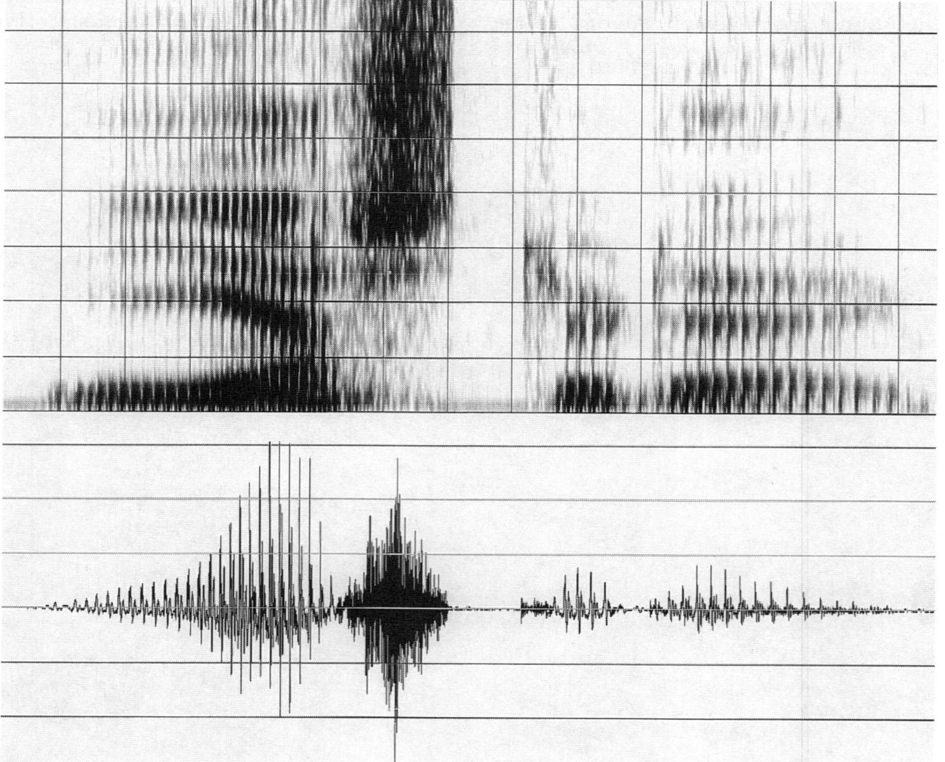

9-4. By examining the spectrogram below, try to determine which of the following words is the subject of analysis: *seeds, keeps, suits, zoos,* or *juice.*

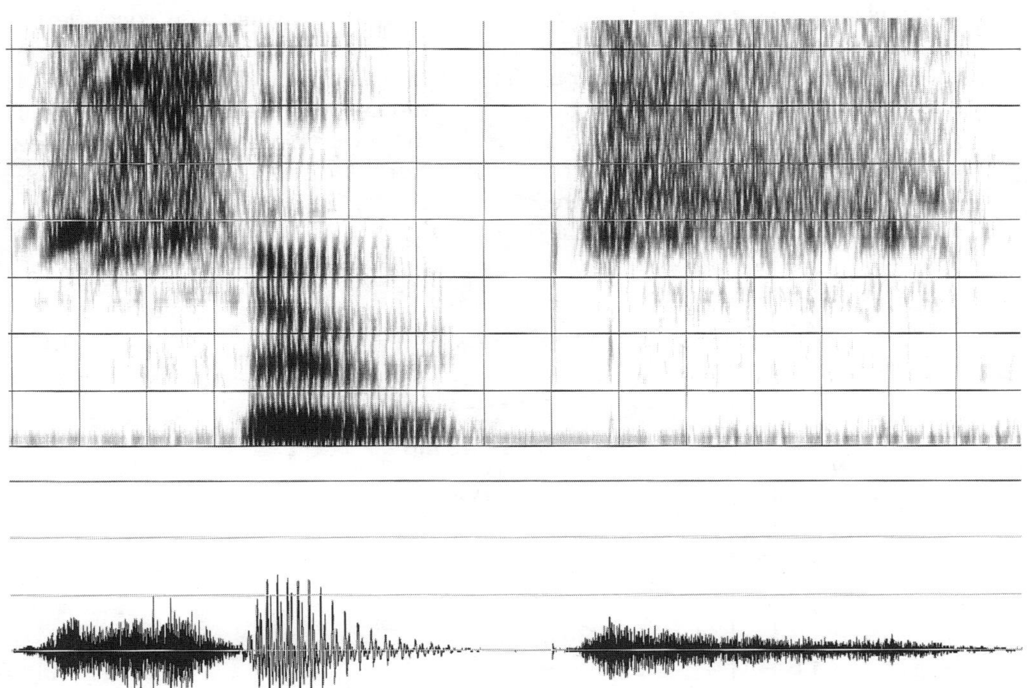

9-5. The top figure below shows the vowel formant regions obtained in a longitudinal study of a male infant. Vowels in babbling and early words were studied at the ages of 8, 12, and 15 months. Measurements of the vowels were used to generate the data shown in this figure. How would you interpret these data in terms of (a) growth of the vocal tract, and (b) acquisition of the vowel system of American English? The bottom figure shows vowel formant data for the twin brother of the infant represented in the top figure. But the boy whose data appear in the bottom figure was born with a profound hearing impairment. Compare the data in the two figures. What would you conclude regarding the effects of hearing loss on early phonetic development? (For a discussion of the acoustic analyses of the vocalizations of this twin pair, see Kent, Netsell, Osberger, and Hustedde, 1987.)

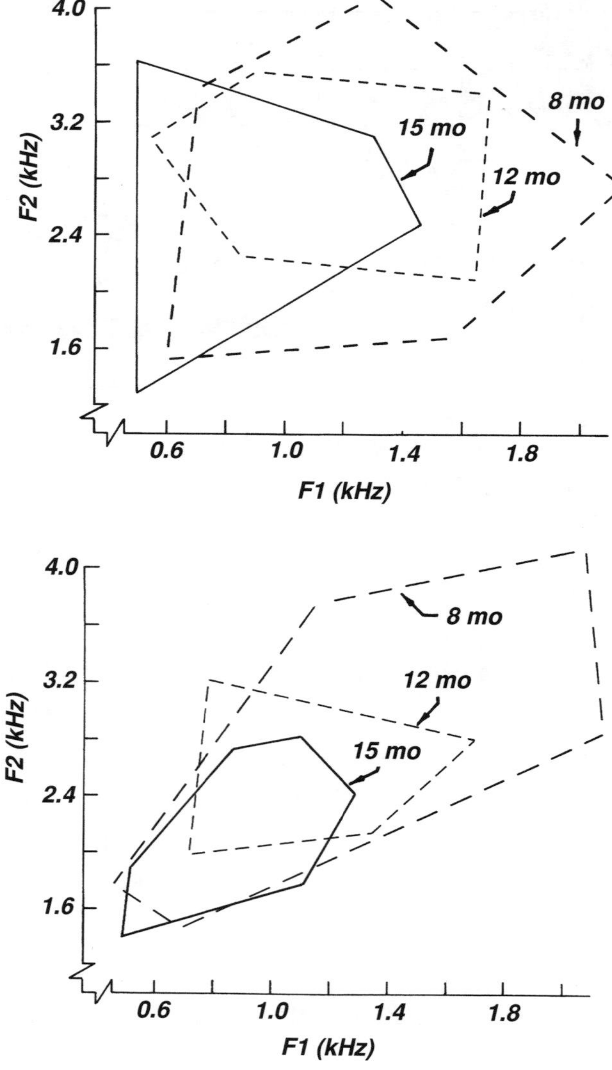

CHAPTER

10

Speech Perception

> ***A word is dead***
> ***When it is said,***
> ***Some say.***
> ***I say it just***
> ***Begins to live***
> ***That day.***
>
> — Emily Dickinson
>
> (From *The Poems of Emily Dickinson,* Thomas H. Johnson, ed. Cambridge, MA: The Belnap Press of Harvard University. Reprinted with permission.)

The world abounds with sounds. In many everyday situations, we find ourselves listening to speech—often trying to understand the speech of one particular person even as other conversations, radio broadcasts, and public address announcements create a sometimes troublesome speech background. How do we understand the speech of other people? How do we select one voice in particular from a crowd of conversing persons? By what processes do we take in the perishable acoustic signal of speech and quickly reach decisions about who said it, what was said, and how it was said? All of these decisions must be made before the speaker produces the next utterance, or before we formulate a response of our own. These are some of the questions that the study of speech perception attempts to answer.

The modern era in the study of speech perception began in the middle of the 20th century with the introduction of machines that conveniently analyzed speech into visible patterns on paper. Although various types of analysis had been around for decades before this time, the earlier techniques were laborious to use and did not always result in easily interpretable representations of speech. But in about 1950, the study of speech was facilitated by two machines that complemented one another and greatly stimulated the scientific study of speech perception. One was the spectrograph discussed in Chapter 9. The other was the **pattern playback**, an instrument that converted visual patterns into speech-like sounds. The spectrograph revealed the acoustic cues for various speech sounds, and the pattern playback enabled the investigator to produce synthetic replicas of speech. The spectrograph was the basic tool of analysis, and the pattern playback was the tool of synthesis.

With advances in technology, both the spectrograph and the pattern playback have been replaced by faster and more sophisticated instruments, but the basic idea of using analysis and synthesis as complementary operations is still a highly productive method in speech science. A great deal has been learned about speech perception by the use of these laboratory tools. This chapter reviews some fundamental discoveries about the perception of speech and the development of theories to account for speech perception.

ACOUSTIC-PERCEPTUAL INVARIANCE IN SPEECH

"It is the immense difference between the physical acoustic signal on the one hand and the perceptual-cognitive world on the other hand that has frustrated theorists and researchers."

(Stephen Handel, *Listening: An Introduction to the Perception of Auditory Events.* Cambridge, MA: Massachusetts Institute of Technology, 1989, p. 265.)

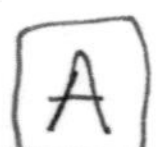

It was noted in Chapter 9 that the acoustic speech signal is highly variable. Any given sound will have a somewhat different acoustic appearance from one production to the next. The variations can be particularly evident when the sound is produced in different phonetic environments (that is, different neighboring sounds) or by different talkers. This variability presents a major problem, because the object of speech perception is to identify phonetic units of some kind. But units must possess some kind of invariance or constancy if they are to be identified. How can the requisite perceptual constancy be achieved if the acoustic properties of individual phonetic events vary across speakers, across conditions such as changes in speaking rate, and even across repetitions of the same sound by the same speaker? In psychology, this is known as the problem of **perceptual constancy** or **perceptual invariance** (Handel, 1989). To account for this problem, five major theoretical directions have been pursued.

Prototypes or Templates

The first theoretical direction relies on **prototypes**, or **templates**. These are exemplars or "ideal forms" of the acoustic pattern for a given phonetic event. These prototypes are representative of expected sound categories. Incoming stimuli are compared against these ideal representations and the closest match is selected. Imagine, for example, that a sound is represented by a particular formant pattern. The template would serve as a reference pattern against which incoming formant patterns would be compared. Figure 10–1 illustrates the basic procedure. The incoming stimuli may be preprocessed or normalized (adjusted to some reference) to facilitate the comparison of stimuli with the prototype. For example, because acoustic properties vary among talkers (as discussed in Chapter 9), normalization can be helpful to eliminate intertalker differences, especially those attributable to age and gender.

Although prototypes have lost some of their popularity in contemporary theories of speech perception, many researchers continue to find them useful. Blumstein and Stevens (1979) proposed that spectral templates for stop bursts could be the basis for the identification of stop consonants from their bursts alone. Examples of spectral templates for bursts were given in Chapter 9. Kuhl, Williams, Lacerda, Stevens, and Lindblom (1992), studying infant speech perception, presented cross-language evidence for templates. The authors of this study referred to the templates as having a **perceptual magnet effect**, in which sounds similar to the prototype are identified with it. In other words, the perceptual magnet "warps" the perceptual space, so that acoustic patterns that are close to the center of a phonetic category (the magnet) are perceived as highly similar. Apparently, this effect occurs in human adults and infants listening to speech sounds, but not for the same sounds in monkeys (Kuhl, 1991). Jusczyk (1993) proposed a model of speech perception in infants that is based on templates. But this is not to say that template recognition is useful only for human speech sounds. The idea also has been applied to nonhuman vocalizations, including birdsongs (Anderson, Dave, & Margoliash, 1996). A major question to be answered about prototypes, or templates, is how the idealized representations come about. How do we know if two sounds A and B are variants of a single prototype or two different prototypes? Possibly, experience with a particular language (or more than one language in the case of children exposed to two or more languages) helps to mold the prototypes, creating perceptual "magnets" that the child uses to organize auditory stimuli.

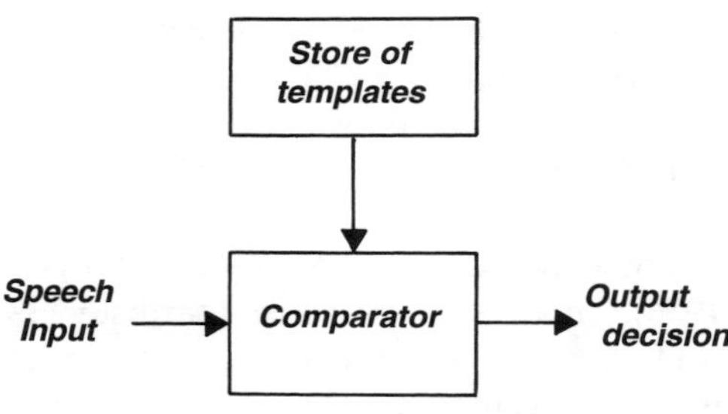

Figure 10–1. Diagram of a process of speech recognition based on templates or exemplars. The speech input is compared with stored templates and the closest match is selected as the decision unit.

Features

The second theoretical alternative is based on **features**. According to feature theory, the various attributes that compose stimuli are identified through a process of abstraction. A number of feature solutions have been proposed for speech perception. Typically, features are considered to be the defining attributes of an element to be recognized. To take a nonspeech example, the following features might be used to recognize a young girl: human, female, young. A change in one feature can change the identified object. For example, a change from female to male changes the identified object from a girl to a boy. A change from young to old changes the identified object from a girl to a woman. In similar fashion, speech sounds can be analyzed in terms of characteristic features. The stop consonant [b], as in *bay*, might be analyzed as having the features stop, voiced, and bilabial. A change in one feature can make a difference in which sound is recognized. For example, a change in voicing (from voiced to voiceless) would change the sound recognized from [b] to [p] (as in *pay*).

In most feature systems proposed for speech sounds, the temporal relations among features are typically neglected, even though timing seems essential to speech. One of the drawbacks to the feature approach is that features are difficult to define and describe. Therefore, the features in many systems are actually a composite of very different kinds of features, some defined at the articulatory level, some at the acoustic level, and some at the perceptual level. One advantage of features is that they often are used in phonological analyses. If the same set of features could be used to account for speech perception and for phonological operations, they would offer both power and economy. That is, a small number of features could be used to account for the formation and recognition of words in a language. The features would be basic components used in language structure and processing.

Is there any evidence that we hear speech in terms of features? One source of evidence is that when listeners try to perceive a distorted speech signal, or try to remember several sounds in a sequence, they often seem to perceive or remember "parts" of the sound. For example, listeners might not respond correctly with *b* when *b* is presented, but they might respond with *p*, which differs from *b* in the single feature of voicing (*b* is voiced and *p* is voiceless), or they might respond with *g*, which differs from *b* in the single feature of place of articulation. This partial perception or recall indicates that listeners analyze sounds in terms of constitutent features. This aspect of speech perception was demonstrated in a classic paper by G. A. Miller and P. E. Nicely (1955). Their work on perceptual confusions among speech sounds has been followed by a large number of experiments that continue to the present. Additional evidence for features came from a research method called selective adaptation (Eimas & Corbit, 1973). But it should not be concluded that there is unanimous support for features among those who study speech perception. For a general discussion of this area of research, see Diehl (1981).

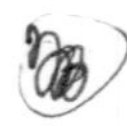

Higher Order Variables

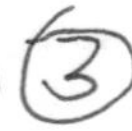

The third kind of theory invokes higher order variables as the means for perceptual constancy. According to this view, acoustic events are uniquely specified by time-varying complex properties. Consistent patterns of energy are thought to occur because they arise from a sound source with self-consistent properties. Consistencies of the source are reflected as consistencies in the acoustic stimulus. Perceptual learning, then, is the discovery of these higher order variables. One example of this approach in speech perception is the vector analysis (or "event perception") proposed by Fowler (1986). This theory proposes that listeners can follow or "hear out" the different articulatory movements that underlie coarticulatory patterns in speech. For example, the listener may be able to hear the acoustic result of tongue or lip movement. However, it is not clear how variables are identified for complex stimuli, and this remains a major problem to be resolved. In some respects, this explanation is consistent with some principles summarized in Chapter 7 for the role of subcortical processing in audition. In that chapter, it is noted that the object of hearing may not be simply to analyze sounds but to identify sound sources.

Innate Systems

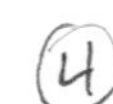

The fourth theoretical approach is based on innate systems. Invariant cues are identified by innate mechanisms. That is, we are simply born with the ability to achieve perceptual constancy. One problem with this theory is how one accounts for the effects of sensory experience. When and how is sensory experience used? In addition, the appeal to innate mechanisms is considered by some to be a weak explanation that begs the question. Proponents of the innate system theory might reply that the innate mechanisms are the result of evolutionary adaptations by which the sensory systems are equipped with the means for reliable perception, even before the individual has substantial sensory experience with the physical world. Still, one would like to explain how the innate mechanisms work: What are the principles? Can they be modeled? Could they be used to develop machines that understand speech? To what extent and by what means are innate mechanisms altered by sensory experience?

Connectionist Networks

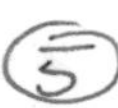

Finally, a recent theoretical direction is known as **connectionist networks**, or **parallel distributed processing** (PDP). The basic assumption is that behavior can be modeled with networks that involve large numbers of interconnected units. These networks are modeled on computers and may involve thousands of units. Some writers view these networks as analogous to neurons, which also have multiple connections. For this reason, the computer networks are sometimes dubbed "neural networks." However, the connectionist networks need not be considered as models of neural networks to be valuable theoretically. Connectionist networks learn patterns that represent the structure of input units, for example, phonetic patterns in speech. The patterns are represented as levels of energy in the connections between nodes. The network "learns" the structure by adjusting energy levels among units until the output of the system matches the input. Critics of this approach question if it really tells us anything about the way humans perceive speech. Proponents of connectionism point to the remarkable success of this procedure in modeling various types of human behavior, including aspects of language. For example, connectionist networks "learning" language patterns sometimes make the same kind of developmental errors committed by children.

EXPERIMENTAL PHENOMENA IN SPEECH PERCEPTION

This section recounts some experimental findings that have been particularly influential in contemporary thinking about speech perception. These phenomena are categorical perception, laterality effects, adaptation effects, and trading relations.

Categorical Perception

Categorical perception is a phenomenon of speech perception that has a long and complex history. Categorical, as opposed to continuous, perception, means that a lis-

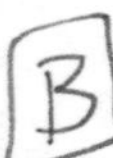

tener categorizes stimuli in such a way that the stimuli within a particular category sound alike. Categorical perception does not simply mean that stimuli can be grouped into categories. Rather, experimental confirmation requires that two general requirements be satisfied. The first requirement is that a continuum of stimuli, varying along some parameter(s), has one or more boundaries that divide the stimuli into perceptual categories. This requirement is demonstrated in an **identification experiment**, which involves the labeling of stimuli. For example, stimuli from a VOT continuum (Figure 10–2) might be labeled as either voiced or voiceless. The second requirement is that the stimuli within a category are poorly discriminated compared to stimuli from different categories. This requirement is demonstrated in a **discrimination experiment**, which involves distinguishing among the various stimuli that form a continuum. For example, using the stimuli in Figure 10–2, the stimuli with VOT values of 40 and 50 ms should be nearly indistinguishable (a near chance level of discrimination), but the stimuli with VOT values of 10 ms and 30 ms should be readily distinguishable. In short, stimuli that are judged to be in the same category are hard to tell apart, whereas stimuli from different categories are readily discriminated.

The concept of categorical perception is by no means unique to speech signals. The same hypothesis can be applied to the perception of colors, for example. The spectrum of colors can be divided into categories such as red, orange, and yellow. But the category of red includes different hues of red. As explained earlier, categorical perception requires not only the demonstration of categorial effects in an identification or labeling experiment, but also predictable variations in the discrimination of stimuli within and across category boundaries. Just because colors can be reliably labeled does not mean that categorical identification has been demonstrated. The next step is to show variations in discrimination related to the presence of category boundaries. The same requirements apply to any number of stimuli, including non-speech sounds.

The categorical perception of speech sounds has assumed a special significance in the history of speech research and has played a major role in theories about speech perception. The early experiments on this phe-

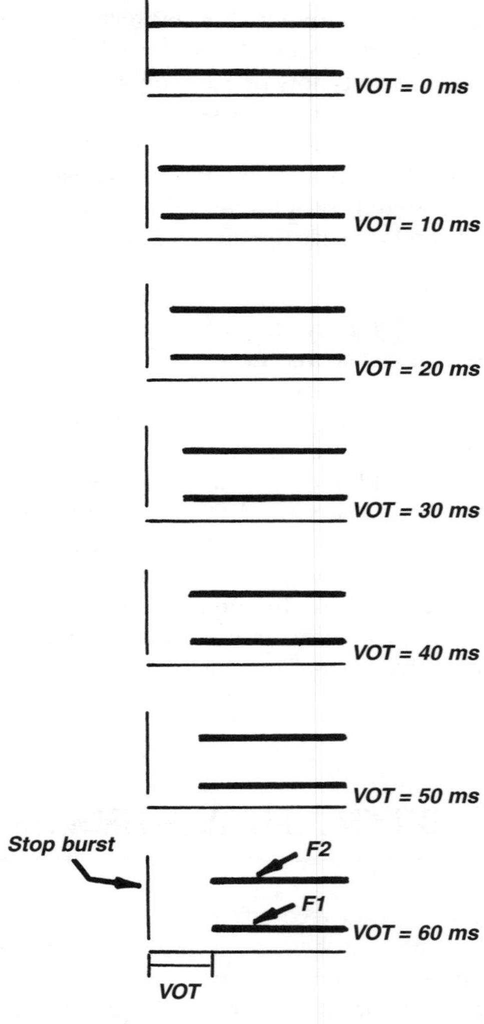

Figure 10–2. A continuum of stimuli that vary in VOT (voice onset time).

nomenon were interpreted to mean that consonant sounds were perceived categorically, but vowel sounds were not. These results contributed to the development of a theory of speech perception considered later in this chapter. Categorical perception has been studied especially for the speech sound continua: voice onset time (VOT), place of articulation, and rise time. VOT will be used as an example in this discussion. As shown in Figure 10–2, a continuum of stimuli can be prepared by techniques such as computer-synthesized speech so that different stimuli have different values of VOT. When the stimuli are presented to listeners for identification, the number of categories depends on the linguistic background of the listeners. For speakers of American English, the different VOT stimuli tend to be heard as one of two categories, a voiced sound like [b] or a voiceless sound like [p]. The identification functions are graphed in Figure 10–3. Notice that [b] judgments predominate for VOT values less than about 20 ms, and that [p] judgments begin to predominate for VOT values higher than 30 ms. In conformity with the definition of categorical perception, a point on the continuum divides the stimuli into voiced and voiceless categories. The boundary region for VOT is about +20 ms, but varies somewhat with factors such as place of consonant articulation and speaking rate. The second part of the experiment is to evaluate listeners' discrimination of the various VOT stimuli. It turns out that listeners do quite well in discriminating stimuli that are selected from the boundary region. They do not do so well in discriminating within-category stimuli such as VOT patterns that are all identified as voiced. In other words, the physical stimuli can be arranged into a small number of categories, and the members of a category are hard to tell apart.

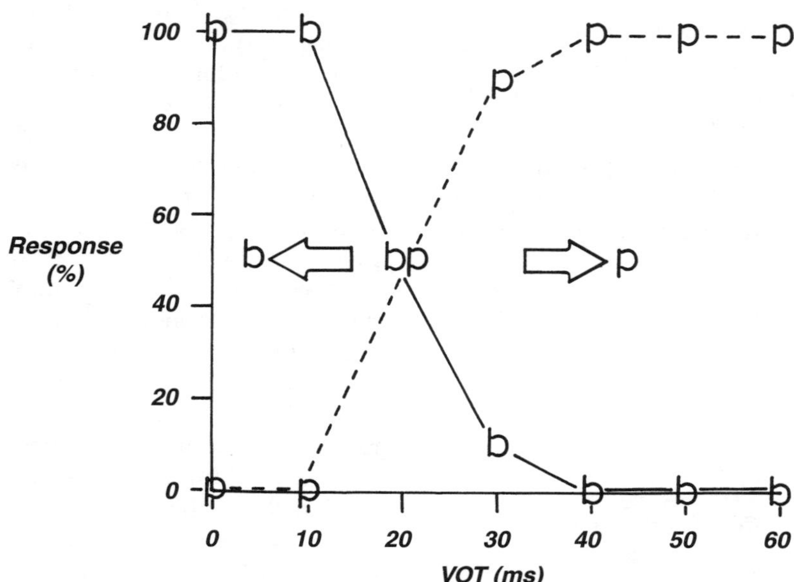

Figure 10–3. Responses of (b) or (p) to the voice-onset stimuli shown in Figure 10–2. The vertical axis is the percentage of (b) or (p) responses, and the horizontal axis is the VOT value. Note the crossover point (phonetic boundary) at about 20 ms.

Research on categorical perception has raised a number of different interpretations of the phenomenon. As noted, the early view was that consonants are perceived categorically, but vowels are not. More recent studies have shown that, under certain conditions, vowels also can be perceived categorically. In addition, a number of questions have been raised about the methods by which categorical perception is demonstrated, and even if the concept as originally defined is valid. These issues go beyond the scope of this book, but Handel (1989) covers several issues regarding the experimental confirmation of categorical perception for speech sounds. His book is a good starting point for a deeper inquiry into this subject.

Research on VOT and related stimuli has addressed a number of issues relevant to the larger discussion of categorical perception for any type of speech feature. A very brief look at various studies on VOT poses the following questions:

1. Is VOT a relevant cue in languages generally, or is it specific to a small number of languages with a certain kind of voicing contrast?
2. Is categorical perception unique to speech stimuli? Is categorical perception acquired by children in the process of language acquisition?
3. Is categorical perception of speech unique to humans?
4. Can lexical and prosodic factors of speech influence aspects of categorical perception?

VOT in Different Languages

Lisker and Abramson's (1970) classic study of voicing in different languages demonstrated that VOT is a useful concept in understanding the voicing contrast of languages with different phonetic categories of voicing. The Lisker and Abramson paper is a good example of cross-language research that points to the possibility of universal properties in the acoustic speech signal. Different languages may depend, to some degree, on common acoustic properties, perhaps reflecting general characteristics of the auditory system. This is not to say that all languages rely on precisely the same acoustic contrasts. It is quite possible that languages differ in the fine details of acoustic cues for phonetic decisions. However, there seems to be merit in the idea that a set of basic acoustic correlates can be identified in cross-linguistic studies.

Categorical Perception of VOT for a Nonspeech Analog

Pisoni (1977) examined the perception of a nonspeech analog to VOT. This analog, called tone-onset time (TOT), is illustrated in Figure 10–4. Notice that the stimulus in question is composed of two tones that can be adjusted to vary in their relative time of onset. The question is whether a categorical response can be demonstrated for the tonal stimuli for onset asynchronies similar to those that occur for VOT. The results showed the existence of categories for TOT at about the same location as seen for VOT, namely, a TOT of either –20 ms or +20 ms. This experiment shows that the categorical perception for VOT may be shared by a nonspeech acoustic continuum. One can therefore question if categorical perception is unique to speech. The identification of **nonspeech analogs** in studies of speech perception is an important arena of speech research. Work of this kind helps to show what, if anything, is unique about the perception of speech compared to the perception of auditory signals in general. A large number of studies have been published in support of the idea that many speech sound discriminations have parallels in the discrimination of nonspeech sounds such as clicks, buzzes, and tones. This re-

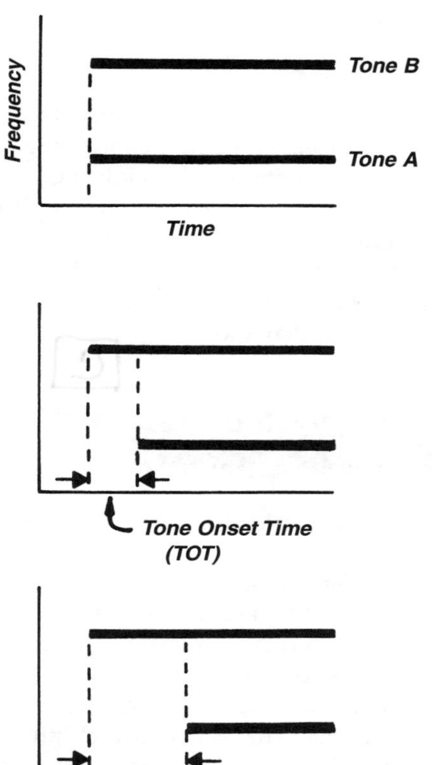

Figure 10–4. A tone-onset time stimulus analogous to the voice-onset time in speech sounds.

search points to an important conclusion: Speech is not necessarily unique in its underlying perceptual phenomena.

Categorical Perception of VOT in Infants

In a seminal study of speech perception in infants, Eimas, Siqueland, Jusczyk, and Vigorito (1971) showed that infants demonstrate categorical effects for VOT stimuli very much like those shown in studies with adults. Of course, the experimenter cannot simply ask infants to identify the stimuli presented to them. The procedure used with infants was an application of heart rate deceleration. When an infant becomes aware of a novel stimulus, the infant's heart rate slows. Therefore, heart rate deceleration can be taken as a sign that an infant has detected a change in environmental stimuli. Eimas et al. applied this concept to speech perception by presenting a stimulus, waiting for the heart rate to stabilize, and then presenting new stimuli that differed in VOT from the first stimulus. When the VOT difference was large enough for the infant to detect the difference, the heart rate slowed. This experiment showed that the boundaries for VOT are present early in life and do not require adultlike language competence. The study by Eimas et al. was a harbinger of a new specialization in speech research, the study of speech perception in infants. This is one of the most exciting areas of contemporary research on speech perception. It is probably fair to state that the bulk of this research confirms the conclusion that newborns are sensitive to many, if not all, of the phonetic contrasts used in the world's languages.

Categorical Perception of VOT in Animals

If infants can perceive VOT categorically, then how about animals? The answer to this question was given for chinchillas in an experiment by Kuhl and Miller (1978). The investigators trained chinchillas to distinguish a prototype of a voiced and voiceless stop consonant. The animals then were tested with a continuum of VOT values. The animals produced categorical effects highly similar to the effects shown by human infants and adults. Apparently, then, categorical perception of speech stimuli is not uniquely a human capability. As far as we know, chinchillas do not produce voiced and voiceless stop consonants. Research on the discrimination of speech and speechlike sounds by animals has raised some important issues, one of which is whether certain acoustic discriminations are based on general characteristics of the mammalian auditory system. But it is not only chinchillas and not even only mammals that can make humanlike speech discriminations. Some birds also can learn to discriminate speech sounds. It appears, then, that many of the phenomena attributed to the perception of speech by humans may be present in some nonhuman species.

Lexical and Speaking Rate Effects on VOT Boundaries

VOT is one attribute of a syllable or word. If decisions about voicing are rigidly based on a particular value for VOT, then these decisions should be unaffected by the lexical properties of an utterance or the speaking rate of the utterance. In other words, certain values of VOT would be rigid and reliable bases of phonetic decisions. An example of a lexical property is whether an utterance is a real word or a nonword. For example, we might ask what happens when listener categories are determined for VOT continua in the real word *dash* and the nonword *tash*? If VOT categories were unaffected by lexical factors, then real words and nonwords would have the same VOT boundaries. However, studies have shown that listeners had a relatively greater range of VOT values for real words than for nonwords, almost as though the acoustic-phonetic space is carved out to facilitate lexical decision making (Ganong, 1980). The general term for this effect is the **lexical identification shift**. The implication is that VOT boundaries are not rigidly fixed, but can be manipulated by linguistic properties. That is, the listener tries to use the acoustic cues to reach lexical decisions, not simply to follow an invariant acoustic mold.

A similar question can be asked about speaking rate. Do VOT boundaries remain invariant in the face of changes in speaking rate? Wayland and Miller (1994) concluded that slowing of the speaking rate for a sentence shifts the locations of best exemplars of VOT ranges for words in the sentence. As the authors state, "sentence-level rate information . . . alters the internal perceptual structure of a phonetic category" (p. 2700).

This brief review of research on VOT illustrates some general issues concerning categorical perception. Although VOT has been illustrated for reasons of simplicity and continuity, the same questions can be asked about other phonetic continua, including those for place of articulation and manner of articulation.

Laterality Effects (Right- or Left-Ear Advantage)

In the real world, the two ears rarely, if ever, receive two different types of stimuli. A sound may be louder in one ear than the other, but the two ears receive a very similar pattern. But in the perception laboratory, it is possible to deliver one stimulus to one ear and another (different) stimulus to the other ear. This is called **dichotic perception**. In a sense, the two ears are placed in competition and the subjects are asked to report what they heard.

For certain stimuli, one ear will outperform the other in tasks of dichotic perception. The ear with better performance (either better overall accuracy of identification, or preferences reported by the subject) is said to have the advantage. A **right-ear advantage** (REA) has been reported for some sounds, particularly stops, whereas a **left-ear advantage** (LEA) has been reported for other sounds, such as tones and steady-state vowels. This laterality effect has been interpreted to mean that some sounds are processed better in one hemisphere, and other sounds are processed better in the other. As explained in Chapter 7, information from the ears goes mostly to the contralateral hemisphere (because there are many more fibers in the contralateral pathway than in the ipsilateral pathway). A right-ear advantage is, therefore, interpreted as a left-hemisphere advantage. Sounds that most reliably have a REA and a presumed left-hemisphere advantage are stop consonants and various other sounds that are brief or dynamic. Sounds that most reliably have a LEA and a presumed right-hemisphere advantage are tones, steady-state vowels, and other stimuli of relatively long duration or invariant acoustic pattern. Because ear effects in speech perception are present in infants (McCain, Studdert-Kennedy, Spieker, & Stern, 1983), laterality seems to be a basic feature of the human brain as a sensory processor.

It should be noted that the laterality effects are often very small, and that not all subjects demonstrate these effects. Although laterality is interesting, there is controversy about the significance of the results in understanding how speech is processed. Some interpretations are considered next, but the reader is cautioned that this topic should be approached with some skepticism.

Possibly, speech perception involves the fusion of information that is preferentially processed in the left and right hemispheres. That is, the left hemisphere presumably has a special advantage in the processing of analytic information, such as the acoustic cues for phonetic events, especially consonants. The right hemisphere may be better at processing melodic information on a longer temporal scale, such as the intonational contours of prosody. These two types of information may be merged following the processing in the respective hemispheres.

Adaptation

Adaptation is a perceptual phenomenon in which repeated exposure to an extreme member of some acoustic continuum causes a shift in a category boundary. For example, repetition of a "strongly" voiceless stop (a stimulus taken from the right-hand side of the VOT continuum in Figure 10–2) causes the voiced-voiceless boundary to shift *toward* the voiceless end of the continuum. In a sense, the auditory system adapts to the repeated stimulus; that is, the stimulus becomes less effective in evoking the phonetic property of "voicelessness."

Trading Relations

As explained in Chapter 9, many speech sounds are associated with two or more acoustic cues. A stop consonant may be associated with a brief silence (the stop gap), a stop burst, and a set for formant transitions. The perceptual system somehow integrates these different cues into a single phonetic percept, such as the stop consonant [t]. Phonetic perception, then, often involves the recognition of different acoustic cues that are interpreted to belong to a single sound. This perceptual unification of acoustic cues is critical to phonemic perception.

It is possible to show a trading relation between the acoustic cues that signal a particular phonetic contrast. For example, the words *witch* and *wish* differ in the final consonant, which is either a fricative or an affricate. As shown in Figure 10–5, the acoustic cues that signal this distinction are the duration of silence and the duration of frication noise, which can be varied independently. Typically, the fricative has a short or nonexistent silence and a relatively long interval of frication. The affricate has a relatively long silence and a relatively shorter interval of frication. The situation becomes more interesting when the fricative or affricate contrast occurs in word-initial position, as in the phrases *say shop* and *say chop*. The distinction is made on the basis of the same two acoustic cues just considered—the duration of silence between the two words and the duration of the frication noise. The longer the silence, the more likely a listener is to hear *say chop*. Lengthening the frication noise increases the likelihood of perception of *say shop*. When

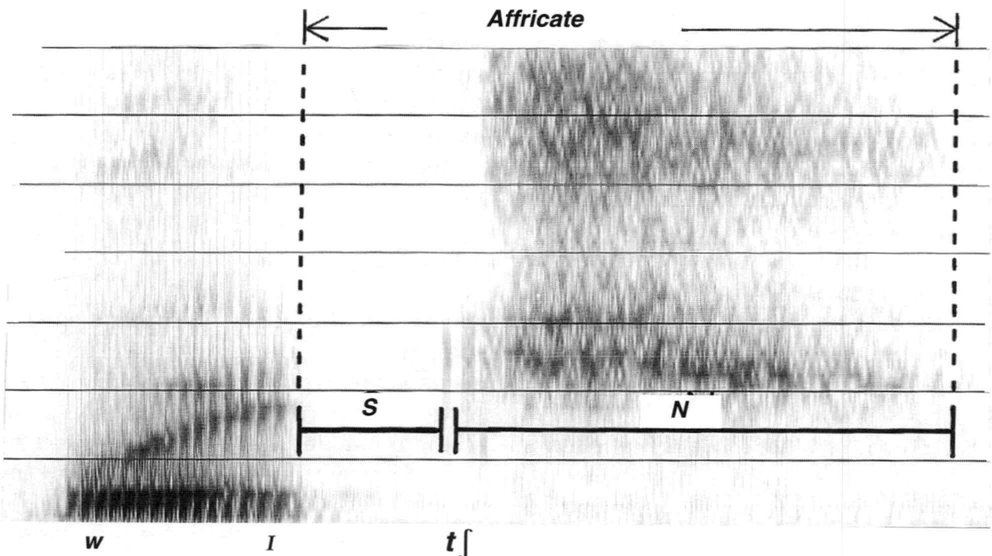

Figure 10–5. Acoustic cues for a fricative-affricate distinction: duration of silence (S) and duration of frication noise (N).

the two cues are varied together, it turns out that they are perceived relationally. That is, the shorter the duration of the frication noise, the shorter the silence needed to hear *say chop* rather than *say shop*. This is a demonstration of trading relations in speech. The existence of trading relations indicates that the listener evaluates two or more cues and makes a relative decision based on their properties (Repp, 1982; Repp, Liberman, Eccardt, & Pesetsky, 1978).

Even though two or more cues may be relevant to a phonetic decision, the cues are not necessarily equal even when the signal is loud and clear. For example, it appears that, in the perception of stop consonants, the burst contains more information about place of consonant production than does the formant transition (Cassidy & Harrington, 1995). This result is rather surprising because the burst is one of the briefest events in speech. Why should the burst be so informative compared to the longer (and typically more intense) formant transitions? One answer was suggested in Chapter 6. The cochlea "functions above all else as a sensitive detector and spectral analyser of brief or transient events" (Masterton, 1992, p. 282). The ear evolved to hear sounds of short duration and to supply the brain with the necessary information to make quick decisions.

Segmentation 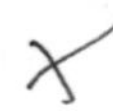

> ***"Speech, as phoneticians well agree, consists of continous streams of sound within breath groups; neither sounds nor words are separated consistently from one another by pauses, but have to be abstracted from the continuum."***
>
> (Kenneth L. Pike, *Phonetics.* Ann Arbor, MI: University of Michigan Press, 1969, p. 42)

The problem of segmentation is a general one in speech perception, but for brevity's sake, only one aspect of this problem is addressed here. Specifically, the problem is word segmentation. As indicated in the quotation that leads this section, the acoustic stream of speech is not marked with definitive word boundaries. The lack of these boundaries was noted in Chapter 9. How, then, does the listener recognize a series of discrete words from an acoustic signal that often blurs the boundaries between linguistic units? Research indicates that the listener relies on a variety of cues to select a set of candidate words. Competition among the candidates then leads to an eventual decision about what words the speaker intended. The shortlist model (Norris, 1994) proposes that competition among candidate words is used for word possibilities that begin at the same point in the signal (e.g., *sack* and *sacrifice* begin with the same syllable) or for word possibilities that begin at different points in the signal (e.g., *mess* and *domestic* both contain the syllable [m ɛ s]).

Some of the acoustic cues available to the listener relate to the metrical structure of the language, that is, to the rhythmic pattern based on stress and other prosodic features. In English and many other languages said to be stress-timed (i.e., the stress pattern regulates temporal structure) most words begin with a strong syllable (a syllable carrying primary stress). Therefore, a strong syllable has a high likelihood of marking word onset.

Another potent cue is the appearance of silence, or pause. Speakers rarely produce a pause within words but they often produce pauses between words. Still another cue is a linguistic concept called **phonotactics**, which refers to the patterns by which phonemes and features can be arranged to form words and syllables. In English, the velar nasal [ŋ] as in *thing* cannot occur in word-initial position. Therefore, if a listener hears this sound, it is fairly safe to assume that it is not the beginning of a word. Another example is that certain phoneme sequences cannot occur in the same syllable. In English, the sequence [dl] cannot occur in the same syllable but it can occur between syllables, as in the word *fiddle*. Listeners may be able to use their knowledge of phonotactic constraints to recognize words in continuous speech. Moreover, certain phonotactic properties may be nearly universal. Kawasaki-Fukumori (1992) proposed an acoustical basis for universal phonotactic constraints according to the principle: The greater the acoustic change from one element to the next within a sequence, the greater the perceptual salience of the change and the more likely that the sequence will be preferred in a language.

Segmentation of the speech stream into discrete words is not a trivial problem. Listeners apparently use several sources of information to choose among the candidate words in a "short list." This is a good point to consider theories of speech perception, that attempt to explain how listeners are able to perceive the acoustic signal of speech.

Auditory Illusions in Speech Perception

The understanding of perceptual systems is informed by both their successes and their failures. Occasionally, our perceptions seem to be mistaken insofar as we reach conclusions that are not consistent with physical reality. This section will consider some auditory illusions that affect speech perception. For a more extensive review of these and related phenomena, see Warren (1996).

Phonemic restoration is the failure of perceivers to recognize that a portion of the speech signal has been replaced by a nonspeech sound. For example, suppose that the underlined sound in the following sentence is replaced by a noise such as a cough or a burst of noise:

Which sound is missing in this sentence?

When the altered sentence is played to listeners, they often are unaware that the [s] sound in the word *missing* has been replaced by another sound. Apparently, the listener restores the missing sound by relying on higher order information such as syntax and semantics. Whether this phenomenon is a success or failure of perception is a matter of interpretation. It might be considered as a failure in that the listener is insensitive to a blatant distortion of the speech signal. But it is a communicative success in that the listener derives the linguistic message despite the alteration. It is probably fortunate that listeners do not always need a high-quality speech signal to understand it. Because we communicate in a world of competing sounds, our speech messages often are obscured by noises. Our ability to understand speech despite these contaminations is part of the robustness of communication.

Verbal transformation is a change in the perception of a speech stimulus when the physical signal is invariant. This phenomenon arises when a listener hears the same word repeated many times in succession. After a number of repetitions, say 40 or 50, the listener often reports a change in the stimulus. For example, in one study, listeners heard the following forms for a stimulus initially heard as *trees: tress, press, stress, dress, tourist, truss, bread, trez, prez, tresh* (Warren, 1996). One interpretation of this effect is that the perceptual system is continually testing new hypotheses against an incoming signal. With repeated presentations of a stimulus, some of the pattern detectors that were initially activated by the pattern lose their sensitivity, perhaps because of an adaptation effect. Other pattern detectors then are more likely to be activated.

THEORIES OF SPEECH PERCEPTION

Several theories of speech perception have been proposed, and it is beyond the scope of this chapter to consider them all in detail. A few selected theories are considered, but first it is helpful to examine some general attributes of theories of speech perception.

Bottom-Up Versus Top-Down Theories

A **bottom-up** theory of perception assumes that the information in the physical signal is essential to, and adequate for, the eventual perceptual decisions to be made. This view also is called **data-driven,** in the sense that the perceptual decision-making process is directed almost entirely by the information obtained from the physical signal. A **top-down** theory of perception takes the view that the decision-making process is highly dependent on higher level sources of information, such as hypotheses generated from linguistic or cognitive operations. This kind of theory often is based on the assumption that analysis of the physical signal is not sufficient to make the requisite perceptual decisions. The top-down kind of theory places less emphasis on an analysis of the physical signal than does a bottom-up kind of theory.

In reality, no theory is exlusively bottom-up or top-down. Every theory of speech perception depends to some degree on an analysis of the physical signal—otherwise, the process would be totally telepathic! And, just about every theory relies on some aspects of higher level information. A strict reliance on bottom-up processing would require a detailed analysis of the acoustic signal and would make it difficult to overcome the frequent corruptions of this signal by noise and other factors. Therefore, bottom-up and top-down are not strictly dichotomous as they describe theories of speech perception. Rather, different theories propose different degrees of reliance on bottom-up or top-down processes. A theory that is classified as bottom-up relies relatively more on processing of the physical signal of speech than does a theory classified as top-down. A theory classified as top-down depends relatively more on sources of higher level information, such as context, syntax, or semantics.

Active Versus Passive Theories

An **active theory** is one that proposes the use of cognitive resources or intellectual energy of some sort. Active theories suppose that perception involves work on the part of the perceiver. For example, the perceiver may generate hypotheses about the phonetic or linguistic interpretation of the speech signal and then test these hypotheses. A **passive theory** is one that does not rely on cognitive resources but rather on passive responses such as thresholds. Passive theories assume that decisions can be made with little or no use of special cognitive operations.

Autonomous Versus Interactive Theories

An **autonomous theory** is based on the idea that perception occurs in a closed system of decision making. All the information needed to reach the required perception decisions is contained in the basic perceptual operations, that is, the substages of perceptual processing. Therefore, there is no need to call on other sources of information such as knowledge of the communicative context or general world knowledge. An **interactive theory** allows that the perceptual decision-making process can and does rely on various sources of information outside the perceptual processor. It allows the substages to interact or to call on other information available to the human perceiver. In the extreme, this kind of theory may call on a perceiver's general experience and full range of intelligence.

These three basic contrasts can be used to group theories of speech perception into related classes. For example, a given theory can be classified as top-down, active, and interactive, whereas another may be essentially bottom-up, passive, and autonomous.

The Motor Theory of Speech Perception

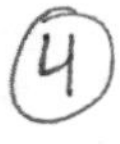

One of the research institutions that has been most influential in speech research is Haskins Laboratories, formerly in New York City and currently in New Haven, Connecticut. Some of the researchers who were part of a highly significant period of research included Frank Cooper, Alvin Liberman, Michael Studdert-Kennedy, and Katharine S. Harris. These and other researchers associated with Haskins Laboratories have contributed many important ideas about speech perception and speech production. A kernel concept has been the idea that the phonetic message is complexly coded in the acoustic signal of speech. This is thought to be one reason why it is difficult to reach a phonetic interpretation from spectrograms or other acoustic displays of the speech signal. Spectrograms are difficult to interpret. Even experts who have devoted years to the study of speech acoustics have to puzzle their way through a spectrogram. In contrast, the auditory message of speech is readily interpreted. Speech is therefore considered to be an **auditory code**.

The 1967 Liberman, Cooper, Shankweiler, and Studdert-Kennedy paper, "Perception of the Speech Code," is a classic treatise on speech perception and is probably the most frequently cited paper on speech perception. This paper puts forth the view that speech is a complex code. Some characteristics of this code are now elaborated.

The acoustic signal of speech represents a substantial restructuring of the phonetic message. Information on successive speech sounds is transmitted in parallel, in a kind of shingling of phonetic features. The parallel transmission permits speech to be understood at rates of up to 30 phonetic segments per second—which is much faster than the ear can follow discrete, sequential units in usual circumstances. That is, when nonspeech sounds are presented at rates of 30 units per second, listeners have extraordinary difficulty in following the sound sequence. Another important property is that phonetic units do not have a one-to-one correspondence with the acoustic signal of speech. Although the acoustic signal is not invariantly related to the phonetic message, the motor commands that control the articulators are invariant. This is the essence of the "motor theory" of speech perception. The theory states that speech is understood in terms of how it is produced; in other words, articulation is the referent for perception. In its extreme form, this theory basically claims that we can perceive speech because we can produce it.

Speech is thought to be perceived with reference to articulation (or in the terms of the revised motor theory, the "gestures" of speech production). The **locus** concept is a way of explaining the acoustic restructuring of speech. A locus is a characteristic acoustic feature that relates to place of articulation. Formant loci are associated with place of articulation. For example, for an adult male speaker, the alveolar place of articulation is associated with a characteristic starting value for F2 of about 1800 Hz. This frequency value of 1800 Hz is the F2-locus for the alveolar place. The speech mode of perception assumes that coded sounds are processed differently from unencoded sounds. Speech is therefore special. Some properties of this purported "special" quality are:

1. The acoustic signal of speech represents a substantial restructuring of the phonetic message.
2. Information on successive speech sounds is transmitted in parallel, in a kind of shingling of phonetic features. At a given instant, the acoustic signal may carry information on more than phoneme.
3. The parallel transmission permits speech to be understood at rates of up to 30 phonetic segments per second.
4. The phonetic units do not have a one-to-one correspondence with the acoustic signal of speech.
5. Although the acoustic signal is not invariantly related to the phonetic message, the motor commands that control the articulators are invariant. This is the *sine qua non* of the "motor theory" of speech perception. The essence of this theory is that speech is understood in terms of how it is produced; in other words, articulation is the referent for perception.

A revised version of the motor theory was described by Liberman and Mattingly (1985). This revised theory responded to criticisms of the orginal theory, but it retains an emphasis on articulatory-perceptual relations. In both its original and revised form, the motor theory of speech perception focuses largely on issues of phonetic identification. It says relatively little about the perception of larger units such as words or phrases, although it does recognize the importance of the syllable as a fundamental unit of perception.

The "speech is special" claim has been the subject of a large number of research papers. This contentious issue cannot be reviewed here in any depth, but the interested reader should consult Cutting and Rosner (1974), Handel (1989), J. D. Miller, Wier, Pastore, Kelly, and Dooling (1976), Pastore, Li, and Layer (1990), and Schouten (1980).

The Logogen Model of Speech Perception

The **logogen** is a neural representation of a word that can be activated by a physical stimulus that matches the stored representation (Morton, 1964). A simple diagram of this model is shown in Figure 10–6. The physical stimulus could be visual (a printed or written word) or auditory (a heard word). The logogen is activated when the stimulus is sufficiently close to the representation. This activation occurs at a certain threshold, which can be influenced by such properties as word familiarity or predictability. The logogen is a passive threshold device: A word is recognized when the physical stimulus is adequate to reach the threshold. Because the logogen depends primarily on an analysis of the physical signal of speech, and, because it makes little use of interactive sources of information, it may be classified as a passive, bottom-up, autonomous theory of speech perception.

The Cohort Theory of Speech Perception

This theory proposes that word recognition is accomplished by detecting the beginning of a spoken word and then selecting all words that share this beginning (Marslen-Wilson, 1980; Marslen-Wilson & Tyler, 1975). For example, if a speaker produces a word beginning with the syllable *cap-*, the listener would select words such as *cap, captain, capsize, captive, caption, capital*, and so on. All of these words with a similar onset portion constitute the **cohort**, or slate, of words from which the right word must be drawn (Figure 10–7). Note that the words do not necessarily share any grammatical or semantic properties. They are similar only in the initial sound pattern. The selection of items in the cohort is said to follow the principle of **bottom-up priority**. Once the cohort has been activated, then unsuitable lexical candidates can be deactivated through the use of additional bottom-up information or syntactic/semantic constraints. Words

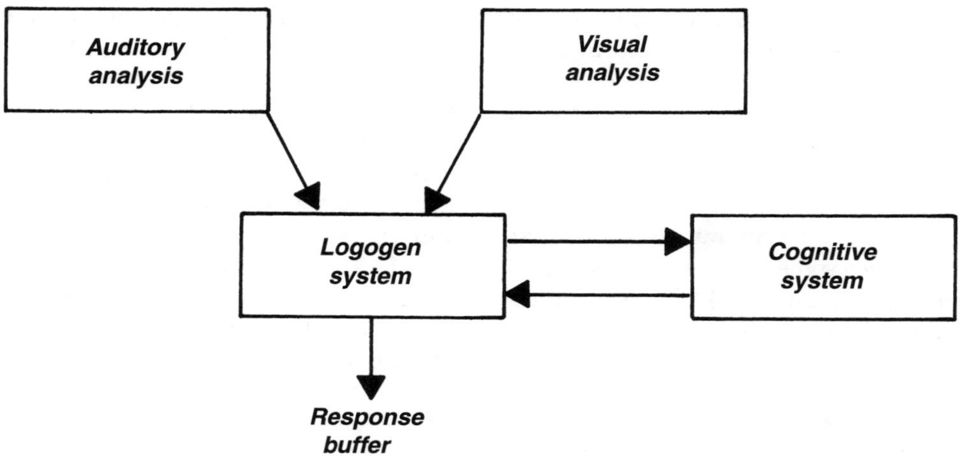

Figure 10–6. The logogen model of speech perception.

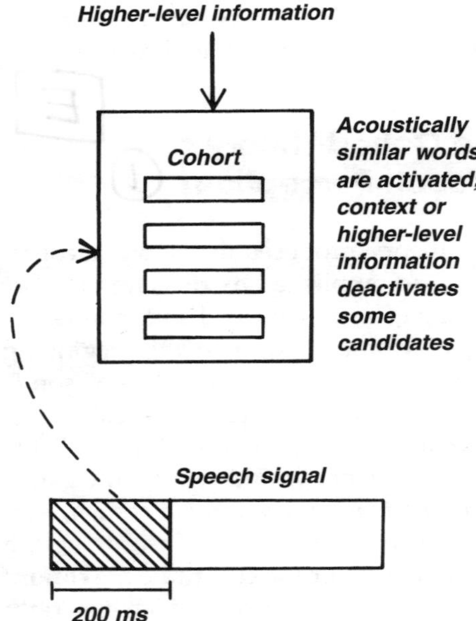

Figure 10–7. The cohort model of word recognition. The initial acoustic segment of a word is used to select acoustically similar items that form a cohort. Context or higher level information can be used to select the correct item from the cohort.

that are similar in their initial portions but differ in later portions can be distinguished at the point at which they diverge. This point is the "uniqueness point." A large number of different words are activated in the initial cohort. But continued processing of the speech waveform eliminates more and more candidates until only the word *captain* remains by the time the last vowel (represented by the alphabet characters *ai*) is reached.

This process may seem strange in that the cohort contains some words that are inappropriate (even implausible) choices given the syntactic and semantic information already available to the listener. But, according to the theory, these words are nonetheless made available for selection. Word candidates are activated in parallel to form the initial cohort. This theory can be described as passive, bottom-up, and autonomous.

The Interactive-Activation Model of Speech Perception

This model is based on a connectionist network model of speech perception (McClelland & Elman, 1986). It uses a variety of processing units, including features, phonemes, and words, all of which are represented at different levels of the network (Figure 10–8). The system is highly interactive. Generally, influences across levels (such as between phonemes and words) are facilitatory, so that activated units on the phoneme level activate units on the word level. But influences within a level tend to be inhibitory, so that activation of one unit on the phoneme level inhibits the activation of a competing phoneme. In an interesting application of this network approach to speech perception in infants, Guenther and Gjaja (1996) demonstrated that the perceptual "magnet" effect emerges as a property of the network exposed to speech stimuli.

Event Perception

The basic contention of event perception theory is that perception informs us about events or objects in the real world. That is, perception is not fundamentally about low-pitched noises, formant patterns, or other components of acoustic analysis. What we need to perceive are the events and objects that populate the world. As applied to speech, this theory means that the listener perceives movements of the tongue, lips, velopharynx, and other articulators (Fowler, 1986). Articulatory movement is an event, and the listener needs to recover this event information from the acoustic signal. Event perception suggests that we hear tongues, lips, and jaws—not phonemes.

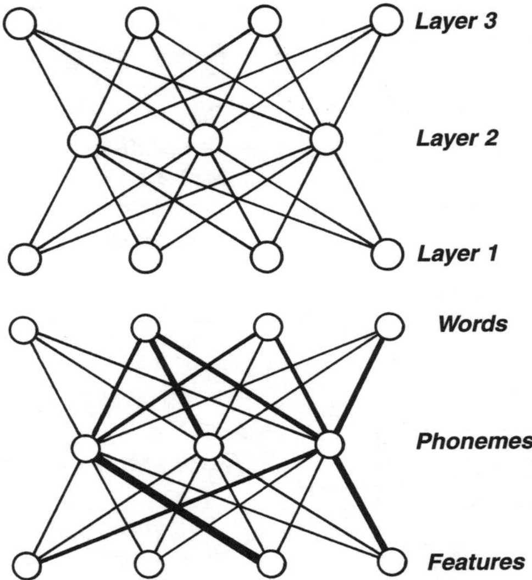

Figure 10–8. Basic aspects of the interactive activation model of speech perception. This model is based on a connectionist network as shown at the top of the illustration. As applied to speech recognition, the layers shown in the top part of the figure can be conceptualized as features, phonemes, and words, as shown in the bottom part of the figure. The lines connecting nodes in the bottom part of the figure represent different weights assigned to the connections. It is through this differential weighting that the network can represent the information presented to the network in the form of input units.

Lexical Neighborhood Activation Model

This model from Luce (1986) proposes that a given word has a similarity neighborhood composed of words that resemble the word in question. Recognition of a word is based on probabilities, namely the probability that the stimulus word was presented compared to the probability that other words in its neighborhood were presented. The frequency of words in a language influences the probabilities as well. For example, when the presented word has a low frequency of occurrence but its neighbors have a high frequency of occurrence, the probability of identifying the stimulus word is relatively low. In contrast, when the presented word has a high frequency of occurrence but its neighbors have a low frequency of occurrence, the probability of identifying the stimulus word is relatively high.

The acoustic-phonetic properties of the stimulus provide the source of information for the initial access to the lexicon. In this respect, the neighborhood activation model is similar to the cohort model. However, it differs from the cohort model in that it uses information about the lexical neighborhood to make predictions about how fast and how accurately words are recognized. The fastest and most accurate recognition is expected for words that have a high frequency of occurrence and small neighborhoods consisting of words with low frequencies of occurrence. The slowest and least accurate recognition is expected for words that have a low frequency of occurrence and large neighborhoods consisting of words with high frequencies of occurrence.

Summary of Theories

Although theories of speech perception and word recognition are diverse in many particulars, several of them have an underlying similarity in their general approach to the problem. This similarity is illustrated in Figure 10–9. The speech signal is first subjected to an acoustic analysis, which yields some kind of initial analysis product, typically an acoustic-phonetic sequence of some sort. This initial product is then compared with or used to activate stored patterns of some kind. These stored patterns could be articulatory referents, a cohort of words, a set of templates, a neigh-

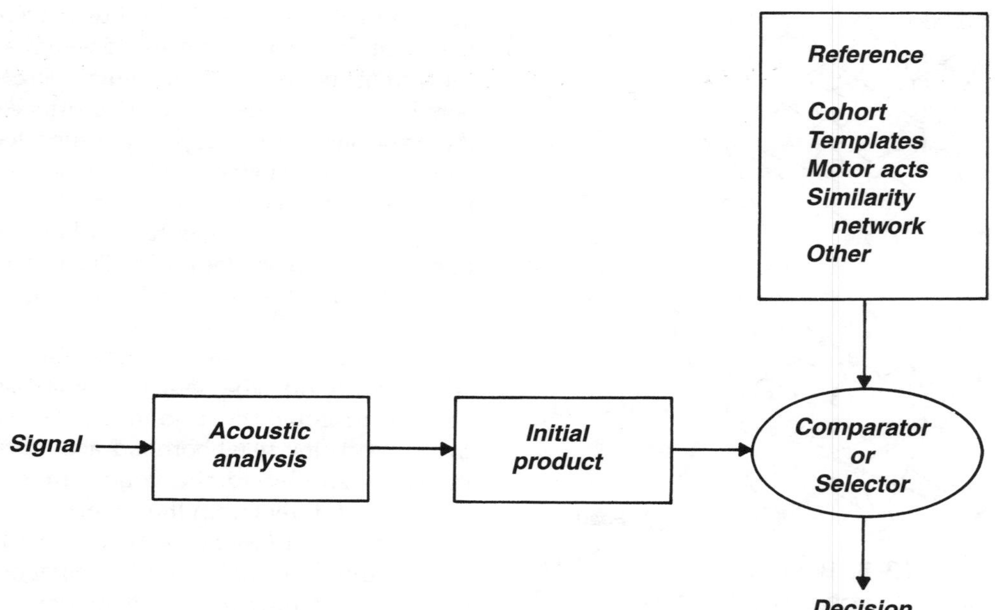

Figure 10–9. The general form of many models of speech perception or word recognition. See text for discussion.

borhood of words, or some other collection. The particular stored pattern that most resembles the initial product determines the perceptual decision. Recognition of a particular word then depends on the quality of information derived from the acoustic analysis, the relative accessibility of the stored references, and the operation of a comparison or selection process. A deficiency or disorder affecting any one of these aspects could interfere with word recognition.

SOME BASIC ISSUES IN SPEECH PERCEPTION

> *"The whole end of speech is to be understood."*
>
> — Confucius

Among the major issues to be resolved in speech perception and word recognition are

- speaker normalization,
- time normalization,
- integrating segmental and suprasegmental information,
- defining the unit(s) of speech perception, and
- cross-modal aspects of speech perception.

Each of these is now considered briefly.

Speaker Normalization

Speaker normalization is the normalization that is needed because of the differences among talkers, especially differences in the acoustic measures of speech such as vowel formant frequencies. As was discussed in Chapter 9, various groups of talkers categorized by sex and age can have rather large differences in the acoustic properties of their speech. To paraphrase Professor Higgins from *My Fair Lady*, one might ask, "Why can't a woman sound more like a man?" (or vice versa). The chief reason, of course, is that the woman has smaller vocal folds and a shorter vocal tract, as discussed in Chapters 4 and 5. As far as speech and voice are concerned, men and women are biologically and acoustically different. The differences in the formant-frequency patterns of vowels have been recognized for many years, but it is not obvious how listeners adjust for these acoustic differences. Speaker normalization is apparently present in infants because they show evidence of recognizing the same phonetic element produced by men or women (Kuhl, 1979). Even though a given vowel produced by a man and a woman has a different acoustic appearance, the infant seems to "know" that it is the same vowel. Therefore, the basic capacity for speaker normalization does not appear to depend on substantial experience with the speech of different talkers, although some refinement of normalization may occur with such experience.

Most solutions of speaker normalization for vowels rely on nonlinear transformations of some kind. Among the solutions proposed in the literature are ratios of formant frequencies, logarithms of formant frequencies, Bark transforms of formant frequencies, or some combination of these, such as logarithms of formant ratios (Kent & Read, 1992). Although a certain degree of normalization ability is evident as early as infancy and although listeners seem quite proficient in perceiving speech produced by different age-sex groups, it appears that normalization requires a listener's cognitive resources. Word recognition performance is poorer for words from a mixed group of talkers than for words produced by a single talker (Pisoni, 1993). In other words, listeners apparently have to make some kind of adjustment for different talkers, and this adjustment is reflected by at least a small reduction in speech recognition.

In the first chapter of this book, reference is made to a proposal by Traunmuller that the speech signal consists of four basic types of information that are woven together. By way of quick review, the four information qualities are:

- **phonetic quality** (the linguistic content of the speech message);
- **affective quality** (paralinguistic emotional quality that accompanies the linguistic message of speech and may contribute to the interpretation of that message);
- **personal quality** (extralinguistic information about the talker, but not the message); and
- **transmittal quality** (perspectival information about the talker's location, including the distance between talker and listener, orientation in space, presence of background noise, and influence of environmental acoustics that may introduce effects such as reverberation).

These four sources of information combine in the production of speech and also in its perception. To explain how these sources are integrated within speech, Traunmuller proposed a modulation theory of speech in which phonetic information is impressed onto speech signals by modulating a personal carrier signal. He hypothesized that the carrier should be understood as a neutral schwalike vowel (that is, a vowel produced with a central tongue articulation) with a relatively low fundamental frequency. Such a carrier involves a static vocal tract posture and a fixed frequency of source excitation. An advantage that this static carrier could hold for speech perception is that the formant and fundamental frequency information could serve the purpose of talker normalization. Both vowel formant information and fundamental frequency information are commonly used in solutions for the speaker normalization problem.

Time Normalization

Time normalization is necessary because different talkers speak at different rates and an individual talker can use different speaking rates on different occasions. Furthermore, articulatory rate may vary substantially within speech streams, such as during a conversation. A talker may have a rapid speaking rate during part of a conversation but then switch to a much slower rate. Dramatic examples of such a change occur when a speaker abruptly swings from a lethargic conversational mood to an agitated state. Hence, normalization is not necessarily a single-setting adjustment for a given situation, but rather a potentially continual adjustment that takes account of moment-to-moment changes in articulatory rate that potentially effects a variety of segmental decisions. (J. A. Miller, 1981).

Different speaking rates are possible because segment durations are flexible. At slow speaking rates, the durations of phonetic segments are relatively long; whereas, at rapid speaking rates, the durations of the same segments become shorter. But, as was noted in Chapter 9, some phonetic decisions seem to depend on durations of acoustic segments. For example, the perception of voiced and voiceless stops in syllable-initial position depends at least partly on differences in VOT. But if VOT varies with speaking rates, then how does a listener maintain a reliable perceptual criterion? As mentioned earlier, Wayland and Miller (1994) concluded that slowing of speaking rate for sentences shifts the locations of the best exemplars of VOT ranges. In other words, the best examples of VOT for voiced and voiceless stops change with speaking rate.

A question that arises is whether speech intelligibility is reduced for speakers who deviate from the typical temporal pattern of normal adult speech. Such speakers may include children and individuals with various communication disorders.

Integrating Segmental and Suprasegmental Information

It is generally agreed that suprasegmental cues of intonation, rhythm, and pausing help the listener segment the incoming speech signal. The problem: How is the suprasegmental information used in conjunction with the segmental information of speech?

Acoustic cues such as f_0, duration, and intensity are thought to be important in signaling suprasegmental structure such as stress and rhythm. But, it also has been argued that stress and rhythm are defined by the overall temporal pattern, such that the acoustic cues are not simply associated with a stress pattern. Perhaps the listener takes account of the basic acoustic cues of f_0, duration, and intensity, but also recognizes the temporal pattern of the utterance.

Grant and Walden (1996) determined the way in which different types of prosodic information are represented in the speech spectrum. The prosodic features they studied were syllable number, syllabic stress, sentence intonation, and phrase boundary location. The importance of particular spectral regions was investigated by the use of different filter conditions in which information in a given spectral region could be passed or eliminated. In general, there was an interaction between filter condition and the recognition of the different prosodic featu[illegible]rication of syllable number and stres[illegible]nefited from information in the high-frequency regions, but intonation patterns were identified successfully from information in low-frequency regions.

What Is the Basic Unit of Perception?

The question in the subheading above might be rephrased as: When we listen to speech, do we analyze it in terms of features, phonemes, syllables, or words? In reviewing the evidence for these different candidates, one author (Sendlemeier, 1995) concluded that all of these units are relevant to speech perception. That is, competent language users can rely on different units, depending on the speech stimuli, the setting, and various factors that influence the predictability of the message. It also may be that listeners of different ages and linguistic competence prefer different sizes of units. For example, there is evidence that young children operate with syllable-sized units, whereas adults are more inclined to extract phoneme-level information (Nittrouer, 1996). The most interesting aspect of perception units may not be which unit is basic, but rather how units of different sizes are integrated in task-dependent speech processing. Infants and young children may be inclined to process speech in terms of syllables because the syllable is a major shaping influence on the speech waveform. Indeed, the ear's sensitivity to amplitude modulation is maximal at the typical syllabic rate of speech (Lauter & Hirsh, 1985). The crests and falls of the acoustic waveform of speech correspond nicely to this basic psychophysical property of the human auditory system.

Cross-Modal Speech Perception

Much of this book emphasizes speech as an acoustic event. It is exclusively an acoustic event when we talk over the telephone or under conditions in which the speaker is invisible to the listener. But, during face-to-face conversations, group discussions, and television broadcasts, speech can be seen as well as heard, with potential for both visual and acoustic cues to be used in speech perception. Of course, lip reading (also known as speech reading) often is used by people with hearing impairment to supplement their reduced auditory capabilities.

But do listeners with normal hearing attend to visual cues in speech? The potential importance of visual cues is demonstrated in a phenomenon known as the **McGurk effect** (MacDonald & McGurk, 1976; McGurk & MacDonald, 1978). This effect was produced in the laboratory by studying different combinations of auditory and visual cues. For example, subjects would view a videotape of a speaker saying the syllable [ba], but would simultaneously hear the acoustic signal for the syllable [da]. In these experiments, a stimulus that was unambiguously identified as [da] in an auditory-only presentation could be heard as [ba] when accompanied by simultaneous video information showing labial closure. Or, when visual information was presented for [b] and aural information was presented simultaneously for [d], the subjects were inclined to hear [g]. That is, their phonetic decision seemed to be a synthesis of the visual and auditory cues. These experiments show that visual information may override or complement auditory information, even if the auditory information is sufficient for reliable phonetic identification in the absence of visual cues. This cross-modal capability also has been studied with synthesized auditory and visual speech (Massaro & Cohen, 1990). With this technique, computers not only sound like talking humans, but they also look the part.

Part of the competence in speech perception is the ability to use cross-modal information. This capability is evident even in infants (Kuhl & Meltzoff, 1982). Perhaps the most remarkable illustration of the perceptual flexibility in speech perception is the Tadoma method discussed in Chapter 1. Users of this method can understand a speaker through tactile information derived by placing a hand over the speaker's face.

LIFE COURSE ISSUES

> ***"[We] found that the manner in which the categorization of information for speech occurs was virtually identical in infant and adult listeners. These findings indicate that the infant possesses finely tuned linguistically-relevant perceptual abilities, which undoubtedly facilitate and shape the task of language acquisition."***
>
> (Joanne L. Miller and Peter D. Eimas, Studies on the Categorization of Speech by Infants. *Cognition*, 1983, *13*. p. 135.)

Speech Perception in Infancy and Childhood

Most of us hear speech in the womb, and studies of neonates have demonstrated that this early auditory experience biases the neonate toward the mother's voice and toward the ambient language. Infants come into the world ready to hear, and they may even be equipped with a "universal phonetic analyzer" that permits them to discriminate just about any of the sounds in the world's languages (Werker & Tees, 1984; Werker & Polka, 1993). By the end of the first year of life, infants have already begun to specialize on the sounds of the mother tongue (Kuhl et al., 1992; Werker & Tees, 1984). By this age, they have lost the discrimination for some foreign sounds. An apparent auditory reorganization has been accomplished. The 1-year-old, who is just beginning to produce single words, has already made a perceptual adaptation to the phonetic system of the parental language. This adaptation went largely unnoticed until innovative researchers turned their attention to the question of how infants hear the sounds of speech.

The ability of infants to discriminate speech sounds is so remarkable that the experimental questions have evolved from "What speech sounds can infants discriminate?" to "What can adults do in the way of speech discrimination that infants cannot do?" But it would be unwise to assume that this precocity in auditory discrimination means that infants hear every bit as well as adults. There is evidence of a continuing refinement in auditory ability. Although the course of this refinement is not well described, it appears that children continue to improve in basic discriminations of frequency, intensity, and duration until the age of about 7 years (Allen & Nelles, 1996; Allen & Wightman, 1992, 1994; Allen, Wightman, Kistler, & Dolan, 1989; Jensen & Neff, 1993; Wightman, Allen, Dolan, Kistler, & Jamieson, 1989). In some studies of children's auditory performance for speech and nonspeech stimuli, the major difference between their performance and that of adults was that the children were much more variable (Allen & Wightman, 1992; Wightman & Allen, 1992). In fact, some investigators drew the conclusion that the major differences could be attributed to attention. Adults pay better attention than children and they therefore demonstrate superior performance overall, even though children can occasionally do as well as adults. We might say that an attending child competes well with the adults, but children may tend not to attend.

Speech Perception, Language Learning, and Education

The attentional factor may interact with other factors to put some children at risk for speech and language disorders. Research evidence indicates that children are less able than adults to discriminate speech in noisy or reverberent environments (Mills, 1975; Neuman & Hochberg, 1983). In addition, children are prone to some diseases that might further disrupt speech perception. For example, recall from Chapter 6 that many children have otitis media (ear infections), which may temporarily produce a hearing loss. Children who have recurrent infections may be at a particular risk for problems in speech perception and perhaps language learning. Clarkson, Eimas, and Marean (1989) used a VOT continuum like that in Figure 10–2 to study speech perception in three groups of children: subjects with normal language and without middle-ear disease, subjects with normal language but with histories of middle-ear disease, and subjects with language impairment and with histories of middle-ear disease. The last group performed significantly more poorly than the other two groups on the perception of sounds varying in VOT. Another study that addresses the effect of otitis media on speech perception examined auditory function in identical twin girls, only one of whom had a significant history of middle-ear disease (Brown, 1994). The girl with the history of otitis media had poorer scores for intelligibility test words than did her twin. Although the exact nature of the perceptual deficit associated with otitis media has not been determined, there is good reason to suspect that it may contribute to language learning difficulties.

Speech perception difficulties also have been suggested as a contributing factor to language disorders in children (Leonard, McGregor, & Allen, 1992; Lubert, 1981; Rom & Leonard, 1990). One hypothesis is that certain grammatical morphemes in English have a low "phonetic substance," that is, they take the form of nonsyllabic consonants (such as the plural morpheme in a word like *dogs* or the past tense morpheme in a word like *talked*) or unstressed syllables (such as the final syllable in a word like *walking*). These grammatical morphemes have reduced auditory salience compared to many other morphemes; that is, they are harder to hear. Consequently, they may pose difficulties in auditory perception, and, if so, the perceptual difficulties may lead to problems in language learning. If we take into account the evidence for poorer attention in children than adults, and the greater difficulty that children appear to have in noisy listening conditions, then the reduced audibility of grammatical morphemes could indeed be one factor that contributes to language impairment in some children. The morphemes related to the syntactic structure of utterances may be heard unreliably by a child engaged in language learning.

Issues in speech perception are highly relevant to learning in the typical classroom environment. This environment is far from ideal as far as speech is concerned (Towne & Anderson, 1997). Consider that in a typical classroom the teacher's speech is about 6 dB more intense than the background noise. This is a marginal signal-to-noise ratio for effective speech communication. The speech signal can be hard to hear above the noise background. If teachers turn their heads away from the class while speaking, or if the noise level increases temporarily, students may miss much of what the teacher is saying. Consider also that the typical classroom has a reverberation time of about 0.45 second, which is an additional obstacle to hearing speech. Next, consider that how well a child can hear a teacher in this classroom is strongly affected by the distance between them. In one study, the percentage of single-syllable words heard by 5- to 7-year-old children with normal hearing varied systematically with the speaker-listener distance: 89% at 6 feet, 55% at 12 feet, and 36% at 24 feet (Crandell & Bess, 1986). The children sitting at a distance of 24 feet from the speaker could hear barely more than one third of the words. It seems likely that many children in typical classrooms find it difficult to hear the teacher at least some of the time. Why don't teachers speak louder to overcome these obstacles? Probably many do, and their increased vocal effort may explain why about 80% of teachers report vocal fatigue and why voice-related problems account for an average of 2 days of sick leave per year (Towne & Anderson, 1997). Noisy reverberent classrooms are a problem for both teachers and students. Fortunately, awareness of this problem is leading to improvements in the design of classrooms, and consideration of amplification systems that will permit all students to hear a teacher. The spoken message is the essential medium of classroom education. The study of speech perception has important applications in this environment that could enhance children's learning and reduce teacher's vocal fatigue.

Speech Perception and Aging

Adults maintain basic speech perception abilities fairly well unless they have a disorder such as hearing loss. As reviewed in Chapter 6, many persons lose some hearing ability with aging, although it is controversial whether the hearing loss is a direct and normal consequence of aging or whether it is the result of cumulative damage from toxins, excessive exposure to noise, poor nutrition, or some other factor. For some, the loss can be severe enough to interfere with speech perception. This is a major concern in the specialty of audiology. As more and more people live to advanced age, the number of individuals with sensory impairments is likely to increase. A significant proportion of the elderly complain of problems with understanding speech, especially in noisy environments.

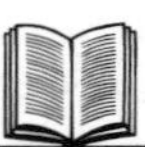

On The Reference Shelf

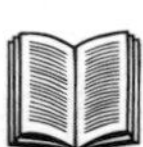

Basic or extended discussions for the reader who seeks more information on topics in speech perception.

Borden, G., Harris, K., & Raphael, L. (1994). *Speech science primer: Physiology, acoustics, and perception of speech* (3rd ed.). Baltimore: Williams & Wilkins.

An introductory text on speech science, this book contains informative summaries on classic studies of speech perception.

Kluender, K. R. (1994). Speech perception as a tractable problem in cognitive science. In M. A. Gernsbacher (Ed.), *Handbook of psycholinguistics* (pp. 173–217). San Diego: Academic Press.

A concise examination of some fundamental issues in speech perception, accompanied by a theoretical interpretation that focuses on information in the physical stimulus of speech.

Liberman, A. M., Cooper, F. S., Shankweiler, D. S., & Studdert-Kennedy, M. (1967). Perception of the speech code. *Psychological Review, 74,* 431–461.

This paper probably is the most frequently cited work on the perception of speech, and perhaps speech in general. This classic paper still serves as a clear exposition on central problems in the study of speech perception. It also presents the essence of the motor theory of perception.

Ryalls, J. (1996). *A basic introduction to speech perception.* San Diego: Singular Publishing Group.

This small book efficiently covers basic experimental and theoretical issues relating to speech perception. It is recommended to the student who wants more introductory-level information on the topic.

Chapter References

Allen, P., & Nelles, J. (1996). Development of auditory information integration abilities. *Journal of the Acoustical Society of America, 100,* 1043–1051.

Allen, P., & Wightman, F. (1992). Spectral pattern discrimination by children. *Journal of Speech and Hearing Research, 35,* 222–233.

Allen, P., & Wightman, F. (1994). Psychometric functions for children's detection of tones in noise. *Journal of Speech and Hearing Research, 37,* 205–215.

Allen, P., Wightman, F., Kistler, D., & Dolan, T. (1989). Frequency resolution in children. *Journal of Speech and Hearing Research, 32,* 317–322.

Anderson, S. E., Dave, A. S., & Margoliash, D. (1996). Template-based automatic recognition of birdsong syllables from continuous recordings. *Journal of the Acoustical Society of America, 100,* 1209–1219.

Blumstein, S. E., & Stevens, K. N. (1979). Acoustic invariance in speech production: Evidence from measurements of the spectral characteristics of stop consonants. *Journal of the Acoustical Society of America, 66,* 1001–1017.

Brown, D. P. (1994). Speech recognition in recurrent otitis media: Results in a set of identical twins. *Journal of the American Academy of Audiology, 5,* 1–6.

Cassidy, S., & Harrington, J. (1995). The place of articulation distinction in voiced stops: Evidence from burst spectra and formant transition. *Phonetica, 52,* 263–284.

Clarkson, R. L., Eimas, P. D., & Marean, G. C. (1989). Speech perception in children with histories of otitis media. *Journal of the Acoustical Society of America, 85,* 926–933.

Crandell, C., & Bess, F. (1986). Speech recognition of children in a "typical" classroom setting. *Asha, 29,* 87.

Cutting, J. E., & Rosner, B. S. (1974). Categories and boundaries in speech and music. *Perception & Psychophysics, 16,* 564–570.

Diehl, R. L. (1981). Feature detectors for speech: A critical appraisal. *Psychological Bulletin, 89,* 1–18.

Eimas, P. D., & Corbit, J. D. (1973). Selective adaptation of linguistic feature detectors. *Cognitive Psychology, 4,* 99–109.

Eimas, P. D., Siqueland, E. R., Jusczyk, P., & Vigorito, J. (1971). Speech perception in infants. *Science, 171,* 303–305.

Fowler, C. (1986). An event approach to the study of speech perception. *Journal of Phonetics, 14,* 3–28.

Ganong, W. F., III (1980). Phonetic categorization in auditory word perception. *Journal of Experimental Psychology: Human Perception and Performance, 6,* 110–125.

Grant, K. W., & Walden, B. E. (1996). Spectral distribution of prosodic information. *Journal of Speech and Hearing Research, 39,* 228–238.

Guenther, F. H., & Gjaja, M. N. (1996). The perceptual magnet effect as an emergent property of neural map formation. *Journal of the Acoustical Society of America, 100,* 1111–1121.

Handel, S. (1989). *Listening: An introduction to the perception of auditory events.* Cambridge, MA: MIT Press.

Jensen, J. K., & Neff, D. L. (1993). Development of basic auditory discrimination in preschool children. *Psychological Science, 4,* 104–107.

Juszcyk, P. (1993). From general to language-specific capacities: The WRAPSA Model of how speech perception develops. *Journal of Phonetics, 21,* 3–28.

Kawasaki-Fukumori, H. (1992). An acoustical basis for universal phonotactic constraints. *Language and Speech, 35,* 73–86.

Kent, R. D., & Read, W. C. (1992). *The acoustic analysis of speech.* San Diego: Singular Publishing Group.

Kuhl, P. K. (1979). Speech perception in early infancy: Perceptual constancy for spectrally dissimilar vowel categories. *Journal of the Acoustical Society of America, 66,* 1668–1679.

Kuhl, P. K. (1991). Human adults and human infants show a "perceptual magnet effect" for the prototypes of speech categories, monkeys do not. *Perception & Psychophysics, 50,* 93–107.

Kuhl, P. K., & Meltzoff, A. N. (1982). The bimodal perception of speech in infancy. *Science, 218,* 1138–1144.

Kuhl, P. K., & Miller, J. D. (1978). Speech perception by the chinchilla: Identification functions for synthetic VOT stimuli. *Journal of the Acoustical Society of America, 63,* 905–917.

Kuhl, P. K., Williams, K. A., Lacerda, F., Stevens, K. N., & Lindblom, B. (1992). Linguistic experience alters phonetic perception in infants by 6 months of age. *Science, 225,* 606–608.

Lauter, J. L., & Hirsh, I. J. (1985). Speech as temporal pattern: A psychoacoustic profile. *Speech Communication, 4,* 41–54.

Leonard, L. B., McGregor, K. K., & Allen, G. D. (1992). Grammatical morphology and speech perception in children with specific language impairment. *Journal of Speech and Hearing Research, 35,* 1076–1085.

Liberman, A. M., Cooper, F. S., Shankweiler, D. S., & Studdert-Kennedy, M. (1967). Perception of the speech code. *Psychological Review, 74,* 431–461.

Liberman, A. M., & Mattingly, I. G. (1985). The motor theory of speech perception revised. *Cognition, 21,* 1–36.

Lisker, L., & Abramson, A. S. (1970). The voicing dimension: Some experiments in comparative phonetics. In *Proceedings of the Sixth International Congress of Phonetic Sciences, Prague, 1967* (pp. 563–567). Prague: Academia.

Lubert, N. (1981). Auditory perceptual impairments in children with specific language disorders: A review of the literature. *Journal of Speech and Hearing Disorders, 46,* 3–99.

Luce, P. A. (1986). *Neighborhoods of words in the mental lexicon.* Unpublished doctoral dissertation, Indiana University, Bloomington.

MacDonald, J., & McGurk, H. (1976). Visual influences on speech perception processes. *Perception and Psychophysics, 24,* 253–257.

Marslen-Wilson, W. D. (1980). The temporal structure of language understanding. *Cognition, 8,* 1–71.

Marslen-Wilson, W. D., & Tyler, L. K. (1975). Processing structure of sentence perception. *Nature, 257,* 784–785.

Massaro, D. W., & Cohen, M. M. (1990). Perception of synthesized audible and visible speech. *Psychological Science, 1,* 55–63.

Masterton, R. B. (1992). Role of the central auditory system in hearing: The new direction. *Trends in Neuroscience, 15,* 280–285.

McCain, K. S., Studdert-Kennedy, M., Spieker, S., & Stern, D. (1983). Infant intermodal speech perception is a left hemisphere function. *Science, 219,* 1347–1349.

McClelland, J., & Elman, J. (1986). The TRACE model of speech perception. *Cognitive Psychology, 18,* 1–86.

McGurk, H., & MacDonald, J. (1978). Hearing lips and seeing voices. *Nature, 264,* 746–748.

Miller, G. A., & Nicely, P. E. (1955). An analysis of perceptual confusions among some English consonants. *Journal of the Acoustical Society of America, 27,* 338–352.

Miller, J. A. (1981). Effects of speaking rate on segmental distinctions. In P. D. Eimas & J. L. Miller (Eds.), *Perspectives on the study of speech* (pp. 39–74). Hillsdale, NJ: Erlbaum Associates.

Miller, J. D., Wier, C. C., Pastore, R., Kelly, W. J., & Dooling, R. J. (1976). Discrimination and labeling of noise–buzz sequences with varying noise-lead times: An example of categorical perception. *Journal of the Acoustical Society of America, 60,* 410–417.

Mills, J. H. (1975). Noise and children: A review of the literature. *Journal of the Acoustical Society of America, 58,* 767–779.

Morton, J. (1964). A model for continuous language behavior. *Language and Speech, 7,* 40–70.

Newman, A. C., & Hochberg, I. (1983). Children's perception of speech in reverberation. *Journal of the Acoustical Society of America, 73,* 2145–2149.

Nittrouer, S. (1996). Discriminability and perceptual weighting of some acoustic cues to speech perception by 3-year-olds. *Journal of Speech and Hearing Research, 39,* 278–297.

Norris, D. (1994). Shortlist: A connectionist model of continuous speech recognition. *Cognition, 52,* 189–234.

Pastore, R. E., Li, X.-F., & Layer, J. (1990). Categorical perception of nonspeech chirps and bleats. *Perception & Psychophysics, 48,* 151–156.

Pisoni, D. B. (1977). Identification and discrimination of the relative onset time of two component tones: Implications for voicing perception in stops. *Journal of the Acoustical Society of America, 61,* 1352–1361.

Pisoni, D. B. (1993). Long term memory in speech perception: Some new findings on talker variability, speaking rate and perceptual learning. *Speech Communication, 13,* 109–125.

Repp, B. H. (1982). Phonetic trading relations and context effects: New experimental evidence for a speech mode of perception. *Pyschological Bulletin, 92,* 81–110.

Repp, B. H., Liberman, A. M., Eccardt, T., & Pesetsky D. (1978). Perceptual integration of acoustic cues for stop, fricative, and affricate manner. *Journal of Experimental Psychology: Human Perception and Performance, 4,* 621–637.

Rom, A., & Leonard, L. B. (1990). Interpreting deficits in grammatical morphology in specifically language-impaired children: Preliminary evidence from Hebrew. *Clinical Linguistics and Phonetics, 4,* 93–105.

Schouten, M. E. H. (1980). The case against a speech mode of perception. *Acta Psychologia, 44,* 71–98.

Sendlemeier, W. G. (1995). Feature, phoneme, syllable or word: How is speech mentally represented? *Phonetica, 52,* 131–143.

Towne, R. M., & Anderson, K. L. (1997, January). The changing sound of education. *Sound and Vibration, 31,* 48–51.

Traunmuller, H. (1994). Conventional, biological, and environmental factors in speech communication: A modulation theory. *Phonetica, 51,* 170–183.

Warren, R. M. (1996). Auditory illusions and perceptual processing of speech. In N. J. Lass (Ed.), *Principles of experimental phonetics* (pp. 435–466). St. Louis: Mosby-Year Book.

Watson, C. S., Qiu, E. W., Chamberlain, M. M., & Li, X. (1996). Auditory and visual speech perception: Confirmation of a modality-independent source of individual differences in speech recognition. *Journal of the Acoustical Society of America, 100,* 1153–1162.

Wayland, S. C., & Miller, J. L. (1994). The influence of sentential speaking rate on the internal structure of phonetic categories. *Journal of the Acoustical Society of America, 95,* 2694–2701.

Werker, J. F, & Polka, L. (1993). Developmental changes in speech perception: New challenges and new directions. *Journal of Phonetics, 21,* 83–101.

Werker, J. F., & Tees, R. C. (1984). Cross-language speech perception: Evidence for perceptual reorganization during the first year of life. *Infant Behavior and Development, 7,* 49–63.

Wightman, F., & Allen, P. (1992). Individual differences in auditory capability among preschool children. In L. A. Werner & E. W. Rubel (Eds.), *Developmental psychoacoustics* (pp. 113–133). Washington, DC: American Psychological Association.

Wightman, F., Allen, P., Dolan, T., Kistler, D., & Jamieson, D. (1989). Temporal resolution in children. *Child Development, 60,* 611–624.

Exercises

10-1. What is meant by the "speech is special" proposal? Describe what it is about speech that is supposed to be special. Explain why this argument is important to understanding speech communication.

10-2. Explain how templates and features differ in theories of speech perception.

10-3. Describe what has been learned about speech perception in infants. What kind of speech perception ability do infants have?

10-4. How does speech perception differ between children and adults? Explain how speech perception may change as a function of maturation.

10-5. Figure 10–10 illustrates the acoustic pattern for seven syllables formed of the stop [d] followed by one of seven different vowels. These are simplified acoustic stimuli in which each syllable pattern is represented by the F1 and F2 structure (consonant-vowel transition and vowel steady state). Note the variability in F2 transition across the syllables. This transition has a variable direction and extent, which may seem puzzling if one attempts to find an invariant acoustic correlate for [d]. How can [d] be identified in the face of this acoustic variability? For one possible answer, assume that the F2 movement always begins at the same F2 frequency value for the consonant and then shifts to the F2 value for the following vowel. Using this assumption, try to infer this starting value, or F2-locus. What frequency value did you infer? Compare your answer with that given in Liberman et al. (1967).

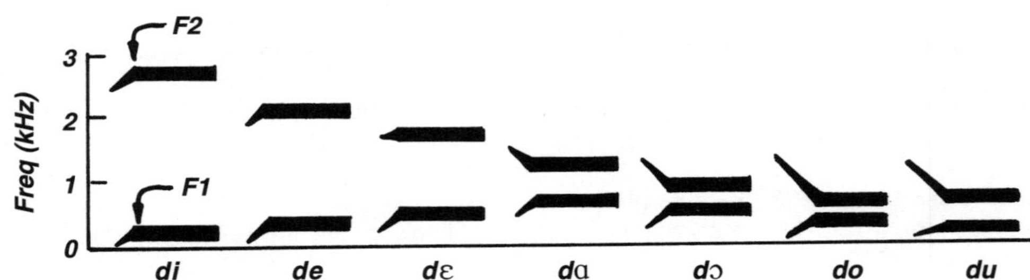

CHAPTER 11

Theories of Speech Production

WHY THEORIES MATTER

Theories are the scientist's way of interpreting facts in an economical and consistent way. A theory can be a powerful explanation because it accounts for the facts about a phenomenon and can be used to make predictions about events that may not yet have been observed experimentally. Progress in science is marked partly by experiments and data collection in general. But it is also marked by the development of new theories, by the rejection of theories that are inadequate to account for the data, and by the modification of theories that account for some but not all of the data. Occasionally, science undergoes a major theoretical shift (a **paradigm shift**, to use the term introduced by Kuhn, 1970). Opinion is divided among philosophers and historians of science as to whether these shifts are abrupt or gradual, but the basic point is that a particular period of science is known by the theories that interpret the known facts and help to direct important new experiments. Therefore, a scientific field is in a very real sense understood by the theories that drive its investigations and interpret its facts.

Theories and data have an interesting relationship. In one sense, theory and data are closely connected, because theories should explain the data and help to guide the collection of important new data. But a particular theory and the data in a scientific field can be severed, as when a critical experiment demonstrates that the standard (accepted) theory cannot account for the new observations. This standard theory is then replaced by an alternative theory that better accounts for the facts of the field.

Introductory texts in fields such as physics, astronomy, sociology, psychology, and economics generally introduce the major theories of the field, if only in broad relief. Speech science books perhaps have been less likely to present the theories of the field. But there are theories to be discussed. Some of them are not merely isolated theories confined to speech phenomena, but rather theories that have counterparts in fields such as physics, biology, and psychology. Much of the real excitement of a science is in its theory. This brief chapter considers theories of speech production. The coverage is limited to a few basic issues. We will not consider theories that have been developed for individual structures or systems, such as the respiratory system, the vocal folds, or the velopharynx. Such specific theories have been developed and many are quite sophisticated, but their discussion goes beyond the purpose of this book. This chapter addresses some of the long-standing basic questions about the overall nature of speech production. The discussion begins with three major problems that theories of speech production should solve.

THE THREE MAJOR PROBLEMS TO BE ACCOUNTED FOR BY A THEORY OF SPEECH PRODUCTION

Of particular importance to theories of speech production are three major problems, as discussed next. These are by no means the only problems to be solved, but these three are especially important, because they are central to the explanation of the organization of speech movements (and, for that matter, many other kinds of skilled movement). These questions are important for understanding the normal speech of the competent adult and also for understanding speech development in children and for the various speech disorders that can affect people of all ages.

> ***"A central debate in speech production research and theory has focused on the problem of the appropriate unit for analysis."***
>
> (A. Smith, "The Control of Orofacial Movements in Speech," *Critical Reviews in Oral Biology and Medicine*, 1992, *3*, p 234.)

Problem 1: Regulating the Serial Order of Speech

Speech typically is conceptualized as a string, or sequence, of elements. The layperson's impression of speech is that it consists of a series of sounds that can be interpreted as higher-level units such as words. Production of the string of sounds involves two fundamental questions: (1) What are the units? and (2) How are they controlled?

The first question is: What are the elements, or basic units, of speech production? Are they phonemes (broad sound classes that do not specify the fine details of a sound's production), allophones (narrow sound classes that represent the influence of phonetic context), syllables (some kind of consonant-vowel organization), demisyllables (parts of syllables), some of these, or all of these? Various conclusions have been reached through different kinds of investigation. Some evidence can be found for just about any unit that has been imagined. Perhaps, though, there is a basic unit, one that is necessarily involved in any organization of speech, even though it may be complemented by other units depending on the nature of the utterance. Many theorists have explicitly or implicitly pointed to the phoneme as such a basic unit. But strong evidence also has been marshalled for the syllable as the basic unit. Others point to evidence that even larger structures, such as the breath group (mentioned in Chapter 4) must be considered. Contention over this question continues, but the evidence strongly points to some minimum unit of production that is either phoneme- or syllable-sized.

A second question pertaining to the control of serial order is: How are the constituent elements regulated? One point of view is that the elements are related to one another in a larger structure, such as a stress grouping defined over a sequence of syllables or words. For example, it has been proposed that in English, syllables tend to occur in an alternating strong-weak (S-W) stress pattern. The word *telephone* has the stress pattern SWS. Several different kinds of structure have been proposed, but some kind of rhythmic grouping generally is suggested.

One way of combining phonetic elements into stress patterns is the **slots and fillers** (Shattuck-Hufnagel, 1979, 1983) or **frame and content** (Davis & MacNeilage, 1995) approach. According to this concept, the stress information for speech production is carried by the slots (or frame). The slots for a given utterance might indicate the number of syllables and their relative stress levels. Taking the word *telephone* as an example, the frame might look something like this:

$$S_{strong} + S_{weak} + S_{strong},$$

where S designates a syllable.

The slots are positions in the syllables to which phonetic elements (the fillers or content) can be assigned. For the word *telephone*, the elements would be assigned as follows:

$$(S_{strong} = [\text{tɛl}]) + (S_{weak} = [\text{ə}]) + (S_{strong} = [\text{fon}]).$$

The slots and fillers concept carries the implication that suprasegmental features, such as stress level and the segmental composition of an utterance, may be somewhat independently determined. This principle finds empirical support in the study of speech errors (Fromkin, 1989; Shattuck-Hufnagel, 1979), such as:

1. "tasted the whole worm" for "wasted the whole term"
2. "piss and stretch" for "pitch and stress"
3. "would you bury me" for "would you marry me"
4. "Nevina, Rado" for "Reno, Nevada"

Many such errors involve the transposition of phonetic elements while preserving the stress pattern of the utterance. In **1.**, the error seems to be a transposition of the initial consonants in the words *wasted* and *term*. The affected syllables have a similar stress level in the utterance. In **2.**, the affected syllables also have a similar stress level, but the transposition involves the syllable-final elements. In **3.**, there is no apparent transposition, but it is significant that the error sound [b] differs from the target sound [m] by a single phonetic feature (nonnasal for nasal). Studies indicate that substitutions of this kind often differ in only a feature or two. Speech errors affecting individual sounds tend to occur between sounds that are phonetically similar. Sometimes a change in a single feature can drastically alter the meaning of an utterance. In **4.**, a complex series of errors can be seen, but it is interesting that the phonemic content is essentially the same in the error and target utterances. The error output is a jumbled version of the phonemes of the intended production. This kind of error pattern is consistent with the idea that the phonetic segments to be produced are stored in a buffer and then retrieved as they are needed to control speech production.

Large numbers of speech errors have been studied with the objective of dissecting them into the underlying organization of speech. Presumably, speech errors occur along the seams of the production process, rather like earthquakes occurring along fault lines. Speech, like the earth's mantle, has plates and slippage zones. Above all, it is clear that speech errors are not random. Rather, they occur in fairly lawful ways, and these consistencies are taken as evidence of the organizational framework of speech.

One implication of the slots and fillers concept is that speech is organized as two parallel streams of organization that are fused in the final production (Figure 11–1). One stream, the slots, carries information on syllable pattern and stress level; the other stream, the fillers, carries information on the phonetic elements that will be inserted into the slots. Mistakes are most likely to occur among syllables with similar levels of stress. This may result from errors in a process that tries to match fillers with slots. When the slots have a similar level of stress, it is easier for the process to make misassignments.

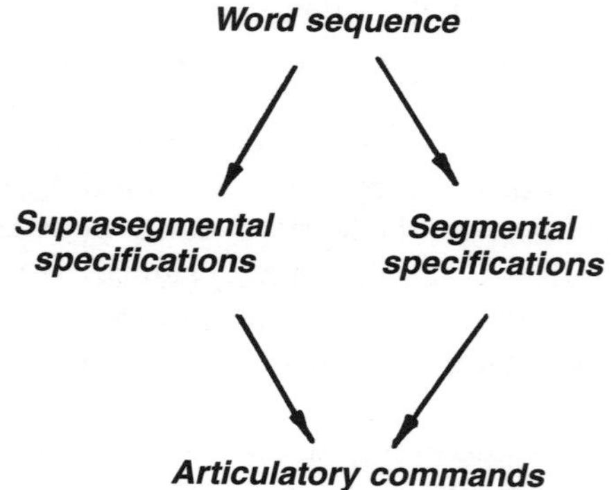

Figure 11–1. A simple version of a model in which suprasegmental information (such as syllable number and stress levels) is combined with segmental (phonetic) information in speech production.

Another factor that predisposes us to make errors is the similarity of the consonant and vowel elements within syllables. Tongue twisters such as "She sells seashells by the seashore" are difficult because of the repetition of a highly similar fricative + vowel combination: *she, sells, sea, shells, sea, shore.* Notice how much less challenging it is to say a more phonetically diverse utterance such as "She buys peanuts by the bandstand."

This model of production also has been used to explain certain aspects of speech development in children, especially the vocalizations in infancy (Davis & MacNeilage, 1995). In this developmental application, the slots are thought to be a frame derived from oscillatory movements of the jaw. As the jaw moves up and down, its movement gives an essential syllabic form to vocalization. Mandibular motion appears early in infancy, which makes this kind of articulatory patterning influential in the infant's first experiences with vocal behavior. The infant starts with this frame (slots) and then inserts phonetic content (fillers). Because of the relatively early neuromuscular maturation of the lips and tongue tip, the most likely phonetic content will be sounds such as [b] and [d]. Therefore, infant babbling takes shape as repetitions of simple syllables: [ba ba ba ba], [de de de de], or [mo mo mo mo]. The phonetic content of babbling is pretty much the same the world over (Locke, 1983), which may indicate that biological universals operate in the earliest stages of sound learning.

Another theoretical controversy surrounds whether feedback is used in any way to regulate the seriation of elements in speech. An early theory of speech production held that speech was controlled like a servosystem in which feedback was used to regulate the articulators (Fairbanks, 1954). Feedback is a signal that returns information from the periphery (e.g., the speech muscles) to the controller that regulates movement. On the issue of feedback, there are two extreme positions, as next discussed.

One perspective of speech organization is that the elements that constitute a particular speech utterance are **preprogrammed**, that is, prepared in advance of actual production by a set of instructions rather like a computer program. The program is then executed by the speech musculature *without* reliance on feedback concerning the movements actually performed. This **programming theory** has been highly influential in the theoretical history of speech production. Perhaps the major weakness of this theory is that it places a tremendous computational burden on the speaker's organizational scheme. There is a great deal to program in speech, and to put everything together in a package of instructions is no mean feat. The opposing theoretical perspective is that **feedback control** is used to confirm the completion of one element and this completion signal triggers the next element. According to this theory, the executive or controller issues instructions and then waits for a signal that the instruction has been completed. A major limitation to **feedback theories** is that the delays in most feedback channels are too long to allow effective control of a motor sequence. If the controller has to wait for a feedback signal before issuing the next motor instruction in a sequence, the whole process depends critically on the feedback delay. It also has been proposed that preprogramming and feedback can be combined by allowing that a basic set of instructions is prepared in advance of movement, but that performance of the set relies on selected feedback signals. The feedback could be sampled only intermittently to check on the overall progress of the motor behavior. Finally, some scientists have advanced a **feedforward theory**, in which advance signals sent to the muscles set the proper conditions for the control of speech movements. Feedforward signals can exert strong regulatory effects on a complex system, but substantial learning is required before these signals can be used reliably.

These issues are discussed in more detail in Kent, Adams, and Turner (1996) and MacNeilage (1970).

Problem 2: Degrees of Freedom

Chapters 3, 4, 5, 6, and 7 discussed the anatomic components of speech and hearing. Readers who needed to memorize the information in those chapters may have been impressed (but perhaps discouraged and frustrated as well) by the large number of bones, muscles, and nerves involved in the act of speaking. The number is impressive in another way as well. A talker must control large numbers of muscles to produce even a relatively simple act of speech, such as asking, "How much of this will be covered on the exam?" This simple question, asked by legions of students each year, contains about 29 phonemes, each of which involves activation of a particular set of muscles in a particular sequence. The initial word *how* is associated with activation of respiratory, laryngeal, and upper airway muscles. Moreover, the tongue, lips, jaw, velum, larynx, and respiratory system each possess several possible types of movement for range, direction, and speed. To complicate matters even more, they can combine in various ways; for example, the lower lip and jaw can move in phase with each other (having the same relative timing) and in the same direction, out of phase with each other (different relative timing) but in the same direction, or in phase with each other, but in opposite directions.

Imagine that it was necessary to teach young children to talk by telling them exactly which muscles to contract, for how long, and how strongly. Even a single word such as *spoon* would involve actions of the respiratory muscles, intrinsic and extrinsic laryngeal muscles, intrinsic and extrinsic tongue muscles, labial muscles, velopharyngeal muscles, and perhaps even the mandibular muscles. If each muscle contraction had to be specified, the production of a single word would entail a rather imposing list of instructions. But suppose instead that one could teach children to speak by using some more general instructions such as "close the lips" and that these general instructions automatically recruited the proper combination of muscle contractions. This is an illustration of the **degrees of freedom** problem. The different movement or muscle-contraction alternatives are called degrees of freedom and the degrees of freedom problem is the control dilemma faced by a system that must regulate all of these variables to accomplish a particular motor response. This problem is by no means unique to speech, as it occurs in almost all coordinated movements of complex muscular systems. Much of human behavior, and animal behavior as well, involves a solution to the degrees of freedom problem.

The challenge to a motor control system is this: How does the control system manage such a large number of degrees of freedom while achieving a desired action? One possibility is that the system expends a great deal of computational effort to control a large number of degrees of freedom. That is, the system deliberately prepares a separate command for each and every muscle involved in each and every movement. An alternative approach is to reduce the total number of degrees of freedom to a more manageable subset. One way of doing so is to combine muscles into **functional collectives**, or **synergies**. The idea is that muscles are controlled *in groups* related to *tasks* or functional objectives, rather than being controlled individually. Examples of functional objectives would be labial closure, vocal fold adduction, or velopharyngeal closure. Labial closure as a general motoric objective could be accomplished by a synergy based on the mandible, lower lip, and upper lip. The concept of synergies is a major tenet of a speech production theory discussed later in this chapter.

Problem 3: The Context-Sensitivity Problem

The third problem is that the production of a sound may vary with the context (neighborhood of other sounds) in which it is produced. In addition, the production of a speech sound is influenced by factors such as speaking rate, stress, and precision of articulation. A given "sound" of speech often can be produced in several different ways. Indeed, the variability of production has been an obstacle in speech research, and much thought and argument has circled the issue of why movements (and even acoustic patterns) have such great variability. This variability of production poses difficult problems for a theory that is based on the idea that a simple library of motor commands is used to generate the movements for individual phonemes.

Different solutions to this problem have been proposed. One of these is to endow the fundamental units of speech production with sensitivity to context. These "context-sensitive allophones" would account for the influences of the sounds that precede and follow a given segment. For example, a given speech segment **x**, that follows segment **y** and precedes segment **z**, could have the phonetic designation $_{y}\mathbf{x}_{z}$, meaning that segment **x** is adjusted to the left- and right-hand segments. A shortcoming to this approach is that coarticulatory influences are not limited to the immediately adjacent phonetic segments but can extend to segments that are at least two or three positions removed. Consequently, the number of context-sensitive allophones required will multiply considerably. The brain may have to store units such as $_{abcd}\mathrm{x}_{efgh}$, that is, element

x adjusted to a preceding sequence **abcd** and a following sequence **efgh**.

Another proposed solution is to allow the contextual influences to arise through specific mechanisms that operate on the control units of speech. One variant of this solution recognizes that units are composed of features. Coarticulation occurs because features can "spread" to adjacent segments so long as these features do not contradict the phonetic requirements of those segments (Daniloff & Hammarberg, 1973). For instance, the feature of lip rounding can spread to earlier segments in a phonetic sequence if those segments do not have a feature of lip retraction. This idea can be illustrated with the word *stew*, transcribed phonetically as [s t u]. The vowel [u] generally is produced with lip rounding. Observations of the articulation of this word have shown that the gesture of lip rounding actually begins during the [s], even though [s] is not typically produced with lip rounding. According to feature spreading concept, the lip rounding can begin early in the phonetic sequence, as long as it does not conflict with the feature specifications of other sounds. Both the [s] and [t] of *stew* can accommodate lip rounding because they are neutral for this feature. The nature of feature spreading can be expressed in a formula that shows how the value of a feature is changed when sounds occur in sequences. Using the example of the word *stew*, the following notation shows that the value of the feature for lip rounding (abbreviated LR and placed in braces) changes from zero (neutral) to positive (lip rounding present) in the sequence [s] + [t] + [u]:

[s] {0LR} + [t] {0LR} + [u] {+LR}

[s] {+LR} + [t] {+LR} + [u] {+LR}

For additional discussion of these issues, see Kent and Minifie (1977).

SELECTED THEORIES OF SPEECH PRODUCTION

Some examples of influential theories are introduced in this section. The theoretical review is by no means exhaustive and is intended only to give a flavor of some major theories.

Stage Theories (Translation Theories)

Stage theories are among the oldest of speech production models, but they have been renewed by fresh ideas that overcome some of the failings of older versions. Stage models have in common the idea that speech is produced by a series of stages (Meyer & Gordon, 1985; Perkell, 1980; Sternberg, Knoll, Monsell, & Wright, 1988; Sternberg, Monsell, Knoll, & Wright, 1978). The result of processing at one stage is passed along to the next stage. One reason for the popularity of these models is that speech seems to involve several different kinds of information, and it is appealing to assign these sources of information to different stages in the production process. Decisions made at one stage are then transferred to another stage, which adds its own set of decisions. The number and type of stages vary among the different stage models, but they typically include stages similar to the following:

1. Segment specification. This stage defines the segments that make up the phonetic message. Different theories typically select syllables, phonemes, or allophones as the segments to be specified. For instance, a phoneme-based model supposes that a sequence of phonemes is the highest stage of control (and probably will be the output of the phonological component of a language system). The segment specification stage is the highest level of motor regulation and frequently is assumed to have a direct interface with the language formulation system. That is, the language component issues an output from which segment specification can be prepared. If one needs to draw a boundary between the processes of language formulation and speech production, it is at this level that the boundary occurs.

2. Feature or goal composition. It is commonly assumed that segments are interpreted as features or as goals. The segment usually is regarded as too abstract to govern the physical processes of speech production. Therefore, the segment is redefined as phonetic features or articulatory goals. For example, the phoneme /p/ may be associated with the features bilabial, stop, voiceless, which suffice to specify actions of the lips and larynx. Several different feature systems have been proposed in the literature on phonetics and phonology. They share the idea that segments are not immediately related to muscular instructions for speech production. Goals specify an articulatory objective, such as closed lips and abducted vocal folds. If features are used in this level, then a stage of feature interpretation intervenes between segment specification and the generation of motor commands. If goals are used, then a stage of goal identification intervenes between segment specification and the generation of motor commands.

3. Motor command generation. Features or goals are used to generate motor instructions to the muscles of speech production. These motor commands regulate the sequence of muscle contractions and also specify the duration and strength of contraction in individual muscles. Motor commands are prepared to accomplish a particular trajectory of movement for each articulator involved in an utterance.

Many stage models also include a level of higher organization that specifies information pertinent to factors such as speaking rate, stress pattern, and other suprasegmental (prosodic) variables. There are strong arguments that speech is governed by a hierarchical structure related to rhythmic or breath-group patterning (Gee & Grosjean, 1983; Martin, 1972).

An example of a stage model with several levels of regulation is shown in Figure 11–2. Certainly, not all stage models share this multileveled organization, but it is shown as an example of the many different structures that might be considered in the regulation of speech production.

A general difficulty in the experimental validation of stage models is that, because the results of one stage are passed on to following stages, it is challenging to demonstrate the reality of any one stage in the sequence. The existence of any single stage is predicated on

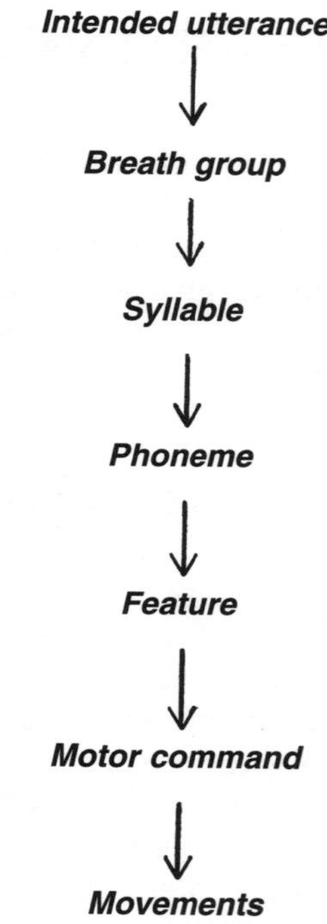

Figure 11–2. An example of a stage model of speech production that has multiple levels of organization.

the existence of others. The stage approach also has been criticized because of the complexity of the decisions involved. Mulder (1983) discusses general issues related to stage models of information processing.

Action Theory (Dynamic Systems Theory)

Action theory is also known as **dynamic systems theory**. The application of this theory to speech was introduced in the 1980s (Fowler, Rubin, Remez, & Turvey, 1980; Kelso, Saltzman, & Tuller, 1986). A basic feature of this theory is that it attempts to avoid the serial levels of control typical of stage theories. According to action theory, the motor act itself is expressed at the level of control. The act to be performed is considered to be task-specific. Particular motor responses are selected to meet the requirements of the task to be performed. Motor control is conceptualized in terms of **coordinative structures** (another term for synergies), which are combinations of muscle contractions that accomplish a particular goal. For example, a coordinative structure that accomplishes closure of the lips might include motor commands to the jaw muscles as well as to muscles of the upper and lower lips. Because the participating muscles are controlled as a set, or collective, that is specific to an intended action, the control system does not have to prepare instructions for individual muscles. Therefore, the degrees of freedom problem is addressed by simplifying the control stategy. Rather than preparing detailed instructions for individual muscles that participate in a motor response, the action theory approach is to perform movements by selection of a suitable coordinative structure, the components of which are constrained to act as a whole in accomplishing a specific task.

Action theory permits flexibility of motor control in the following ways. First, the component motor responses in a coordinative structure can be adjusted as needed to meet the requirements of a particular task. Say, for example, that the task to be performed is closure of the lips. This objective can be accomplished through various means, as readers can demonstrate to themselves. First, if the jaw is immobile, then the muscles of the upper and lower lips can effect labial closure. To demonstrate this, hold your jaw in a mid-open position and close your lips together while holding the jaw in fixed position. Second, if the jaw is free to move, then the jaw muscles cooperate with the lip muscles to achieve closure of the lips. To demonstrate this possibility, begin with your jaw in a wide-open position and then allow your jaw and lips to move together to accomplish bilabial closure. Third, if the lips are inactive, the jaw can work by itself to bring the lips into a closed state. To demonstrate this third possibility, begin with your jaw in a wide-open position and then, while trying to keep your lips in an inactive, relaxed state, close your jaw vigorously. Most individuals succeed in bring the lips together.

A second way that action theory affords flexibility is that the magnitudes of the motor responses are scaled to meet the demands of various speaking conditions, especially speaking rate and stress. The extent of an articulatory movement for a given phonetic requirement tends to be larger for slow speaking rates and heavy stress. Inversely, the extent of a movement tends to be smaller for rapid speaking rates and light stress. In action theory, **order variables** regulate the magnitude of the movements in a coordinative structure. In this way, a coordinative structure can satisfy the same phonetic task, such as lip closure, with varying amounts of movement. By analogy, a person who is writing a word on a sheet of paper can make the loops and lines larger or smaller while preserving the basic pattern of muscle contraction in the hands and fingers. Order variables adjust the magnitude of movement required for suprasegmental aspects of speech.

A related theory is the **gestural theory of phonology** (Browman & Goldstein, 1986).

This theory borrows some fundamental concepts from dynamic systems theory, and makes an explicit connection to the phonological component of language by assuming that phonology is encoded in terms of abstract gestures. An example of a gesture is a movement of the tongue to a high position in the oral cavity. A gesture-based phonology would avoid the kind of translation that more traditional phonologies require, such as a translation from phonemes to features to articulatory movements. In gestural theory, the gesture is the primitive (basic element) of the phonological system, and phonological patterns are described in terms of interactions among gestures. Advocates of this theory contend that it offers an economical explanation of a number of phonological patterns in the world's languages and also has implications for the study of phonological development in children. An appealing aspect of gestural theory is that it can be implemented as a computer model to include specification of movements and the resulting acoustic signal. Saltzman and Munhall (1989) describe a model of the gestural regulation of vocal tract movements.

Figure 11–3 shows how concepts from gestural theory can be used to produce a gestural or motor score (set of instructions to

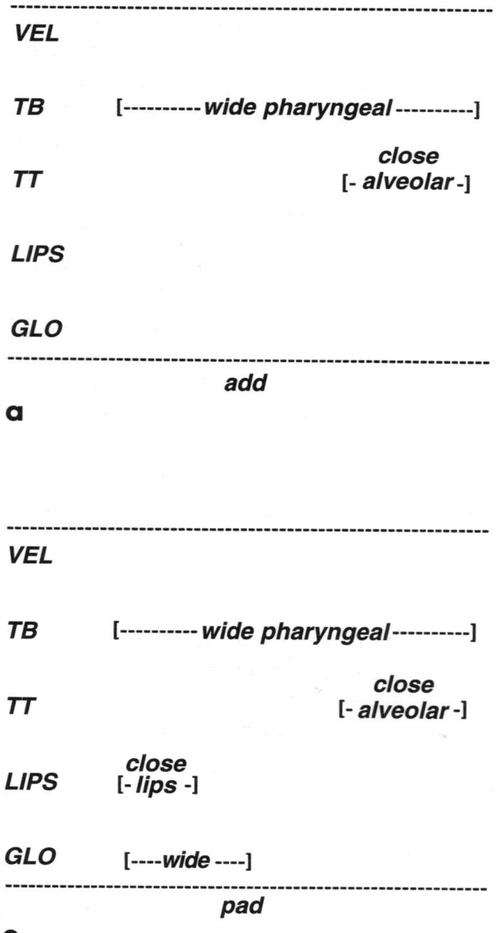

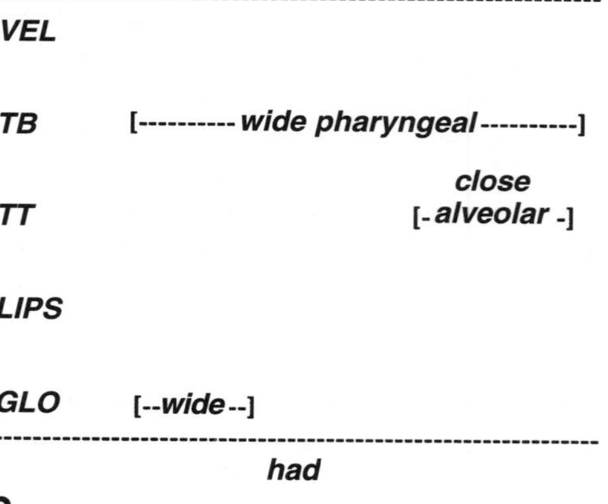

Figure 11–3. Examples of gestural or motor scores used in gestural phonology. The gestures are shown in brackets and the horizontal position of the brackets for a given gesture indicates the relative timing of that gesture in the score. VEL = velum; TB = tongue body, TT = tongue tip, LIPS = upper and lower lips, and GLO = glottis. **a.** Score for the word *add*, with gestures specified for the tongue body and tongue tip. **b.** Score for the word *had*, with gestures specified for the tongue body, tongue tip, and glottis. **c.** Score for the word *pad*, with gestures specified for the tongue body, tongue tip, glottis, and lips.

the muscles) for speech production. Each score depicts the gestures needed for production of a particular phonetic sequence. The three parts of the illustration pertain to the words *add, had,* and *pad*. The word *add* (Figure 11–3a) contains the front vowel [æ], which is produced with a wide pharynx. Therefore, the gesture [wide pharyngeal] specifies the general tongue body (TB) position for the vowel. The final consonant [d] requires a lingua-alveolar constriction of the tongue tip (TT), which is indicated by the gesture [close alveolar]. As can be seen in Figure 11–3b, the gestural score for the word *had* is similar to that for the word *add*, but specifies an initial voiceless interval for the initial [h] by means of the gesture [wide] for the glottis (GLO). Finally, in Figure 11–3c, the score for the word *pad* is similar to that for the word *had*, except for the additional requirement of a bilabial closure. Therefore, the gesture [close lips] is added to the score, at about the same time as the gesture for a wide glottis. The relative timing of the gestures in a score can produce different phonetic sequences.

Action theory or dynamic systems theory has swept over many disciplines, including movement science, physical therapy, speech science, and subdisciplines of psychology. It has had deep impact on theoretical issues, and also on practical matters such as designing an optimum program for retraining of movements in individuals with neurological disorders.

Some problems and weaknesses in the application of action theory to speech have been discussed by Nolan (1982) and Wilson and Morton (1990).

Connectionist Theories

Connectionist networks, also known as distributed parallel processing, are built of numerous highly interconnected nodes. Sometimes these networks are called **neural networks** because of their presumed similarity to neural circuits. An example of this general approach is discussed for speech perception in Chapter 10. Network modeling of speech production has been done by Dell (1986), Jordan (1991), and Guenther (1994, 1995). These networks are called *massively parallel* in recognition of the large number of elements that make up the network. Figure 11–4 is an example of a very simple network, consisting of two layers, input units and output units. Each of the nodes representing the input can be connected to the nodes representing the output, and the signals that pass along these connections assume various weightings. In a common application of this kind of network, a task to be learned is introduced to the network through its input units. For example, if we wanted to teach the system to say the word *spoon*, we might use as input units the phonetic symbols [s p u n]. The network is then given a chance to "learn" the task by adjusting the internal weights of

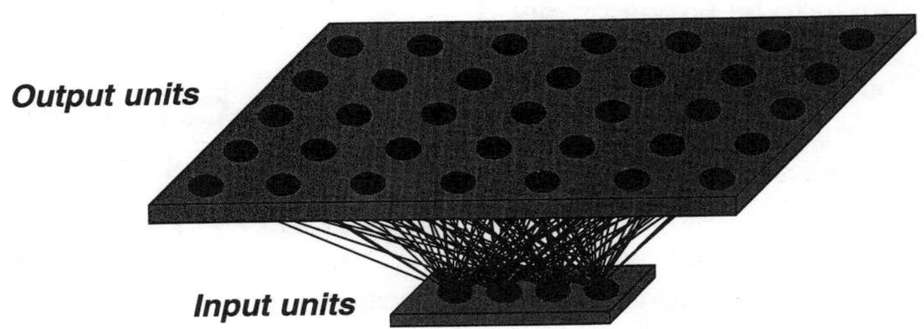

Figure 11–4. Example of a two-layer connectionist network with input units and output units.

its connections until the output units give a satisfactory match to the input units. The computer programs that accomplish this objective can run for several hours to resolve complex problems. Actual networks used for modeling these complex processes are much more elaborate than the simple example shown in Figure 11–4, but the operation is essentially the same. More elaborate network solutions may use three or more levels of units.

Connectionist networks have attracted a great deal of interest because they have successfully modeled a number of complex processes and systems, including aspects of grammar, speech perception, and speech production. In speech production applications, these networks have shown coarticulatory effects like those in natural speech, even though the experimenter did not deliberately program the system with coarticulation rules. That is, the system "learned" coarticulation by weighting its network connections in accord with structure in the input. It also appears that these networks can address important problems in speech acquisition and the effects of speaking rate (Guenther, 1994, 1995).

Connectionist networks are extremely powerful and are capable of modeling a number of problems in human behavior. A major challenge is to demonstrate that these models provide important insights into how humans actually solve these problems. It is possible for a modeling system to be too powerful, because it can reach a solution for any problem that is given to it. Such a system cannot be shown to be wrong or ineffective. One way of making networks more similar to actual biological or psychological systems is to constrain the networks with properties of the systems to be modeled. For example, a network model of speech production might be equipped with constraints related to muscular actions.

Hanson and Burr (1990) offer a very useful analysis of what connectionist networks learn, and Massaro (1988) discusses some of the limitations of this modelling approach. Pinker and Meher (1988) is a valuable source for an examination of general issues in connectionist modeling.

Quantal Theory

Quantal theory addresses the relation between vocal tract configuration and acoustic output (Stevens, 1972, 1989). Similar work has been done by Carré and Mrayati (1990). A basic tenet of the theory is that this relation is nonlinear. Sometimes a relatively large change in articulation has very little effect on the acoustic output. But other small changes in articulation have major acoustic consequences. Therefore, speakers discover that articulatory movements are not equal in their acoustic consequence. This discovery would have important implications in controlling the movements of speech. Configurations that tolerate some variability in placement without seriously altering the acoustic signal might be preferred for the phonetic systems of natural languages. These configurations would enable us to speak rapidly, to coarticulate, and to make small errors in articulatory placement without interfering with the transmission of phonetic information. Quantal theory does not explain all of the problems in speech production, but it may offer some important principles about how a speaker controls the vocal tract to produce desired acoustic effects. X-ray studies of configurations in speech production have been interpreted to show support for the quantal theory (Wood, 1979).

Linguistic-Communicative Theories of Speech: H & H Theory

These theories have to do with global issues of speech production related to the linguistic and communicative functions of speech. These theories are not directly concerned with how speech movements are controlled but rather with how the linguistic intentions or communicative goals of the speaker lead to overall settings of speech production. For example, psycholinguists have observed for many years that speakers possess different styles or registers of speech. A speaker can be formal on one occasion, but casual on another. Similarly, a speaker can strive for highly intelligible speech on one occasion, but be content with a very relaxed slurred style on another. Part of the normal competence of an adult speaker is the ability to adapt speaking patterns to different situations and tasks. We consider only one theory under this heading.

Lindblom (1990) proposed a theory, the **H & H theory** (for **hyperspeech** and **hypospeech**), which states that speech production is a balance between two opposing sets of demands. One set of demands is for intelligible speech, that is, efforts to ensure the perceptual adequacy of the speech signal. The other set of demands relates to economy of physiological effort, that is, making speech articulation as easy as possible to save energy. An individual speaker in a particular communicative setting controls speech production along a continuum of hyperspeech to hypospeech. This perspective implies that utterances will vary as the circumstances of communication differ. The "same" phonetic message will be produced in different ways depending on the speaker's intention and evaluation of the communicative setting.

Hyperspeech is described as "output-oriented" because the underlying control is purposive and prospectively organized. Hyperspeech ensures that speech sound discriminations can be heard by a listener. The emphasis is on the quality of output in an effort to ensure that intelligible speech is produced. Hypospeech is "system-oriented" insofar as it tries to achieve a low-cost form of regulation. Hypospeech tends to reduce the energy costs of speech production and it therefore can reduce the discriminability of the speech output. When factors such as context or topic familiarity can be relied on to ensure successful transmission of the intended message, speakers are expected to use hypospeech (or, more accurately, to move toward the hypospeech side of the hypospeech-hyperspeech continuum) in accord with the principle of economy of effort. The output-oriented aspects of hyperspeech that emphasize speech sound discriminability conflict with the system-oriented aspects of hypospeech that seek to conserve energy. It is not possible to satisfy the requirements of hyperspeech and hypospeech simultaneously. A major implication of the H & H theory is that a speaker does not rely on an invariant regulatory process, but rather selects a regulatory process that is adjusted to the demands of the communicative situation. It is assumed that speakers are flexible and adaptive. We can communicate under various conditions of interference with listeners of varying sensory or linguistic competence and by making deliberate efforts to adjust our speaking style to social and personal parameters. The H & H theory draws attention to this fundamental property of speech.

CONCLUSION

This brief and selective look at theoretical issues in speech production is intended not so much to give definitive answers as it is to define persistent questions. Science proceeds in the face of unsettled issues, and speech scientists have labored for decades without reaching consensus on some of the difficult and deep questions. But progress has been made. The process of speech is not easily understood. Theories help the scientist to ask the questions that are most important. They also help to organize the accepted facts into a coherent understanding. Discussions of theories help to sharpen our understanding of an area of science. In addition, a theory of speech production can have important implications for understanding speech development in children, various kinds of speech disorders, and the development of speech technologies (discussed in Chapter 12). Answers to fundamental questions about speech, such as "What is the basic unit of speech production," would have important implications for understanding speech development and speech disorders, and for defining the relationship between processes of language formulation and processes of speech production.

On The Reference Shelf

Recommended to readers who seek additional information on topics introduced in this chapter.

Levelt, W. J. M. (1989). *Speaking: From intention to articulation*. Cambridge, MA: MIT Press.
A discussion of the numerous processes involved in speaking. This book gives one of the most comprehensive accounts of the act of speaking, from the intention to speak to the movements of the speech organs.

Lofqvist, A. (1997). Theories and models of speech production. In W. J. Hardcastle & J. Laver (Eds.), *The handbook of phonetic sciences* (pp. 405–426). Oxford, England: Blackwell.
A concise review of major directions in the modeling of the movements of speech production.

Fujimura, O. (1990). Methods and goals of speech production research. *Language and Speech, 33*, 195–258.
A brisk survey of the field, by one of its most prominent investigators.

Kent, R. D., Adams, S. G., & Turner, G. (1996). Models of speech production. In N. J. Lass (Ed.), *Principles of experimental phonetics*. St. Louis: Mosby.
A survey of theories and models of speech production.

Smith, A. (1992). The control of orofacial movements in speech. *Critical Reviews in Oral Biology and Medicine, 3*, 233–267.
A concise but enlightening discussion of how speech movements are regulated.

Chapter References

Browman, C., & Goldstein, L. (1986). Towards an articulatory phonology. *Phonology Yearbook, 3*, 219–252.

Carré, R., & Mrayati, M. (1990). Articulatory-acoustic-phonetic relations and modelling, regions and modes. In W. J. Hardcastle & A. Marchal (Eds.), *Speech production and speech modelling* (pp. 211–240). Dordrecht, Netherlands: Kluwer Academic Publishers.

Daniloff, R. G., & Hammarberg, R. E. (1973). On defining coarticulation. *Journal of Phonetics, 1*, 239–248.

Davis, B. L., & MacNeilage, P. F. (1995). The articulatory basis of babbling. *Journal of Speech and Hearing Research, 38*, 1199–1211.

Dell, G. S. (1986). A spreading-activation theory of retrieval in sentence production. *Psychological Review, 93*, 283–321.

Fairbanks, G. (1954). Systematic research in experimental phonetics, I: A theory of the speech mechanism as a servosystem. *Journal of Speech and Hearing Disorders, 19,* 133–139.

Fowler, C. A. (1980). Coarticulation and theories of extrinsic timing. *Journal of Phonetics, 8,* 113–133.

Fowler, C., Rubin, P., Remez, R. E., & Turvey, M. T. (1980). Implications for speech production of a general theory of action. In B. Butterworth (Ed.), *Speech production* (Vol. 1, pp. 373–420). New York: Academic Press.

Fromkin, V. A. (1989). Grammatical aspects of speech errors. In F. J. Newmeyer (Ed.), *Linguistics: The Cambridge Survey. I. Linguistic theory: Extensions and implications* (pp. 117–138). Cambridge, UK: Cambridge University Press.

Gee, J. P., & Grosjean, F. (1983). Performance structures: A psycholinguistic and linguistic appraisal. *Cognitive Psychology, 15,* 411–458.

Guenther, F. H. (1994). A neural network model of speech acquisition and motor equivalent speech production. *Biological Cybernetics, 72,* 43–53.

Guenther, F. H. (1995). Speech sound acquisition, coarticulation, and rate effects in a neural network model of speech production. *Psychological Review, 102,* 594–621.

Hanson, S. J., & Burr, D. J. (1990). What connectionist models learn: Learning and representation in connectionist networks. *Behavioral and Brain Sciences, 13,* 471–518.

Jordan, M. I. (1991). Serial order: A parallel distributed processing approach. In J. L. Elman & D. E. Rumelhard (Eds.), *Advances in connectionist theory: Speech* (pp. 214–249). Hillsdale, NJ: Erlbaum.

Kelso, J. A. S., Saltzman, E. L., & Tuller, B. (1986). The dynamical perspective on speech production: Data and theory. *Journal of Phonetics, 14,* 29–59.

Kent, R. D., Adams, S. G., & Turner, G. (1996). Models of speech production. In N. J. Lass (Ed.), *Principles of experimental phonetics* (pp. 3–45). St. Louis: Mosby.

Kent, R. D., & Minifie, F. D. (1977). Coarticulation in recent speech production models. *Journal of Phonetics, 5,* 115–133.

Kuhn, T. (1970). *The structure of scientific revolutions* (2nd ed.). Chicago: University of Chicago Press.

Lindblom, B. (1990). Explaining phonetic variation: A sketch of the H & H theory. In W. J. Hardcastle & A. Marchal (Eds.), *Speech production and speech modelling* (pp. 403–439). Dordrecht, Netherlands: Kluwer Academic Publishers.

Locke, J. (1983). *Phonological acquisition and change.* New York: Academic Press.

Lofqvist, A. (1990). Speech as audible gestures. In W. J. Hardcastle & A. Marchal (Eds.), *Speech production and speech modelling* (pp. 289–322). Dordrecht, Netherlands: Kluwer Academic Publishers.

MacNeilage, P. (1970). Motor control of serial ordering of speech. *Psychological Review, 77,* 182–196.

Martin, J. G. (1972). Rhythmic (hierarchial) versus serial structure in speech and other behavior. *Psychological Review, 79,* 487–509.

Massaro, D. W. (1988). Some criticisms of connectionist models of human performance. *Journal of Memory and Language, 27,* 213–234.

Meyer, D. E., & Gordon, P. C. (1985). Speech production: Motor programming of phonetic features. *Journal of Memory and Language, 24,* 3–26.

Mulder, G. (1983). The information processing paradigm: Concepts, methods and limitations. *Journal of Child Psychology and Psychiatry, 24,* 19–35.

Nolan, F. J. (1982). The role of action theory in the description of speech production. *Linguistics, 20,* 287–308.

Perkell, J. S. (1980). Phonetic features and the physiology of speech production. In B. Butterworth (Ed.), *Language production* (Vol. 1, pp. 337–372). New York: Academic Press.

Pinker, S., & Mehler, J. (Eds.) (1988). *Connections and symbols.* Cambridge, MA: MIT Press.

Saltzman, E. L., & Munhall, K. G. (1989). A dynamical approach to gestural patterning in speech production. *Ecological Psychology, 1,* 333–382.

Shattuck-Hufnagel, S. (1979). Speech errors as evidence for a serial-ordering mechanism in sentence production. In W. Cooper & E. Walker (Eds.), *Sentence processing.* Hillsdale, NJ: Erlbaum.

Shattuck-Hufnagel, S. (1983). In P. F. MacNeilage (Ed.), *The production of speech* (pp. 109–136). New York: Springer-Verlag.

Sternberg, S., Knoll, R. L., Monsell, S., & Wright, C. E. (1988). Motor programs and hierarchical organization in the control of rapid speech. *Phonetica, 45,* 172–197.

Sternberg, S., Monsell, S., Knoll, R. L., & Wright, C. E. (1978). The latency and duration of rapid movement sequences: Comparison of speech and typewriting. In G. E. Stelmach (Ed.), *Information processing in motor control and learning* (pp. 117–152). New York: Academic Press.

Stevens, K. N. (1972). The quantal nature of speech: Evidence from articulatory-acoustic data. In P. B. Denes & E. E. Davis (Eds.), *Human communication: A unified view* (pp. 51–66). New York: McGraw-Hill.

Stevens, K. N. (1989). On the quantal nature of speech. *Journal of Phonetics, 17*, 3–46.

Wilson, W. R., & Morton, K. (1990). Reconsideration of the action-theory perspective on speech motor control. *Clinical Linguistics and Phonetics, 4*, 341–362.

Wood, S. (1979). A radiographic analysis of constriction locations for vowels. *Journal of Phonetics, 7*, 25–43.

Exercises

11-1. Select one of the theories discussed in this chapter and read one or more of the papers cited as sources. Try to identify the strengths and weaknesses of the theory. What is your own opinion of the theory?

11-2. Construct your own stage model of speech production, incorporating what you believe to be the major aspects in the control of speech. For example, you might start with a breath group at the top level and work down through progressive levels to the movement of individual articulators. Try to develop a model that specifies the information needed to produce speech.

11-3. The "degrees of freedom" problem can be applied quite generally to human behavior. Describe how this problem applies to the following: reaching for a book on a high shelf, picking up a cup and drinking from it, writing a word on a blackboard, and catching a thrown object with both hands.

11-4. As an example of the "context sensitivity" problem, describe how the phonetic element represented by the alphabetic character *n* would be distinctively produced in the following words: *answer, anthem, snow,* and *sneak.* **Hint:** the phonetic element [n] can be produced as an alveolar, a dental, a lip-rounded consonant, or a lip-retracted consonant.

11-5. Using the scores in Figure 11–3 as a guide, make up a gestural score for the words *pan* and *ban*. **Hint:** a nasal consonant requires a gesture for lowered velum, and a voiced consonant cannot be produced with a wide glottis.

CHAPTER

12

Applied Speech Sciences

> ***"A science of communication, like all other science, must consist of . . . a set of scientific symbols. The peculiar aspect of a science of communication is that its scientific symbols refer to other symbols. It uses language to talk about language, and it is somewhat puzzling that new symbols about old symbols could clarify the problem in any way."***
>
> (George A. Miller: *Language and communication*. New York: McGraw-Hill, 1951, p. 2.)

This chapter explores selected applications of speech science. Some applications pertain to speech technologies, such as producing and recognizing speech by computer. Other applications have to do with the use of speech as evidence in criminal investigations, such as identifying individuals from recordings of their voices. Still other applications involve studying, assessing, or treating disorders of communication. These application areas are briefly reviewed as examples of the ways in which speech science has produced practical benefits to individuals and to society. Basic research on speech has been the foundation for these applications. Basic and applied research often interact, such that discoveries in either domain can stimulate progress in the other. If truth is the goal of science, then it is unlikely that truth comes in two kinds, one basic and one applied. Rather, truth is a single whole that can be approached in different ways.

Because this chapter surveys a broad territory, the treatment of each topic is necessarily brief, but references are suggested for readers who want a deeper coverage. The primary purpose of this chapter is to give an idea of the range of applications in speech science.

HUMAN-MACHINE SPEECH COMMUNICATION

> ***"If computers could recognize and understand speech, there would be a revolution in the way in which humans use computers."***
>
> (D. Kewley-Port, Speech recognition, in A. Syrdal, R. Bennett, & S. Greenspan (Eds.), *Applied speech technology*. Boca Raton, Florida: CRC Press, p. 343.)

> ***"Voice communication with machines is no longer a dream but a reality. The tremendous progress that has been accomplished has come about as a result of solving successfully some of the fundamental problems caused by the immense variability present in the speech signal."***
>
> (B. S. Atal: Speech recognition by machines. In K. Elenius & P. Branderud (Eds.), *Proceedings of the XIIIthe International Congress of Phonetic Sciences (ICPhS 95)*. Stockholm: International Congress of Phonetic Sciences, 1995, p. 496.)

One way of humanizing technology is to give technology human attributes, one of which is speech. Although people can effectively use devices such as a keyboard, a pointer, or a mouse to communicate with machines, many users would prefer to talk to their machines. Talking is natural, easy, and probably much less likely to cause repetition-use syndromes such as carpal tunnel syndrome. Working for hours at a keyboard can be fatiguing and, over the course of weeks, can result in painful conditions that are not always easily treated. Speaking poses fewer risks and is a comfortable activity for most people.

There has long been a fascination with the idea of animals, machines, or nonliving objects that can understand and produce speech. In the folktale, "Ali Baba and the Forty Thieves," Ali Baba secretly watches a band of thieves gain entry to their riches-laden cave with the simple command, "Open Sesame." When the thieves depart, Ali Baba uses the same words to open the cave and discover the gold and treasures it contains. The spacecraft computer in the science fantasy film *2001: A Space Odyssey* was named HAL and it could carry on human-like conversations with the crew members. (HAL was also proficient in speech reading and was able to understand what the crew members were saying just by observing the movements of their mouths.) Improvements in speech synthesis and automatic speech recognition are bringing to reality the kind of human-machine speech communications that were imagined in the film. Today's children may very well become adults who will find it quite routine to communicate with computers using conversational speech. Machines that understand human speech and speak in response reflect accumulated scientific and technical progress in speech communication. These machines have a variety of practical applications in business, science, education, and entertainment.

DIGITAL SPEECH CODING

Most of the technologies discussed in this section are based on digital speech coding, some basic aspects of which are covered in Chapter 9. The information in this section is a basic overview of speech synthesis and automatic speech recognition. Recent comprehensive treatments of these issues are available in Roe and Wilpon (1994) and Syrdal, Bennett, and Greenspan (1995).

Speech Synthesis

Speech synthesis, or the production of speech by machine, can be accomplished in different ways, but three of the most important are: **copy synthesis**, **articulatory synthesis**, and **terminal analog synthesis**. The last two are sometimes grouped together under the name, **synthesis by rule**, because the procedure involves a set of rules that control the components of the synthesizer. In contrast, copy synthesis can work essentially as a procedure of looking up the desired information in a library of speech units. Each of these is now summarized.

Copy synthesis works by combining stored patterns to make longer utterances. Various kinds of stored patterns have been used. These include words, numbers, syllables, and demisyllables (basically, half-syllables that can be combined to form words). An advantage to this kind of synthesis is that if suitable patterns have been stored, then production of connected speech patterns is relatively easy. A major difficulty has been in the selection of the right kind of stored units. Although each kind of unit can be satisfactory under certain conditions, it is not clear that any single unit works well all of the time. For some applications, this method is simple and highly effective. For example, if the application requires generation of a spoken series of numbers, like telephone numbers, then storage of digits can be quite successful. But generation of narrative information, such as a story or conversation, is much more challenging with this approach.

One of the most promising directions, **diphone synthesis**, operates on stored units that extend from the steady-state portion of one sound to the steady-state portion of the following sound. For example, the syllable *seek* ([sik]) could be composed by combining the [si] diphone with the [ik] diphone; [sik] = [si] + [ik]. An advantage of this approach is that many aspects of coarticulation are intrinsic to the stored units. A disadvantage is that this approach requires a large number of stored units. This disadvantage diminishes in importance as computers gain in speed and memory size. Diphone synthesis has been used successfully in some personal computer systems and is the basis of the synthesized voices in MacinTalk™.

Articulatory synthesis, also called a **transmission-line analog**, is a model of the physiology of human speech and includes components that resemble human articulators. Therefore, the articulatory synthesizer may have a tongue, jaw, lower lip, and other "articulators," each of which can be controlled to produce humanlike speech patterns. This kind of synthesizer is really like a mechanical talker, although in practice the vocal tract organs are usually modeled in a computer. The ultimate success of this approach rests on a good understanding of speech physiology. If the model is based on a clumsy model of the tongue, its intended lingual articulation may fall short of humanlike speech. One of the earliest speech synthesizers was an articulatory synthesizer. This early model, developed by Wolfgang von Kempelen in the 18th century, used a bellows for the lungs, a vibrating reed for the voice source, narrow pipes to generate turbulence, and a flexible rubber apparatus for the vocal tract. The basic components match the three major subsystems of speech production: respiratory system (the bellows), laryngeal system (the vibrating reed), and the upper airway (the narrow tubes and the simulated vocal tract).

The young Alexander Graham Bell saw a reconstruction of von Kempelen's speaking machine and became fascinated with the prospect of creating his own device to make speech sounds. Working with his brother Melville and with advice from his father, Bell made a model of the vocal organs that reportedly could be made to produce vowels and nasals. This early experience with speech may have had some influence on Bell's later experiments, including the work that produced the telephone. Bell's telephone is considered by some to be the most valuable patent ever issued. This invention permitted communication at a distance and therefore greatly enhanced the power of human speech.

Modern systems use computer models of the speech systems. The acoustic output of the models is generated with articulatory-acoustic formulas. The vocal tract model and the acoustic formulas are entirely computer programs. All that is needed for sound output is a speaker.

Finally, terminal-analog synthesis attempts to produce satisfactory replicas of the end product of speech, the acoustic signal. These synthesizers do not model speech physiology per se but rather depend on energy sources and resonators controlled to produce acoustic patterns like those of natural speech. A major type of terminal-analog synthesizer is known as a **formant synthesizer**, so called because it produces speech largely by specifying the formants of a modeled utterance. This kind of synthesizer is in widespread use today, but the quality of speech varies considerably across the various systems. The best of them produce speech that is highly intelligible and has a fairly natural quality. Moreover, some systems allow selection of different speaking rates and even different voices (child, woman, man). The DECTalk™ system is a good example of a formant-based speech synthesizer.

Figure 12–1 shows the basic components of a typical speech synthesizer based on a source/system model. An impulse train generator coupled to a glottal pulse model supplies voicing excitation. The impulse train is basically a series of pulses that mimic the fundamental frequency of vocal fold vibration. The glottal pulse model shapes the pulses to produce the desired spectrum (like the source spectrum discussed in Chapter 9). A random noise generator provides the source energy for stop bursts and frication segments. The capability for voiced/unvoiced mixture can be used to produce voiced fricatives. The vocal tract model can be developed according to the general properties described in Chapter 9.

Terminal analog synthesizers are commonly used in the most popular systems for personal and commercial use. Considerable progress has been made in producing speech that is fairly intelligible and natural.

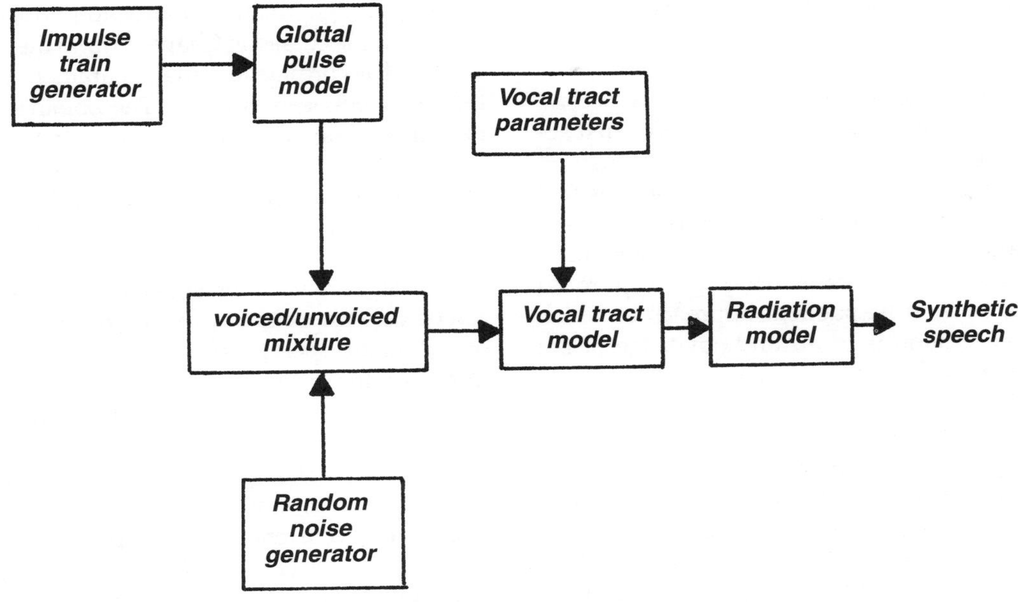

Figure 12–1. Speech synthesizer based on source-system model of speech production.

But most systems cannot compare with natural speech in either their intelligibility or their quality. Studies of word recognition generally show that natural speech is considerably more intelligible to listeners than the synthetic speech produced by almost any commercially available system (Greene, Logan, & Pisoni, 1986; Hoover, Reichle, Van Tassell, & Cole, 1987; Mitchell & Adkins, 1989; Mirenda & Beukelman, 1987, 1990). However, DECTalk™ is one of the most intelligible synthesizers across major units of speech—word, sentence, and paragraph.

In summary, several techniques have been developed for speech synthesis. A good indication of the progress in this field is the improving intelligibility and naturalness of the speech that is produced. Certainly, there is room for improvement, but if the rate of progress over the last two decades is an indication of what the future may hold, then it is highly likely that within a few years, speech synthesizers will produce speech that is barely distinguishable from natural speech. Moreover, future systems for speech synthesis may permit flexible and convenient regulation of speaking rates, emotional attributes, and voice quality.

Automatic Speech Recognition

Automatic speech recognition, also called machine speech recognition, is the technology by which machines can recognize speech. In their most elaborate and refined manifestation, these machines might even be called **speech understanding systems**, for they can derive linguistic interpretations—and maybe even affective interpretations—of some utterances. Speech recognition systems vary greatly in their capability. Some can recognize only digits spoken by one speaker, others might recognize a vocabulary of 500 words produced by a small group of speakers, and still others have the capability to recognize over a thousand words spoken by a rather large sample of speakers of either sex and varying age.

Automatic speech recognition is accomplished in three primary ways. The first approach uses statistical techniques of pattern recognition. The recognition system is first "trained" on a set of speech data that enables the system to learn important regularities about the signal. The second approach is an acoustic-phonetic approach in which recognition is based on knowledge of the relationship between acoustic patterns and phonetic structures. The third approach uses artificial neural networks (connectionist networks). The networks are trained on a data set until satisfactory performance is demonstrated. It is also possible to combine these methods, for example, a statistical pattern recognition can be combined with information on acoustic-phonetic relations.

The basic components of a typical speech recognition system are shown in Figure 12–2. The speech input, as might be obtained from a microphone, is first digitized (analog to digital conversion; A-to-D conversion, as discussed in Chapter 9) and then analyzed according to certain parameters that vary between systems. The obtained parameters are compared to stored reference patterns. If a suitable match is found, then a positive decision is made and the corresponding text is selected for output.

Statistical properties of spoken language can be very important factors in the design of automatic speech recognition systems. Consider, for example, just two statistical properties of speech: the relative frequency of occurrence of individual speech sounds and the sequential probabilities between sounds. Some sounds that have a high frequency of occurrence are the phonemes /n t s r/. Dewey (1923) reported that these four consonant phonemes accounted for 25% of all phoneme occurrences in his speech samples. In a study by Mines, Hanson, and Shoup (1978), half of all phoneme occurrences were accounted for by just ten phonemes: /ə n t ɪ s r i l d ɛ/. As might be inferred from these phoneme listings, the

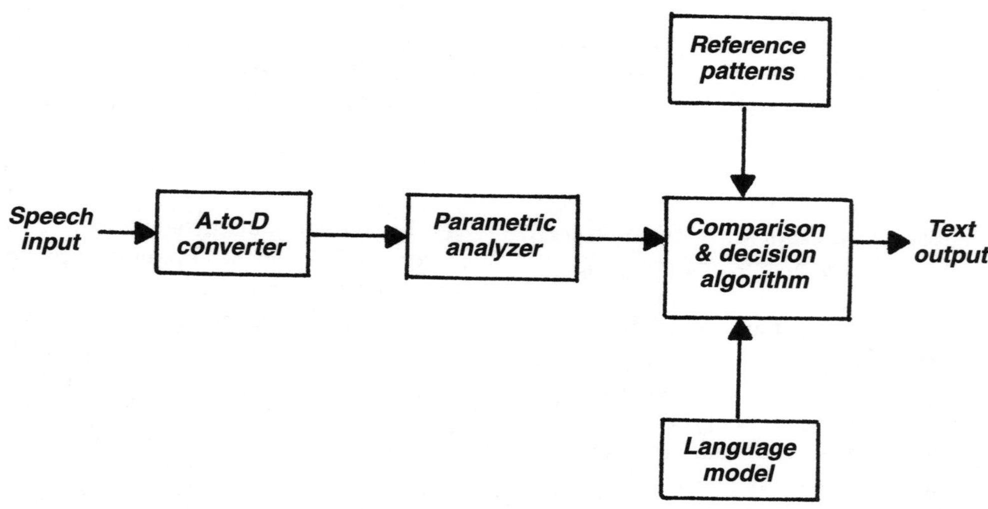

Figure 12–2. Typical speech recognition system.

majority of consonant and vowel occurrences are produced at the front of the mouth. Among consonants, the dental and alveolar places of production account for 80% of consonant occurrences (Mines et al., 1978). Any speaker who has had a painful injury to the tip of the tongue probably can testify to the frequent use of the lingua-dental and lingua-alveolar places of consonant production.

Regarding sequential or transitional statistics, some phoneme sequences are much more likely to occur than others. The most frequently occurring consonant clusters are pairs of sounds that share an alveolar place of articulation but differ in manner. As an example of sequential probabilities, try to guess the phoneme constituents of a CCVC (consonant + consonant + vowel + consonant) word for which three phonemes are provided:

d ___ ɑ p

Note that some consonants can be eliminated from consideration immediately. For example, it is not possible to form an acceptable syllable-initial consonant cluster with the forms /dl/, /dg/, /dm/, and /dt/. By the simple process of elimination, you probably can identify the missing phoneme as /r/ to form the word *drop*.

Similar statistical properties pertain to other levels of language structure, including the frequencies of occurrence of individual words and the probabilities of transitions between words. These properties are powerful constraints on spoken language, and they can be used to good advantage by automatic speech recognition systems.

One of the most important developments in automatic speech recognition was the use of **hidden Markov models** (HHM). Although the discussion of these models goes beyond the scope of this basic text, a few general remarks can be made. A primary point is that these models are probabilistic decision-making procedures. That is, they operate statistically on sequences in speech. They are related to **Markov chains**, which are a number of states with transitions among them. A simple Markov chain might consist of three states represented by the numerals **1**, **2**, and **3**. Each of these states can be associated with a symbol, say **A**, **B**, and **C**, for the simple three-state system. The transitions between states are associated with a probability, for example, a probability $\mathbf{a}_{1,2}$ that represents the probability between states 1 and 2. A transition between any two states yields a symbol output. For example, a transition between states **1** and **2** might be associated with the symbol output **AB**. The Markov chain outputs symbols as transitions are made between states. Hidden Markov models are similar to Markov chains, except the output symbols of hidden Markov models are themselves probabilistic. That is, for any given state, it is assumed that all output symbols are possible, with each having its own probability. What does this have to do with speech recognition? Imagine that the output symbols associated with the HMM are short-term spectra of speech (templates). These templates can be used to identify the sounds in the acoustic signal. The process is probabilistic but it has been the basis for substantial progress in automatic speech recognition.

In summary, automatic speech recognition has been marked by rapid advances. Although current systems do not have the capability to recognize unrestricted vocabularies spoken by a diverse sample of speakers, it appears that the likelihood for improvement is considerable, especially as systems for recognition incorporate refined statistical strategies coupled with linguistic knowledge.

Speech Technology and the Future of Communication

The telephone revolutionized human communication, permitting spoken language to travel over vast distances. On the horizon as this text is written is a world with increasingly powerful systems for communication. One advance is computer telephony integration (CTI). This is any system that uses a computer to enhance or control telephones. Because telephone service is widely available and because computers offer fast and efficient performance, their integration should make it possible to place powerful communication systems in homes, schools, and the workplace. Early versions of CTI systems enabled automated phone conversations, with such options as placing an outbound call, monitoring and logging calls, sending an e-mail message, and retrieving and sending data (e.g., fax-on-demand). But the capabilities of CTI systems can go well beyond that early stage.

Although the telephone may seem ubiquitous, it has not always been available in remote areas. Regions that do not have service from the telephone industry at present may in the future be connected worldwide by satellite communications. With a portable telephone, a caller can use satellite communications to place a call from anywhere in the world to anywhere else in the world. This capability would greatly extend the sphere of spoken language.

> *"By the year 2001, speech synthesis and recognition systems are expected to play important roles in advanced user-friendly human-machine interfaces . . . Services using these systems will include database access and management, various order-made services, dictation and editing, electronic secretarial assistance, robots (e.g., the computer HAL in* **2001—A Space Odyssey**), *automatic interpreting (translating) telephony, security control, and aids for the handicapped (e.g., reading aids for the blind and speaking aids for the vocally handicapped)"*
>
> (S. Furui: Toward the Ultimate Synthesis/Recognition System. In D. B. Roe & J. G. Wilpon (Eds.), *Voice Communication Between Humans and Machines.* Washington, DC: National Academy Press, 1994, p. 450.)

FORENSICS

The word *forensics* has two general meanings, one having to do with courts of justice and the other with public debate or discussion. It is the first meaning that is dealt with here. The field of forensic science pertains to the investigation of criminal evidence, including fingerprints, DNA, serology (blood), firearms, photographs, shoe prints, tire treads, and voiceprints. As noted in Chapter 1, speech is at once public and individual. We can understand speech produced by the competent users of a language, but we also can recognize individual speakers. It is the possibility of speaker identification that contributes to one realm of forensic science. The objective is to identify a subject from his or her speech patterns, especially when recordings have been made of that person's speech. This field of investigation is known generally as speaker identification. As an example of its application, in 1971 the Army Mathematics Research Center at the University of Wisconsin-Madison was bombed, apparently as a protest against the war in Vietnam. The evening that the bomb was ignited, the police station received an anonymous call warning that a bomb was set to go off. A recording was made of the call and it was hoped that it could be used as evidence to prosecute the responsible parties. Recordings of threats, obscene messages, or verbal harrassment are potentially useful to law enforcement agencies in identifying and prosecuting guilty parties.

Speaker identification is accomplished by three major approaches: listening (aural recognition), machine (automatic recognition), and visual examination of spectrograms. The common laboratory method relies on the preparation of spectrograms (or voiceprints), which are used to search for similarities in the acoustic patterns of a suspect's speech and the speech obtained as criminal evidence. For example, if recordings are made of an individual who makes obscene or threatening phone calls, the recordings are then analyzed and compared against the speech patterns of a suspect.

Speaker identification is based on two primary sources of differences among speakers: (1) anatomic differences in the size and shape of the speech organs and (2) subtle differences in how speech sounds are made by different people. The former are called **physiological differences** and the latter **behavioral differences**. Differences between individual speakers are a combination of the physiological and behavioral factors. But speech is affected by a large number of variables, including a person's emotional state, health status, use of intoxicants, loudness and rate of speech, and even the transmission pathway from which a recording is eventually obtained (recall the four types of information reviewed at the beginning of Chapter 1). Moreover, a speaker may intentionally try to disguise his or her voice, and some disguises are quite effective. Speaker identification can be a difficult process, one in which a variety of factors may have to be considered (Bolt et al., 1979; Gruber & Poza, 1995; Kent & Chial, in press; Nolan, 1997; Tosi, 1979). It is doubtful that speaker identification from spectrograms could ever be as accurate as identification of individuals from fingerprints. However, speaker identification may be useful as one form of evidence in identifying criminal suspects.

The major parameters used in speaker identification by acoustic methods can be divided into two major classes, voice source parameters and vocal tract resonance parameters (Kuwabara & Sagisaka, 1995), as discussed below.

Voice Source Parameters

These parameters include: average vocal fundamental frequency, the time-frequency pattern of fundamental frequency (fundamental frequency contour), fluctuations in fundamental frequency, and glottal wave shape. All of these pertain to properties of the laryngeal source, as discussed in Chapters 4 and 9.

Vocal Tract Resonance Parameters

These parameters include: shape of the spectral envelope, absolute values of the formant frequencies, the time-frequency patterns of the formant frequencies (formant tracks), the long-term average spectrum (LTAS), and formant bandwidths. These properties are related to topics covered in Chapter 9.

Summary

Voiceprints are a method of speaker identification in which spectrograms are used to match samples of speech, usually a sample recorded in connection with a criminal activity and a subsequent sample recorded from a suspect. Because the speech signal is influenced by a host of personal, environmental, and transmission variables, voiceprints are not like fingerprints in their potential to identify one individual among thousands or millions. However, voiceprints may be useful in narrowing the number of suspects in a criminal investigation.

SPEECH, LANGUAGE, AND HEARING DISORDERS

Speech is a robust human function. Most children acquire speech quite readily, and although they may have certain immature patterns of articulation during their early years, they are adequately intelligible even to strangers. Speech, once acquired, is a lifelong faculty for most people and is frequently one of the last significant actions on the deathbed (think of the references to "last words," "deathbed confession," "making peace," and "saying the final goodbye"). However, for some children, speech is not easily acquired and may be limited in its communicative success. And for some adults, speech is difficult to produce and may be hard for others to understand. It has been estimated that in the United States, 6% of children in grades 1–12 have a speech disorder of some kind (National Institute of Neurological and Communicative Disorders and Stroke, 1991, 1992, 1993). The same report estimates that 10–15% of preschool children have speech disorders.

The academic discipline that studies speech, language, and hearing disorders is quite young. It is identified by names such as speech pathology and audiology, speech-language pathology and audiology, communicative disorders, communication sciences and disorders, and audiology and speech sciences. The historic academic roots of this discipline can be traced to the University of Wisconsin in 1914. At that time, the School of Public Speaking offered a new program of coursework in an area of study called Speech Correction. In 1920, the department was renamed the Department of Speech. The first doctoral degree in Speech Correction was awarded to Sara Stinchfield in 1922.

Another important foundation was in the third decade of the 20th century. A principal architect of this new field was Carl Emil Seashore, dean of the Graduate College and head of the Department of Psychology at the University of Iowa. Seashore's vision for a new academic field was really an interdisciplinary program. The first doctoral graduate was highly influential in the further development of speech-language pathology and audiology. His identity is revealed in the following excerpt.

> ***"That student was Lee Edward Travis. It is probably essentially true that he was the first individual in the world to be trained by clearly conscious design at the doctoral level for the definite and specific professional objective of working experimentally and clinically with speech and hearing disorders. [After summarizing the major events in Travis's life, the author goes on to explain the basic philosophy underlying the origins of speech-language***
>
> ***(continued)***

> *pathology and audiology. Importantly, the origin is in a laboratory that Travis established at the University of Iowa.] The fact that the program began substantially with the building of a laboratory was aptly symbolic of the fundamental Seashorian thinking that has so deeply affected the work in speech pathology and audiology at Iowa from the beginning. Dean Seashore's point of view . . . was that before a service can be rendered men and women must be properly trained to render it, before they can be properly trained there must be dependable knowledge and methods to be imparted to them, and before there can be dependable knowledge and methods there must be scientific research. In other words, there must be productive laboratories before there can be worthwhile classrooms, and there must be worthwhile classrooms before there can be effective clinics."*
>
> (Wendell Johnson: The Time, the Place, and the Problem. In W. Johnson & R. R. Leuteneggar, *Stuttering in Children and Adults,* University of Minnesota Press, Minneapolis, 1955, p. 7.)

Disorders of speech can be classified according to the major groups:

- voice disorders,
- neurogenic speech disorders,
- structural speech disorders,
- phonological disorders,
- fluency disorders, and
- speech disorders associated with hearing impairment.

These major groups are discussed in the following sections with an eye toward the application of speech science.

Voice Disorders

Chapter 3 discussed the specialized structure of the human vocal folds, which appear to be highly adapted for the kind of adjustments needed for speech and song. Disorders of voice arise from a variety of reasons, including vocal abuse (excessive or unusual use of the larynx), toxins that damage the laryngeal tissue, benign or cancerous growths of the vocal folds or other laryngeal structures, neurological disease that impairs neural regulation of the larynx, trauma (such as physical injury from a blow to the larynx), and perhaps changes associated with aging. Voice disorders are estimated to affect 10% of the population in the United States. According to Pannbacker and Middleton (1994), various studies of the prevalence and incidence of voice disorders in school-aged children report figures in the range of 6.0 to 23.4%.

The larynx is relatively inaccessible to direct observation. It is therefore difficult to ascertain the status of the laryngeal tissues without special procedures. Considerable progress has been made in the development of acoustic and physiologic techniques to assess laryngeal status and function. Techniques that permit visual examination of the vocal folds include videostrobscopy, as discussed in Chapter 4. This technique is highly valuable in the examination of diseased or disordered vocal folds and is a major source of information on laryngeal pathology. Aerodynamic recordings also are used in the clinical examination of the larynx. For example, excessive levels of airflow during phonation may indicate an inefficient phonatory function related to disease. Acoustic techniques also have been of great interest, especially because they are noninvasive and therefore do not pose major risks or discomfort to the subjects being examined.

Although no single technique provides all of the desired information about voice disorders, a combination of two or more techniques can be quite powerful. Perceptual assessment is easily done and therefore is commonly used in conjunction with other methods. A limitation to perceptual assessment alone is that perceptual ratings of voice disorder often lack the desired degree of validity and reliability (Kent, 1996). Stroboscopic and acoustic methods also can be combined in many situations and they are often complementary in the information they provide. Because stroboscopy relies on a kind of averaging process to derive the slow-motion images of vocal fold vibration, it can neglect some cycle-to-cycle information. Acoustic procedures can be quite sensitive to cycle-to-cycle variations and therefore provide information that may be lost in a stroboscopic procedure such as videostroboscopy. A book that provides an extensive discussion of voice disorders is Aronson's (1990) *Clinical Voice Disorders*.

Neurogenic Speech Disorders

These are impairments of speech that result from neurologic disease, damage, or maldevelopment. There are two primary types of neurogenic speech disorder: **dysarthria** and **apraxia of speech**. Dysarthria is a disorder of speech that is associated with slowness, weakness, or incoordination of speech movements. The underlying problem is one that affects virtually all movements of the affected muscles. Therefore, disorders of feeding and swallowing often partner the disorder of speech. The nature of the speech impairment takes different forms with different types of neurologic dysfunction. An experienced speech-language pathologist can distinguish varieties of dysarthria that are associated with different underlying neurologic disorders. An influential classification system based on perceptual judgments of dysarthria was introduced by specialists at the Mayo Clinic in 1969 (Darley, Aronson, & Brown, 1969a, 1969b). Dysarthrias can cause signficant reductions in intelligibility and can also result in severe quality disorders, such as hoarseness or nasality. Among the most severe types of dysarthria are those that affect all three subsystems of speech production, respiratory, laryngeal, and upper airway.

Apraxia of speech (also called verbal dyspraxia or verbal apraxia) is a relatively rare disorder that especially affects the sequencing of movements in speech, even though the muscles do not appear to be weak, slow, or incoordinated (as they do in the dysarthrias). Literally, apraxia means a loss of skill. What seems to be lost in apraxia of speech is the skilled control of sequences of speech sounds. Individuals with apraxia of speech typically have a slow, groping, effortful articulation and tend to produce errors that are judged to be substitutions, deletions, and distortions of phoneme-sized elements. For example, a person with apraxia of speech might say "dornaro" for "tornado." A similar disorder that affects children is known as **developmental apraxia of speech**.

Modern methods for studying speech are providing an improved understanding of neurogenic speech disorders. Acoustic and physiologic studies of dysarthria have been helpful in showing the relative degree of impairment in the respiratory, laryngeal, and upper airway systems. In addition, recent research has begun to demonstrate how specific control problems of different structures, such as the velopharynx, relate to reduced intelligibility or impaired quality.

Acoustic and physiologic studies have helped to shape a new understanding of apraxia of speech. The original understanding of this disorder emphasized the sound substitutions that are judged to occur with high frequency. These errors were interpreted to mean that apraxia of speech is a disorder that affects the selection and sequencing of phonemes. But acoustic and physiologic investigations revealed a variety of sequencing problems, including subtle errors in the control of individual movements. It appears, then, that apraxia of speech affects several aspects of speech production and is not an isolated problem at the level of phonemic organization.

A recent comprehensive account of neurogenic speech disorders is Duffy's *Motor Speech Disorders* (1995). It is recommended to the reader who wants detailed information on the neurogenic disorders of speech.

Structural Speech Disorders

These disorders are associated with abnormalities of the physical structures of speech. They include a variety of problems of an altered or abnormal anatomy. The general term **anomaly** covers these various conditions. Congenital disorders are those in which the anomaly is present at birth. Another term for anomaly is **dysmorphology** (the prefix *dys-* means poor and *morphology* means shape). A congenital craniofacial dysmorphology that can severely affect speech development is **cleft palate**, which results from an imcomplete fusion of the hard or soft palate in the embryonic stages of development. A brief review of the relevant embryology is given in Chapter 14. Cleft palate may be accompanied by cleft lip, or either condition may occur separately. Sometimes only the uvula is affected, resulting in a **bifid uvula**. This condition is important clinically because some individuals with a bifid uvula have a submucosal cleft of the palate. Figure 12–3 shows schematic drawings of a bifid uvula, cleft of the lip, and cleft of the palate. Clefting of the lip and/or palate occurs in approximately 1 of every 750 live births in the United States (McWilliams, Morris, & Shelton, 1990). The risk increases as the age of the mother increases. Cleft palate causes difficulties in both feeding and speech. Sur-

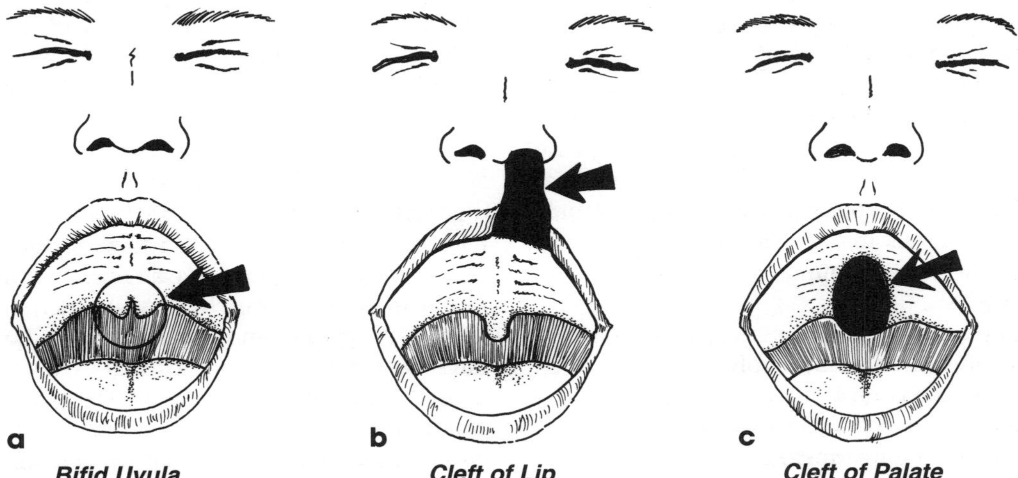

Figure 12–3. Patterns of clefting of lip and palate. Area of cleft is outlined with thick line. Examples: **a** = cleft of uvula (bifid uvula), **b** = cleft of lip only, and **c** = cleft of palate only. In **b** and **c**, the cleft region is indicated by darkened areas.

gical repair early in the child's life often can correct major features of the problem, especially as they affect oral functions for feeding and speaking.

Structural disorders also can occur as the consequence of trauma (physical injury), as in the case of automobile accidents. Some structural disorders are the outcome of surgical procedures, such as resection of the tongue in individuals with lingual cancer. The compensatory abilities of many people with these disorders is testimony to the robustness of speech. One man who lost virtually all of his tongue, part of his jaw, and all of his teeth was nonetheless capable of fairly intelligible conversational speech. His successful compensation is evidence of the remarkable power of reorganization of the motor processes of speech. To be sure, there are limitations to compensation, which is why reconstructive surgery and prosthetic management may be necessary to restore speech in persons with structural disorders. Reconstructive surgery attempts to repair significant anomalies (to close openings, to bring structures into proper relationship, or to give structures a suitable shape or size). Prosthetic management involves the use of artificial implants or other assistive devices. For example, a **palatal lift** is a device that supports the soft palate in a semi-elevated position, so that velopharyngeal closure is facilitated. Tongue prostheses have been designed for individuals who have lost a significant part of the tongue. Although the prosthesis does not possess the normal muscular properties of the tongue, it provides a bulk that enables the production of certain speech sounds.

The assessment and management of structural disorders can involve a variety of issues. The complexity is exemplified in the congenital condition of cleft lip and cleft palate. The treatment of children with this disorder typically requires a team approach, in which a number of specialists from different fields coordinate their talents to help the child. Among the specialists that may be represented on a cleft palate team are speech-language pathologists, oral or plastic surgeons, otolaryngologists, dentists, prosthodontists, and psychologists. The scope of the treatment process as it relates to communication is reviewed in several valuable texts, including *Communicative Disorders Related to Cleft Lip and Palate* (Bzoch, 1989) and *Cleft Palate Speech* (McWilliams et al., 1990).

Phonological Disorders

Phonological disorders in children are rather common and typically constitute a major part of the caseload of a speech-language clinician working in the schools. A developmental phonological disorder may be defined as a phonological system that develops more slowly than is typical or develops in atypical ways. This disorder typically is recognized by the presence of speech sound errors for which no immediate structural or neurological origin can be determined. Phonology is the part of language that is concerned with speech sounds and the assembly of these sounds into words. Children with phonological disorders have difficulties with this part of language. Although the great majority of developmental phonological disorders have an unknown cause, progress has been made in identifying possible subtypes of children who are phonologically disordered or speech-delayed, including some who have a genetic predisposition, others who have had a significant medical history of otitis media, some who may have a neurological impairment resulting in developmental apraxia of speech, and, finally, some who have developmental psychosocial involvements (Shriberg, 1982, 1994, 1997). Many children will outgrow the disorder, but others continue to be hampered by it, and still others may suffer from related, long-term disabilities, such as a reading problem. The relation between phonological disorders in children and reading disabilities later in life are considered in a later section.

The study of phonological disorders has long been the province of the ear. Clinicians use their auditory skills to identify speech sound errors and to discern progress in the correction of these errors. However, acoustic methods are increasingly used, especially in the laboratory setting, but also to a limited degree in the clinical setting. One of the attractions of acoustic analysis is that it can demonstrate acoustical differences in sound patterns that are not always perceptible even by experienced clinicians (Weismer, Dinnsen, & Elbert, 1981). In their book on articulation and phonological disorders, Bernthal and Bankson (1993, p. 241) state, "While acoustic analysis is primarily a research tool to supplement perceptual analysis, the time is fast approaching when clinicians will have inexpensive technology available for doing selected acoustic measurements."

Fluency Disorders

Stuttering, or fluency disorder, can arise at any age, but the great majority of individuals with the developmental form of stuttering are identified in the preschool years. Stuttering often is diagnosed when children are in a highly active phase of speech and language development. Research indicates that 75% of the risk for stuttering occurs by the age of 3½ years (Yairi & Ambrose, 1992a, 1992b). The prevalence of stuttering has been estimated to be about 1% of school-aged children worldwide (Peters & Guitar, 1991). Stuttering takes several forms, primarily part-word or whole-word repetitions, pauses, and sound prolongations. Some of the symptoms are less obvious. For example, a stutterer may circumlocute, meaning the substitution of words on which fluency is likely for words on which fluency is less likely. Many stutterers can predict the words on which they will stutter, so circumlocution is one means of dealing with expected dysfluency. Stuttering symptoms have been shown to interact with a variety of motor, linguistic, psychological, and sociological factors. Some conditions may be called fluency-inducing, because they seem to facilitate fluent speech. Other factors are dysfluency-inducing, because they have the opposite effect. Some fluency-inducing conditions are: reading material that has already been read several times (an example of **adaptation**), speaking to a pet, and choral speaking. Some dysfluency-inducing conditions are: reading an unfamiliar and complicated text, speaking before a large audience, and addressing an unfriendly audience.

Although most stuttering occurs in children and has an onset before the age of 4 years, stuttering also can appear in adults, often in association with neurological disorders (Rosenbek, Messert, Collins, & Wertz, 1978; Ringo & Dietrich, 1995). Stuttering associated with neurological disorders has been termed **neurogenic stuttering**. Ringo and Dietrich (1995) concluded that the acquired, or neurogenic, form of stuttering differs from the more typical developmental form of stuttering in several ways:

1. Neurogenic stutterers tend to stutter on grammatical words (e.g., prepositions and conjunctions) as well as substantive words (e.g., nouns and verbs). Developmental stuttering is associated with a greater likelihood of dysfluency on substantive words.
2. Neurogenic stutterers do not exhibit anxiety about their stuttering, which is quite unlike the usual circumstance in developmental stuttering.
3. In neurogenic stuttering, dysfluencies are not limited to initial syllables, as is often the case in developmental stuttering.
4. Secondary symptomatology is relatively infrequent in neurogenic stuttering but common in developmental stuttering.

5. Adaptation effects are not as pronounced in neurogenic as in developmental stuttering.

The cause of stuttering is controversial, and a number of theories of its etiology have been advanced. Possibly, subtypes of stuttering should be recognized, taking into account factors such as a family history of stuttering (which may indicate a genetic component) and head injury (which may indicate a neurologic abnormality). Motor issues have been emphasized in one major strand of contemporary research. Accordingly, there has been increased interest in acoustic and physiologic investigations of this disorder. These new data sources are particularly important for answering questions such as:

1. Is there a primary laryngeal focus to stuttering? Some authorities believe that reflex mechanisms in the larynx are a major feature in stuttering and therefore direct therapeutic efforts to facilitate an easy onset of phonation.
2. Are moments of stuttering associated with incoordinations of speech movements as a causal or precipitating factor?
3. Is stuttering correlated with unusual patterns of hemispheric activation? An idea that can be traced back to the 1930s is that stutterers have an anomalous hemispheric control of speech production. Recent brain imaging studies are adding valuable new information to this possibility, but it is difficult to determine if anomalous hemispheric activation is the *cause* of stuttering or an *effect* of experiences with stuttering.
4. Is it possible to distinguish children who will spontaneously recover from stuttering from those who will not?

Because acoustic and physiologic techniques have been used mainly in the study of adult speech, their application to children's speech often requires innovation and adaptation. Much has been accomplished in this regard, and these efforts have cleared the way for new research directions.

A number of other disorders of fluency are recognized by clinicians. One of these, **palilalia**, is the compulsive repetition of linguistic elements, typically words or phrases. Unlike stuttering, in which the utterance-initial position is most vulnerable to dysfluency, palilalia usually involves reiterations at the middle and end of utterances. The following is a response from a subject with palilalia who was asked to repeat the sentence, *The barn swallow captured a plump worm*:

> The barn swallow, the barn swallows, swallows, swallows, captured, captured, barn swallows, swallows captured a plump, captured a plump, captured a plump, a plump, a plump, a plump worm, worm, worm, worm, worm.

Speech Disorders Associated with Hearing Impairment

We learn speech by hearing the spoken language of others and by hearing our own attempts at speech. The importance of auditory information in learning speech is profound. Most individuals born deaf never acquire spoken language as a reliable and successful means of communication. Studies have shown that normal-hearing individuals can understand only about 20% of speech produced by children with profound hearing impairment (Smith, 1975). This is not to say that individuals who are deaf cannot acquire intelligible speech, for some do. But the great majority do not. Absence or distortion of the auditory speech signal presents a serious obstacle to the learning of spoken language. Auditory patterns are the primary source of information by which children learn spoken language. Audition continues to be important as a feedback channel. Acquired deafness in adults can result in impaired speech articulation, especially for fricative consonants.

The speech difficulties often associated with severe hearing loss have been studied by acoustic and physiologic methods. Acoustic studies have shown that vowel formant regions for different vowels produced by deaf speakers are: (a) more centralized than in the speech of talkers with hearing, (b) may overlap considerably so that acoustic contrasts among vowels are reduced, and (c) tend to be more variable than in the speech of talkers with hearing (Angelocci, Kopp, & Holbrook, 1964; Osberger, Levitt, & Slosberg, 1979). The effects of hearing impairment on vowel production may emerge even in the babbling vocalizations during the first year of life (Kent, Netsell, Osberger, & Hustedde, 1987; see the exercises in Chapter 9).

One of the applications of speech science in aiding persons with auditory impairment is the design of improved hearing aids. New designs include digital hearing aids that offer highly selective amplification and control over various aspects of sound quality (e.g., feedback reduction and automatic gain control). In addition, progress has been made in developing a system that permits the user to convert the rate of a speech signal in real time (Miyasaki, Nakamura, Seiyama, Imai, & Takagi, 1996). For listeners who have difficulty in processing speech when presented at its normal rate, this technology enables an adjustment of speech rate to slower values. The portable system slows the rate of speech by prolonging the durations of steady state segments such as pauses and vowels. The hearing aid of the future may be a combination of these various types of signal processing.

Specific Language Impairment

Strictly speaking, **specific language impairment** is not a speech disorder, but rather a language disorder. That is, it is commonly assumed that the essense of the disorder is an impairment of language processes, perhaps involving semantics, syntax, or some other component of language. However, some studies indicate that aspects of speech may relate to specific language impairment. One example of recent evidence is work showing that children with specific language impairment have a temporal processing deficit, and perhaps even more specifically, an auditory temporal processing deficit. This idea was given new force by studies showing that children with specific language impairment benefitted from training on acoustically altered speech stimuli (Merzenich et al., 1996; Tallal et al., 1996). The stimuli were first lengthened and then the transitional elements were amplified. The effect of these changes was to increase the salience of the dynamic aspects of speech related primarily to consonants. The outcome of the training was improved performance in both speech discrimination and language comprehension.

These experiments could mean that at least some children with specific language impairment have an underlying difficulty with the perception of speech. Further research with additional control conditions is needed to test this idea, but it is an interesting example of the potentially intimate connections between speech and language.

DIALECT AND NON-NATIVE LANGUAGES

For most people, learning a non-native language (abbreviated L2 for second language) is a challenging task. One has to learn the vocabulary, grammar, phonology, and phonetic characteristics of the new language. Although each of these can be difficult to master, it is the sound patterns of the new language that present some of the most persistent difficulties. With sufficient study and practice, many adults can do quite well in learning a new vocabulary and a new grammar. But the great majority will never speak the new language without a telltale accent, a kind of phonetic imprint of the first-learned language. When someone is described as having a "foreign accent," it is usually the sound pattern that is the basis for the identification of accent. Many adults who attempt to learn a new language will have a lifelong foreign accent in that language, no matter how long they speak it, even if it becomes their most frequently used language.

Interestingly, the likelihood of acquiring an accent-free L2 increases if the L2 is learned early in childhood. Age of learning appears to be one of the best predictors (and perhaps the single best predictor) of whether a person will learn the L2 without an L1 accent. A practical implication of this finding is that L2 instruction should commence during childhood if the objective is to learn a nativelike production of the L2. A theoretical implication is that the processes of phonologic or phonetic learning undergo an essential change between early childhood and puberty. Flexibility in L2 learning seems to diminish considerably during this period, and the reduced flexibility may reflect change in the neural representation of language.

Where does the difficulty in learning L2 sound patterns arise? Although the difficulty may be based on both perceptual and productive limitations, much of the current research focuses on perceptual limitations. The speech learning model (SLM), proposed by Flege (1997, in press) states that experience with sounds in the L1 generates a perceptual grid through which sounds in the L2 are discriminated. That is, the L1 sounds create a set of phonetic-perceptual biases that are strongly resistant to change. A similar perspective on the difficulty of learning L2 sounds was taken by Best (1993, 1994).

The perceptual-limitation hypothesis is used to explain why some L2 sounds are more easily learned than others. Among the L2 sounds that are most difficult to learn are those that occur in the close acoustic neighborhood of L1 sounds. Figure 12–4 shows an hypothetical example of vowel sounds in L1 (represented by the uppercase symbols A, B, C, and D) and vowel sounds in L2 (represented by the lowercase symbols a, b, c, and d). It is expected from the SLM theory that the L2 vowel "a" would be difficult to discriminate because it is near (hence similar but not identical to) the L1 vowel "A." However, L2 vowels that do not occur proximal to L1 vowels should be relatively easy to discriminate. For example, discrimination and learning are expected to be fairly easy for the L2 vowel "b" because it lies in a region of the acoustic-perceptual space that is not occupied by a vowel from L1.

The examples discussed pertain to vowels, but the SLM theory makes similar predictions for consonants. For instance, it would be predicted that L1 and L2 consonants that have similar VOT values would be more difficult to discriminate than L1 and L2 consonants that have dissimilar VOT values.

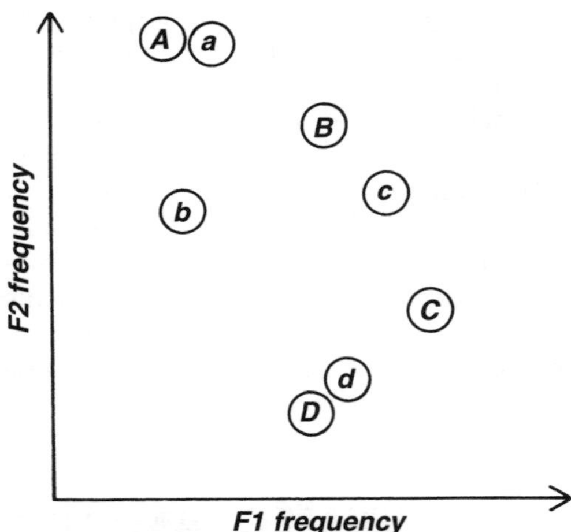

Figure 12–4. Vowel formant (F1–F2) plot showing a hypothetical example of vowel sounds in L1 (represented by the uppercase symbols A, B, C, and D) and vowel sounds in L2 (represented by the lowercase symbols a, b, c, and d). See text for discussion.

DYSLEXIA

Dyslexia is a reading disability. What does reading have to do with speech? According to some dyslexia specialists, there may be a very strong relationship, at least in certain types of dyslexia. Actually, the definition of dyslexia is somewhat complicated and there is some disagreement among authorities (Stanovich, 1994). But the basic idea is that dyslexia is a reading disability that cannot be explained by low intelligence, obvious sensory deficit (such as a visual impairment), or lack of educational opportunities. That is, the deficit in reading seems to stem from a problem with some skill or cognitive process that is specific and essential to reading. The prevalence of dyslexia is approximately 5%, with roughly four times as many boys as girls being diagosed with the condition (Badian, 1984; Jorm, Share, McLean, & Matthews, 1986). (It is interesting to compare this percentage with the sex ratios for speech and language disorders reviewed in Chapter 1.)

The primary point of this discussion is to introduce the possibility that at least some dyslexias may be rooted in a prior phonological disorder. Some authorities on dyslexia have concluded that phonological awareness (awareness of the segmental structure of language) is a prerequisite to the rapid acquisition of reading skill. In fact, one of the most distinctive indicators of the phonological difficulties that many people with dyslexia have is a problem in naming **pseudowords** (wordlike forms that do not actually occur in the language) (Rack, Snowling, & Olson, 1992). Many people with dyslexia experience considerable difficulty reading words like *phex, noufle,* and *shawnger*. For this reason, dyslexia relates to general issues in the acquisition of speech and language. Possibly, some factors that contribute to dyslexia come about well before a child seriously takes on the task of learning to read. One major theory of dyslexia is that the disorder results from deficits in phonological processing (Siegel, 1993; Stanovich, 1993). This theory proposes a very strong link between learning to read and early experiences with phonological development.

Dyslexia is surrounded by several controversies, one of which holds particular relevance to issues in this book. Some scientists have proposed a connection between dyslexia and deficits in auditory temporal perception (Farmer & Klein, 1995; Tallal, 1980, Tallal, Miller, & Fitch, 1993). The basic idea is that speech perception requires rapid auditory temporal processing. A disability in this ability can lead to phonological impairments, as are observed in some individuals with dyslexia. However, the evidence for the association between impaired auditory temporal processing and dyslexia is not conclusive (Studdert-Kennedy & Mody, 1995).

SPEECH AND PSYCHIATRY

A number of psychiatric disorders can be accompanied by, or characterized by, unusual patterns of spoken language or by a distinctive voice quality. Some disorders for which speech has been studied include: schizophrenia, depression, infantile autism, and manic disorder. The literature on this subject is decidedly complicated, and no attempt at a summary will be made here. Readers who want to delve into this topic may find Darby (1981) a good starting point.

SPEECH IN ART AND CULTURE

> **Socrates:** *Rhetoric is like medicine.*
>
> **Phaedrus:** *How so?*
>
> **Socrates:** *Why, because medicine has to define the nature of the body and rhetoric of the soul—if we would proceed, not empirically but scientifically, in the one case to impart health and strength by giving medicine and food, in the other to implant the conviction or virtue which you desire, by the right application of words and training.*
>
> —Plato, in *Phaedrus*

This book emphasizes the speech *sciences*, but it should be mentioned at least briefly that speech can be entertaining, informative, and enlightening. Speech can be a form of art, as in the case of the polished monologue. Speech is, along with music, the sound of a culture. The power of speech is illustrated by the phenomenon of the guest speaker: organizations, agencies, clubs, and assemblies of all kinds invite speakers to address them. There is a general desire to hear the voice of the famous, the powerful, the attractive, and even the despised. Cultures everywhere celebrate the spoken word. The technologies of communication have made it possible for one individual to speak at one instant to an audience of millions. Rhetoric is an ancient skill, but one that is constantly renewed by our need to nurture the human soul. The science and technologies of speech can enhance the artistic and cultural aspects of speech. For example, acoustic analyses can be applied to famous speeches to document the modulations of voice that stirred the listeners. Or, modern methods of digital speech processing can be used to create digital recordings of messages for long-term storage and easy retrieval of a high-fidelity signal.

The methods of speech science can be used to study some of the problems in sociolinguistics, or social patterns in language usage. As one example, acoustic analysis has been applied to study speech patterns in bilingual individuals. Labov (1986) reported from one such analysis that a second-generation Puerto Rican woman living in Philadelphia had three norms for vowel production: a target influenced by Spanish, a target typical of speakers living in Philadelphia, and a target described as "overcorrected" and maximally opposed to the Spanish target. Acoustic studies offer a quantification and sensitivity that may be difficult to accomplish with perceptual analyses of speech.

CONCLUSION

This chapter is a brief sampling of major areas of applied speech science. Perhaps the major thing to be said is that speech science has manifold applications made possible by research into the basic processes of speech production and perception. With the rapid growth and refinement of speech technologies such as speech coding, speech synthesis, and automatic speech recognition, it is likely that these technologies will soon affect the day-to-day life of nearly all citizens in modern societies. Speech science also finds applications in forensics and language learning. Finally, applied speech science has been a fundamental tool for the investigation of communication disorders and for the development of assessment and treatment procedures.

On The Reference Shelf

Recommended to readers who seek deeper or extended discussions. Most of these references are not directly cited in this chapter, but they are highly useful source materials.

Edwards, A. D. N. (1991). *Speech synthesis: Technology for disabled people*. London: Paul Chapman Publishing, Ltd.

A good introduction to the ways in which synthetic speech can be used by people with disabilities.

Flanagan, J. L. (1972). Voices of men and machines. *Journal of the Acoustical Society of America, 51,* 1375–1387.

An interesting review of accomplishments in synthetic speech.

Minifie, F. D (1994). *Introduction to communication sciences and disorders*. San Diego: Singular Publishing Group.

This broad-based introduction to the field of communication disorders includes 16 chapters contributed by well-known scholars and scientists.

Poulos, M. G., & Webster, W. G., (1991). Family history as a basis for subgrouping people who stutter. *Journal of Speech and Hearing Research, 34,* 5–10.

This paper is a good example of the search for factors that might relate to a communication disorder.

Rabiner, L. R. (1995). The impact of voice processing on modern telecommunications. *Speech Communication, 17,* 217–226.

A brief, highly informative account of how speech technologies are changing telecommunication.

Roe, D. B., & Wilpon, G. (Eds.). (1994). *Voice communication between humans and machines.* Washington, DC: National Academy Press.

This compendium is suited for the reader who seeks a broad but fairly deep discussion of the various uses of human-machine voice communication.

Syrdal, A., Bennett, R., & Greenspan, S. (1995). *Applied speech technology*. Boca Raton, FL: CRC Press.

This book explores several facets of speech communication technology. It is highly recommended to the reader who wants a broad sweep of this rapidly expanding field.

Chapter References

Angelocci, A. A., Kopp, G. A., & Holbrook, A. (1964). The vowel formants of deaf and normal-hearing eleven- to fourteen-year-old boys. *Journal of Speech and Hearing Disorders, 29*, 156–170.

Aronson, A. E. (1990). *Clinical voice disorders* (3rd ed.). New York: Thieme, Inc.

Badian, N. A. (1984). Reading disability in an epidemiological context: Incidence and environmental correlates. *Journal of Learning Disabilities, 17*, 129–136.

Bernthal, J. E., & Bankson, N. W. (1993). *Articulation and phonological disorders* (3rd ed). Englewood Cliffs, NJ: Prentice-Hall.

Best, C. T. (1993). Emergence of language-specific constraints in perception of non-native speech: A window on early phonological development. In B. De Boysson-Bardies, S. de Schonen, P. Jusczyk, P. MacNeilage, & J. Morton (Eds.), *Developmental neurocognition: Speech and face processing in the first year of life* (pp. 289–304). Dordrecht, The Netherlands: Kluwer Academic Publishers.

Best, C. T. (1994). The emergence of native-language phonological influences in infants: A perceptual assimilation model. In J. C. Goodman & H. C. Nusbaum (Eds.), *The development of speech perception: The transition from speech sounds to spoken words*. Cambridge, MA: MIT Press.

Bolt, R. H., Cooper, F. S., Green, D. M., Hamlet, S. L., Hogan, D. L., McKnight, J. G., Pickett, J. M., Tosi, O., & Underwood, B. D. (1979). *On the theory and practice of voice identification*. Washington, DC: National Academy of Sciences.

Bzoch, K. R. (1989). (Ed.). *Communicative disorders related to cleft lip and palate* (3rd ed.). Boston: Little, Brown.

Darby, J. K. (1981). *Speech evaluation in psychiatry*. New York: Grune & Stratton.

Darley, F. L., Aronson, A. E., & Brown, J. R. (1969a). Cluster of deviant speech dimensions in the dysarthrias. *Journal of Speech and Hearing Research, 12*, 462–496.

Darley, F. L., Aronson, A. E., & Brown, J. R. (1969b). Differential diagnostic patterns of dysarthria. *Journal of Speech and Hearing Research, 12*, 249–269.

Dewey, G. (1923). *Relative frequency of English speech sounds*. Cambridge, MA: Harvard University Press.

Duffy, J. R. (1995). *Motor speech disorders: Substrates, differential diagnosis, and management*. St. Louis: Mosby.

Farmer, M. E., & Klein, R. M. (1995). The evidence for a temporal processing deficit linked to dyslexia: A review. *Psychonomic Bulletin & Review, 2*, 460–493.

Flege, J. E. (1987). The production of "new" and "similar" phones in a foreign language: Evidence for the effect of equivalence classification. *Journal of Phonetics, 15*, 47–65.

Flege, J. E. (in press). Second-language learning: Theory, findings, and problems. In W. Strange (Ed.), *Speech perception and linguistic experience: Theoretical and methodological issues*. Timonium, MD: York Press.

Greene, B. G., Logan, J. S., & Pisoni, D. B. (1986). Perception of synthetic speech produced automatically by rule: Intelligibility of eight text-to-speech systems. *Behavior Research Methods, Instruments, and Computers, 18*, 100–107.

Gruber, J. S., & Poza, F. (1995). Voicegram identification evidence. *American Jurisprudence Trials, 1*.

Hoover, J., Reichle, J., Van Tassell, D., & Cole, D. (1987). The intelligibility of synthetic speech: Echo II vs. Votrax. *Journal of Speech and Hearing Research, 30*, 425–431.

Jorm, A. F., Share, D. L., McLean, R., & Matthews, D. (1986). Cognitive factors at school entry predictive of specific reading retardation and general reading backwardness: A research note. *Journal of Child Psychology and Psychiatry and Allied Disciplines, 27*, 45–54.

Kent, R. D. (1996). Hearing and believing: Some limits to the auditory-perceptual assessment of speech and voice disorders. *American Journal of Speech-Language Pathology, 7*, 7–23.

Kent, R. D., & Chial, M. R. (in press). Voice spectrography ("Voiceprints"). In D. L. Faigman, D. Kaye, M. J. Saks, & J. Sanders (Eds.), *Scientific evidence reference manual*. St.Paul, MN: West Publishing Co.

Kent, R. D., Netsell, R., Osberger, M. J., & Hustedde, C. G. (1987). Phonetic development in twins who differ in auditory function. *Journal of Speech and Hearing Disorders, 52*, 64–75.

Kuwabara, H., & Sagisaka, Y. (1995). Acoustic characteristics of speaker individuality: Control and conversion. *Speech Communication, 16*, 165–173.

Labov, W. (1986). Sources of variability inherent in the speech process. In J. S. Perkell & D. H. Klatt (Eds.), *Invariance and variability in speech processes* (pp. 402–425). Hillsdale, NJ: Erlbaum.

McWilliams, B. J., Morris, H. L., & Shelton, R. L. (1990). *Cleft palate speech* (2nd ed.). Philadelphia: B. C. Decker.

Merzenich, M. M., Jenkins, W. M., Johnston, P., Schreiner, C., Miller, S. L., & Tallal, P. (1996). Temporal processing deficits of language-impaired children ameliorated by training. *Science, 271*, 77–81.

Mines, M., Hanson, B., & Shoup, J. (1978). Frequency of occurrence of phonemes in conversational English. *Language and Speech, 21*, 221–241.

Mirenda, P., & Beukelman, D. R. (1987). A comparison of speech synthesis intelligibility with listeners from three age groups. *Augmentative and Alternative Communication, 3*, 120–128.

Mirenda, P., & Beukelman, D. R. (1990). A comparison of intelligibility among natural speech and seven speech synthesizers with listeners from three age groups. *Augmentative and Alternative Communication, 6*, 61–68.

Mitchell, P. R., & Adkins, C. P. (1988 or 1989). A comparison of single word intelligibility of two voice output communication aids. *Augmentative and Alternative Communication, 5*, 84–88.

Miyasaki, E., Nakamura, A., Seiyama, N., Imai, A., & Takagi, T. (1996). A new technology to compensate degeneration of hearing intelligibility for elderly listeners: Development of a portable real-time speech rate conversion system [Abstract]. *Journal of the Acoustical Society of America, 100*, 2740.

National Institute on Deafness and Other Communication Disorders. (1991, 1992, 1993). *National Strategic Research Plan*. (NIH Publication No. 95–3711.). Washington, DC: U.S. Department of Health and Human Services, Public Health Service, National Institutes of Health.

Nolan. F. (1997). Speaker recognition and forensic phonetics. In W. J. Hardcastle & J. Laver (Eds.), *The handbook of phonetic sciences* (pp. 744–767). Cambridge, MA: Blackwell.

Osberger, M. J., Levitt, H., & Slosberg, R. (1979). Acoustic characteristics of correctly produced vowels. [Abstract.] *Journal of the Acoustical Society of America, 66*, 13.

Pannbacker, M. H., & Middleton, G. F. (1994). Voice disorders. In S. Adler & D. A. King (Eds.), *Oral communication problems in children and adolescents* (pp. 103–140). Boston: Allyn & Bacon.

Peters, T. J., & Guitar, B. (1991). *Stuttering: An integrated approach to its nature and treatment*. Baltimore: Williams & Wilkins.

Rack, J. P., Snowling, M. J., & Olson, R. K. (1992). The nonword reading deficit in developmental dyslexia: A review. *Reading Research Quarterly, 27*, 28–53.

Ringo, C. C., & Dietrich, S. (1995). Neurogenic stuttering: An analysis and critique. *Journal of Medical Speech-Language Pathology, 2*, 111–122.

Rosenbek, J., Messert, B., Collins, M., & Wertz, R. (1978). Stuttering following brain damage. *Brain and Language, 6*, 82–96.

Shriberg, L. D. (1982). Toward classification of developmental phonological disorders. In N. J. Lass (Ed.), *Speech and language: Advances in basic research and practice* (Vol. 8; pp. 2–18). New York: Academic Press.

Shriberg, L. D. (1994). Five subtypes of developmental phonological disorders. *Clinics in Communication Disorders, 4*, 38–53.

Shriberg, L. D. (1997). Developmental phonological disorder(s): One or many? In B. W. Hodson & M. L. Edwards (Eds.), *Perspectives in applied phonology* (pp. 105–127). Gaithersburg, MD: Aspen Press.

Siegel, L. S. (1993). Phonological processing deficits as the basis of a reading disability. *Developmental Review, 13*, 246–257.

Smith, C. R. (1975). Residual hearing and speech production in deaf children. *Journal of Speech and Hearing Research, 18*, 795–811.

Stanovich, K. E. (1993). A model for studies of reading disabilities. *Developmental Review, 13*, 225–245.

Stanovich, K. E. (1994). Annotation: Does dyslexia exist? *Journal of Child Psychology, 35*, 579–595.

Studdert-Kennedy, M., & Mody, M. (1995). Auditory temporal perception deficits in the reading–impaired: A critical review of the evidence. *Psychonomic Bulletin and Review, 2*, 508–514.

Tallal, P. (1980). Auditory temporal perception, phonics and reading disabilities in children. *Brain and Language, 9*, 182–198.

Tallal, P., Miller, S. L., Bedi, G., Byma, G., Wang, X., Nagarajan, S. S., Schreiner, C., Jenkins, W. M., & Merzenich, M. M. (1996). Language comprehension in language-learning impaired children improved with acoustically modified speech. *Science, 271,* 81–84.

Tallal, P., Miller, S., & Fitch, R. H. (1993). Neurobiological basis of speech: The case for the preeminence of temporal processing. In P. Tallal, A. M. Galaburda, R. R. Llinas, & C. von Euler (Eds.), *Temporal information processing in the nervous system* (Annals of the New York Academy of Sciences, Vol. 82, pp. 27–47). New York: New York Academy of Sciences.

Tosi, O. (1979). *Voice identification: Theory and legal applications.* Baltimore: University Park Press.

Weismer, G., Dinnsen, D., & Elbert, M. (1981). A study of the voicing distinction associated with omitted, word-final stops. *Journal of Speech and Hearing Disorders, 46,* 320–327.

Yairi, E., & Ambrose, N. A. (1992a). A longitudinal study of stuttering in children: A preliminary report. *Journal of Speech and Hearing Research, 35,* 755–760.

Yairi, E., & Ambrose, N. A. (1992b). Onset of stuttering in preschool children: Selected factors. *Journal of Speech and Hearing Research, 35,* 782–788.

Exercises

12-1. Examine Figure 12–1 and explain how the components of this model relate to the source-filter theory of speech production introduced in Chapter 9.

12-2. Examine Figure 12–2 and explain how the components of this model compare with the models of human speech perception discussed in Chapter 10.

12-3. This is an exercise in imagination. Try to think of various ways in which the integration of telephony and computers could be used to advantage for both personal and business use.

12-4. Synthesized speech can be evaluated in several ways. One way emphasized in this chapter is its intelligibility. Recalling the sources of information in speech introduced in Chapter 1, explain how the following three sources might be applied to the evaluation of synthesized speech: phonetic quality, affective quality, and personal quality.

12-5. Discuss how the methods of speech science can be applied to the study of disorders of speech, voice, and language. Cite at least three specific examples of these disorders.

CHAPTER 13

The Evolution of Speech

> ***"Biochemical analysis reveals that humans and chimpanzees share more than 99% of their genetic material, and are more closely related to each other than, say, the horse and the zebra. If these close relatives did not invent language on their own, perhaps they could learn one of ours. Yet all early attempts to teach the chimpanzee to speak were completely unsuccessful."***
>
> (W. S.-Y. Wang, *Human communication: Language and its psychobiological bases.* San Francisco: W.H. Freeman and Co., 1982, p. 3.)

Humans, or the species *homo sapiens* ("man the wise"), have been on earth since 100,000 years ago, or perhaps 500,000 years ago, or perhaps even before that. Authorities differ on which number is correct, primarily because of a disagreement on whether modern humans should be defined to include only anatomically modern people (which gives rise to the figure of 100,000 years), or should be expanded to include more primitive species such as the Neanderthals (in which case the age of our species is on the order of a half a million years and maybe older). Figure 13–1 shows a diagrammatric representation of the evolution of the primates. The primates are divided into two major groups, the *prosimians* (lower primates) and the *anthropoids* (higher primates). The prosimians predate the anthropoids by about 35 million years. A present-day representative of the prosimian is the lemur. The anthropoids are represented today by the New World and Old World monkeys, the apes, and humans.

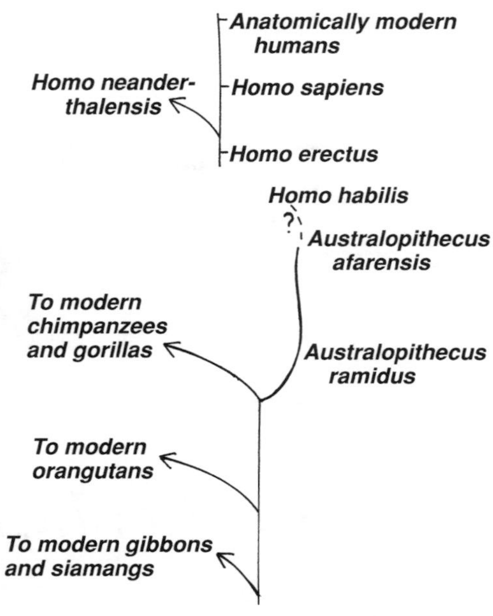

Figure 13–1. Diagram of the evolution of the primates.

> ***"The clearest differences between the pongid [e.g., orangutan] and hominid [chimps, gorillas, and humans] lineages lie in anatomical features that reflect intelligence, the existence of language, tool use, diet and masticatory habits, and locomotion."***
>
> (Shipman, P., Climbing the family tree: What makes a hominid a hominid? *The Journal of NIH Research*, 1995, *7*, 50–55.)

Evolutionary landmarks that distinguish the hominids from other species and humans from other hominids are largely fossil remains that testify to a large brain, employment of language, use of tools, a small snout, and bipedal locomotion. Among the distinguishing anatomic features of humans are large brains (and therefore a large cranium to enclose the large mass of neural matter, especially the interneurons), a small snout (not so effective as a large snout for chewing hard materials but more suited to accommodate a vocal tract with a large phonetic repertoire), a shortened, widened pelvis (adapted to walking on two legs), and hands designed to afford a precision grasp.

These features form a backdrop for an inquiry into language origins. This is a deep and difficult question, but one that may be of ultimate significance in understanding what humans are and how they differ from nonhumans. The following sections explore this issue.

LANGUAGE, SPEECH, AND EVOLUTION

> *"Harry Jerison calls language the 'Rolls-Royce of brain adaptations.' I think he is right, for this particular kind of information processing is a luxury item, afforded to no species other than our own."*
>
> (Dean Falk, *Braindance.* New York: Henry Holt & Co., 1992, p. 184.)

The debate continues as to whether humans are alone in the animal kingdom in having the capacity for language. New fuel for the debate comes from Savage-Rumbaugh's (1994) descriptions of Kanzi, a chimpanzee who reportedly learns and manipulates arbitrary symbols called lexigrams. Skeptics argue that Kanzi and other nonhuman primates who exhibit symbol learning, may in fact acquire lexical items, like nouns, adjectives and verbs, but do not acquire grammatical items, like prepositions, relatives, and determiners. (See Bickerton, 1990, for a discussion.) The debate over language notwithstanding, agreement is general that nonhuman primates do not speak. *Spoken language* seems to be the unique province of humans. Still, we should be careful not to define language, spoken or otherwise, in such a rigid fashion that its uniqueness to humans is assured by mere definition rather than thoughtful examination of the issues. Our inquiry should accept a broad definition of language, and should at least consider the hypothesis that human language may be built on precursor faculties.

WHY IS SPEECH UNIQUE TO HUMANS (ASSUMING THAT IT IS)?

> *"The question of how and why an anthropoid began to speak is central to all our efforts to understand man and his evolution."*
>
> (Elaine Morgan, *The aquatic man.* New York: Stein & Day; 1982, p. 94.)

The British scholar Dennis Fry gave a sharp focus to the talking faculty of humans by renaming our species *Homo loquens* ("man the talker") as opposed to *Homo sapiens* ("man the wise"). Why do humans alone have the capacity to speak? The explanations that have been proposed fall mainly into the following categories: (a) only humans possess a vocal tract that is suitable for the production of phonetically diverse sounds; (b) humans alone have the brain size needed for the capacity of language; (c) unlike any other species, humans have a neural organization that allows for the cerebral representation of vocalization, thus placing sound and thought in the same neural domain; and (d) humans are unique in several features including, at the minimum, their skull structure, vocal tract anatomy, and a neural organization that supports syntax (or, alternatively, the acquisition and transfer of information).

Differences in Vocal Tract Anatomy

The vocal tract of humans is distinct from that of any other living creature. As was discussed in earlier chapters, the human has a distinctive right-angled craniovertebral junction, which gives the vocal tract its own right-angled appearance (Figure 13–2). The human larynx sits relatively low in the neck and is associated with a deep pharynx and an epiglottis that is well separated from the velopharynx. The snout is relatively short in comparison with nonhuman primates. What value do these anatomic features have? In particular, would they have evolutionary value in the survival of the human species? Lieberman (1992) believed they do, and argued specifically that "natural selection for the ability to produce the vowel sounds [i]

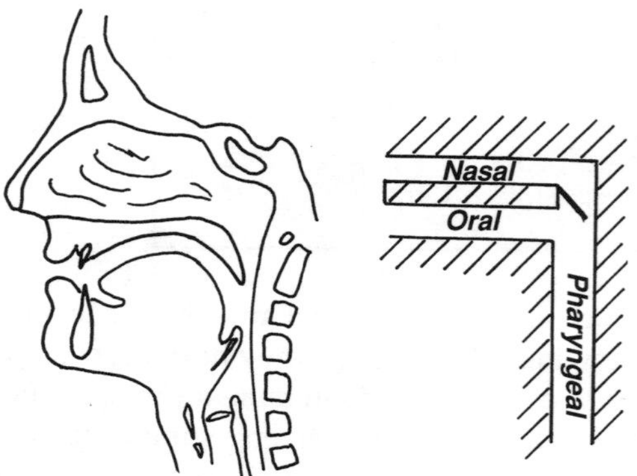

Figure 13–2. The right-angled configuration of the human vocal tract.

[as in *he*] and [u] [as in *who*] played a part in the evolution of the human supralaryngeal vocal tract" (p. 62). These vowels are thought to be important because they help to define the maximal formant-frequency range of human speech, that is, they represent a potential for acoustic contrastivity.

The evolutionary value of speech must have been great, for the adaptations of the vocal tract came at some cost, including reduced chewing capacity (because of the smaller snout and therefore shorter jaw), higher risk of aspiration and choking (because of separation of the epiglottis and palate), and risk of impacted wisdom teeth (because the small jaw does not leave adquate space for the most posterior molars). Evolution is not progression toward a perfect ideal but rather a series of trade-offs. As Nesse and Williams (1994) expressed it, "The human body is neither fragile nor robust, neither perfect nor pointlessly flawed. Like all products of organic evolution, it is a bundle of compromises, each offering an advantage—at a price" (p. 38). The supreme price is paid annually by hundreds of people who choke to death. One of these was the eminent speech scientist, Grant Fairbanks, who choked on a piece of meat.

The vocal tract argument is rather difficult to evaluate because the evidence is incomplete. One form of evidence lies in the various attempts that have been made to teach animals to produce speechlike sounds. One of the most persistent of these speech training experiences produced very limited results: sounds that resembled *cup* and *papa*, for example (Hayes & Hayes, 1951). From computer modeling studies, it appears that nonhuman primates might be able to produce nasalized vowels somewhat like the human vowels in *hit*, *hood*, *hate*, and *hat*, and consonants resembling the human consonants [t] as *till*, [d] as in *dill*, [b] as in *bill*, and [p] as in *pill*. Lieberman (1991) discusses this issue in some detail, and his book is a good source for additional information.

It should be noted that facsimiles of human speech can be produced with sound-producing organs that are very much different from the human vocal tract. Mynah birds and gray African parrots can produce sounds that are remarkably like human speech, but the vocal faculty in these birds is accomplished with an organ called the *syrinx*, which consists largely of membranes.

McCrone (1991) suggested that the human vocal tract offers not only the advantage of producing a range of sounds, but also the capability for speaking quickly. For superior communication ability, the vocal tract should ensure a high rate of communicative events. Of course, it is not sufficient that the same sound can be produced repetitively at a fast rate, for example, *ta ta ta ta ta*. Ideally, it should be possible to produce different sounds (phonetically contrastive acoustic events) at a high rate with some kind of coherence that enables their perception against background noises. An outstanding accomplishment of the human vocal system is its ability to generate a rapid succession of distinct sounds that cohere together as an utterance readily identified with a common source, the speaker. This signal carries the potential to transmit the four kinds of information mentioned in the beginning of Chapter 1: phonetic quality, affective quality, personal quality, and transmittal quality. These are conveyed essentially in parallel and with a fairly brisk rate of information exchange.

Differences in Brain Size

Perhaps language demands a large brain. Therefore, only a species that has an adequate volume of neural tissue could acquire language, whether spoken, written, or signed. As a first step in evaluating this argument, we might consider evidence that the size of the vocal repertoire in any species is proportional to the size of the brain. Birds are a good species to study for this purpose because various species of birds differ in the size of their song repertoire and the complexity of their songs. Scientists have studied these different birdsongs and also have examined the size of the neural components that control song production. The question is: Do birds with large song repertories or complex songs have proportionately larger volumes of neural tissue that regulate song production? The answer, according to Arnold (1992) and DeVoogd, Krebs, Healy, and Purvis (1993), is affirmative. Although additional studies are needed to confirm this conclusion, we can conclude at least tentatively that there is a correlation between the number of signals that an animal can produce and the volume of neural tissue that regulates signaling. But even if this assertion is true, it is a large jump from birdsong to human language.

Humans have relatively large brains. One means of comparing brain size among different animals is to compute the *encephalization quotient*, which is the ratio of brain size to body size (recall that *encephalon* means brain, or, more literally, "in the head"). The average animal has an encephalization quotient of 1. Humans have a quotient of about 3, meaning that humans have a brain that is three times larger than the brain of an average primate of similar size. Perhaps the relatively large size of the human brain underlies the special faculty of language. The great relative size of the human brain is about the only feature that stands out in comparisons with other species. Other proposed differences, such as a relatively large neocortex and association cortex, a relatively large cerebellum, and a left-right hemispheric asymmetry, do not distinguish humans from at least a few other species (Le May & Geschwind, 1975; Passingham, 1973).

It has in fact been suggested that a certain minimum brain size is needed before human faculties such as spoken language can emerge. The thinking seems to be that the demands of language require a rather massive amount of neural tissue. The counter-evidence to this proposal was supplied by Lenneberg (1964) with reference to a condition called nanocephalic dwarfism ("bird-headed" dwarfs). Nanocephalic dwarfs are like miniatures of typically sized humans. Unlike most other individuals of exceptionally small size, they have the same skeletal proportions as humans of average size. Thus, they have a brain-body weight ratio like that of regularly sized humans. However, their brain weights are more like those of a newborn (300–400 grams, as compared to 1200–1500 grams for average adults). The relevant question is: Do nanocephalic dwarfs develop spoken language? The answer, according to Lenneberg, is: "All of them acquire the rudiments of language, including speaking and understanding, and the majority master the verbal skills at least as well as a normal 5-year-old child" (Lenneberg, p. 84). It appears that absolute brain size is not a good criterion for the emergence of spoken language but perhaps relative brain size is.

Another way of comparing nervous system development among species is to determine the ratio of interneurons (the neurons that make up the CNS) to the peripheral (sensory and motor) neurons. Rats have about 20 interneurons for every peripheral neuron. Humans have about 20,000 interneurons for each peripheral neuron. The vast difference in the interneuron to peripheral neuron ratio is important because, "The larger the ratio, the greater the possibilities for manipulating and comparing information" (Wills, 1993, p. 262.). An enormous pool of interneurons may be the neural advantage that enabled humans to gain linguistic hegemony over all other species.

A related question is: Why did the human brain grow so much? Did it grow to serve functions such as language? A major difficulty in answering this question is that it is easy to fall into a trap of circularity: language requires a large brain; therefore, humans grew large brains because they were needed for language. Is it possible that large brains occurred for other reasons, and that language was a by-product? One proposal along this line was advanced by Falk (1990, 1992) in the **radiator theory of hominid brain evolution**. This theory is based on the idea that brains are highly sensitive to heat. The argument is that many human ancesters had small brains because they lacked the ability to cool cranial blood adequately. But with bipedalism (walking on two legs), circumstances changed. The first change was a rearrangement of cranial blood vessels to counteract the effects of gravity in bipedalism. The second change was that bipedalism permitted geographic mobility to human ancesters. Presumably, these creatures went to savanna habitats that were often hot. The hotter the climate, the greater the need for cooling of the cranial blood. Better circulation led to larger brain size. But other scientists have put forth an essentially opposite theory: As our ancestors moved into colder, more challenging climates, they needed larger brains for survival skills.

Of course, many other ideas have been proposed to account for the growth of the human brain. Especially prominent are suggestions that the brain became large in humans because of activities such as toolmaking, survival in a dangerous world, or communication among members of a group. Perhaps no single explanation will suffice. Brain growth may have been the result of several factors. It is possible that as the brain increased in size for any single reason (e.g., tool making) this increased capacity led to other behaviors (e.g. social interaction facilitated by tool making), which themselves contributed to further increases in brain size.

Differences in Neural Organization

This explanation holds that the way in which information is organized neurally is the key to spoken language. The essential requirement is that speech as a motor activity is represented in the cerebral cortex (the ultimate expression of encephalization). In contrast, the sounds used by animals do not have a cerebral representation, at least not one that compares with that in humans.

Some experimental results that bear on this question were obtained from efforts to simulate parts of the exposed brain in humans and animals. The classic studies of brain stimulation in humans were conducted by Penfield and Roberts (1959). A more recent practitioner of the technique is Ojemann (1983), who stimulated the exposed cerebral cortex in persons undergoing neurosurgery for epilepsy. Of particular relevance are attempts to stimulate the presumed motor centers of speech. The results were to evoke simple vocalizations and to disrupt ongoing vocalizations, but such stimulation has not elicited words or even well-formed syllables. The corresponding studies on animals have been much more successful in evoking species-specific calls. For example, stimulation of the limbic system and various diencephalic structures can elicit nearly the entire sound repertoire of monkeys (Larson, 1988). It should also be noted that the repertoire of sounds in nonhuman species is quite small and learning plays a small or doubtful role in the acquisition of the species-typical sounds except in some songbirds. In contrast, human languages have large sound repertoires that must be learned by each individual speaker.

Jurgens (1992) proposed an evolutionary scheme for vocalization based on three subsystems, as follows:

Subsystem I. The basic capability is the coordination of respiratory, laryngeal and upper-airway actions to produce vocalization. The neural support for this subsystem includes the reticular formation and phonation-related motor and sensory nuclei of the brain stem and spinal cord. This subsystem may possess the subroutines needed for genetically preprogrammed vocal patterns.

Subsystem II. This subsystem initiates vocal utterances and selects among fixed vocal patterns. It has a more complex neural organization based on three levels: The lowest level consists of the periaqueductal gray and neighboring neural structures. The middle level involves subcortical limbic structures including the hypothalamus, midline thalamus, amygdala, and septum. These structures participate in the regulation of emotion and also serve to relate external stimuli to internal stimuli geared to motivation. The highest level involves the anterior cingulate cortex, which serves to exercise voluntary control over emotional states.

Subsystem III. This is composed of the motor cortex and its primary input and output structures, cerebellum, ventrolateral thalamus, primary somatosensory cortex, putamen, nucleus ruber and pyramidal tract. This subsystem regulates voluntary fine control over vocal patterns.

The interaction of these three subsystems is schematized in Figure 13–3. Because each subsystem is composed of several neural structures, the entire system of neural regulation is complex. Notice the similarity to the large-scale distributed networks discussed in Chapter 7.

A variant of the brain-organization explanation is that the human brain is both large

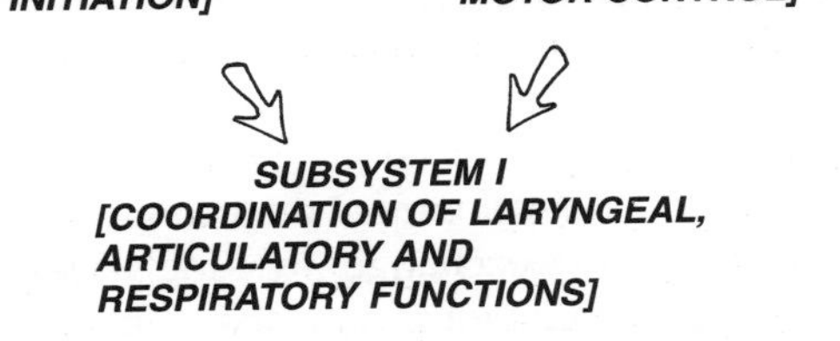

Figure 13–3. Jurgens' (1992) evolutionary scheme for the control of vocalization based on three subsystems.

and slow to develop. In contrast to the nonhuman primates, humans undergo a substantial amount of brain development after birth, so that neural connections are formed in parallel with early life experiences. This developmental pattern is called **neoteny**, literally "holding on to youth." The human infant is slower to develop than most other species, and this maintenance of the juvenile condition offers unique opportunities for the imprinting of experience on brain development (and also for a prolonged period of parental and societal instruction). Nonhuman primates depend much more on automatic or instinctive neural systems that are largely formed before birth. But the connections in human brains are formed in good measure during interactions with the environment. This explanation is by no means explicit to speech, but perhaps speech is just one example of the fruits that come with a retarded brain development, retarded, that is, in respect to the timeline of birth and life experience. Human brains are wired for spoken language even as language in its more abstract form develops in concert with human experience. In this view, the uniqueness of speech to humans is part of a more general uniqueness, in which a delayed timetable of brain development allows the brain to be formed by the potentially rich lessons of behavioral interaction with the environment.

Multiple-Factor Theories

Information-based Theories

One view of language is that its origins lie in the evolution of information transfer. A proponent of this idea is King (1994), who argues that language should be understood as a gradual development on a continuum of information exchange. In King's view, language developed as a means of *information donation*, such as occurs when an older member offers information to a younger member, and *information acquisition*, such as occurs when a younger member receives the information and stores it for subsequent use. According to the continuum perspective, language did not appear all at once, but rather was a late stage in a continuum process of information exchange. The origin of language therefore would have to be understood against the gradual and essentially continuous changes that gave rise to modern humans. These may include the factors considered in the previous discussion. But one more factor should be thrown in the mix—manual gestures.

Gestures

Manual gestures may be a part of the evolutionary background of spoken language. As McNeill (1992) discusses, there are some interesting relations between gestures and speech. Gestures are used only during speech, and therefore constitute a parallel channel of communication. Gestures and speech are semantically and pragmatically coexpressive, reflecting cognitive overlap in their information sources. A synchrony obtains between gestures and speech, such that they are deployed in a fixed temporal pattern. Speech is timed such that certain words occur with certain parts of a manual gesture. Gestures and speech have a mutual development in children, and they break down together in disorders such as aphasia. Some authors maintain that language began as manual gestures. This may be so. But the question then becomes, as Kendon (1991) puts it, "If language began as gesture, why did it not stay that way?" Speech must offer some extraordinary advantages to make it the first choice in virtually every human culture capable of hearing its sounds. (Chapter 1 considers some of the advantages that speech holds.)

This is not to say that gesture and speech are incompatible. As indicated in the previous paragraph, McNeill (1992) noted some important relations and similarities between gesture and speech. Their similarity may be expressed more pointedly by describing them both as *gesture*. Manual gesture is gesture by hand; speech is gesture by vocal apparatus. This comment recalls the discussion of gestures from Chapter 11. And, in fact, the same basic idea of speech as gesture has been proposed as a unifying concept in the origin of language. According to Armstrong, Stokoe and Wilcox in their book, *Gesture and the Nature of Language*, all language, spoken or signed, is articulatory gesture.

Bickerton's Three-Factor Theory

Bickerton (1990) identified three major distinguishing features of humans that may define the boundary conditions of language. The three are: neural organization suitable for the appearance of syntax, a modified skull, and a restructured vocal tract. He suggested that some single genetic mutation might have been sufficient to produce a creature with this triple of attributes. Pinker (1994) dismissed this suggestion by comparing it with the possibility that an exploding airliner might come together in the form of a submarine. But, in fairness to Bickerton, it should be noted that he does allow that some other factor, as yet unidentified, could account for all three changes. The thrust of Bickerton's thesis seems to be that human language is the product of at least three evolutionary developments. Whether by happy evolutionary coincidence or by some mutual explanatory factor, these three attributes came together as the biological foundations for language. Possibly, one of them alone would have given humans a linguistic capability. For example, if syntactization occurred in the absence of a restructured vocal tract, then perhaps language would have emerged as a manual system, like the sign languages used by the deaf. But if syntactization appeared at about the same time as changes in the skull and its constituent vocal tract, then our ancestors may have been inspired to harness vocalization to syntax. The advantages of spoken communication would have been considerable. For example, speech allows communication while the hands are otherwise occupied and does not depend on the full visibility of the communication partner.

Edelman's Three-Factor Account of Speech

Edelman (1987) proposed three evolutionary anatomical adaptations for speech. The first is a set of changes in the basicranium related to bipedalism. The alteration of the basicranium led to a reshaping of the supralaryngeal tract and various adjustments of the vocal folds, as described elsewhere in this book. These changes permitted an expanded repertoire of sounds. The second adaptation was the development of cortical regions, especially Broca's and Wernicke's areas, that "were responsible for the production and categorization of phonetic structures that involve coarticulation in speech" (Edelman, 1987, p. 174). The involvement of these cortical regions in the categorization and recategorization of the gestures in speech contributed to the formation of a phonetically specialized memory. The third adaptation was the connection of the phonetically related cortical regions to other areas associated with functions such as the planning of motor sequences, auditory perception, and concept formation. These neural connections gave considerable power to phonetic expressivity, placing it at the confluence of rich informational systems.

Edelman's proposal emphasizes the coemergence of a human vocal tract and neural systems capable of coordinating sensory, motor, and conceptual information.

Morgan's Aquatic Theory

Morgan (1982) argued that some aspects of human evolution might be explained by a phase in which our ancesters lived an aquatic life. This is not necessarily to say that our ancestors spent most of the day in water, swimming like fish or frogs, but rather to say that at least a significant portion of time was spent in watery environments—perhaps to reach different places by swimming, to search for aquatic food sources, to escape land-dwelling predators, or to seek relief from the heat. Morgan points out that humans have a number of physical characteristics consistent with life in the water, including: hairless skin, subcutaneous fat, ventro-ventral copulation, and a capability to close off the nasal cavity from the larynx. These are physical features fairly common to creatures that spend much of their time in the water. They are not so common to land-dwelling creatures.

The last of these, velopharyngeal closure, is relevant to speculations on the origin of speech. Humans who dive into the water "hold their breath" by closing the velopharynx. This action prevents water that has entered the nasal cavity from reaching the larynx and respiratory airway. Unlike some aquatic creatures, humans cannot close their nostrils to prevent entry of water. If swimming and diving were in fact important activities in early human evolution, then velopharyngeal closure would have had pronounced survival value. A secondary benefit would have accrued to vocal communication. Presumably, human ancestors with the ability to close the velopharynx would have discovered that a closed velopharynx enabled loud calls for signaling or threatening. This is true because nasally transmitted sound is absorbed by the tissues of the nasal cavities (as discussed in Chapter 9). To be loud, our ancestors would have relied on orally radiated sound. They might also have discovered the phonetic value of using both oral and nasal sounds, which increases the potential phonetic repertoire. By this argument, speech would have been a secondary benefit of velopharyngeal closure.

Other modifications of the vocal tract could have arisen from behavior-induced modifications. Morgan (1982) noted that bipedalism may tend to produce a lowering of the larynx. As the larynx descends, the pharynx lengthens and the vocal tract assumes its modern form. Therefore, sound-making capability would have increased. These arguments are suggested to show that a number of sequential adjustments may have contributed to the evolution of humans and human speech.

Grooming and Gossip

Dunbar (1996) proposed a theory that language evolved among hominids as an inexpensive and particularly efficient form of grooming. Grooming maintains social cohesion, and its social value may be reflected in the fact that some nonhuman primates devote as much as 20% of their waking hours to this activity. Presumably, this is far more effort than is needed for hygiene alone. It takes only so much time to remove the insects and other material from a partner's hair. Grooming may be an important social interaction that promotes bonds among members of a group. But manual grooming probably has diminishing effectiveness as group size increases. That is, with larger groups, it is very challenging to use manual grooming to preserve social order. The individual is faced with the problem of having only two hands but many allied members of the group who are candidates for grooming. Manual grooming may have been inadequate when there were too many individuals and too many potential conflicts to resolve. Language, then, may have emerged as a kind of "vocal grooming." Language has a particular power in that it may have extended the effects of grooming to several members at once. Dunbar's theory discounts the evolutionary emergence of language for problem solving and information exchange. In his theory, language appeared as a form of auditory social comfort. Presumably, the sound signals of language had a grooming benefit that could not be attained by visual hand gestures. Therefore, spoken language was a preferred form of social grooming. One vocal member could soothe several members of a group at once. Grooming led to gossip (so the theory goes), and the more elegant uses of language came only later.

Multiple Factors and Gradualism

Although some writers suppose that speech appeared quite suddenly in recent evolution, Wills (1993) argued that the evolutionary process leading to speech was very gradual. Speech may be the result of manifold evolutionary changes that spanned a long interval. Furthermore, it may be misleading to seek the roots of speech and language in a singular evolutionary change. Wills (1993) remarked that, "The evolution of language is inseparable from the evolution of the many other capabilities of our minds that have made us uniquely human" (p. 297).

Leakey (1994) elaborated on the two major conceptions of the evolutionary origins of language. The conception that regards language as uniquely human, possibly an outgrowth of enlarged brains, often is associated with the belief that language evolved recently and quickly. The second conception, that language evolved from various capacities, leads to the belief that language evolved earlier and rather slowly. Leakey discusses various interpretations of how language relates to other human capabilities and activities, including artistic expression, burial of the dead, technological innovation, regional differences in culture, long-distance contacts, population of groups that live together, use of raw materials in technology, social interaction, and imposition of order. It is not clear if language was an outgrowth of these factors or a faculty that codeveloped with them as a facilitating agent. The evidence for language origins is at best indirect, given that "Words do not fossilize" (Leakey, 1994, p. 127).

Compared to other mammals, humans are very slow to mature and therefore supremely define the phenomenon of neoteny. Much of our brain development occurs outside the womb and therefore in concert with our exploration of the world. Therefore, experience has a strong opportunity to shape brain development. Humans also have the greatest longevity among mammals. Threescore and ten is Methuselan by mammalian standards, as most mammals have lifespans of less than 30 years. The oldest living humans on record have attained an age of about 120 years, compared to a maximum of about 80 years estimated for elephants and blue whales. Longevity is perhaps necessary but not sufficient for accumulated wisdom. Humans also possess the largest relative brain size of all species. The brain, with its extraordinary population of interneurons, has immense capacity for information and for learning from experience. These three factors—neoteny, longevity, and big brain—may be closely related in setting the conditions for the intellectual prowess of humans. Speech and language are products of this prowess. Speech may have been selected as the preferred modality of language as the human vocal tract took form, perhaps through forces not initially connected with language at all. For example, bipedalism may have led to alterations of the vocal tract that enhanced the capability to produce oral sounds.

Paul Broca, whose contributions to the localization of brain functions were briefly noted in Chapter 7, was the founder of French anthropology and an avid student of Darwin. This section closes with a comment from Broca on the study of evolution.

> ***"We are much too fearful of losing the noble halo which we so fondly drape around our cradle. Personally, I am not obsessed by this fear. I am not one to despise upstarts or find more merit in rising than in descending."***
>
> (Quoted by F. Schiller, *Paul Broca: Founder of French anthropology, explorer of the brain.* Oxford, England: Oxford University Press, 1992, p. 222.)

ASYMMETRY OF LANGUAGE REPRESENTATION

Birds and humans share some interesting similarities in regard to vocal communication. As noted in Chapter 6, both species are precocious in auditory development. The human fetus hears in the womb, and some birds hear while in the egg. Humans and many birds are ready to receive auditory information early in life. Another similarity is that both species are highly lateralized in the neural regulation of vocal communication. This lateralization is often cited as a major factor in accounting for proficiency in producing and receiving sound signals. Hemispheric asymmetry for language has been demonstrated in a large number of studies. Right-handed individuals almost invariably have a left-hemisphere dominance for language. Left-handed persons have either right- or left-hemisphere dominance, with some studies indicating a statistical advantage for the left. However, this is not to say that language is necessarily and exclusively represented in one hemisphere. The nondominant right hemisphere in right-handers does possess at least a limited language ability.

A fundamental question is why is asymmetry should be desirable at all. Kertesz (1989) considered this question and discussed the relative advantages of symmetric versus asymmetric representation. He noted that a purely symmetrical structure is likely to result in a duplicative representation. Therefore, an exactly symmetrical brain would favor an equal language representation in both hemispheres. One advantage to this representation is resistance to damage: if one hemisphere is damaged, the other can take over. An asymmetrical representation offers the advantage of a greater adaptability based on complementary functions. An example of complementary functions for speech could be segmental (phonetic) versus suprasegmental (prosodic) processing. Much of the evidence on laterality for language is consistent with a left-hemisphere advantage for segmental processing, such as determining the consonants in a word. Other evidence points to an advantage of the right (nondominant) hemisphere for the processing of speech melody (intonation), emotion, and discourse structure. Asymmetry allows each hemisphere to operate on the type of information for which it is best suited. The left hemisphere seems to be especially good at analyzing fine temporal structure, such as the acoustic cues of phonemes. The right hemisphere is better at processing information that is distributed over longer time intervals, such as the intonational structure of a sentence.

This lateral complementarity of the hemispheres could reduce errors by separating basic types of information in the initial cerebral processing. That is, if segmental processing is done mainly in the left hemisphere while suprasegmental processing is accomplished chiefly in the right, their mutual interference would be minimized. But the fibers that connect the two hemispheres, such as the corpus callosum, would then permit an adaptable integration of the two types of information sources. The design of the brain need not be dichotomous. It could allow for a general asymmetry while affording some degree of shared representation (hence redundancy). As will be discussed later in this chapter, female brains may be different from male brains in having a greater degree of redundant bilateral representation.

Asymmetry might also be advantageous for the control of rapid, precise movements such as those for speech. Peters (1992) commented that a bilateral representation of speech motor control would require a highly reliable interhemispheric coordination to insure synchrony of movements in the bilateral speech muscles. That is, bilateral representation would essentially create a situation of two masters who must work in perfect unison. But a unilateral representation would put control in one cerebral region, thereby ensuring precise actions of the speech muscles.

Various theories of the evolutionary origins of asymmetry have been advanced. A complete review of these theories is not possible here, but brief comments will be given on some of these theories. LeDoux (1982) believed that asymmetry for language might be based on the functions of the inferior parietal cortex. He argued that the inferior parietal cortex of one hemisphere evolved to provide fine control of dexterity at the expense of spatial ability. If the right hand is preferred for dexterous tasks, then the left-hemisphere inferior parietal cortex would be the primary seat of dexterity. The inferior parietal cortex of the other (right) hemisphere evolved to regulate spatial behavior. The two areas working together would give the organism good dexterity but also an effective representation of spatial information. Presumably, language was drawn towards the left inferior parietal cortex because of the gestural phase in language evolution. It has often been proposed that manual operations (reaching, throwing, manipulating foods) controlled by the left hemisphere set the stage for language mechanisms.

A preference for right-handedness and specialization of the left hemisphere for language frequently have been invoked as critical features in human evolution. It has been noted by many scientists that there seems to be evolutionary progression of vocal control along the neuraxis. In less evolved species, the neural control of vocalization seems to reside in subcortical structures. But primates possess a neural control for vocalization at the level of the cingulate gyrus, a structure of the limbic system. Humans alone have genuine voluntary control for vocalization at the level of the cerebral cortex. Perhaps this difference helps to explain why chimpanzees can learn to communicate using sign language or plastic tokens, but achieve little in the way of vocal communication that resembles human speech.

The evolutionary study of language in relation to handedness has stumbled over the the apparent lack of hand preference in nonhuman primates. Why do humans show a distinct hand preference but apes, gorillas, and chimpanzees do not? By careful observations of nonhuman primates, MacNeilage and colleagues (MacNeilage, 1987; MacNeilage, Studdert-Kennedy, & Lindblom, 1987, 1993) shed some new light on this issue. They discovered, like many other observers, that nonhuman primates use the two hands about equally often. However, they also discovered that hand selection in nonhuman primates is task-dependent. The animals tend to reach with the left, but prefer to manipulate objects with the right. It was concluded that handedness is rooted in postural actions. Prosimians prefer the left hand for reaching but the right hand for postural support. These hand specializations presumably give rise to corresponding specializations in the contralateral hemispheres. Therefore, the right hemisphere is specialized for visual-spatial information (relating body position to the spatial environment), whereas the left hemisphere is specialized for the use of information concerned with posture and position. This left hemisphere specialization might have attracted language, on the assumption that similar regulatory principles apply to language as to removing the seeds from a pod. For other speculations on handedness and language, see Calvin (1983).

From the discussion to this point, it might seem that the plan of evolution is to make one hemisphere dominant for language. But the story is not quite so simple. As noted, the nondominant hemisphere has capabilities of its own (for further discussion, see Code, 1997). Furthermore, women appear to have a more bilateral language representation than men. This topic is considered in the following section.

Evolutionary Determinants of Gender-based Language Variations

In addition to the foregoing speculations on the evolutionary foundations of language in the most general sense, many authors have sought evolutionary explanations for variations in language behavior, such as differences in language usage between males and females. One hazard in this thinking is that it tends to embrace stereotypes about men's and women's behaviors. Although men and women may be different along certain behavioral dimensions, it is well to remember that differences among the individuals within either sex can be very large compared to some of the purported differences in mean abilities between men and women. Small differences in the average performance of a population can wither in the face of large individual differences. With this caveat in mind, let us consider briefly some hypotheses about sex differences in spoken language that may have evolutionary origins.

Joseph (1993) advanced an evolutionary basis for the supposed tendency of males to be strong silent types and of females to be garrulous social beings. Males, he points out, have typically been the hunters. As such, they developed skills and behavior patterns suited to the hunt. In particular, the prowess and success of the male hunters depended on keen visual-spatial skills, enforced silence to avoid detection by the prey, and large-muscle strength to wield hunting implements and to carry home the rewards of the hunt. Although men may talk of their exploits after the hunt is finished, the hunt itself was necessarily conducted largely in silence. The !Kung people of Africa are a good example of the silent male hunter (Morgan, 1982). Females have more often assumed roles of caregivers to offspring and gatherers of food such as berries, roots, and nuts. These activities could be accompanied by vocal communication, and, in fact, may have been facilitated by it. Sounds would ensure that the group would stay safely together and that their efforts would be effectively coordinated. And, of course, vocalizations would not scare away the plants to be gathered. Therefore, women were more inclined to use vocal communication as a continuous part of their daily life. Verbalization would have been a daylong accompaniment to nearly all activities. The evolutionary argument based on these differences is, of course, that men are less likely than women to engage in speech as an accompaniment to daily activities. The stereotype of men as the strong silent types would by this argument have evolutionary footing.

Sex differences in the use of speech may be related to sex differences in brain activity that occur during verbal activities. Recordings of brain activity during tasks such as word recognition and word generation show that men tend to use the left-hemisphere rather exclusively, whereas women tend to activate regions in both hemispheres (Shaywitz et al., 1995). Language in males may be a more localized and more lateralized neural function than in women. This more concentrated representation in males comes with a certain disadvantage in that men are not as likely as women to recover from strokes that affect the language areas of the brain. The more widely distributed a function is in its neural representation, the less likely that function is to be devastated by circumscribed damage, as might happen in a stroke. It also has been suggested that males are more likely to stutter because of sex differences in the neural representation of speech. (See Chapter 1 for a discussion of sex differences in speech and language disorders.) Is there any advantage to a restricted language representation? Perhaps not in itself, but segregation of function may be part of a more general plan of neural assignment in which neural representations are somewhat isolated to maintain their integrity in the face of multiple demands on neural tissue. Also, it has been suggested that a major reason for specialized cortical processing areas is to reduce interhemispheric conduction delay (Ringo, Doty, DeMenter, & Simard, 1994). That is, it takes time to transfer information from one hemisphere to the other, so rapidity of information processing may be facilitated by restricting the processing to one hemisphere.

Perhaps the restricted language representation is a price that males pay for their relatively superior performance on visual-spatial tasks. Males may have learned to inhibit right-hemispere language functions to give this hemisphere a privileged role in visual-spatial activities that make for a successful hunt, a victorious battle with enemies, or more extensive environmental exploration. Regarding the last of these, Gaulin (1996) proposed an evolutionary model to account for sex-related differences in spatial ability. Possibly, male and female patterns of hemispheric activity are caused by the effects of hormones on the developing brain. Fetal exposure to androgens (male hormones) may lead to improved spatial ability (Gaulin, 1996) but decreased verbal ability (Geschwind & Galaburda, 1987; Marx, 1982). Verbal ability may also contrast with mathematical ability, and it is interesting that results of an EEG study of mathematically precocious individuals indicate enhanced activation of the right hemisphere (O'Boyle, Alexander, & Persson, 1991).

Arguments over sexual superiority frequently miss the point that each sex may have its own particular advantages—however small—in various realms. The two general areas often emphasized in research on gender differences in humans are verbal ability (Hyde & Linn, 1988) and mathematical ability (Hyde, Fennema, & Lamon, 1990). It is well to remember that brains are not one-dimensional. Neither sex is consistently superior and some of the differences observed at the population level are small compared to the wide variations among individuals. This is not to deny that males and females differ in various aspects of speech and language. Some differences are culturally determined. Other differences may be rooted in biology and are therefore immutable in the ordinary course of events.

EVOLUTION: A POSTSCRIPT

This chapter has emphasized evolution because it is the primary theoretical basis for conjectures on the development of spoken language. But evolution is not a monolithic theory, for it contains its own controversies and differences of opinion. Although there is a tendency to consider Darwin's contributions as a single evolutionary theory, Mayr (1985) analyzed Darwin's work as consisting of five separate theories, each of which had its own scientific legacy. The five subtheories are as follows: (a) the theory of evolution *per se*, or the idea of a descent with modification; (b) the theory of common ancestry; (c) the theory of gradualism, or modification by small increments; (d) the theory of multiplication of species by division of lineages; and (e) the theory of natural selection, or the process by which some variations are maintained and others are lost.

To consider the evolutionary theory further, we might ask: Is the evolution of the human species complete? Some take the position that it is. In their view, humans have evolved about as much as they ever will. We as a species are complete. But others contend that evolution is always in progress, and that contemporary humans are just another point on the evolutionary path. Generally, evolution is studied retrospectively, by tracing developments and their presumed adaptive value. A prospective view would be to imagine what kind of evolutionary adaptations would favor the survival and success of the human species. For example, if language is a major evolutionary triumph, then may language itself be evolving to a more efficient, more powerful form? What could such a form be?

In his *Critique of Judgment* (1790), Kant wrote of humans as those "that were able to believe themselves the final end of creation." Do today's humans mark an end or a continuation? Darwin himself wrote hopefully on the matter of human evolution:

> Man may be excused for feeling some pride at having risen, though not through his own exertions, to the very summit of the organic scale; and the fact of having thus risen, instead of having been aboriginally placed there, may give him hope for a still higher destiny in the distant future. [Charles Darwin, *The Descent of Man*, New York: AMS Press, 1971, p. 405.]

On The Reference Shelf

Recommended as general discussions of the evolution of speech and language.

Aitchison, J. (1996). *The seeds of speech*. Cambridge, England: Cambridge University Press.
A contemporary review of ideas on the evolution of speech.

Hauser, M. D. (1996). *The evolution of communication*. Cambridge, MA: MIT Press.
A scholarly examination of various lines of evidence on how communication evolved.

Joseph, R. (1993). *The naked neuron*. New York: Plenum Press.
An informative account of evolution and the brain, with commentary on language.

Leakey, R. ((1994). *The origin of humankind*. New York: Basic Books.
A readable account, highly suited for the general reader.

Lieberman, P. (1991). *Uniquely human*. Cambridge, MA: Harvard University Press.
The author advances his own theory on what makes humans unique.

Pinker, S. (1994). *The language instinct*. New York: William Morrow and Company.
This popular book, written in a generally entertaining style, addresses the notion that language is in our genes.

Wills, Christopher (1993). *The runaway brain*. New York: Basic Books.
A neuroscientist considers issues in brain evolution in this thoughtful and clearly written book.

Chapter References

Armstrong, D. F., Stokoe, W. F., & Wilcox, S. E. (1995). *Gesture and the nature of language*. Cambridge, England: Cambridge University Press.

Arnold, A. P. (1992). Developmental plasticity in neural circuits controlling birdsong: Sexual differentiation and the neural basis of learning. *Journal of Neurobiology*, *23*, 1506–1528.

Bickerton, D. (1990). *Language and species*. Chicago: University of Chicago Press.

Calvin, W. H. (1983). *The throwing madonna: Essays on the brain*. New York: McGraw-Hill.

Campbell, J. (1982). *Grammatical man*. New York: Simon & Schuster.

Code, C. (1997). Can the right hemisphere speak? *Brain and Language, 57*, 38–59.

DeVoogd, T. J., Krebs, J. R., Healy, S. D., & Purvis, A. (1993). Relations between song repertoire size and the volume of brain nuclei related to song: Comparative evolutionary analyses amongst oscine birds. *Proceedings of the Royal Society, London, 254*, 75–82.

Dunbar, R. (1996). *Grooming, gossip, and the evolution of language*. Cambridge, MA: Harvard University Press.

Edelman, G. (1989). *The remembered present: A biological theory of consciousness*. New York: Basic Books.

Falk, C. (1990). Brain evolution in *Homo*: The "radiator" theory. *Behavioral and Brain Sciences, 13*, 333–381.

Falk, D. (1992). *Braindance*. New York: Henry Holt and Company.

Gaulin, S. J. C. (1996). Does evolutionary theory predict sex differences in the brain? In M. S. Gazzaniga (Ed.), *The cognitive neurosciences* (pp. 1211–1225). Cambridge, MA: MIT Press.

Geschwind, N., & Galaburda, A. M. (1987). *Cerebral lateralization: Biological mechanisms, associations, and pathology*. Cambridge, MA: MIT Press.

Hayes, K. J., & Hayes, C. (1951). The intellectual development of a home-raised chimpanzee. *Proceedings of the American Philosophical Society, 95*, 105–109.

Hyde, J., & Linn, M. C. (1988). Gender differences in verbal ability: A meta-analysis. *Psychological Bulletin, 104*, 53–69.

Hyde, J., Fennema, E., & Lamon, S. J. (1990). Gender differences in mathematics performance: A meta-analysis. *Psychological Bulletin, 107*, 139–155.

Joseph, R. (1993). *The naked neuron*. New York: Plenum Press.

Jurgens, U. (1992). On the neurobiology of vocal communication. In H. Papousek, U. Jurgens, and M. Papousek (Eds.), *Nonverbal vocal communication* (pp. 31–42). Cambridge, UK: Cambridge University Press.

Kant, I. (1790). *Kritik der Urteilskraft*. Trans. by W. S. Pluhar (1987) *Critique of judgment*. Indianapolis, IN: Hackett Publications Company.

Kendon, A. (1991). Some considerations for a theory of language origins. *Man, 26*, 199–221.

Kertesz, A. (1989). Hemispheric dominance: Its development and relation to speech disorders. *Folia Phoniatrica, 41*, 61–88.

King B. J. (1994). *The information continuum. Evolution of social information transfer in monkeys, apes and hominids*. Santa Fe, NM: School of American Research Press. (Distributed by University of Washington Press.)

Larson, C. R. (1988). Brain mechanisms involved in the control of vocalization. *Journal of Voice, 2*, 301–311.

Ledoux, J. E. (1982). Neuroevolutionary mechanisms of cerebral asymmetry in man. *Brain, Behavior and Evolution, 20*, 196–212.

LeMay, M., & Geschwind, N. (1975). Hemispheric differences in the brains of Great Apes. *Brain, Behavior and Evolution, 11*, 48–52.

Lenneberg, E. (1964). A biological perspective of language. In E. Lenneberg (Ed.), *New directions in the study of language* (pp. 65–88). Cambridge, MA: MIT Press.

Lieberman, P. (1991). *Uniquely human*. Cambridge, MA: Harvard University Press.

MacNeilage, P.F. (1987). The evolution of hemispheric specialization for manual function and language. In S. P. Wise (Ed.), *Higher brain functions* (pp. 285–309). New York: John Wiley and Sons.

MacNeilage, P. F., Studdert-Kennedy, M. G., and Lindblom, B. (1987). Primate handedness reconsidered. *Behavioral and Brain Sciences, 10*, 247–303.

MacNeilage, P. F., Studdert-Kennedy, M. G., & Lindblom, B. (1993, January/February). Hand signals. *The Sciences*. 53, 32–37.

Marx, J. L. (1982). Autoimmunity in left-handers. *Science, 217*, 141–144.

Mayr, E. (1982). *The growth of biological thought: Diversity, evolution, and inheritance*. Cambridge, MA: Belknap Press.

McCrone, J. (1991). *The ape that spoke*. New York: William Morrow & Co.

McNeill, D. (1992). *Hand and mind: What gestures reveal about thought*. Chicago: University of Chicago Press.

Montagu, A. (1989). *Growing young*. Granby, MA: Bergin & Garvey Publishers.

Morgan, E. (1982). *The aquatic man*. New York: Stein & Day.

Nesse, R. M., & Williams, G. (1994, November/December). Nothing to sneeze at. *The Sciences, 34*, 34–38.

O'Boyle, M., Alexander, J. E., & Persson, C. (1991). Enhanced right hemisphere activation in the mathematically precocious: A preliminary EEG investigation. *Brain and Cognition, 17*, 138–153.

Passingham, R. E. (1973). Anatomical differences between the neocortex of man and other primates. *Brain, Behavior, and Evolution, 7*, 337–359.

Peters, M. (1992). Cerebral asymmetry for speech and the asymmetry in the path lengths for the right and left recurrent nerves. *Brain and Language, 43*, 349–352.

Pinker, S. (1994). *The language instinct*. New York: William Morrow and Company.

Popescu, P. (1996). *Almost Adam*. New York: Avon Books.

Ringo, J. L., Doty, R. W., DeMenter, S., & Simard, P. Y. (1994). Time is of the essence: A conjecture that hemispheric specialization arises from interhemispheric conduction delay. *Cerebral Cortex, 4*, 331–337.

Shaywitz, B. A., Shaywitz, S. E., Pugh, K. R., Constable, R. T., Skudlarski, P., Fulbright, R. K., Bronen, R. A., Fletcher, J. M., Shankweiler, D. P., & Katz, L. (1995). Sex differences in the functional organization of the brain for language. *Nature, 373*, 607–609.

Savage-Rumbaugh, E. S. (1994). *Kanzi: The ape at the brink of the human mind*. New York: John Wiley and Sons.

Wills, Christopher (1993). *The runaway brain*. New York: Basic Books.

Exercises

12-1. Speech apparently is unique to humans, although some authorities argue that language may not be unique to our species. This chapter considers several major reasons why speech could be a uniquely human faculty. Discuss whether some or all of these reasons also could be used to defend the assertion that language is unique to humans. In framing your answer, you will need to make a clear distinction between language and speech. **Hint:** speech is one of several possible modalities of language.

12-2. What is meant by the statement, "Evolutionary progress is marked by encephalization and lateralization"? Discuss how this statement pertains to the neural representation of speech and language.

12-3. Select any book on evolution or anthropology that contains information on speech or language. What is the major contention of the author(s) on this subject? Do you agree or disagree with this position? Explain your answer.

12-4. Suppose that an anthropologist discovers a remarkably intact fossilized skull of a prehistoric human-like specimen. The anthropologist is greatly excited over this discovery and exclaims, "This ancester was surely capable of speech!" Explain what kind of features might have led to this conclusion.

12-5. In his book *Almost Adam*, Petru Popescu imagined what it might be like if protohumans were discovered in an isolated region of Africa. He describes how these creatures might live and act, including the pattern of their vocalizations. For those who like to read fiction with some factual references, this book may be both entertaining and informative. The question to those who read it is: What is the author's conception of communicative ability in these protohumans? Specifically, what is the repertoire of sounds? What scientific evidence may be the basis for his speculations on this matter?

CHAPTER

14

The Embryology of the Speech Organs

> *"I am fearfully and wonderfully made."*
>
> (Psalms 139:4)

Before the mother-to-be may realize that she is pregnant, events are rapidly unfolding that eventually will give shape to the various organs of the new body developing within her. *Embryology*, the biological specialty that studies the animal embryo, covers the development of an organism from the fertilized egg, to the formation of an embryo, to the growth of the fetus. A critical scientific advance that led to rapid progress in this field was the introduction of the **cell theory** in 1838 by Matthias Jakob Schleiden. Theodor Schwann, after whom the Schwann cells (Chapter 7) are named, confirmed Schleiden's work 1 year later. With the discovery of this theory, embryology could proceed from the principle that cell division is a primary means for the development of tissues and organs. The division of cells produces a sufficient quantity of cells that can eventually differentiate to form organs of the body.

The basic processes of embryology are **cytogenesis**, **histogenesis**, and **organogenesis**. Cytogenesis is the origin of cells through multiplication, differentiation, and, in some cases, programmed death. Histogenesis is the origin of tissues, accomplished by the processes of orientation, interconnection, and migration of cells. Organogenesis is the origin of organs and involves especially the blending of tissues into organ systems.

At its minimum, the study of embryology is relevant to understanding how the organs of the body take form. The information presented in this chapter pertains primarily to the organs previously mentioned in this book, especially the organs that constitute the respiratory system, laryngeal system, upper airway system, auditory system, and the nervous system. In addition to its value in understanding normal anatomy and physiology, embryology is the basis for conceptualizing a variety of disorders and abnormalities that arise before birth. Because many of these conditions are named after events and structures that occur in embryological development, a basic knowledge of embryology is helpful in evaluating clinical information about dysmorphologies such as cleft lip and palate. In addition, more than one quarter of the Mendelian syndromes (genetic disorders) in humans have some manifestation in the craniofacial system. Craniofacial dysmorphologies, therefore, figure prominently in the identification of these syndromes.

The abbreviated account that follows summarizes the calendar of human embryology, with a special emphasis on the brain and the organs of speech and hearing. Detailed information is available from sources listed under On the Reference Shelf.

EMBRYONIC AND FETAL CHRONOLOGY

Conception to 1 Month Gestational Age

Conception is the fertilization of an egg by a sperm. It marks the beginning of development and is the reference point for **gestational age** (GA). Gestation is pregnancy and GA is age postfertilization. Conception produces a single cell that contains chromosomes from both parents (23 chromosomal pairs from the mother and 23 pairs from the father). The male and female germ cells are called **gametes**. The result of their nuclear fusion is called a **zygote**. This microscopic entity is equipped with the genetic blueprint needed to form a unique human body. The early stages of this process are illustrated in Figure 14–1. The fertilized egg is called an **ovum**. This single cell divides to form two cells, each of which divides in turn to form two other cells, and so on, until at about the 4th or 5th day postconception, some 64 or so cells are clustered in a berrylike ball called the **morula**. No differentiation of cells is apparent at this time. The raspberrylike structure is simply a sphere of similar cells. As the morula grows, it moves through the Fallopian tube on its journey to the uterus. At about the 5th day, the morula enters the uterus. It is ready to begin its temporary residence in the womb.

> ***"In the universe of the womb, the real drama of creation begins when the embryo is almost two weeks old. Driven by unseen forces, entire sheets of cells begin to expand or contract, slide past one another, and fold in on themselves in a feverish attempt to start a life."***
>
> (G. Eichele, "Budding thoughts." *The Sciences,* 1992, January/February, 32, pp. 30–36.)

In 1 or 2 more days, as the cells attach to the uterus, the morula is transformed to a **blastocyst** (also called a **blastula)**, which is a fluid-filled sphere that contains a cluster of cells at one end (Figure 14–1). This cluster, called the **polar mass,** will soon give rise to the first differentiated cells. These cells are part of the **embryonic disk**, which forms in about 10 to 13 days postconception. The **amniotic cavity** also develops at this time. Differentiation of cells occurs by a process

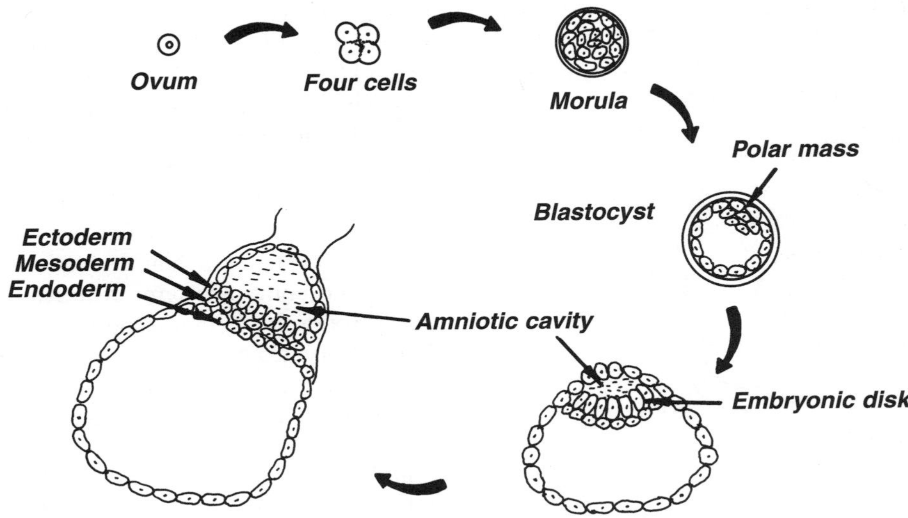

Figure 14–1. Early embryonic events: ovum, four-cell stage, morula, blastula, and lamination to form the endoderm, mesoderm, and ectoderm.

called **lamination** (layering) that initially produces two distinct layers, the **ectoderm** and **endoderm**. A third middle layer, the **mesoderm**, soon follows. These three layers, shown in Figure 14–1, are the precursors of the major organs of the body. The endoderm gives rise to specialized cells that eventually become the visceral organs (e.g., the digestive tract and lungs). The mesoderm produces cells that differentiate into bones, muscles, connective tissues, blood, and blood vessels. The ectoderm leads to the development of several organs, especially the nervous system, certain mucous membranes, and the epidermis, or skin. The common embryonic origin of organs such as the nervous system and epidermis is helpful in understanding certain diseases that affect both of these systems.

At about 18 days, the mother may notice that menstruation is late. This is generally the earliest time at which pregnancy is suspected. A new stage commences in embryonic development: the **neurula** stage. This stage is the beginning of an identifiable nervous system and is diagrammatically summarized in Figure 14–2. The single layer of ectodermal cells first forms a **neural plate**, or sheet of cells. A depression called the **neural groove** forms within the plate. The plate then rolls up around the groove to form the **neural tube**. The **neural folds** that form the tube close initially in a region corresponding to the lower cervical and upper thoracic divisions of the nervous system. The last regions to close are the openings at either end of the tube. These rostral and caudal openings are called **neuropores**. The fusion of the neuropores marks the end of neurulation. The entire process, lasting about 10 days, results in the early formation of a neuraxis. A defect in the neural tube is called a **dysraphia**. One example of a neural tube defect is the condition of **spina bifida**. Babies born with spina bifida often survive, but may have serious disabilities. Other forms of dysraphia may threaten the life of the embryo.

At the end of the 3rd week GA, there is an initial segmentation of the neural tube into the **prosencephalon** (forebrain), **mesencephalon** (midbrain), and **rhombencephalon** (hindbrain), as illustrated in Figure 14–3. The mesencephalon was introduced in

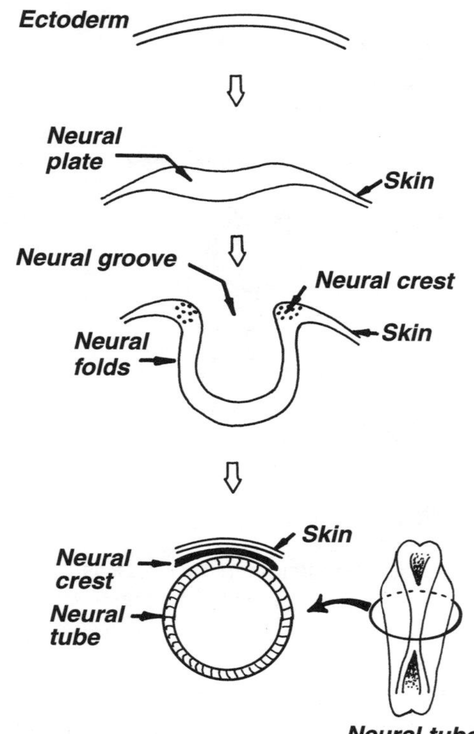

Figure 14–2. Process of neurulation, that is, formation of the neural tube. The ectoderm forms a neural plate containing a small groove. The plate folds around the groove to form a tube. After closure of the tube, the skin and neural crest lie outside the neuraxis (CNS).

Chapter 7. The prosencephalon is a rostral swelling of the tube that eventually will give rise to the telencephalon and diencephalon (Figure 14–3). The rhombencephalon is a caudal swelling that is the precursor of the metencephalon and myelencephalon (Figure 14–3). These early brain segments prefigure the central nervous system. The **cephalic fold** also appears as the consequence of a flexing of the embryo. This flexing is evident in Figure 14–3.

At about this same time of 3 weeks GA, the embryo has five U-shaped arches called the **branchial arches** (Figure 14–4). Situated behind these arches are the primitive oral cavity and digestive tract. The arches are numbered I, II, III, IV, and V, proceeding inferiorly. The first two arches are also called the **mandibular arch** and **hyoid arch**, respectively. The branchial arches give rise to a number of structures of the larynx and upper airway, some of which are listed in Table 14–1. The branchial derivation helps to explain some anatomic features of the adult. For example, cranial nerve V (trigeminal) innervates both the muscles of mastication and the tensor tympani of the middle ear (as noted in Chapter 7). This innervation pattern is consistent with the derivation of both the mandible and the malleus (on which the tensor tympani inserts) from the first branchial arch. A primitive oral cavity called the **stomodeum** (oral pit), appears as a small slit between the bulbous frontal process and the mandibular arch. The embryo's face at 4 weeks has the appearance shown in Figure 14–5.

The 4th week GA is the typical date at which pregnancy is confirmed. The embryo is about 3 or 4 mm long. It has a neural tube, a primitive face, the buds of the primary bronchi of the respiratory system, a rudimentary epiglottis, and an otic plate that will develop into the ear. Until the 4th or 5th week, the primitive mouth (stomodeum) has been separated from the foregut by a **buccopharyngeal membrane**. As this membrane ruptures, an open passage is created between the mouth and foregut. The heart begins to beat at the end of the first month GA. Oxygen from the mother's blood diffuses across a membrane to reach the blood in the embryo. From now until birth, the growing organism derives its nutrition from the mother's blood flowing through the placenta. But the embryo produces its own blood cells, and there is no mixture of maternal and embryonic blood. Oxygenation of the fetal blood is aided by the special properties of fetal hemoglobin, which has a strong affinity for oxygen.

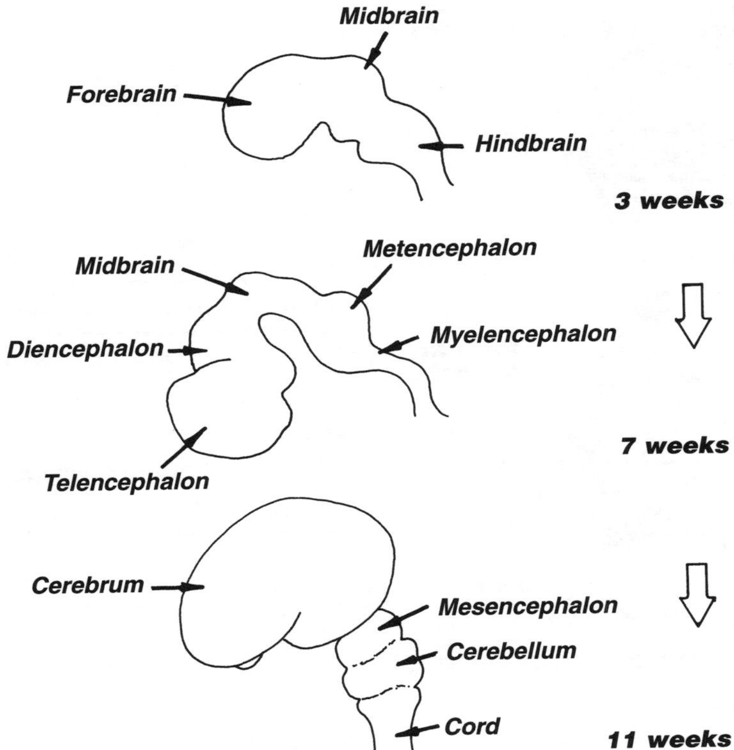

Figure 14–3. Appearance of the brain at 3, 7, and 11 weeks, showing divisions that appear at various times. Note the appearance of the cephalic flexion, or bending of the head of the embryo.

1st Month to End of 3rd Month

At either the 5th week or 9th week GA, there is a change in developmental designation from embryo to fetus. Some authorities use the figure of 5 weeks, others the figure of 9 weeks. Still others prefer a physical measure such as the crown-rump distance (a suitable measure of length because the fetus typically has a sitting posture). For convenience, the discussion in this book uses gestational age.

By the 6th week GA, five segments are evident in the neural tube (Figure 14–3). These are the same divisions introduced in Chapter 7: telencephalon, diencephalon, metencephalon, mesencephalon, and myelencephalon. The appearance of these segments is accompanied by the essential formation of the ventricular system. Table 14–2 shows the correspondence between brain structures and divisions of the ventricular system. Abnormalities in development of the ventricular system can result in **hydrocephalus**, or dilation of all or part of the ventricular system. The internal capsule has appeared and the meninges are being defined, beginning with the pia and dura mater. During this period, the muscles are

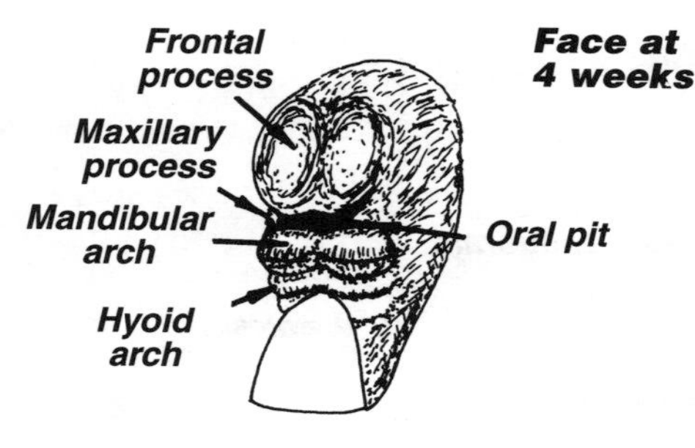

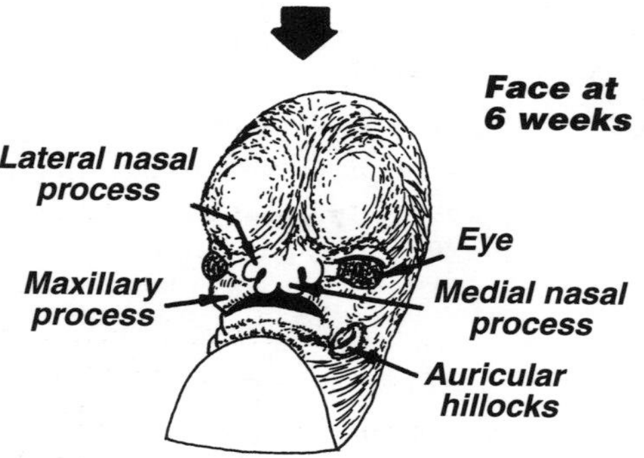

Figure 14–4. Appearance of the face at 4 and 6 weeks.

Table 14–1. Derivation of various structures from the five branchial arches.

Arch	Derived Structures
I	Mandible, malleus, incus
II	Body of hyoid bone, stapes
III	Major horns of hyoid bone
IV	Thyroid cartilage
V	Arytenoid cartilage

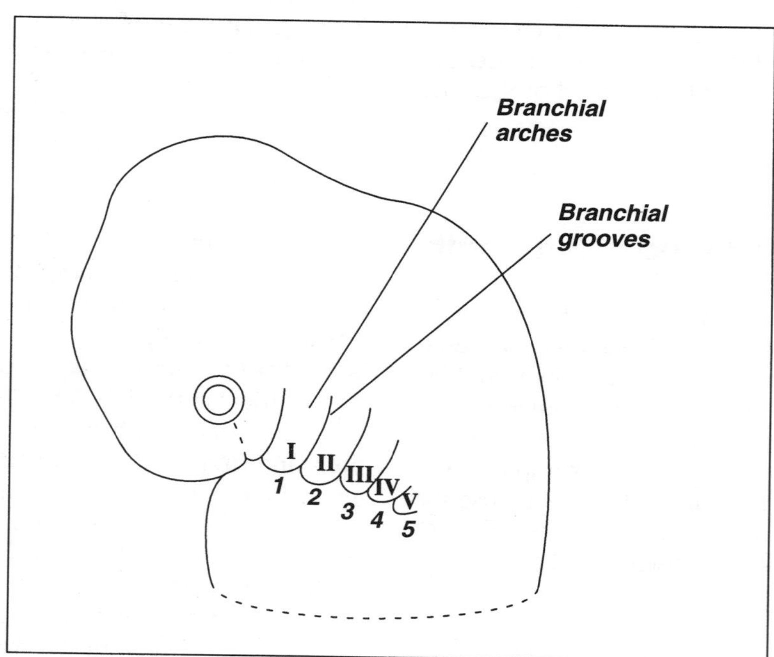

Figure 14–5. The branchial arches.

Table 14–2. Correspondence between divisions of the brain and parts of the ventricular system.

Brain Division	Ventricle
Telencephalon	Lateral ventricles
Diencephalon	Third ventricle
Mesencephalon	Cerebral aqueduct
Metencephalon	Rostral part of fourth ventricle
Myelencephalon	Caudal part of fourth ventricle

beginning to be controlled by the brain. Fetal movements now occur. By the end of the 2nd month, the external genitalia are evident, and testosterone secretions are beginning to produce male adaptations from the basic female form. That is, all embryos begin as female, and the male sex is basically an adaptation of the female plan. The fetus is about 3 cm long, or a little more than 1 inch.

At this stage of development, the face is beginning to take form through the merging and fusion of five processes: one frontonasal (sometimes called simply frontal), two maxillary, and two mandibular (Figure 14–6a). The paired maxillary and mandibular processes merge at midline and fuse to form a unitary structure (Figure 14–6b and 14–6c). Failure of the processes to merge and fuse can result in conditions such as cleft palate. The cleft appears as a congenital fissure (a) in the median line of the palate, (b) lateral to the premaxillary process, or (c) both of these. By about the end of the 6th week, the face is acquiring essential features such as the eyes, mouth, and nose (Figure 14–5). The nose begins as olfactory pits in the frontonasal process. As the frontonasal process grows downward, it is divided by the olfactory pits into the **median nasal processes** and **lateral nasal processes**. The lateral processes eventually form the alar cartilages of the nose and, by union with the maxillary processes, also form the midface area inferior to the eyes (the infraorbital face region). The downward growth of the median nasal process gives rise to the **globular process**, which in turn produces the primary palate.

Between the 7th and 9th weeks, the mandible grows considerably in length and width and gains neuromotor control that permits it to swing to an open position. This development of the mandible permits the tongue to descend from the nasal cavity (Figure 14–7). With the tongue out of the way, the palatal shelves, which had been perpendicular to the tongue (Figure 14–7), assume a more horizontal position and begin to join (Figure 14–8). The hard palate achieves complete closure at about 8 or 9 weeks. Its final unitary form is the result of fusion of the two maxillary processes and the medial nasal process (Figure 14–9). That is, three embryologic tissues become one. The soft palate closes as far as the uvula at about the 10th week. Swallowing is now possible. The lungs have assumed a lobulated appearance. Beginning at about 8 weeks GA and continuing until the 16th week, the bronchial tree undergoes its dichotomous branching (as discussed in Chapter 4) to produce a progressively bifurcated airway in each lung.

If a cleft of the palate is going to develop, it will begin during the period between the 7th and 11th week, when the palate normally is closing. In a condition called **Pierre Robin syndrome**, the mandible does not develop properly and therefore does not swing open to allow the tongue to descend

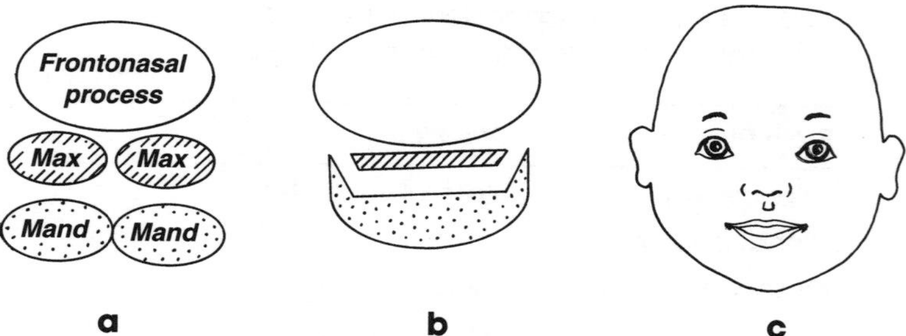

Figure 14-6. Schematic illustration of the formation of the face: **a.** The 5 embryonic processes—one frontonasal, two maxillary (Max), and two mandibular (Mand). **b.** Merging of the paired maxillary and mandibular processes. **c.** Basic plan of infantile face.

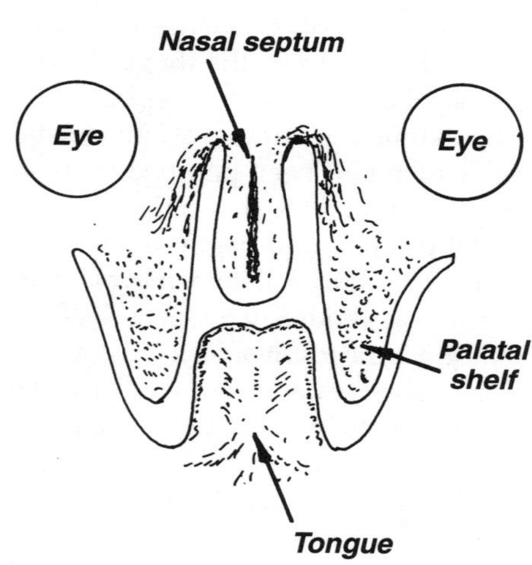

Figure 14-7. Schematic drawing of the arrangement of nasal septum, palatal shelves, and tongue in an embryo of about 8 weeks GA.

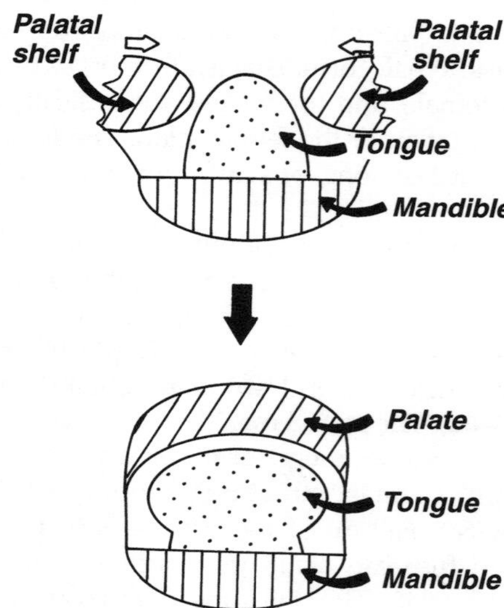

Figure 14-8. Schematic drawing of formation of distinct oral and nasal cavities as the tongue descends from the nasal cavity and the palatal shelves move toward midline closure.

into the oral cavity. The persistent elevation of the tongue prevents closure of the palate. Consequently, the child is born with mandibular hypoplasia (a small, underdeveloped mandible) and a cleft palate.

Advancing to the 3rd month GA, inspection of the fetus shows the brain to resemble a miniature boxing glove, owing largely to the appearance of the lateral (sylvian) fissure (Figure 14–10). The fetal brain now weighs about 10 grams and neurons are being added at the rate of about 2,000/sec. The most common time for miscarriage is 10 weeks GA. Apparently, the failure of critical organs to develop properly results in a

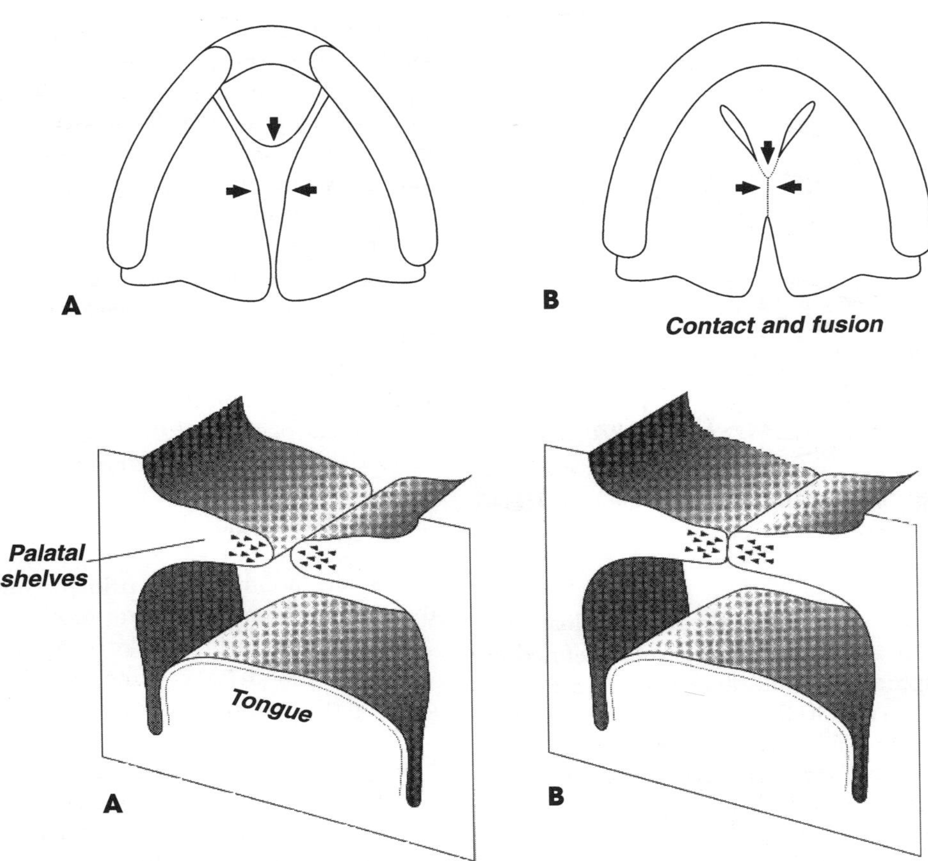

Figure 14–9. Formation of hard palate: **A.** The paired maxillary processes and median nasal process grow toward one another. **B.** Contact and fusion.

fetal crisis. By the end of the 3rd month, most of the bones have centers of ossification, the fingers and toes are taking form, and the external genitalia assume male or female characteristics. Also by this time, the soft palate has been completely formed. The first trimester of pregnancy is critical to the basic plan of the face.

During the 3rd month the opening to the developing larynx is created by resorption of a membrane formed by epithelial tissue. In cases of incomplete resorption, the persistence of the membrane may result in **laryngeal webs** or certain kinds of **papillae** on the vocal folds of the newborn. Surgery may be required to correct these problems.

4th Month to 6th Month

At the 4th month GA (the beginning of the second trimester of pregnancy), the lateral fissure of the brain is readily detectable. Myelination begins in the dorsal and ventral roots of the spinal cord. Many reflexes appear, along with frowning and thumb sucking. The nostrils are open, and there is a continuous passage from nose to lungs. The ossification of the ossicles begins. By the end of the 4th month, the fetus is about 15 cm (6 inches) long and weighs about 110 gm.

At the 5th month GA, the brain is only about 5 cm in length but the full complement of neurons already is present. From

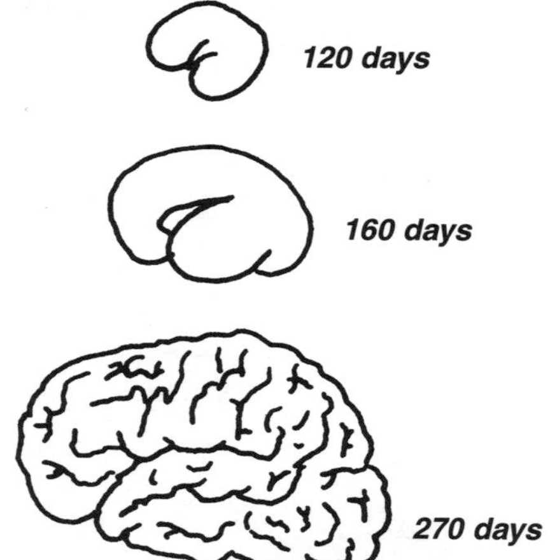

Figure 14–10. The brain at 110, 150, and 270 days GA.

this point, neurons begin to be lost, not added. However, the glial cells (defined in Chapter 7) are multiplying rapidly and continue to add to their number well after the neurons have ceased to proliferate. Fetal hiccoughs may begin. During the 5th or 6th month, the body is covered by a downy hair called **lanugo**. The ear is essentially structurally complete, and the fetus is beginning to hear sounds (see Chapter 6). In another 2 or 3 weeks, myelin can be observed in cranial nerve VIII.

Beginning at about the 24th week, the lung grows until it fills the thoracic cavity. Also, the gas-exchange units of the lungs take form. But the lungs are filled with fluid and have no respiratory function in the fetus.

At the 6th month GA, the fetus has the capability for hand grip. The fetal eyelids open and close. The brain weighs about 200 grams, or less than one-half a pound. The fetus has a body length of about 30 cm and weighs about 625 gm.

7th Month to Birth

At the 7th month GA (the beginning of the final trimester), the eye's retinal layers are completed, and the eyes are no longer covered by the pupillary membrane. The legal right of the fetus to a separate existence is often recognized after 29 weeks. A fetus born at this age may be capable of life outside the womb. It is about 40 cm long and weighs more than 1 kg. The brain weighs about 200 gm. The skin has a ruddy and wrinkled appearance and is covered by a white substance called the **vernix** (a combination of epithelial cells, lanugo hairs, and glandular secretions). The lip epithelium is well developed, and the larynx is assuming its neonatal position at the level of the 6th cervical vertebrae. The fetus has both a grasp reflex (closure of the hand in response to tactile stimulation) and a Moro (startle) reflex.

At the 8th month GA, all primary sulci of the cerebral hemispheres are formed (Figure 14–10). The wrinkled skin evident during the 7th month has become smoother because of deposits of subcutaneous fat.

Finally, at the 9th month GA, the fetal brain weighs about 350 to 400 gm (12 ounces, or just short of a pound). This is about one third of its eventual adult weight. With birth, the fetal stage of development comes to a close and is followed by the neonatal, or newborn, stage.

Neonatal Stage

Birth requires critical adaptations of the respiratory system, which served no role in gas exchange during fetal life. Within a few seconds, the lungs must inflate and serve the ventilatory requirements of the newborn. The fetus derives all of its oxygen from the placenta. Because the fetal and maternal blood do not mix, oxygen from the mother's blood diffuses into the fetal blood. As noted earlier, this process is aided by special properties of fetal hemoglobin, which has a stronger affinity for oxygen than does adult hemoglobin. Until birth, the venous return does not pass through the fetal lung but rather passes through an opening in the heart called the **foramen**

Table 14–3. The Apgar score for neonatal assessment. Points are added in each category, for a maximum score of 10. If a score of 8–10 is achieved at 1 or 5 minutes after birth, active rescuscitation usually is not required.

	Apgar Score		
Sign	**0**	**1**	**2**
Heart rate	Absent	Less than 100 beats/min	More than 100 beats/min
Respiratory effort	Absent	Weak cry	Strong cry
Muscle tone	Limp	Some flexion	Good flexion
Reflex irritability	No response	Some motion	Good motion
Color	Blue or pale	Body pink, extremities blue	Pink

ovale (oval window). Diversion of blood through this opening in the atrial septum ceases at birth so that the lung receives all venous return. The fetal circulatory system also has an opening between the aorta and the pulmonary artery that allows venous blood entering the right ventricle to flow into the systemic circulation. This opening, called the **ductus arteriosus**, normally closes within a few days after birth. Also within a few weeks after birth, infant hemoglobin is gradually replaced by adult hemoglobin, and alveoli begin to develop rapidly in the lungs (this process of alveolarization continues until the age of about 8 years).

The status of the newborn typically is assessed with the **Apgar score**, a 10-point scale based on five characteristics listed in Table 14–3. Each characteristic is rated as a 0, 1, or 2. An Apgar score of 8 or less is an indication that the newborn may require medical assistance. This score is based on readily observable features that signal important information about the neonate's health status. It is typically the first examination in a person's life.

CONCLUSION

This final chapter of the book ends with a beginning—the neonate about to start on the path to spoken language. The infant begins to acquire speech even as the anatomic systems of speech are being formed and remodeled. Speech as a modality of language (i.e., a means of expressing language) will be learned along with language itself. The relation between speech and language is sufficiently close that some people think of them as being one and the same. If all goes well in a child's development, he or she will use speech easily and naturally. Speech will be a lifelong companion and valuable servant. It may seem like a part of the self. Although speech is especially suited for communication with others, many people on occasion speak even to themselves when no one else is around to listen. To be sure, speech is public for the most part. But it also has a private value, one that reflects our sense of self. It establishes us in a community of collegial speakers, even as it distinguishes us from all others.

"In his whole life man achieves nothing so great and so wonderful as what he achieved when he learned to talk."

(Otto Jespersen)

"The self is surrounded by mirrors of language."

(Hans Hormann)

"Language most shows a man; speak that I may see thee."

(Ben Jonson)

"Speech is civilization itself. The word, even the most contradictory word, preserves contact. It is silence which isolates.

(Thomas Mann)

"Language, as well as the faculty of speech, was the immediate gift of God"

(Noah Webster)

On The Reference Shelf

The following sources of information were used in preparation of this chapter; they are recommended as additional reading.

Avery J. K. (Ed.). (1994). *Oral development and histology*. New York: Thieme Medical Publishers.
Comprehensive discussions of histology and general growth processes.

Bzoch, K. R. (Ed.). (1989). *Communicative disorders related to cleft lip and palate*. Boston: College-Hill Press.
Useful information on development of the craniofacial system in relation to cleft lip and palate.

DeMyer, W. (1988). *Neuroanatomy*. (The National Medical Series for Independent Study). New York: John Wiley.
Includes a summary of embryology of the nervous system.

Leff, A. R., & Schumacker, P. T. (1993). *Respiratory physiology: Basics and applications*. Philadelphia: W. B. Saunders.
A compact and informative text on the subject; Chapter 10 deals with lung growth and development.

Lemire, R. J., Loeser, J. D., Leech, R. W., & Alvord, E. C. (1975). *Normal and abnormal development of the human nervous system*. Hagerstown, MD: Harper & Row.
Detailed information on normal and abnormal development of the nervous system.

Zemlin, W. R. (1988). *Speech and hearing science: Anatomy and physiology* (3rd ed.). Englewood Cliffs, NJ: Prentice-Hall.
A good source for embryology of the speech and hearing organs.

Exercises

14-1. Assuming that 8 or 9 weeks GA is the dividing point between embryo and fetus, describe the status of the human face and nervous system at the close of the embryonic period.

14-2. Explain why cleft lip and palate occur in the first trimester of pregnancy. Also explain why clefting may take different forms, such as cleft of the lip only, cleft of lip and palate, a unilateral cleft, or a bilateral cleft.

14-3. Babies born prematurely at 7 months GA may survive. Describe the general developmental status of the fetus at this age.

14-4. What is the general developmental status of the nervous system at birth? How does its general appearance, size, and neuronal population compare with the nervous system in an adult?

14-5. Draw a sketch of the mandible, the three ossicles, the hyoid bone, and the thyroid and arytenoid cartilages. Then, referring to the information in Table 14–1, use five different colors to show the branchial arch derivation of each structure. For example, the hyoid would have two different colors, as would the ossicular chain.

Glossary

a- not, without, lacking.

ab- away from.

abdomen the part of the body situated between the thorax and pelvis; the diaphragm separates the thoracic and abdominal cavities.

abduct to draw away from midline.

acoustic reflex a bilateral reflex of the stapedius muscle in the middle ear; it is activated by sounds of high intensity and reduces the transmission of energy into the inner ear.

acoustics the branch of physics that deals with the study of sound.

action potential (AP) electrical potential generated by a wave of depolarization at the surface of a nerve or muscle tissue.

ad- (consonant assimilates to initial consonant of roots beginning with c, f, g, p, s, or t) to, toward.

adduct to draw toward midline.

adenoids enlarged or hypertrophied pharyngeal tonsil.

adenoidectomy surgical removal of adenoids.

aer- or **aero-** pertaining to air.

afferent carrying toward, especially the center; afferent nerves are generally sensory and carry information toward the CNS.

affricate a speech sound characterized by an articulatory closure (stop phase) followed by a noise interval (frication phase).

agonist a muscle whose action is opposite to another muscle, the antagonist.

airflow the volume of air moved in a unit of time, e.g., milliliters per second or liters per minute.

air pressure force of air per unit area, measured in pascals.

air volume quantity of air contained in a vessel, usually measured in liters or milliters in human physiology.

ala- winglike.

alveolar pressure air pressure within the alveoli (terminal sacs) of the lungs.

alveolus a small cavity or pit.

amplitude magnitude; excursion of movement.

ampulla flasklike structure or dilation of a tube; a part of the vestibular mechanism.

amygdaloid almond-shaped.

an- *see* **a-**.

ana- up, again.

anastomosis communication between vessels or structures.

anatomical position the body in upright posture, with arms at the side and palms facing forward. This is a standard position for anatomic reference.

angio- pertaining to blood vessels.

anion an ion carrying a negative charge.

anlage the foundation for a subsequent development; in embryology, the earliest recognizable appearance of a developing part or organ.

annular ring-shaped.

anomaly a deviation from typical structure or pattern; abnormality.

ansa loop or arc.

antagonist a muscle that opposes action of another (**the agonist**).

ante- front, before.

anti- against.

antiformant *see* **antiresonance**.

antiresonance a resonance phenomenon in which energy transmission is impeded; compare with **resonance**.

anthropology the study of prehistoric humans.

aperiodic not periodic, irregular.

apex peak or top.

aphasia an impairment of language related to neurologic disease or damage.

aphonia loss or absence of voice; compare with **dysphonia**.

apo- away from, or derived from.

aponeurosis sheetlike connective tissue that attaches muscle to bone.

apposition a fitting together.

approximate to bring together, draw near.

arch-, archi- beginning, origin.

arcuate arched, bow-shaped.

articulation in anatomy, a joint or juncture of bones; in speech, the movement and positioning of the speech organs in sound production.

articulators the speech organs involved in sound production, typically reserved for structures of the vocal tract (tongue, lips, jaw, palate).

articulatory model a model that accounts for the movements of speech.

articulatory synthesis a type of speech synthesis (machine-generated speech) in which the organs of the vocal tract are simulated and controlled to produce speechlike patterns.

association fibers fibers that connect two regions of the cerebral cortex in one hemisphere.

attractors a concept used in dynamic systems theory to account for transitions and stabilities in motor behaviors. Three major types are point attractors, limit cycle attractors, and strange attractors.

automatic speech recognition the recognition of speech by machine.

axon the process of a neuron that usually is efferent in function.

bandwidth a range or span of frequencies.

Bark scale a nonlinear transformation of frequency based on the psychophysical properties of human audition.

basal nuclei (basal ganglia) subcortical masses of neuronal cell bodies, including the caudate, putamen, and globus pallidus. They are involved especially in motor functions.

basilar membrane a membrane of the cochlear duct, forming the floor of the organ of Corti.

belly the fleshy portion of a muscle.

Bernoulli force or effect a decrease in pressure at a constricted region of a tube that results from increased velocity of fluid while a constant volume flow is maintained.

bi- two.

bifurcate to divide into two branches.

bilateral pertaining to both sides.

blade a wide, flat structure; a division of the tongue just posterior to the tip and anterior to the dorsum.

blastocyst a hollow ball of cells.

blastula a hollow ball of cells.

bolus a ball or mass of masticated food prepared to be swallowed; a quantity of liquid ready to be swallowed.

bone hard supportive tissue of the body made of various minerals.

branchial pertaining to the embryonic gill arches.

breath group the syllabic pattern produced on one exhalation.

Broca's area Brodmann area 44, located on the inferior margin of the frontal lobe of the brain, considered to be important in the expression of spoken language; named after Paul Broca.

Brodmann's areas regions of the cerebral cortex, assigned distinctive numbers by

Brodmann to reflect differences in cellular structure.
bronch- windpipe.
bronchiole the smallest division of the bronchial tree.
bronchus the primary division of the trachea, leading to the lungs on either side.
bucc- pertaining to the cheek.
bulb, bulbar pertaining to the brainstem.
calcify to harden through the deposit of calcium salts.
callosum hard.
calvarium skullcap.
canal a passageway or duct.
capillary slender blood vessel; the interface between the arterial and venous circulatory systems.
caput the head.
cartilage a flexible, nonvascular connective tissue; the three kinds of cartilage are hyaline cartilage, fibrocartilage, and elastic cartilage.
caudal toward the tail or coccyx.
cementum thin layer of bone that lines the insertion of teeth into the alveolus.
central nervous system the division of the nervous system that consists of the brain and spinal cord.
cephalo- pertaining to the head.
cerumen a water-soluble waxlike substance secreted by cells in the external canal of the ear.
cervical pertaining to the neck.
choana a funnellike opening or channel.
chondral pertaining to cartilage.
cilia slender hairlike projections of cells that are capable of a rhythmic beating motion.
cingulum a girdle or zone.
cleft palate a congenital fissure in the roof of the mouth.
co- together.
coarticulation an event in speech production in which adjustments of the speech production system are made simultaneously for two or more speech sounds. Typically, coarticulation is defined for articulatory adjustments that reflect the properties of at least two phonemes.
coccyx the most inferior portion of the vertebral column, having roughly the shape of a cuckoo's beak.
cochlea snail shell; the inner ear.
cochlear duct the membranous labyrinth within the cochlea that contains the organ of Corti; also called the cochlear partition.
cohort in speech perception, a set of words that share a word-initial acoustic sequence.
collagen white fibers of the corium of the skin, tendon, and other connective tissues.
colliculus a small elevation; hillock.
com- together.
commissure a joining together, as in the commissural nerve fibers that join the right and left cerebral hemispheres.
con- with, together.
concha shelllike structure.
condyle rounded prominence on a bone; the process of the mandible that inserts into the temporomandibular joint.
congenital present at birth.
contra- opposite.
contalateral pertaining to the other side.
copy synthesis a type of speech synthesis (machine-generated speech) in which stored copies of speech segments are retrieved and assembled to form an utterance.
cornu horn.
corona crown.
corpus body.
coronal plane a vertical plane that divides a structure into front and back portions.
corpus callosum a band of white fibers that connects the right and left cerebral hemispheres; a commissure.
cortex outer covering or layer.
cost- rib.
coupling interaction between two or more systems.
cranial nerves the 12 pairs of peripheral nerves that emerge from the base of the brain.

cranium portion of the skull that contains the brain.

crest ridge, bony prominence.

crypt pitlike depression or tubular recess.

-cule denoting something small.

cut- skin.

cyst-, cysto- pertaining to sac or bladder.

cyto-, cyt- pertaining to cell.

cytology the science dealing with the structure of cells.

cytoplasm the protoplasm of a cell, excluding that of the nucleus.

damping rate of absorption of sound energy.

decibel a logarithmic unit used for the measurement of sound intensity or pressure.

deciduous temporary, shedding.

decussate to cross over.

deglutition swallowing.

degrees of freedom the number of independently controllable elements in a system.

de- down, from, negative.

dendrite the process of a neuron that serves an afferent function; it receives input from other neurons or sensory receptors.

dent-, dentate pertaining to tooth or teeth.

derm- skin.

dermatome a region or strip of skin innervated by a given spinal nerve.

dextro-, dextr- pertaining to the right side.

di- two, twice.

dia-, di- through, between.

dialect a variation of a language, distinguished by patterns of phonology, morphology, or syntax.

diaphragm a partition separating two cavities; the large, dome-shaped muscle that separates the thoracic and abdominal cavities.

diastema a space between two teeth.

digitate possessing fingerlike projections.

digitize to convert from analog (continuous) form to digital (discrete) form.

dilate to expand or enlarge.

diphone a segment of speech that represents the interval from the middle of one sound to the middle of a following sound; i.e., it begins and ends with a steady-state and includes a transition between two given sounds.

dis-, di-, dif- away, negative, apart.

diphthong a class of speech sound formed of two vowels that occur within a single syllable. The first vowel is called the onglide and the second, the offglide.

discrimination task in speech perception, a procedure designed to assess listeners' ability to discriminate, or tell apart, stimuli. Labeling or categorization of stimuli is not required.

distal away from the body or from the medial axis.

distend to swell or stretch out.

dorsal toward the backbone.

duct a tube, especially for the passage of secretions or excretions.

dyne a unit of force; defined as the force required to accelerate during 1 second a mass of 1 gram to a velocity of cm per second.

dys- diseased, faulty, bad.

dysphonia an impairment of voice or phonation.

e- out from.

ec- out of.

ecto- situated on the outside or surface.

edema abnormal collection of fluid in a tissue, swelling.

edentulous toothless.

efferent conduction away from a central point; toward the effectors (muscles or glands).

elastic cartilage flexible, nonvascular connective tissue that does not ossify with age.

elasticity the property of returning to the original state following deformation.

electromotility change of shape under electrical stimulation.

embryo early developing stage of an organism; in humans, the development period between the 2nd and 8th weeks of gestation.

eminence projection or prominence.

en-, em- in.

encephalo- brain (literally, within the head).
endolymph the fluid contained in the membranous labyrinth of the inner ear.
ento- within or inner.
ep-, epi- upon or above some other thing.
error rate in automatic speech recognition, the accuracy of speech recognition, typically expressed as the percentage of words correctly identified.
eustachian tube the narrow passage that connects the middle ear and the nasopharynx; also called the auditory tube.
eversion turning outward.
ex- out of, toward the surface.
extension straightening out from a flexed position.
external auditory meatus the canal that leads from the auricle to the tympanic membrane.
extra- outside.
facet small surface.
fasciculus small bundle.
features in phonetics, distinctive properties of sounds.
feedback a signal that is returned from the periphery to a central controller; often used to increase stability in a system.
fetus the developing organism after the embryonic period and before birth.
filter a device or system that has a frequency-selective transmission of energy.
fissure relatively deep groove.
flexion act of bending.
foramen natural opening or passage.
formant resonance of the vocal tract.
formant frequency center frequency of a formant.
formant synthesis a type of speech synthesis (machine-generated speech) in which resonators are controlled to produce formantlike patterns.
formant transition a change in formant frequency, especially in relation to consonant-vowel or vowel-consonant sequences.
Fourier transform a mathematical tool that relates time-domain (waveform) and frequency-domain (spectrum) representations of signals. It is based on the idea that any signal can be decomposed into a set of sinusoid waves.
fossa depression, pit.
fovea pit.
fractal a geometric pattern that can be scaled at various sizes and multiply combined to form a complex structure.
frenum, frenulum a fold of skin or mucous membrane that restricts the range of movement of a structure.
frication the generation of noise through the turbulent flow of air through a constricted region.
fricative a class of speech sounds characterized by noise energy.
frontal anterior, or pertaining to the forehead.
funiculus small, cordlike structure.
fundamental frequency the lowest frequency of vibration in a harmonic series.
fusiform spindle-shaped.
gamete a sexual germ cell, either the female ovum or male sperm cell.
gangli-, ganglio- knotlike.
ganglion a mass of nerve cell bodies lying (usually) outside the central nervous system.
genu knee.
gene the biological unit of inheritance; a gene specifies a protein or enzyme.
genetic inherited.
genio- pertaining to the chin.
gestation pregnancy.
gingiva gums.
gland a cell, tissue, or organ that produces a substance that is used elsewhere in the body.
-glia gluelike substance or structure; a support structure in the central nervous system.
glide a class of speech sound that has a gradual articulatory movement; sometimes called a semivowel.
glosso-, gloss- pertaining to the tongue.
glottal volume velocity the flow of air through the glottis during phonation.
glottis the space between the vocal folds, typically measured as width or area.

gnatho-, gnath- pertaining to the jaw.

gnomic having the same shape under changes in size.

gray matter a population of cell bodies of neurons.

gyrus a fold in the cerebral cortex; a convolution.

hamulus hook-shaped.

harmonics the partials of a complex sound, having frequencies that are integral multiples of the fundamental frequency.

head an enlargement at one end of a bone.

hemi- half.

hemo-, hema- pertaining to blood.

hertz (Hz) the symbol for cycle per second, named after the physicist Heinrich Hertz.

hetero-, heter- other, different.

hiatus a large opening.

hidden Markov model a mathematical model consisting of (1) a finite set of states, (2) transition probabilities between the states, (3) a finite set of possible outcomes, and (4) a probability distribution over the set of outcomes associated with each state. Similar to a Markov model except that in a hidden Markov model, the states are not directly associated with outcomes, but rather with probabilities.

homeo- same or constant.

hominids any of a family (*hominidae*) of bipedal primate mammals including modern humans and immediate ancesters.

homunculus a little man or person.

hyaline cartilage a type of tough, nonvascular connective tissue that may be converted to bone in adulthood.

hydrodynamics the study of fluids under pressure.

hydrostat a fluid-filled muscular organ that forms its own skeletal support by the selective contraction of certain muscle fibers.

hyper- over, above.

hypo- under, beneath, deficient.

identification task in speech perception, a procedure designed to assess listener's ability to label, or identify, speech sounds.

idio- peculiar, distinct.

idiopathic cause unknown.

ilium broad superior part of the hipbone.

imaging techniques procedures that produce pictures of internal structures of the body.

impulse a stimulus carried by a nerve fiber; wave of depolarization.

in-, im- 1. in, into. 2. not.

inferior lower or located beneath, toward the feet.

infra- below, beneath.

inguino-, inguin- pertaining to the groin.

inhibit to arrest or repress.

innervation distribution of nerves to a part of the body; route of neural regulation.

innominate nameless.

insertion the region where a muscle or its tendon attaches to a bone that is moved by contraction of the muscle.

in situ in position.

intensity measure of energy flow per unit of area per unit of time.

inter- between, among, together.

interface 1. a surface that is the common boundary between two parts or spaces. 2. a point of connection between two processes or operations.

internal away from the outside, toward the inside.

internuncial a connecting or intervening medium; in the nervous system, refers to the neurons of the CNS.

intonation the pattern of fundamental frequency over an utterance, especially a phrase or sentence.

intra- within.

intrinsic inherent, situated within.

intro- inside, within.

inversion the turning inward of a structure or part.

in vivo the living state.

ion an electrically charged atom or group of atoms.

ipsi- self.

ipsilateral situated or pertaining to the same side.

iso- equal.

-itis inflammation.
keratinized possessing a horny layer of flattened cells containing keratin.
kerato- pertaining to horny tissue or the cornea.
kilo- thousand.
kinesthesia the sensation of movement.
kyto- pertaining to cell.
labio- pertaining to lips.
labiodental pertaining to lips and teeth.
labryinth complex maze of passages; the inner ear including the cochlea and vestibular system.
lacri- pertaining to tears.
lacto- pertaining to milk.
lacuna a small cavity or pit.
lal-, lala-, lalo- pertaining to speech or babbling.
lamella thin plate or scale.
lamina thin plate or layer.
laminar, laminated composed of layers.
laminar flow a type of airflow in which the air moves in smooth layers.
laryngo- pertaining to larynx.
lateral a class of speech sounds produced with a midline obstruction that causes sound to be emitted laterally (to one or both sides).
latero- pertaining to the side.
lemma husk.
lemniscus a fiber tract of the central nervous system.
lenticular lens-shaped.
leuco- white.
levator something that elevates or raises.
ligament a band of fibrous connective tissue that links bones or maintains organs in position.
limbus the border of a structure.
limbic bordering.
lingua- pertaining to the tongue.
lingula small tongue-shaped structure.
lipid a fat or fatlike substance that is water insoluble.
liquid a phonetic term for the rhotics (r-sounds) and laterals.
lobe a division of an organ, usually demarcated by fissures or constrictions.
locus place.
locus theory the theory that places of articulation are identified with a particular value of a formant frequency.
logarithm the exponent indicating the power to which a base must be raised to equal a given number. Commonly used bases are 10 and the natural number *e*.
logo- pertaining to speech or words.
logogen in speech perception, a theoretical passive sensing device that is associated with each word in a mental lexicon. Activation of a logogen is the means to recognition of a particular word.
loudness the psychoacoustic attribute of the magnitude of a sound, as might be scaled on a dimension ranging from soft to loud; it relates most closely to the intensity of a sound.
lumbar pertaining to loin.
lumen light; the opening within a tube.
lymph a transparent, yellowish fluid that transports waste from the blood.
macro- large.
macula a stain or spot.
mal- defective, bad, wrong.
malleus (from the Latin for *hammer*) the largest of the auditory ossicles, which attaches to the tympanic membrane and incus.
malocclusion any deviation from a normal or typical occlusion of the teeth.
mammo- pertaining to breast.
mandible lower jaw.
manubrium (from the Latin for *handle*) the upper portion of the sternum.
Markov model a network model of states and transitions in which the transitions between states are associated with probabilities of occurrence.
masseter chewer.
mastication chewing.
mater mother.
matrix the location on which something is formed, or the substance from which it develops.
maxilla the upper jaw.
maximum phonation time the maximum time over which phonation can be sustained.

meatus an opening or canal.
mechanoreceptors sensory receptors that respond to mechanical stimulation, such as pressure or deformation.
medial toward the axis, near the midline.
mediastinum generally, the median partition between divisions of an organ; the visceral organs located between the pleural sacs.
medulla the innermost part of an organ or structure.
mega-, **megalo-** of great size.
membrane a thin layer of tissue that lines cavities, divides spaces, or binds structures.
membranous glottis the anterior portion of the length of the glottis that is not adjacent to cartilaginous tissue.
meningeo- pertaining to membranes, especially the meninges that cover the central nervous system.
mental 1. pertaining to the mind. 2. pertaining to the chin.
mental lexicon a speaker's knowledge about words, including sounds, meanings, and grammatical roles.
mesencephalon midbrain.
meso-, **mes-** middle or intermediate.
meta-, **met-** after, beyond, accompanying.
metencephalon the region of the brainstem associated with the pons and the cerebellar peduncles.
micro-, **micr-** of small size.
mio- less.
minute volume the amount of air exchanged by an organism in one minute.
mitochondria intracellular structures that provide energy for the cell.
modality one of the sensory qualities, such as taste, smell, or hearing.
modulate to alter the intensity, frequency, or quality of some stimulus.
molar used for grinding; the three most posterior teeth of the permanent (adult) dentition.
mono- single.
morph-, **morpho-** pertaining to form.
morphology in biology, the study of form and structure; in linguistics, the study of word formations.
morula a solid ball of cells, resembling a mulberry.
motor control theory (or model) a theory of how movements are regulated for a given behavior.
motor strip the precentral gyrus of the frontal lobe (Brodmann area 4), associated with voluntary motor action.
motor theory a theory of speech perception based on the idea that speech is perceived in reference to the motor processes (articulations) by which it is produced.
motor unit the motor fibers innervated by a single axon.
muco-, **muc-** pertaining to mucus or mucous membrane.
mucosal wave a wavelike motion of the vocal fold cover that occurs during vibration of the folds; related to the vertical phase difference in vocal fold vibration.
mucous (adjective) pertaining to mucus.
mucus viscous secretion of mucous glands.
multi- many or much.
myelencephalon the medulla oblongata.
myelin the white fatty covering on the large axons of a neuron.
myelo-, **myel-** pertaining to marrow, myelin, or the spinal cord.
mylo-, **myo-**, **my-** pertaining to muscle.
myxo- pertaining to mucus or slime.
naris (plural **nares**) one of the orifices of the nasal cavity; nostril.
nasal a class of speech sound involving radiation of sound energy through the nasal cavities, with or without an accompanying oral radiation of energy.
nasal formant a low-frequency resonance associated with transmission of energy through the nasal tract.
neck a constricted portion of a structure or vessel.
necro- pertaining to death.
neo-, **ne-** new or strange.

neonatal pertaining to the first 4 weeks after birth; newborn.
neoplasm abnormal new growth, tumor.
neural, neuro-, neur- pertaining to nerves or nervous system.
neurology the study of the nervous system and its disorders.
neuron a nerve cell, the basic unit of the nervous system.
nigra black.
noci- to harm or injure.
node a knot, knob or swelling.
nodule a small node.
nomenclature a system of names or terms.
non- absence.
notch an indentation.
nucleus 1. the part of a cell that contains the genetic material. 2. an aggregation of nerve cells, especially in the central nervous system (compare with **ganglion**).
ob- against, in front of, toward.
oblique inclined, diagonal.
obstruent a class of nonasal speech sound made with a radical obstruction of the vocal tract; the obstruents include stops, fricatives, and affricates.
occlusion generally, closure or contact; in dentistry, the closing pattern of the masticatory surfaces of the upper and lower teeth.
octave an interval corresponding to a frequency ratio of 2 to 1 between two sounds.
odonto- pertaining to tooth or teeth.
olfactory pertaining to the sense of smell.
oligo- small or deficiency.
omo- pertaining to shoulder.
ontogeny the development or course of development of an individual organism.
operculum lip or flap.
orbicular circular or rounded.
organ of Corti the sensory organ of hearing located within the cochlear duct and containing the hair cells.
origin the place of attachment of a muscle which is relatively fixed when the muscle contracts; compare with **insertion**.
oro- pertaining to mouth.
osseus composed of bone.
ossicular chain the three bones of the middle ear: malleus, incus, and stapes.
osteo- pertaining to bone.
otitis an inflammation of the ear.
otitis media an inflammation of the middle ear.
otoacoustic emission (**OEA**) energy emitted from the ear during the transduction of acoustic energy to neural impulses.
otology the medical specialty that deals with the ear.
otorhinolaryngology the medical specialty that deals with the ear, nose, and throat.
oval window the membrane between middle ear and the inner ear into which the footplate of the stapes inserts.
ovum egg.
palato- pertaining to the roof of the mouth.
pallidus pale.
palpate to examine manually.
pan all.
parietal forming or located on a wall.
parietal pleura inner surface of thoracic cavity.
pars part of a structure or area.
Passavant's ridge (or **pad**) a muscular bulge that projects from the posterior nasopharyngeal wall to assist velopharyngeal closure.
patent open.
patho- pertaining to disease.
pectoral pertaining to the chest or breast.
pedia, ped- pertaining to child.
pedo- 1. pertaining to child. 2. pertaining to foot.
peduncle a small foot or stalk.
per- throughout, completely.
peri- around.
perilymph the fluid in the space between the membranous and osseous labyrinths of the inner ear.
period the time required for one complete cycle of vibration.

periodic regular in occurrence, predictably recurring.

periodontal the tissues that surround and protect the teeth.

peripheral toward the outward surface or region.

peripheral nervous system the division of the nervous system that lies outside the brain and spinal cord; includes the cranial and spinal nerves.

-phage, **-phagia** eating.

phase transition a qualitative change in the behavior of a system.

phonation vibration of the vocal folds to produce sound.

phone an individual sound of speech; an elementary sound unit.

phoneme the smallest sound unit in a language that distinguishes words.

phono-, **phon-** pertaining to sound, especially speech or voice.

physics the science that deals with the laws of nature, especially forces and the composition of matter.

physiology the science that deals with the functions of living organisms and their components.

pia soft, tender, delicate.

pineal shaped like a pine cone.

pinna a feather or winglike structure; the prominent part of the outer ear attached to either side of the head.

pit a depression or indentation, usually small.

pitch a psychaoustic quality that is usually scaled from low to high; it relates most closely, but not exclusively, to the frequency of vibration of a sound.

placenta an uterine vascular tissue that allows diffusive exchange of respiratory and nutritive products between the maternal and fetal blood.

plane generally, a flat surface; in anatomy, a two-dimensional surface that either intersects the body or is tangential to it.

plate a flat structure, especially a thin bony layer.

pleura the serous membrane that lines the thoracic cavity and surrounds the lungs.

plexus a network of interconnecting nerves or vessels.

pneumo- pertaining to air or to lungs.

pneumotachograph a device used to measure the volume rate of airflow.

pocket a saclike space.

poly- many or much.

polymorphous having various forms.

pons a bridge of tissue between two organs.

pore small opening.

post- behind or after.

post-synaptic neuron the neuron that receives an input across the synaptic cleft.

posterior toward the back.

pre- before.

pressure force per unit area measured at a given point.

pro- before, in front of.

process in general, an operation or event; in anatomy, a projection or prominence.

prone the posture of lying face down.

proprioception the awareness of the body's position, including posture, movement, and orientation in space.

prosencephalon the division of the central nervous system that includes the telencephalon and diencephalon.

proso- forward or anterior.

prosody the component of speech that includes melody, rhythm, stress pattern, and intonation; the complement to the phonetic (segmental) component.

prosthesis an artificial replacement for a missing or dysfunctional part.

proto-, **prot-** first.

protoplasm the basic substance of a cell.

prototype in perception, an ideal instance or exemplar of a perceptual category.

protuberance a projecting part or prominence.

proximal nearest; closer to the body from a given point of reference.

pseudo- false.

puberty the period of development in which sexual maturation and rapid growth occur.

pyriform pear-shaped.

quadri- four.

radiation characteristic a property in acoustics that relates to the dispersion of sound from a sound source; a baffle effect.

ramus branch or division.

raphe a seam or ridge formed at the line of union of two symmetrical halves of a structure.

re- back, again, contrary.

recess small cavity.

rectus straight.

reflex an involuntary motor act.

resonance the condition of a vibrating system that is driven by a periodic force at the natural frequency of the system. Under this condition, the amplitude of vibration can become very large.

resorb to absorb again.

respiration the process by which gases are exchanged between an organism and its environment.

reticular netlike.

retract to draw back, shorten.

Reynold's number a dimensionless number used as an index of turbulence in fluid flow.

raphy seam or suture.

rhino-, rhin- pertaining to or resembling the nose.

rhombencephalon the division of the central nervous system that includes the metencephalon and myelencephalon.

rhythm the temporal or stress pattern of speech.

rima glottidis glottis; the space between the vocal folds.

root the part of a structure hidden within other tissues.

ridge an elevation or crest.

rostral 1. beaklike. 2. toward the head.

ruga (plural. **rugae**) a wrinkle or fold.

saccule small sac.

saggital 1. arrow-shaped. 2. pertaining to the anterior-posterior plane of the body, or the plane that divides the body into right and left parts.

saliva a fluid secreted within the mouth to lubricate the bolus for swallowing and to maintain moisture within the oral cavity. Saliva is typically clear, slightly alkaline, and somewhat viscous.

sampling the process of making a series of measurements from a continuous (analog) signal.

sampling rate the rate at which a signal or process is sampled; in digital processing of speech, the sampling rate specifies the intervals at which the analog waveform is converted to digital form.

segmentation the delineation of successive sound segments in a speech signal.

sensory strip the postcentral gyrus of the parietal lobe, associated with somatosensory function (Brodmann areas 1, 2, and 3).

sexual dimorphism male-female differences in structure or form.

sinus cavity.

smooth muscle visceral muscle.

somatic pertaining to the body.

somatic growth growth pattern of body in general.

somatic muscle skeletal (striated) muscle.

special senses the qualities of taste, smell, vision, hearing, and balance.

spectrum an analysis of sound energy in terms of the magnitude (and sometimes phase) of its frequency components.

spectrogram a type of short-term running spectrum in which sounds are analyzed in a three-dimensional pattern of time, frequency, and amplitude.

speech mode that concept that speech is perceived in a special mode, unlike that for nonspeech signals.

spinal nerves the 31 pairs of peripheral nerves that emerge from the spinal cord.

sterno- pertaining to sternum.

stoma-, stomato- pertaining to mouth.

stop a class of nonnasal speech sound characterized by a complete obstruction of the vocal tract; also called a plosive.

strain deformation resulting from stress.

strain gauge a transducer that converts mechanical displacement into electrical signals.

stria line or streak.

striated striped.

strident in phonetics, a fricative with intense noise energy.
stylo-, styl- pertaining to the styloid process of the temporal bone.
sub- under, beneath, deficient.
sulcus furrow or groove.
super- above, excessive.
superficial at or toward the surface.
supine the posterior of lying on the back.
supra- above, over, upon.
surface wave a wave that moves along a surface; the vertical-phase difference observed on the vocal fold during vibration.
suture a line of junction between two parts.
syllable a unit of speech consisting of either a single vowel (or a syllabic consonant) or a vowel and one or more consonants associated with it. The syllable is often used to describe patterns of stress and timing in speech.
sym- with, together.
symphysis a region of union between two structures.
syn- together.
synapse the site of interneuronal communication; a functional gap between adjacent neurons.
synchrondrosis a cartilaginous articulation that is converted to bone before adulthood.
syndrome a set of symptons that occur together.
synovial fluid a clear fluid secreted by the membranes in an articular capsule.
synthesize 1. to combine separate elements into a whole. 2. produce speech by artificial means.
systemic pertaining to the body as a whole.
tag flaplike attachment or appendage.
tectorial membrane the membrane that forms the roof of the organ of Corti (compare with **basilar membrane**).
tectum rooflike structure.
tegmen a roof or cover.
tele- pertaining to distant or the end.
telencephalon the division of the central nervous system corresponding to the cerebral hemispheres.
telephony any device that permits speech communication over long distances.
template a pattern.
tendon nonelastic band of connective tissue by which muscle is attached to bone.
tensor a muscle that tenses.
tetra- four.
thoraco- pertaining to chest.
thorax the part of the body superior to the diaphragm and inferior to the neck; the chest.
tissue a population of cells with a similar structure and function.
tonsil a mass of lymph nodes and associated tissues embedded in the pharyngeal mucosa.
tonus a continuous state of slight muscle contraction.
torque a rotatory force.
torsion twisting.
torso the trunk of the body.
torus rounded ridge or protuberance.
trachea the ringed tube that connects the larynx with the bronchi.
tract a bundle of nerve fibers with a shared origin, termination, and function.
trans- across, beyond, through.
transverse crosswise; at right angles to the longitudinal plane.
tri- three.
turbulence a flow condition in which rotating elements of varying pressure and velocity are formed; condition under which noise is generated by an airstream.
tympanic membrane ear drum, the membrane separating the outer and middle ears.
ultra- excess.
un- not.
uni- one.
utero pertaining to the uterus.
utricle 1. a small sac. 2. a division of the vestibular system.
uvula the small appendage suspended from the soft palate.
vallecula a small depression.
vasculature the blood vessels and circulating blood system.

vein a vessel that returns blood to the heart.

velopharyngeal port the passage that connects the oral and nasal cavities.

velum soft palate.

ventro-, ventri- pertaining to the belly, or anterior part of the body.

vesicle a small fluid-filled sac.

vestibule a cavity that serves as an entrance to a canal.

villi slender process on a membrane's surface.

viscera the soft organs in the cavities of the body.

visceral pleura the outer surface of the lung.

vital capacity the maximum amount of air that can be exhaled following a maximal inhalation.

vocal fundamental frequency the primary frequency of vibration of the vocal folds during phonation.

vocal tract model a model that pertains to the shaping of the vocal tract for the production of speech sounds.

voice bar a low-frequency band on a spectrogram that represents the energy of the fundamental frequency of phonation.

voice onset time the time between the release of an articulatory constriction and the onset of voicing.

volume velocity a measure of airflow that takes account of both amount and speed of air.

Waldeyer's ring a ring of lymphatic (tonsillar) tissue at the oral-pharyngeal-nasal junction.

wave a propagation of a disturbance through a medium.

waveform a graph of amplitude versus time.

wavelength the distance that a periodic signal travels in one complete cycle of vibration.

xiphoid sword-shaped; the bony inferior extension of the sternum.

zygote the cell resulting from the union of two cells.

APPENDIX

Answers to Selected Exercises

Exercise 5-7

1 Levator labii superioris alaeque nasi
2 Levator labii superioris
3 Levator anguli oris
4 Buccinator
5 Mentalis
6 Depressor labii inferioris
7 Depressor anguli oris
8 Platysma
9 Masseter
10 Temporalis
11 Zygomaticus major
12 Zygomaticus minor
13 Sternocleidomastoid

Exercise 5-8

1 Musculus uvulae
2 Palatopharyngeus
3 Internal pterygoid (deep head)
4 Internal pterygoid (superficial head)
5 External pterygoid (upper head)
6 Masseter
7 Styloglossus
8 Stylohyoid
9 Stylopharyngeus
10 Posterior belly of digastric
11 Sternocleidomastoid

Exercise 6–1

It may help to arrange the structures in order of their participation in the process of audition. The sequence is:

pinna
external auditory meatus
tympanic membrane
malleus
incus
stapes
oval window
organ of Corti

With this sequence, explain how each structure is involved, beginning with the outer ear, proceeding to the middle ear, and concluding with the inner ear.

Exercise 7-1

telencephalon
diencephalon
mesencephalon
metencephalon
myelencephalon
cerebral hemispheres
thalamus and hypothalamus
midbrain
pons
medulla oblongata

Exercise 7-3

k	cortex of temporal lobe
i	pons
c	insula
b	Sylvian (lateral) fissure
d	corpus callosum
g	thalamus
f	cerebral acqueduct
j	cerebellum
e	lateral ventricle
h	cerebral peduncle
a	median longitudinal fissure

Index

A

B

C

D

E

F

I

K

L

M

N

O

P

Q

R

S

T

U

W

X

Z

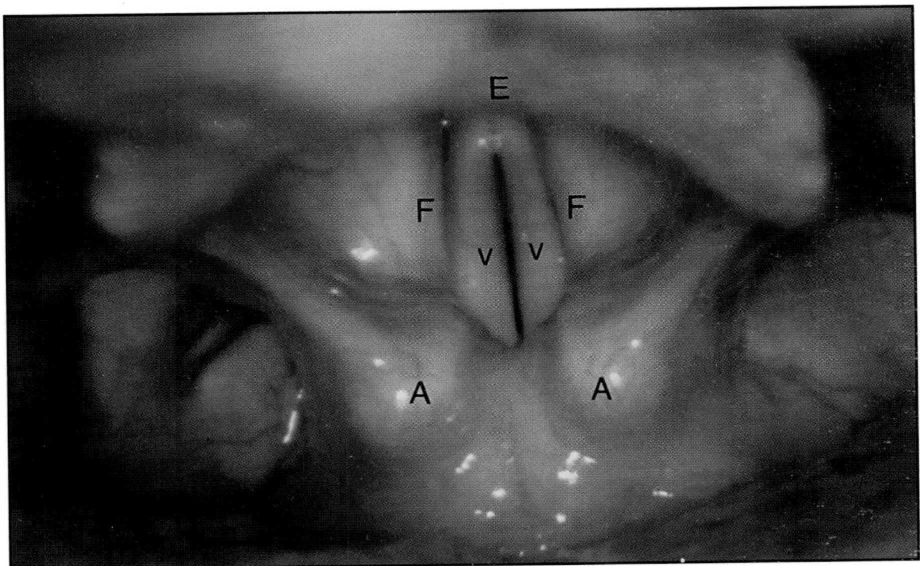

PLATE 1. Photograph of normal larynx showing vocal folds (V), false vocal folds (F), arytenoids (A), and epiglottis (E). (From Physical Examination by R. T. Satloff, 1997, p. 210. In R. T. Sataloff, *Professional Voice: The Art and Science of Clinical Care,* 2 ed. Copyright 1997 Singular Publishing Group, Inc. Reprinted with permission.)

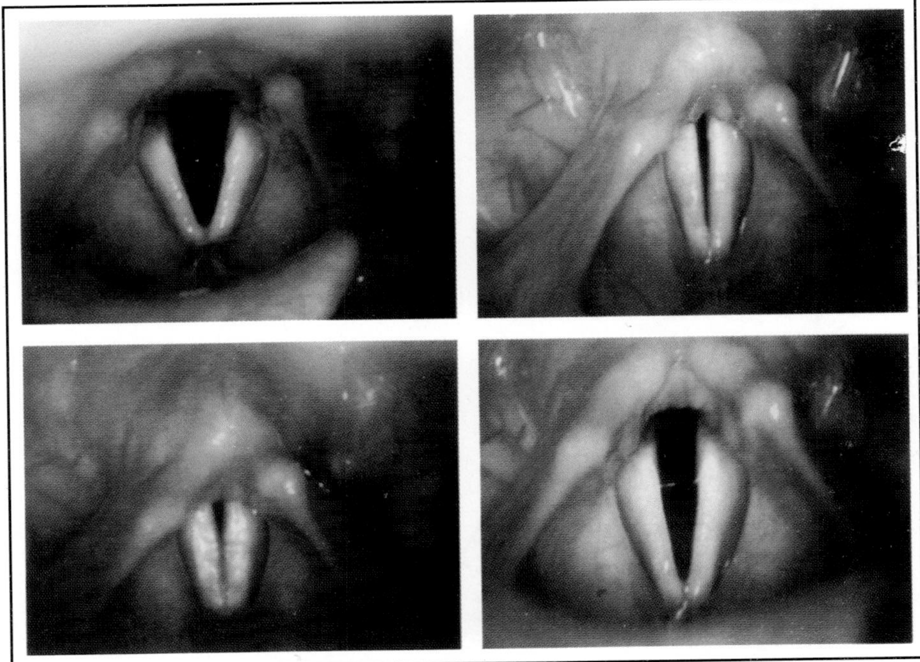

PLATE 2. The normal vocal fold: during breathing (*top left*), starting phonation (*top right*), end of phonation (*bottom left*), and breathing (*bottom right*). (From *Atlas of Laser Voice Surgery* by J. Abitbol, 1995, p. 46. Copyright 1995 Singular Publishing Group, Inc. Reprinted with permission.)

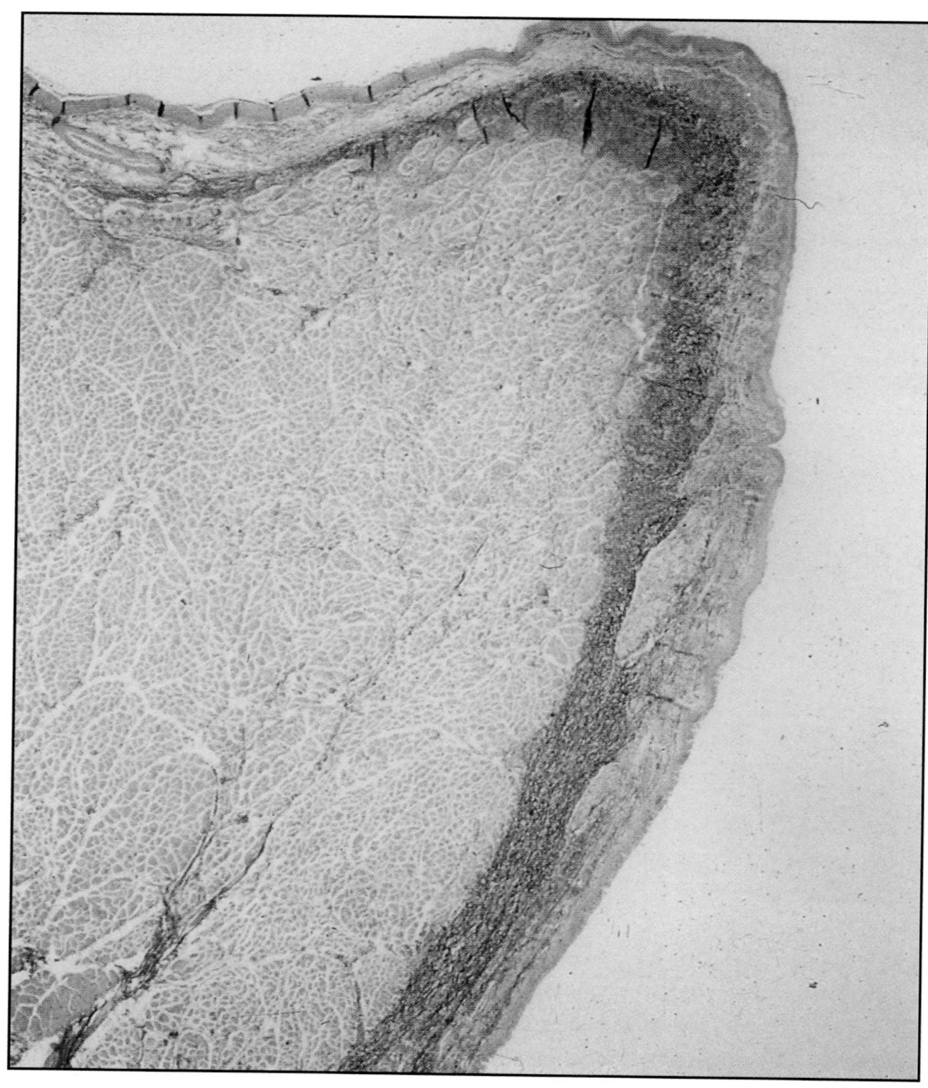

PLATE 3. AC5 coronal section of the midportion of the membraneous vocal fold (From *Histological Color Atlas of the Human Larynx* by M. Hirano and K. Sato, 1993, p. 45. Copyright 1993 by Singular Publishing Group, Inc. Reprinted with permission.)

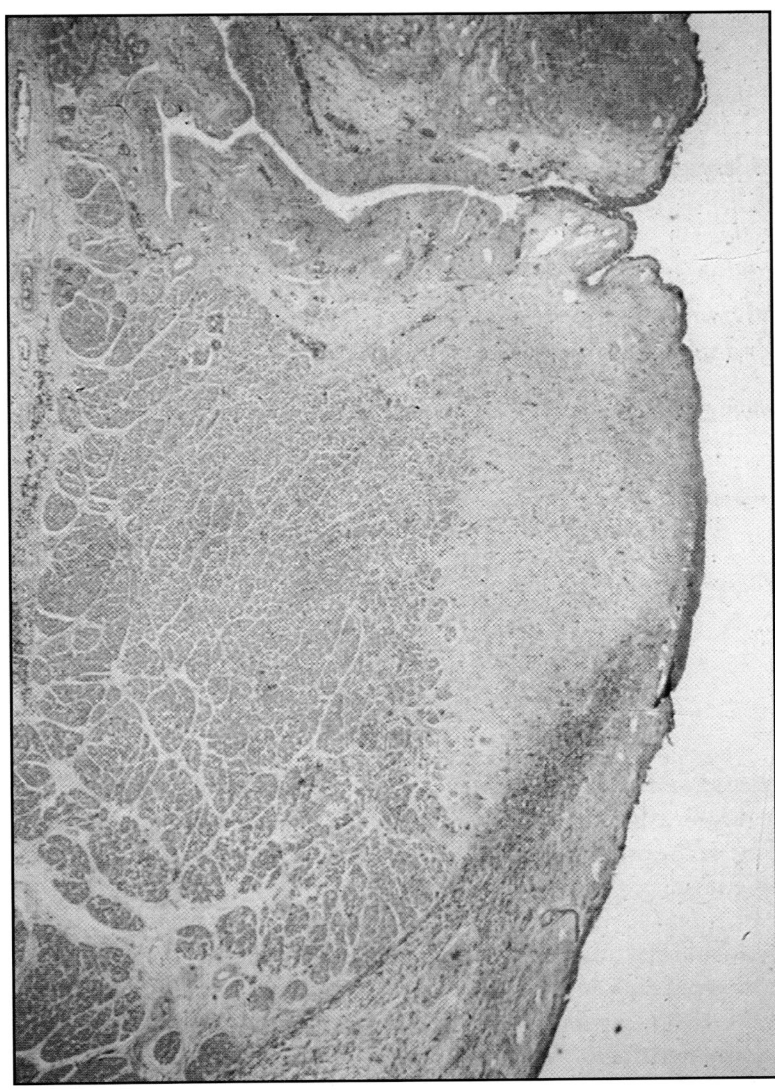

PLATE 4. NC5 coronal section of the midportion of the membraneous vocal fold (From *Histological Color Atlas of the Human Larynx* by M. Hirano and K. Sato, 1993, p. 92. Copyright 1993 by Singular Publishing Group, Inc. Reprinted with permission.)

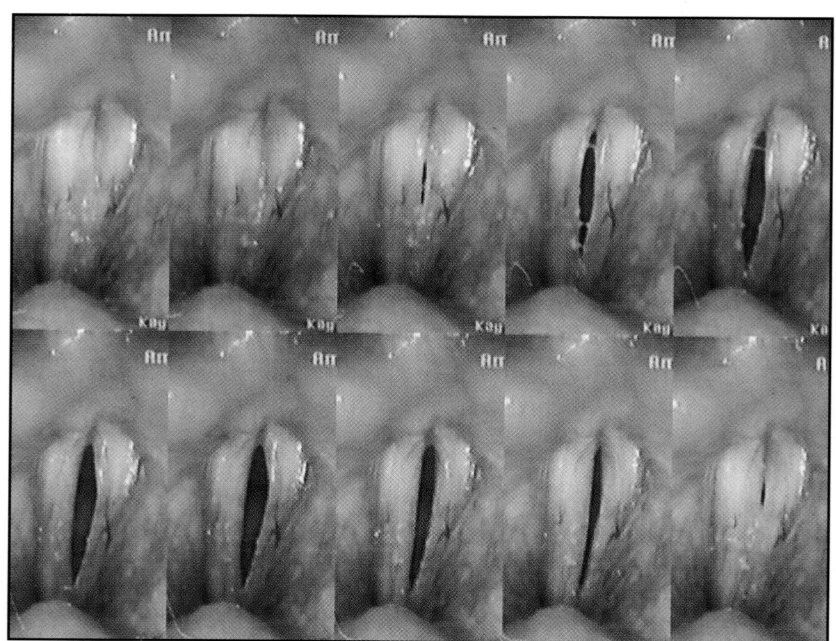

PLATE 5. Videoprint from the Kay Elemetrics stroboscopy system. This special feature automatically captures the vocal folds at 36° intervals and prints ten images (360°) simulating the behavior of a complete glottic cycle. This feature can be very helpful in illustrating asymmetries. (From The Clinical Voice Laboratory by R. T. Sataloff, J. Reinhardt, K. A. Heuer, M. M. Baroody, R. K. Rulnick, and M. Hawkshaw, 1997, p. 226. In R. T. Sataloff, ed. *Professional Voice: The Art and Science of Clinical Care.* Copyright 1997 Singular Publishing Group, Inc.)

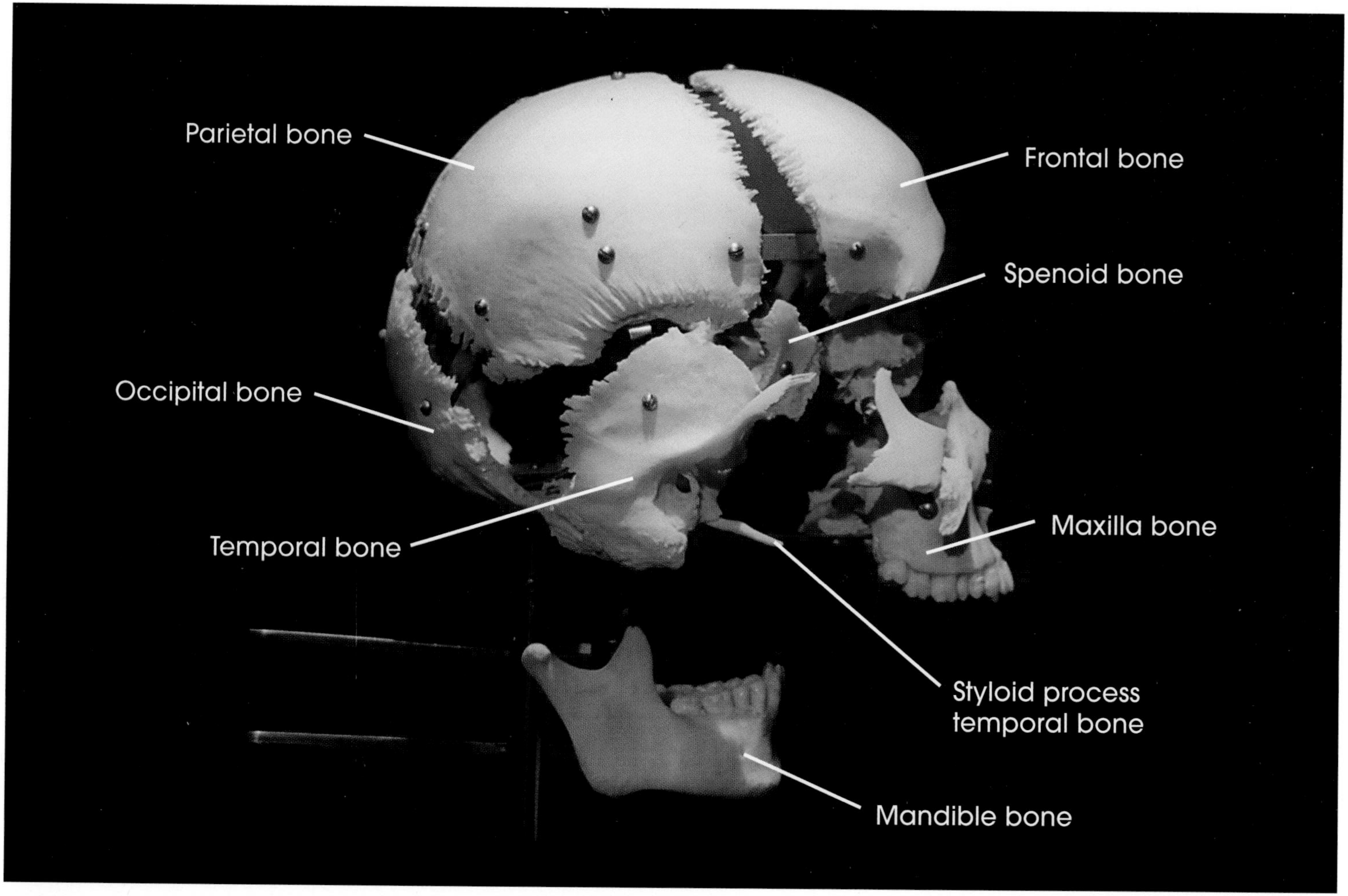

PLATE 6. Disarticulated skull and facial skeleton, right lateral view.

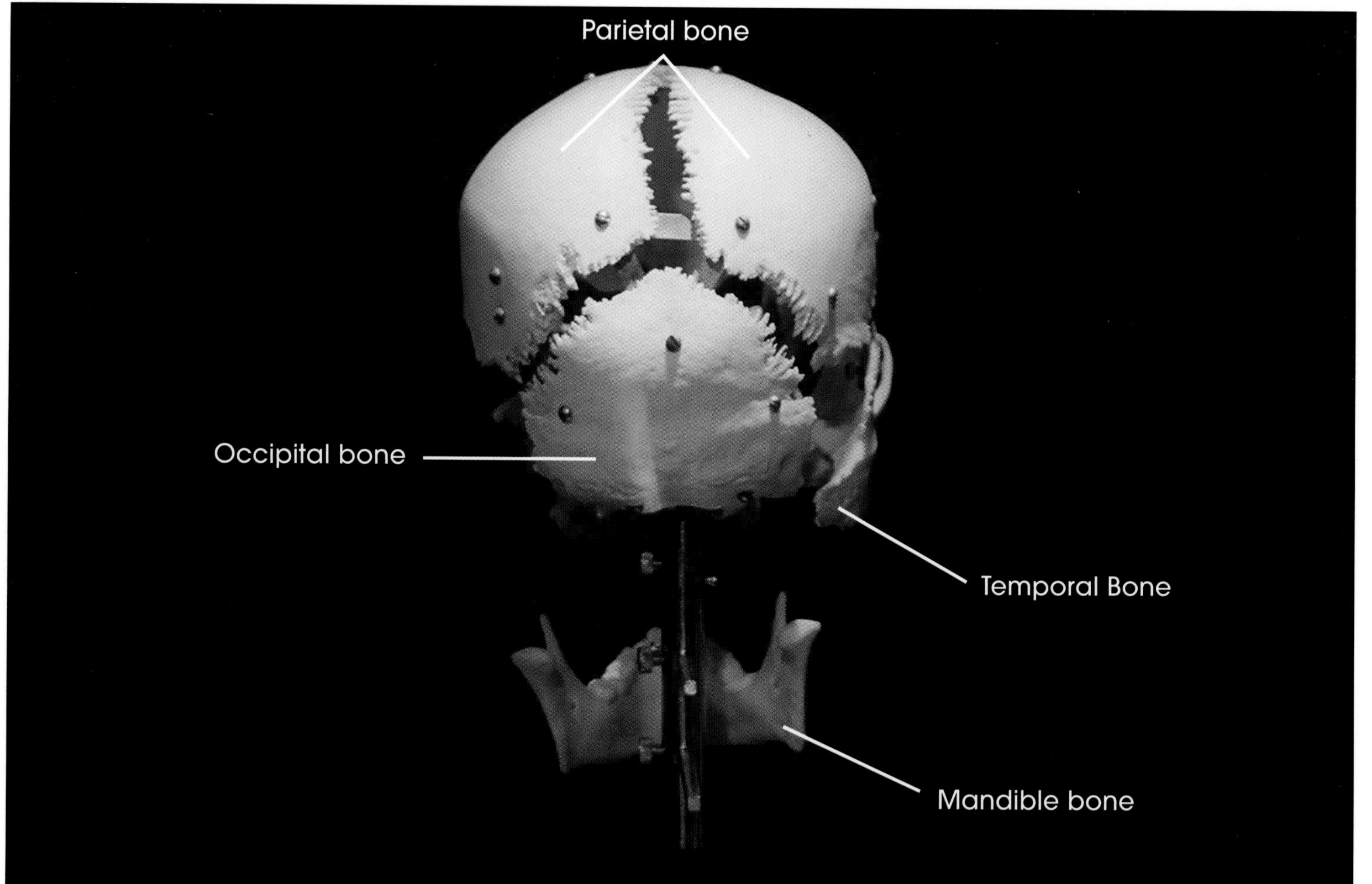

PLATE 7. Disarticulated skull and facial skeleton, posterior view.

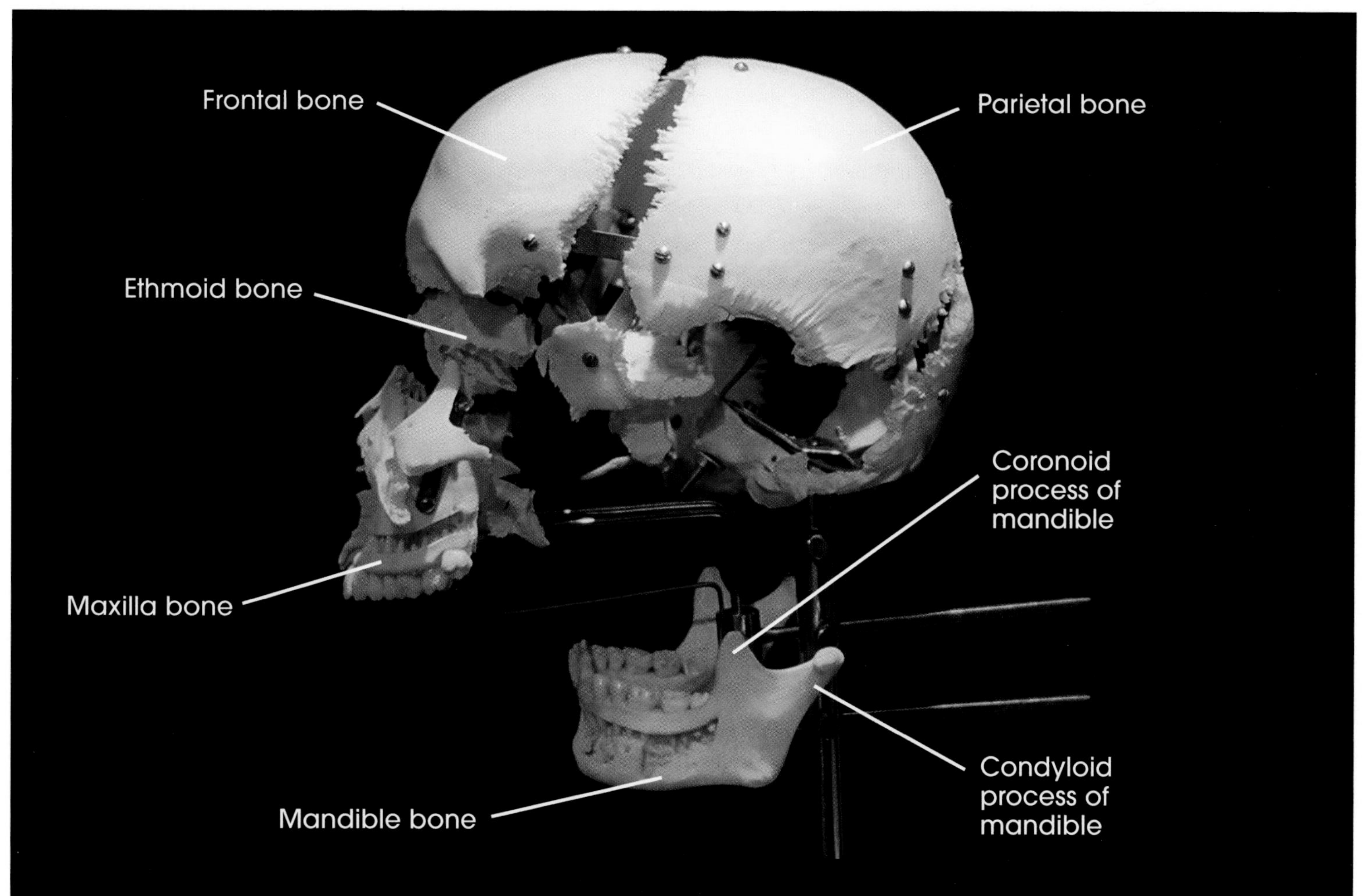

PLATE 8. Disarticulated skull and facial skeleton, left lateral view.

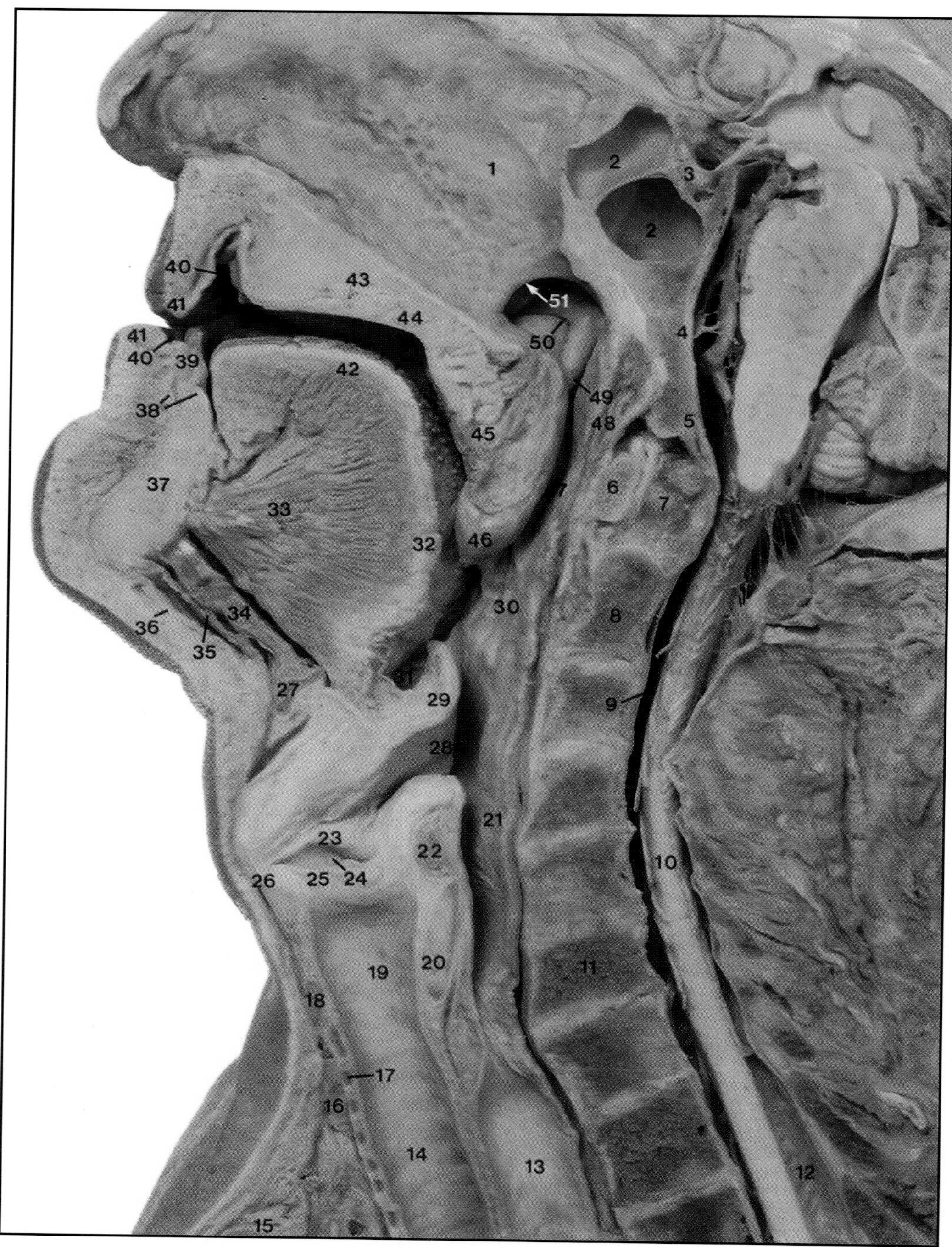

PLATE 9. Upper airway (vocal tract) anatomy, as seen in a dissection of the human head. (From *A Colour Atlas of Head and Neck Anatomy* by R. M. H. McMinn, R. T. Hutchings, & B. M. Logan, 1981, p. 136. London: Wolfe Medical Publications. Reprinted with permission. R. T. Hutchins photo.)

The mouth, palate, pharynx and larynx

The right half of a sagittal section of the lower part of the head and neck, slightly to the left of the midline

KEY:

1 Nasal septum
2 Sphenoidal sinus
3 Pituitary gland
4 Clivus
5 Anterior margin of foramen magnum
6 Anterior arch of atlas
7 Dens of axis
8 Body of axis
9 Spinal subarachnoid space
10 Spinal cord
11 Body of sixth cervical vertebra
12 Subarachnoid septum
13 Oesophagus
14 Trachea
15 Jugular notch of manubrium of sternum
16 Isthmus of thyroid gland
17 Second tracheal ring
18 Arch of cricoid cartilage
19 Lower part of larynx
20 Lamina of cricoid cartilage
21 Laryngeal part of pharynx
22 Transverse arytenoid muscle
23 Vestibular fold
24 Ventricle of larynx
25 Vocal fold (vocal cord)
26 Lamina of thyroid cartilage
27 Body of hyoid bone
28 Aryepiglottic fold
29 Epiglottis and epiglottic cartilage
30 Oral part of pharynx
31 Vallecula
32 Postsulcal part of dorsum of tongue
33 Genioglossus
34 Geniohyoid
35 Mylohyoid
36 Platysma
37 Body of mandible
38 Gingiva
39 Left lower central incisor tooth
40 Vestibule of mouth
41 Lip
42 Presulcal part of dorsum of tongue
43 Hard palate
44 Palatal glands in mucoperiosteum
45 Soft palate
46 Uvula
47 Nasal part of pharynx
48 Pharyngeal tonsil
49 Pharyngeal recess
50 Opening of auditory tube
51 Posterior nasal aperture (choana)

- The hyoid bone lies at the level of the third cervical vertebra.
- The thyroid cartilage lies at the level of the fourth and fifth cervical vertebrae.
- The cricoid cartilage lies at the level of the sixth cervical vertebra.
- The isthmus of the thyroid gland lies opposite the second, third and fourth tracheal rings.

- When enlarged the lymphoid tissue of the pharyngeal tonsil becomes known as the adenoids.

- The mouth or oral cavity consists of the vestibule and the oral cavity proper.
- The vestibule of the mouth is the narrow space bounded on the outer side by the lips and cheeks, and inside by the gingivae (gums) and teeth.
- The oral cavity proper is bounded at each side and in front by the alveolar arches with the teeth and gingivae; at the back it communicates with the oral part of the pharynx by the oropharyngeal isthmus which lies between the palatoglossal arches. (The tonsils which lie behind the palatoglossal arches are therefore in the oral part of the pharynx, not in the mouth).

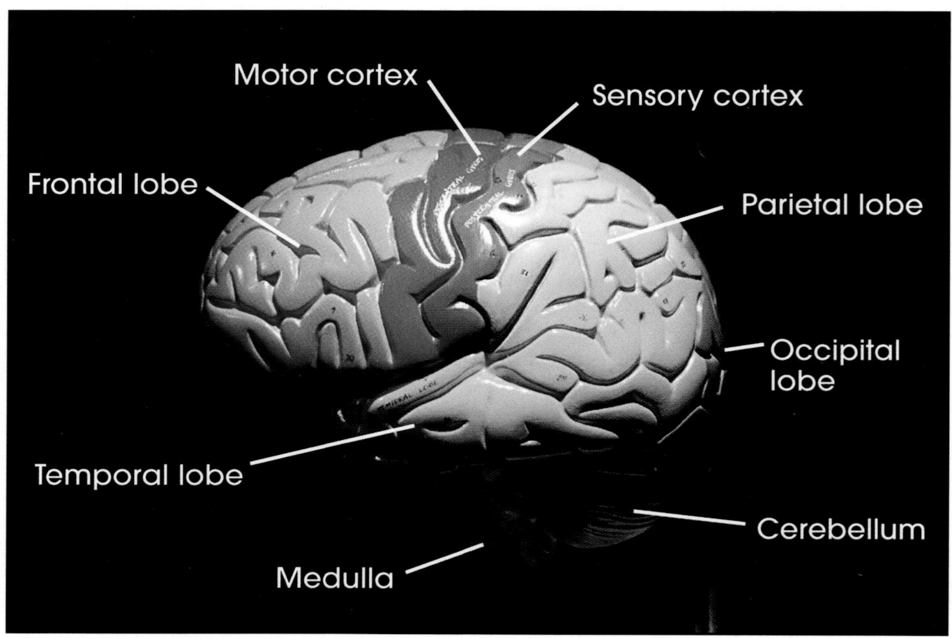

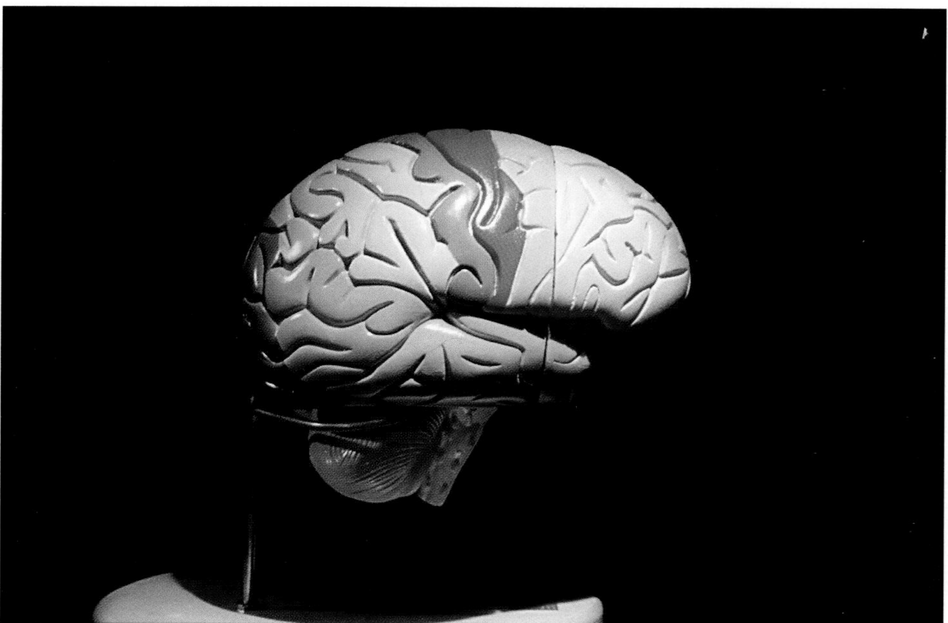

PLATE 10. Models of the brain with colored regions of left (top) and right (bottom) hemispheres.

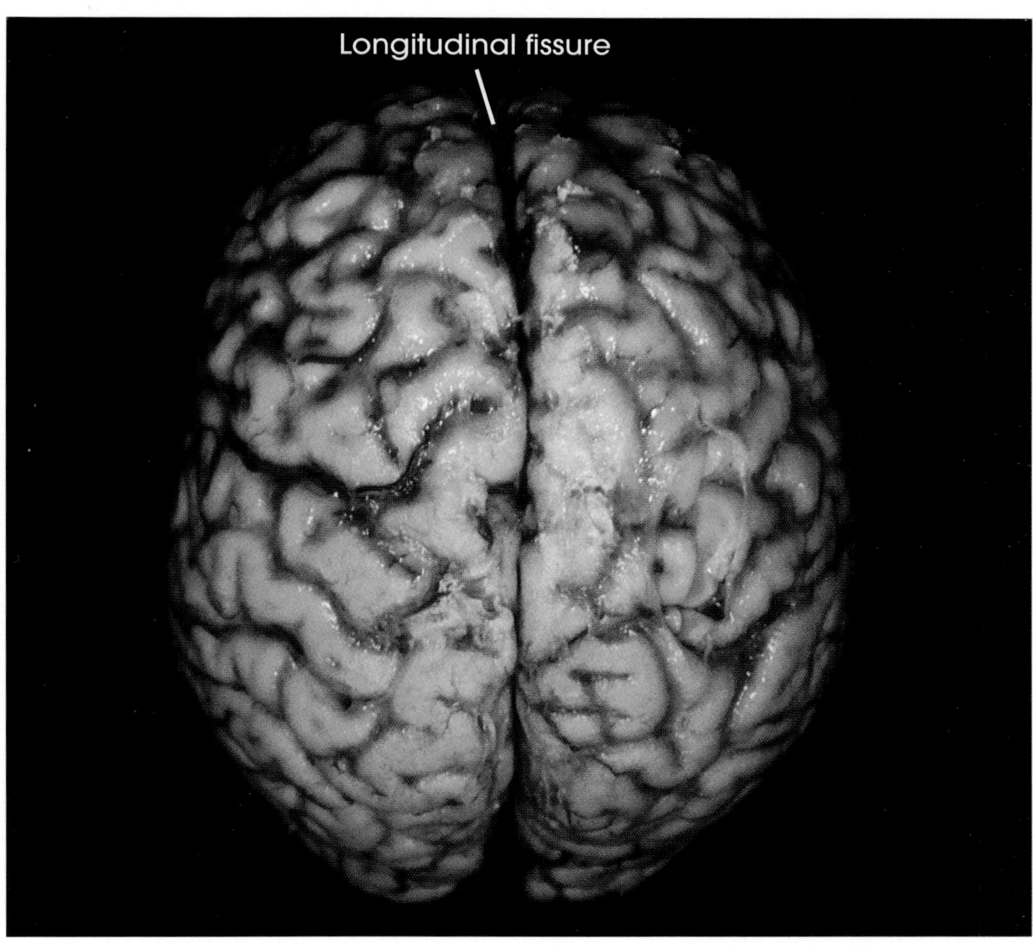

PLATE 11. Superior view of cerebral hemispheres.

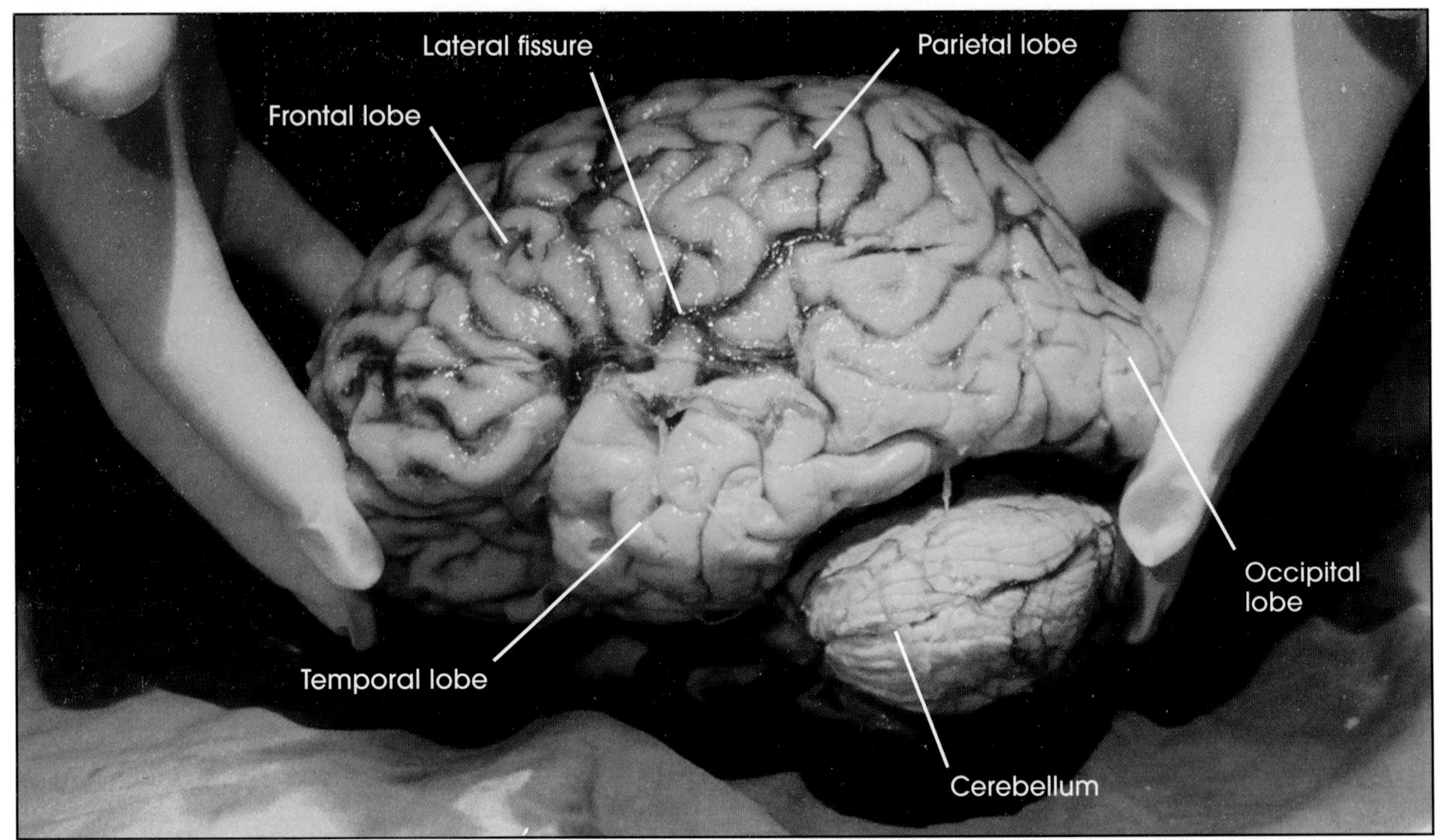

PLATE 12. Lateral view of cerebral hemispheres.